Chronic Renal Disease

Causes, Complications, and Treatment

Chronic Renal Disease

Causes, Complications, and Treatment

Edited by

Nancy Boucot Cummings, M.D.

National Institutes of Health
Bethesda, Maryland

and

Saulo Klahr, M.D.

Washington University School of Medicine
St. Louis, Missouri

PLENUM MEDICAL BOOK COMPANY
New York and London

Library of Congress Cataloging in Publication Data

Main entry under title:

Chronic renal disease.

"This book is an outgrowth of the issues addressed by participants at a number of NIH conferences held in the 1980s"—Pref.

Includes bibliographies and index.

1. Renal insufficiency—Congresses. 2. Renal insufficiency in children—Congresses. 3. Chronic disease—Congresses. I. Cummings, Nancy B. II. Klahr, Saulo. III. National Institutes of Health (U.S.) [DNLM: 1. Kidney Failure, Chronic—congresses. WJ 342 C5565]

RC918.R4C58 1985 616.6′1 84-24904

ISBN 0-306-41764-2

233 Spring Street, New York, N.Y. 10013

Plenum Medical Book Company is an imprint of Plenum Publishing Corporation

Printed in the United States of America

Preface

Chronic renal disease has received increasing attention and concern since the passage in 1972 of PL 92-603, which provided coverage for end-stage renal disease (ESRD) treatment by the federal government. The human and economic costs of the ESRD program serve to emphasize the need to prevent or to arrest those diseases resulting in chronic renal failure, since none of the available treatments is without complications and/or side effects. The ESRD program, the only federal one that provides coverage for a catastrophic illness for almost the entire population (those qualifying under Social Security), cost almost $2 billion in 1983. The escalating costs of the ESRD program are attributed to the increasing number of patients requiring treatment and have focused concerns of the United States Government, both Congress and the administration, on ESRD.

The National Institutes of Health (NIH), especially the Kidney, Urology, and Hematology Division of the National Institutes of Arthritis, Diabetes, and Digestive and Kidney Diseases (NIADDK), supports a sizable research program that bears on chronic renal disease and in association with this has sponsored many conferences and workshops on research on and causes and complications of chronic renal failure. This book is an outgrowth of the issues addressed by participants at a number of NIH conferences held in the 1980s.

Diseases affecting the kidney vary in their pathogenic and histologic detail and in their rate of progression, but they all result in similar alterations in renal function and cause a common constellation of chemical and physiologic abnormalities. The hallmark of chronic renal disease is a progressive decrease in glomerular filtration rate.

Various mechanisms are responsible for kidney injury and ultimately for chronic renal disease. These include abnormal immunologic processes, disturbances in coagulation, infection, biochemical and metabolic disturbances, vascular disorders, congenital abnormalities, obstruction to urine flow, neoplasia, and trauma. Each of these mechanisms may interact with one or more of the other mechanisms to cause advancing renal disease. Progressive kidney disease may occur as a consequence of diseases in which the kidney is primarily involved and in which the presenting features are usually those of renal disease. Kidney disease also can occur during the course of systemic diseases (diabetes, hypertension) and intoxications in which renal failure may be a presenting feature.

Although adequate data are not available about the incidence of ESRD in North America, mortality figures suggest that there is an incidence of about 200 cases per million population. These figures vary according to geographic area and in relation to the proportion of blacks in the population. The incidence of renal disease in blacks is higher than that in whites (possibly related to the higher incidence of hypertension in the black population).

In diseases of the kidney characterized by irreversible injury, once a critical level of renal functional deterioration is reached, progression to ESRD invariably occurs even if the initiating event or condition has resolved or has been eradicated. Immunopathogenic mechanisms probably account for most forms of primary glomerular disease in humans. Although immunologic events and the mediators of glomerular damage that they induce may be responsible for initiating most glomerular diseases, certain clinical and experimental observations suggest that the rate of progression of these diseases is influenced by several nonimmunologic factors. The understanding of and ability to manipulate factors responsible for progression of renal disease have been quite limited. Although ideally therapeutic efforts should be directed to preventing the development or to arresting the progression of renal disease, only two modalities of effective treatment are available for the patient with ESRD. These modalities are kidney transplantation and dialysis (either peritoneal or hemodialysis). Currently about 75,000 patients are undergoing dialysis in the United States and about 5000 renal transplants are performed annually. Ideally major efforts should be directed toward prevention of the occurrence of renal disease or progression of the disease once it has developed. However, dialysis and transplantation remain the major modalities for treatment of ESRD. Considerable effort has been devoted to understanding the problems and complications that occur in patients treated by hemodialysis, peritoneal dialysis, and/or transplantation.

This book is divided into four major sections. The first section describes studies about the pathogenesis of renal disease. This section is divided into two major areas: one about research trends in glomerular diseases, the most frequent cause of ESRD, and the other about cystic diseases of the kidney, an area that has not been well studied. Cystic diseases of the kidney, particularly polycystic kidney disease, may affect as many as 250,000 Americans and may account for 10–12% of the patients with ESRD treated by dialysis or transplantation. The second section of this book, "Recent Advances on Some Complications of Chronic Renal Failure," focuses attention on three general areas: renal osteodystrophy and the neurologic and cardiovascular complications of renal failure. The latter are the major cause of mortality in patients with ESRD and/or those undergoing dialysis. The third major section of this book is devoted to the unique problems of the child with renal failure. Extrapolation of information about chronic renal failure and its rate of progression and treatment obtained in adults to children is not warranted. In children with ESRD, problems with growth, caloric intake, and mental retardation are of major importance. The technical problems of treating children differ markedly from those in adults and are unique problems. Section IV addresses selected aspects of therapy in the patient with renal failure. It includes discussions of the use of drugs, the acute problems that develop during hemodialysis, the control of treatment morbidity and uremic toxicity by hemodialysis and hemofiltration therapy, the use of transplantation and adequate immunosuppression, and nutritional therapy in chronic renal failure. It has become evident in recent years, particularly from studies in experimental animals, that dietary manipulations may influence the rate of progression of chronic renal failure. If this proves to be so, dietary manipulations may prove effective in delaying or even halting the progression of renal disease in humans.

It is hoped that these chapters will prove useful to readers by helping them develop a better understanding of these aspects of the pathogenesis, progression, complications, and treatment of chronic renal disease.

Nancy Boucot Cummings, M.D.
Saulo Klahr, M.D.

Bethesda, Maryland
St. Louis, Missouri

Contents

I. STUDIES OF PATHOGENESIS OF RENAL DISEASE

Research Trends in Glomerular Diseases

Cystic Diseases of the Kidney

I

STUDIES OF PATHOGENESIS OF RENAL DISEASE

Research Trends in Glomerular Diseases

1

A Personal Perspective on the State of the Art in Research in Glomerulonephritis

Richard J. Glassock

During the 20 years in which I have been personally involved in research on glomerulonephritis, the field has undergone a remarkable transformation. From the initial probing excursions into the pathogenesis of glomerulonephritis in the early 1960s a highly sophisticated discipline has arisen. Wide application of electron microscopic and immunofluorescent techniques to human biopsy material has taught us much, focused our interest on aberrant immune processes, and brought an ever-increasing complexity to the classification of human glomerular diseases. Paradigms developed during this period have, after a time of widespread acceptance, recently shown unmistakable signs of being replaced by a new and more richly varied set of dogmas. To the clinician, not directly involved in research in this area, the field seems to be ever more populated with an often bewildering variety of spontaneous and induced models of glomerular disease in experimental animals. However, experimental approaches in animals have been the bedrock of investigation into the pathogenesis of glomerulonephritis, and this work has taught us much about the ways in which aberrant immune processes bring about glomerular injury and the factors that mediate the injury itself. Highly sophisticated procedures such as direct micropuncture of glomerular capillaries and even isolated perfusion of individual glomeruli, tissue culture and cell cloning of glomerular constituents, receptor binding and enzyme kinetics, and very recently the development of monoclonal antibodies as probes of glomerular structure promise to add exciting new

Richard J. Glassock • Department of Medicine, UCLA School of Medicine, and Department of Medicine, Harbor–UCLA Medical Center, Torrance, California 90509.

dimensions to our understanding of a structure that less than a decade ago was viewed as only a passive ultrafilter serving primarily to provide a rich supply of water and ions to the tubules for reabsorption.

Thus, the glomerulus is now known to be a site of production of several humoral substances and to be highly responsive to the action of additional substances reaching it via the bloodstream. The glomerular capillary wall is now known, or thought, to consist of a dozen or more discrete antigenic substances, some of which are important in conferring a strong negative charge on the glomerular capillary wall, which in turn is vital to the molecular permselectivity attributes of the filter. The emerging complexity of the cellular, biochemical, and molecular structure of the glomerulus has been reviewed by Dr. Gary E. Striker of the Department of Pathology at the University of Washington. Dr. Striker and his colleagues have contributed much to our current understanding in this rapidly evolving area.

Not surprisingly, diseases of the glomerulus may arise spontaneously or can be experimentally induced by the interaction of a circulating antibody with one or more of the antigenic constituents of the glomerulus. The distribution, density, and anatomic location of these antigenic constituents greatly influence the character of the resulting disease. In addition, antigens not normally native to the glomerulus may be artifically planted in this site and serve as a nidus for a potentially injurious local immune reaction. These events may provide useful new insights into the relationship between glomerular disease and environmental factors. Dr. Curtis B. Wilson of the Research Institute of Scripps Clinic in La Jolla, California, one of the foremost renal immunopathologists in the world, has reviewed the state of the art in this area.

By virtue of the special hemodynamic and biophysical attributes of the glomerular capillaries and the lymphaticlike channels of the mesangium, the glomerulus is quite vulnerable to deposition from the circulation of a variety of substances, including circulating aggregates of antigen and antibody, so-called immune complexes. Since the pioneering work of Germuth and Dixon and colleagues, it has been recognized that such immune complexes may participate in the generation of disorders of glomerular structure and function. Although the true nature of these immune complexes is by and large unknown in human disease, much has been learned through experimental work about the molecular and local factors influencing their deposition in tissues, including glomeruli, and about the processes that govern their traffic through and removal from the glomerulus. These have been reviewed by Dr. Mart Mannik of the Division of Rheumatology at the University of Washington. Dr. Mannik has long been involved in fundamental research on the kinetics of immune complex disease and has made many original contributions in this field.

The common pathways by which immune processes result in tissue injury are being delineated. The separate and interdependent roles of complement, polymorphonuclear leukocytes, monocytes, platelets, coagulation, and kinins are being more precisely defined. One emerging area of great interest is the role of mononuclear cells in tissue injury.

Many other aspects of glomerular disease could also have been selected for discussion, such as immunogenetics and the role of the major histocompatibility complex in determining the predisposition to glomerular disease or the role of viruses in glomerular disease, to name a few. The topics discussed represent areas of intense interest with potential practical value in the detection, prevention, and treatment of human glomerular disease. Each chapter provides an overview of the field, emphasizing the author's own contributions as well as major unresolved problem areas and promising future directions for research. It is hoped that this brief glimpse of research in the field of glomerulonephritis will stimulate additional original and creative approaches to the problem.

2

Biosynthesis and Immunochemical Localization of Glomerular Components

Gary E. Striker, Federico M. Farin, Paul D. Killen, and Jeffrey F. Bonadio

The molecular composition of the glomerulus became a target of interest when Masugi (1934) first demonstrated that immunization of animals with kidney tissue resulted in a diffuse glomerular lesion. The search for the nephritogenic antigen, although not yet complete, has provided the impetus for many studies of glomerular structure and function. The importance of understanding the sites of synthesis and degradation of matrix constituents relates to (1) normal glomerular structure and function, (2) localization and disposition of immune deposits, (3) immunogenicity of individual components (i.e., cellular and humoral responses to glomerular constituents), and (4) genetic or acquired diseases resulting in an accumulation of abnormal matrix constituents resulting in loss of function—chronic glomerulonephritis.

The following discussion highlights only a few of the past studies, focusing instead on current data and new directions. The major emphasis will be on normal glomerular structure and function, since there is little information on matrix composition in genetic and acquired forms of chronic glomerular diseases and others in this volume will be covering topics related to immunogenicity of individual components and the localization of immune deposits.

1. Structure of the Glomerulus

1.1. Origin of Cells

The glomerular visceral epithelial cells are derived from metanephric mesenchyme. They arise from an S-shaped indentation of a cystic structure which is the origin of the primitive nephron. *In vivo* the indentation carries along endothelium and perivascular cells. Utilizing a system developed by Grobstein, Bernstein *et al.* (1981) have demonstrated that the visceral

Gary E. Striker, Federico M. Farin, Paul D. Killen, and Jeffrey F. Bonadio • Department of Pathology, University of Washington, Seattle, Washington 98195.

epithelium develops an arborized structure resembling a mature glomerulus, including pedicels. Furthermore, there is an adjacent lamina rara externa and a lamina dense. These data provide strong evidence that the vascular and epithelial components of the glomerulus may respond to independent stimuli.

Vernier and Birch-Anderson (1963) demonstrated that the vascular indentation of the primitive glomerulus arises from the adjacent mesenchyme. The endothelium had an adjacent basal lamina which fused, at the periphery, with the lamina densa of the visceral epithelial cell. The third glomerular cell type, the mesangial cell, has been shown to enter the glomerulus along with the endothelial cell. The mesangial cell has been shown to be in communication with smooth muscle cells, and recently Barajas (1979) has postulated that their physiologic function is to regulate glomerular blood flow.

1.2. Matrix

As pointed out previously, the peripheral basal lamina can be seen to result from fusion of a basal lamina from glomerular visceral epithelial cells and ingrowing endothelial cells. The role that each cell plays in synthesis of the fused structure is not clear. We studied the developing kidney with affinity-purified antibodies to collagen types I, III, and IV and to two other basal lamina components, laminin and a heparan-sulfate-containing proteoglycan. We found that the fused basal lamina stained positively for type IV collagen, the proteoglycan, and laminin. The basal lamina of the rounded structure into which the glomerular tufts were invaginating also stained positively for these elements. The interstitium of the kidney contained antigens recognized by antibody to type III collagen. In the nephrogenic zone we were unable to demonstrate positive staining with antibodies either to the helical domain of type I collagen or to type I procollagen.

In collaboration with Dr. Jay Bernstein we were able to further dissect the origin of molecular structure of the basal lamina. In this *in vitro* model notochord and primitive renal tissue are on opposing sides of a millipore filter in organ culture. Glomerular development proceeds to formation of a complex, folded structure. Podocytes develop into branched structures with mature pedicels and filtration slit membranes. There is an adjacent basal lamina. Immunocytochemical staining reveals that this basal lamina contains collagen (type IV), laminin, and the basal lamina proteoglycan. Interestingly, this development proceeds in the absence of penetration of the stalk by endothelial or mesangial cells. Thus, not only does glomerular development proceed in the absence of the associated vasculature, but it appears that the visceral epithelial cell can synthesize and deposit the components of the adjacent basal lamina.

1.3. Peripheral Vascular Loop Segment

There are three components of the *basement membrane:* the visceral epithelial cell layer, the basal lamina, and the endothelial cell layer. The basal lamina zone consists of the lamina rara externa, the lamina densa, and the lamina rara interna.

1.3.1. Visceral Epithelial Cell Layer

The *epithelial cell* has relatively few *in vivo* markers. It has a dense glycocalyx, and several techniques have been used to demonstrate surface receptors for C3b (Shin *et al.*, 1977). Its role in the synthesis of the basal lamina was alluded to previously. We have isolated these cells *in vitro* and shown that they retain their surface C3b receptors (Killen and Striker, 1979). We have not been able to consistently demonstrate a response of these cells to mitogens derived from macrophages or platelets. They synthesize type IV collagen which exists as a dimer of high-molecular-weight procollagen chains (Crouch and Bornstein, 1979). The chain composition was estimated to be $[\alpha 1]_2\ \alpha 2$ by SDS polyacrylamide gel electrophoresis with a molecular weight of 178,000. The epithelial cells also synthesized proteoglycans.

The major glycosaminoglycan retained in the cell layer was heparan sulfate (Striker *et al.*, 1980). The medium contained both heparan sulfate and chondroitin 4,6-sulfate. Recently it was found that the medium proteoglycans consisted of two molecular species which could be isolated by chromatography on DE52 cellulose (F. M. Farin and G. E. Striker, unpublished). It remains to be seen whether the two different glycosaminoglycans segregate on the individual proteoglycans or exist as a mixture or both. Visceral epithelial cells *in vitro* also synthesize a high-molecular-weight glycoprotein (Killen and Striker, 1979). Approximately 60% is absorbed to a gelatin-sepharose column and precipitable by affinity-purified antibody to plasma fibronectin. A smaller fraction is precipitable by antibody to laminin (kindly provided by Dr. George Martin, National Institute of Dental Research). These data on fibronectin synthesis cannot be used to shed light on the controversy of whether this material is present on the peripheral vascular loop because epithelial cells have been shown to synthesize fibronectin *in vitro* when they are dividing. However, upon reaching confluence they switch to the synthesis of laminin.

1.3.2. Basal Lamina

The *basal lamina* has been shown to contain sialoglycoproteins (Mohos and Skoza, 1969), principally in the lamina rara externa. Recently, using histochemical techniques and specific digestion methods, Kanwar and Farquhar (1979a,b) have shown that the basal lamina contains heparan sulfate as its major glycosaminoglycan. They were also able to demonstrate synthesis of a proteoglycan containing heparan by perfusing a kidney with ^{25}S and analyzing isolated glomeruli. Since the pioneering studies, first of Krakower and Greenspan (1951) and then of Kefalides and Winzler (1966), many investigators have reported on the isolation and characterization of the collagenous composition of the whole glomerular matrix. These studies have depended on enzymatic degradation of the intact structure for isolation of the collagen chains (Kefalides and Winzler, 1966). Since these studies have begun, it has become clear that type IV collagen is less resistant to proteolysis than other collagen types (Crouch and Bornstein, 1979), that the α2 chain is more easily degraded than the α1 monomer (Sage *et al.*, 1979), and that there are a number of specific degradation products (Daniels and Chu, 1975; Tryggvason *et al.*, 1980). In addition to these disclaimers, it should be recognized that analyses of whole glomeruli include the mesangial region as well as the peripheral vascular loop. There is reason to believe from biosynthetic (Striker *et al.*, 1976) and immunohistologic data (Scheinman *et al.*, 1980) that this region contains other collagen types. Immunohistologic studies demonstrate that the peripheral basal lamina contains type IV collagen (Scheinman *et al.*, 1980). There is a controversy about whether fibronectin is located in this region (Courtnoy *et al.*, 1980).

1.3.3. Endothelium

The *endothelial cell* can be identified *in vivo* and *in vitro* because of its cellular content of factor VIII antigen (Jaffe *et al.*, 1973) and surface localization of angiotensin-converting enzyme (Johnson and Erdos, 1978). Sage *et al.* (1979) have recently shown that these cells synthesize collagen types III and IV. They also identified a new collagen type which was relatively sensitive to proteases, including thrombin. Gamse *et al.* (1978) showed that these cells synthesized several glycosaminoglycans *in vitro*, including heparan. Recently, Jaffe *et al.* (1973) demonstrated that endothelial cells isolated from human umbilical vein synthesize fibronectin and suggested that they were the source of plasma fibronectin. The isolation and propagation of glomerular endothelial cells have recently been reported (Striker *et al.*, 1984a). Cells containing factor VIII antigen can often be found in primary isolates of glomerular cells; however, they can only be successfully passaged in the presence of plasma-derived growth factor.

1.4. The Mesangium

The *mesangium* is bounded by the lamina densa on one aspect and the endothelium on the other. The cellular composition is of at least two types. One is derived from the primitive mesenchyme and resembles a smooth muscle cell morphologically (Yamada, 1955). This cell, in common with many mesenchymal cells, will endocytose adjacent macromolecules (Farquhar *et al.*, 1961). It also responds to mitogens derived from platelets and macrophages with brisk proliferative response (Striker *et al.*, 1980). The other cell derives from the circulation and appears to be the principal cell responsible for the phagocytosis of material deposited in the glomerulus (Striker *et al.*, 1979). The mesangial matrix can be differentiated from the lamina densa *in vivo* by guanidine treatment (Huang, 1979). By immunofluorescence microscopy types IV and V collagen have been localized to this region (Scheinman *et al.*, 1980). Mesangial cells have been shown to localize injected angiotensin II to their surface *in vivo* and to contract in response to this substance *in vitro* (Ausiello *et al.*, 1980; Sraer *et al.*, 1974). We have isolated the contractile mesangial cell *in vitro* and studied its biosynthetic products (Striker *et al.*, 1980; Killen and Striker, 1979). Collagen types I, III, and IV were identified. Compared to smooth-muscle cells isolated from the accompanying renal artery, mesangial cells synthesized more of both types III and IV collagen. The total amount of collagen synthesized per cell was similar to the arterial cell and considerably greater than the visceral epithelial cell. Like this latter cell type, mesangial cells also synthesized fibronectin and laminin. Their glycosaminoglycan pattern was much more complex. Dermatan, chondroitin 4,6, and heparan sulfates were all present in medium and cell layer. From these *in vitro* data it was suspected that type I collagen would be found in the mesangium; however, this was not the case in normal glomeruli.

2. Future Directions

There remains a considerable body of information about the normal glomerulus which is either unclear or unknown. The *in vitro* studies of the biosynthesis of matrix constituents have barely begun, and nothing is known about its turnover. Furthermore, only isolated cells or organ cultures have been examined. Specific mixing experiments have not been conducted.

The influence of inflammatory cells and their mediators on matrix synthesis and degradation should be investigated. Neutrophils (Gader *et al.*, 1980; Mainardi *et al.*, 1980) and macrophages (Werb *et al.*, 1980) contain proteolytic enzymes, including collagenases, which can degrade matrix constituents.

In addition to these *in vitro* studies, the composition of the matrix in clinical renal disease should be further examined utilizing the probes now available (Striker *et al.*, 1984b).

Finally, the effect of specific alterations in matrix components might yield useful information on the localization of material deposited in glomeruli.

References

Ausiello, D. A., Kreisberg, J. I., Roy, C., and Karnovsky, M. J., 1980, Contraction of cultured rat glomerular cells of apparent mesangial origin after stimulation with angiotensin II and arginine vasopressin, *Am. J. Physiol.* **65:**756.

Barajas, L., 1979, Anatomy of the juxtaglomerular apparatus, *Am. J. Physiol.* **237**(5):F343.

Bernstein, J., Cheng, F., and Roszka, J., 1981, Glomerular differentiation in metanephric culture, *Lab. Invest.* **45:**183.

Courtnoy, P. J., Kanwar, Y. S., and Farquhar, M. G., 1980, Fibronectin localization in the rat glomerulus, *J. Cell. Biol.* **87:**691.

Crouch, E., and Bornstein, P., 1979, Characterization of a type IV procollagen synthesized by human amniotic fluid cells in culture, *J. Biol. Chem.* **254:**4197.

Daniels, J. R., and Chu, G. M., 1975, Basement membrane collagen of the renal glomerulus, *J. Biol. Chem.* **250:**3531.

Farquhar, M. G., Wissig, S. L., and Palade, G. L., 1961, Glomerular permeability I. Ferritin transfer across the normal glomerular capillary wall, *J. Exp. Med.* **113:**47.

Gader, J. E., Fells, G. A., Wright, D. G., and Crystal, R. G., 1980, Human neutrophil elastase functions as a type III collagen "collagenase," *Biochem. Biophys. Res. Commun.* **95:**1815.

Gamse, G., Fromme, H. G., and Kresse, H., 1978, Metabolism of sulfated glycosaminoglycans in cultured endothelial cells and smooth muscle cells from bovine aorta, *Biochim. Biophys. Acta* **544:**514.

Huang, T. W., 1979, Basal lamina heterogeneity in the glomerular tufts of human kidneys, *J. Exp. Med.* **149:**1450.

Jaffe, E. A., Hoyer, L. W. and Nachman, R. L., 1973, Synthesis of antihemophilic factor antigen by cultured human endothelial cells, *J. Clin. Invest.* **52:**2757.

Johnson, A. R., and Erdos, E. G., 1978, Activities of enzymes in human pulmonary endothelial cells in culture, *Circulation* Suppl. **II:**108.

Kanwar, Y. S., and Farquhar, M., 1979a, Anionic sites in the glomerular basement membrane, *J. Cell. Biol.* **81:**137.

Kanwar, Y. S., and Farquhar, M., 1979b, Presence of heparan sulfate in the glomerular basement membrane, *Proc. Natl. Acad. Sci. USA* **76:**1303.

Kefalides, N. A., and Winzler, R. J., 1966, The chemistry of glomerular basement membrane and its relation to collagen, *Biochemistry* **5:**702.

Killen, P. D., and Striker, G. E., 1979, Human glomerular visceral epithelial cells synthesize a basal lamina collagen *in vitro, Proc. Natl. Acad. Sci. USA* **76:**3518.

Krakower, C. A., and Greenspan, S. A., 1951, Localization of nephrotoxic antigen within isolated renal glomerulus, *Arch. Pathol.* **51:**629.

Mainardi, C. L., Dixit, S. N., and Kang, A. H., 1980, Degradation of type IV (basement membrane) collagen by a proteinase isolated from human polymorphonuclear leukocyte granules, *J. Biol. Chem.* **255:**5435.

Masugi, M., 1934, Uber die experimentelle Glomerulonephritis durch das spezifische Antinierenserum. Ein Beitrag zur Pathogenese der diffusen Glomerulonephritis, *Beitr. z. path. Anat. u. z. allg. Path.* **92:**429.

Mohos, S. C., and Skoza, L., 1969, Further characterization of sialoglycoprotein glomerular antigen, *Fed. Proc.* **28:**364.

Sage, H., Crouch, E., and Bornstein, P., 1979, Collagen synthesis by bovine aortic endothelial cells in culture, *Biochemistry* **24:**5433.

Scheinman, J. I., Foidart, J., and Michael, A. F., 1980, The immunohistology of glomerular antigens V. The collagenous antigens of the glomerulus, *Lab. Invest.* **43:**373.

Shin, M. L., Gelfand, R. B., Nagle, J. R., Green, C. I., and Frank, M. M., 1977, Localization of receptors for activated complement on visceral epithelial cells of the human renal glomerulus, *J. Immunol.* **118:**869.

Sraer, J. D., Sraer, J., Ardaillou, R., and Mimouni, M., 1974, Evidence for renal glomerular receptors for angiotensin II, *Kidney Int.* **6:**241.

Striker, G. E., Savin, V., Agodoa, L., and Killen, P., 1976, Glomerular cells *in vitro, Contrib. Neph.* **2:**25.

Striker, G. E., Mannik, M., and Tung, M. Y., 1979, Role of marrow-derived monocytes and mesangial cells in removal of immune complexes in renal glomeruli, *J. Exp. Med.* **149:**127.

Striker, G. E., Killen, P. D., and Farin, F. M., 1980, Human glomerular cells *in vitro*: Isolation and characterization, *Transplant. Proc.* **12**(3):88.

Striker, G. E., Soderland, C., Bower-Pope, D. F., Gown, A. M., Schmer, G., Johnson, A., Suchtel, D., Ross, R., and Striker, L. J., 1984a, Isolation, characterization, and propagation *in vitro* of human glomerular endothelial cells, *J. Exp. Med.* **160:**323.

Striker, L. M.-M., Killen, P. D., Chi, E., and Striker, G. E., 1984b, The composition of glomerulosclerosis. I. Studies in focal sclerosis, crescentic glomerulonephritis, and membranoproliferative glomerulonephritis, *Lab. Invest.* **51:**181.

Tryggvason, K., Robey, P. G., and Martin, G. R., 1980, Biosynthesis of type IV procollagens, *Biochemistry* **19:**1284.

Vernier, R. L., and Birch–Anderson, A., 1963, Studies of the human fetal kidney. Permeability characteristics of the developing glomerulus, *J. Ultrastruct. Res.* **8:**66.

Werb, Z., Banda, M. J., and Jones, P. A., 1980, Degradation of connective tissue matrices by macrophages, *J. Exp. Med.* **152:**1340.

Yamada, E., 1955, The fine structure of the renal glomerulus of the mouse, *J. Biophys. Biochem. Cytol.* **1:**551.

3

The Role of Fixed (Native) and Planted Antigens in Glomerular Disease

Curtis B. Wilson

The humoral mechanisms of immunologic injury causing glomerulonephritis (GN) and potentially tubulointerstitial nephritis can be classified on the basis of the solubility of the antigens involved (Table 1) (Wilson and Dixon, 1981) Soluble antigens in circulating or extravascular fluids, upon reaction with antibody, lead to immune complex (IC) formation. Circulating IC can attain widespread vascular deposition, or their localization may be confined primarily to the glomerulus, which appears to be a particularly susceptible site. Circulating IC can form involving exogenous antigens, generally from infectious agents, or endogenous antigens, such as nuclear materials or tumor-associated antigens (Wilson and Dixon, 1981). IC formation also occurs extravascularly, as in the Arthus reaction (Cochrane and Janoff, 1974), in experimental thyroiditis (Clagett *et al.*, 1974), and in some tubulointerstitial renal diseases in which tubular antigens, including Tamm–Horsfall protein, have been implicated (Unanue *et al.*, 1967; Hoyer, 1980).

Antibodies can also react directly with insoluble (kidney-fixed) antigens (Table 1) (Wilson, 1979; Wilson and Dixon, 1979; Couser and Salant, 1980). Tissue-fixed antigens may be either structural components of the kidney, such as glomerular basement membrane (GBM) and other non-GBM capillary wall materials, or substances from some extrarenal source that are trapped or planted within the glomerulus or potentially other renal structures. Once an immune reaction has occurred and antibody has deposited in the glomerulus or extraglomerular renal tissue by either mechanism, mediation systems are brought into play, leading to tissue injury. Depletion studies have clearly

Curtis B. Wilson • Department of Immunopathology, Research Institute of Scripps Clinic, La Jolla, California 92037. This is publication No. 2411 from the Department of Immunopathology, Research Institute of Scripps Clinic, 10666 North Torrey Pines Road, La Jolla, California 92037. This work was supported in part by United States Public Health Service Grants AM-20043, AM-18626, and AI-07007; and Biomedical Research Support Grant RRO-5514.

Table 1. Categorization of Antibody-Induced Renal Injury Based on the Solubility and Location of the Antigens Involved

Antibodies reactive with soluble antigens
- Soluble antigens in the circulation
  - Circulating immune complex disease
    - Exogenous antigens—e.g., drugs, microbial antigens
    - Endogenous antigens—e.g., nuclear proteins, tumor antigens
- Soluble antigens in the extravascular fluids
  - Extravascular immune complex disease
    - Experimental models—Arthus reaction, tubular antigens

Antibodies reactive with insoluble or tissue-fixed antigens
- Structural antigens of the kidney
  - Classic basement membrane antigens
    - GBM antigens
    - TBM antigens
  - Other nonclassical glomerular capillary wall antigens
    - Experimental models—glomerular antigens in rats (Heymann's nephritis), rabbits

Exogenous or endogenous antigens trapped or "planted" in the kidney
- Experimental models—e.g., immunoglobulin, immune complexes, mesangial deposits, charged molecules, lectins, ?bacterial products, ?DNA

shown a role for complement, polymorphonuclear leukocytes (Cochrane, 1978), and recently monocytes/macrophages (Schreiner *et al.*, 1978; Holdsworth *et al.*, 1981) in certain stages of glomerular damage in experimental animals.

1. *Nephritogenic Basement Membrane Antigens*

1.1. *Experimental Anti-Basement Membrane Antibody Diseases*

Of tissue-fixed antigens that react deleteriously with antibody, the GBM has been recognized as a nephritogenic antigen from experiments dating back through the work of Masugi in the 1930's to the original observation of Lindemann in 1900, who showed the nephrotoxicity of heterologous antikidney antisera (Unanue and Dixon, 1967). More recently, tubular basement membrane (TBM) has been shown to be the nephrotogenic antigen in certain forms of tubulointerstitial nephritis (Andres and McCluskey, 1975; Wilson and Dixon, 1981). Experimentally, heterologous anti-GBM antibody-induced GN occurs in two phases. The first or immediate phase is produced when a sufficient amount of antibody is administered. In the rat, this takes about 75 μg of antibody per gram of kidney (Unanue and Dixon, 1965a). Seven to ten days after administration of the antibody, a second, autologous or delayed phase occurs when the host makes an immune response to the foreign or planted immunoglobulin that is bound to its glomerulus (Unanue and Dixon, 1965b). This phase of injury is the classic example of a planted antigen leading to glomerular injury.

Table 2. Anti-Basement Membrane Antibody Diseases in Man

Anti-GBM antibodies are associated with:
- Combined pulmonary hemorrhage and glomerulonephritis (Goodpasture's syndrome)
- Severe, often rapidly progressive glomerulonephritis
- Occasionally milder, sometimes remitting forms of glomerulonephritis
- Pulmonary hemorrhage presenting as idiopathic pulmonary hemosiderosis
- Recurrent or *de novo* glomerulonephritis after transplantation

Anti-TBM antibodies are associated with:
- Tubulointerstitial nephritis
  - Complicating anti-GBM glomerulonephritis
  - Complicating immune complex glomerulonephritis
  - Some drug-associated tubulointerstitial nephritis
  - Rarely primary tubulointerstitial nephritis
  - Recurrent or *de novo* tubulointerstitial nephritis after transplantation

Other anti-basement membrane antibodies may be responsible for:
- Choroid plexus injury
- Intestinal injury

Several models of both anti-GBM and anti-TBM antibody-induced diseases have been produced in experimental animals by active immunization with GBM, GBM-like antigens isolated from the urine, or TBM (Wilson and Dixon, 1981). For example, sheep immunized with GBM in adjuvant develop a fulminant proliferative GN, with immunologic evidence of anti-GBM antibodies bound to the GBM (Steblay, 1962). Furthermore, anti-GBM antibodies recovered from their circulations transfer the disease to normal sheep (Lerner and Dixon, 1966).

1.2. Anti-Basement Membrane Antibody Diseases in Man

In 1967, Lerner and associates demonstrated the immunopathologic role of anti-GBM antibodies in a series of patients with GN and linear deposits of IgG along their GBMs (Lerner *et al.*, 1967). Anti-GBM antibodies, either obtained from the circulations of these patients or eluted (acid pH) from their renal homogenates, were capable of transferring GN to subhuman primates. The immunopathogenicity of anti-GBM antibodies in human GN was further confirmed when glomerular injury recurred in a renal transplant placed in one of these patients who had demonstrable circulating anti-GBM antibodies. With the help of many collaborators located around the United States and abroad, we have been able to identify almost 700 patients with anti-GBM antibodies. As the series grows, an increasingly larger spectrum of clinical manifestations emerges (Table 2). About 61% of the patients have a condition called Goodpasture's syndrome, consisting of pulmonary hemorrhage and GN. About 37% have GN alone, and 2% have their clinical disease confined to the lung. GN is often rapidly progressive but may be milder and self-remitting. Anti-TBM antibodies accompany the anti-GBM antibodies in about 70% of instances (Lehman *et al.*, 1975). At least two types of anti-TBM antibodies are associated with anti-GBM disease, one reacting with the TBM of only a few tubules and the other reacting diffusely with the TBM of all cortical nephrons. Anti-TBM antibodies also occasionally complicate IC-induced GN and drug-related renal injury, for example, in association with methicillin-related tubulointerstitial nephritis (Border *et al.*, 1974). There are also a few patients who may have primary tubulointerstitial anti-TBM disease (Andres and McCluskey, 1975; Wilson and Dixon, 1981). The choroid plexus basement membrane is an occasional additional site for the reaction of anti-basement membrane antibodies (Wilson and Dixon, 1981). We have seen one patient with intractable diarrhea and nephrotic syndrome who had anti-basement membrane antibodies that reacted with the basement membrane of the jejunum in addition to the TBM (Wilson and Dixon, 1981). Even transplanted kidneys may provide a reactive site, and a complication of this surgical procedure is the recurrence or *de novo* production of both anti-GBM and anti-TBM antibodies (Wilson and Dixon, 1973).

Very little is known about the stimuli that initiate spontaneous autoimmune anti-GBM antibody responses. Since the anti-GBM antibody response is usually transient, the stimulus may also be short-lived. Although no obvious stimulus has been identified as common to an appreciable number of patients, some possible stimuli, such as influenza A2 infection, hydrocarbon solvent and drug exposure, and renal injury, are associated temporally with the onset of disease in a few patients (Beirne and Brennan, 1972; Wilson and Dixon, 1973; Border *et al.*, 1974; Beirne *et al.*, 1977). Occasionally, immunologic renal injury can precede the formation of anti-GBM antibodies, as in membranous GN (Klassen *et al.*, 1974) or systemic lupus erythematosus (Wilson and Dixon, 1981). We have three patients in our series who have developed anti-GBM antibody after treatment of Hodgkin's disease or other lymphomas. Others have noted this association (Kleinknecht *et al.*, 1979). It may be that stroma of the lymph node, particularly after treatment with radiation for lymphoma, may in some way induce anti-GBM antibodies in occasional patients much as lymphoid stroma induced anti-GBM antibodies in anti-lymphocyte globulin preparations some years ago (Wilson *et al.*, 1971). Differences in basement membrane antigens also occur between individuals, which, as will be discussed later, have contributed to the formation of anti-GBM and/or anti-TBM antibodies after renal transplantation (Wilson, 1980a). Basement membrane antigens are also present in the urine (and serum) (McPhaul and Dixon, 1969; Willoughby and Dixon, 1970). When concentrated and reinjected, the urinary antigens can induce nephritogenic anti-GBM antibodies in experimental animals (Lerner and Dixon, 1968). Similar antigens conceivably could lead to induction of anti-basement membrane antibodies in man.

Several years ago, we developed a radioimmunoassay for anti-GBM antibodies utilizing as an antigen a collagenase-solubilized GBM preparation (Wilson *et al.*, 1974a). Other assays are available for the same purpose but involve somewhat different methods of GBM antigen solubilization (reviewed in Wilson and Dixon, 1981). The collagenase-solubilized GBM antigen blocks the reaction of anti-GBM antibodies with basement membranes detectable by indirect immunofluorescence, suggesting that the antigen mixture contains most, if not all, the relevant nephritogenic GBM antigens. Th antigen is nephritogenic in animal studies.

The reactive antigen can be characterized by polyacrylamide gel electrophoresis (PAGE) (Holdsworth *et al.*, 1979). When the immune precipitates of human anti-GBM antibodies and collagenase-solubilized antigens are analyzed by PAGE, two peaks of reactivity having molecular weights of approximately 54,000 and 27,000 are identified. These reactive peaks have about an 80% homology on peptide map analysis. Some reactive material does not enter the gel. It is possible to isolate the reactive antigen peaks by immunoabsorption. Amino acid analysis of the material purified by immunoabsorption reveals that there is no hydroxyproline or hydroxylysine, indicating its noncollagenous nature. The antigenic mixture has significant amino acid differences from the whole isolated GBM, having considerably more serine, glutamic acid, and lysine, and less proline, valine, methionine, isoleucine, leucine, tyrosine, phenylalanine, and arginine. Qualitative assessment of the carbohydrate content of the reactive materials suggests a heteropolysaccharide content. It is possible to obtain fractions that are enriched for either the 54,000- or the 27,000-molecular-weight peaks. Although all sera with anti-GBM antibodies react with both fractions, most sera bind better to the fraction enriched for the 54,000-molecular-weight peak. Samples from a few patients react preferentially with the fraction enriched for the 27,000-molecular-weight material, and several sera react similarly with both fractions. Thus, individuals vary somewhat in reactivity, which may allow for further subdivision of the anti-GBM antibody patient population.

The immunoabsorbent-purified GBM antigen material detects anti-basement membrane antibodies in almost all patients who have other immunopathologic features of anti-basement membrane antibody disease (Wilson, 1980b). There is little quantitative difference in the levels of antibody binding between patients with Goodpasture's syndrome and those with anti-GBM antibody-induced GN alone, implying that the different clinical presentations are not related to the quantities of anti-GBM antibody detected. For positive identification, serum must be obtained early in the course of disease, since the production of circulating anti-GBM antibody is transient, disappearing within a mean duration of about 15 months (range 1–58 months). We have seen one woman who had three bouts of Goodpasture's syndrome over an 11-year period, with reasonable documentation of anti-GBM antibodies during the first and last episodes (Dahlberg *et al.*, 1978). Some differences in the anti-basement membrane antibodies of patients with Goodpasture's syndrome and those with GN alone are suggested by the relative extent of nonrenal basement membrane reactivity demonstrated some years ago by using immunofluorescence (McPhaul and Dixon, 1970). We have just completed a survey of circulating anti-lung basement membrane antibodies in 60 patients with anti-GBM antibody-induced Goodpasture's syndrome compared to 60 patients with anti-GBM antibody-induced GN only. Samples from patients with Goodpasture's syndrome reacted with lung basement membrane antigens, as tested by indirect immunofluorescence, much more frequently than did those with GN alone. Since the clinical division between the two groups is rather arbitrary, some of the overlap may reflect incorrect clinical classification.

The observation that anti-GBM antibody production is transient (Wilson and Dixon, 1973) has generated enthusiasm for aggressive treatment to hasten the decline of antibody production and remove antibody already present in the circulation. This is done with immunosuppressive regimens—including steroids, cyclophosphamide, and other immunosuppressive drugs—and plasma exchange to remove 4–5 liters of plasma every day, replacing the plasma volume with physiologic fluids that do not contain antibody (Lockwood *et al.*, 1975; Johnson *et al.*, 1978). Individual episodes of pulmonary hemorrhage do not correlate well with levels of detected anti-GBM antibody. For many patients, clinical problems such as infection and physiologic disturbances, as in fluid overload (Rees *et al.*, 1977; Johnson *et al.*, 1978), bring on a bout of pulmonary hemorrhage which can be very severe and actually life-threatening, although generally short-lived. At the moment, combined plasma exchange and plasmapheresis therapy are in favor (Lockwood *et al.*, 1979). Evaluation must await carefully controlled clinical trials which are in progress (Johnson *et al.*, 1979). In the most advanced trial, some improvement has been noted in patients treated with immunosuppressive regimens and plasmapheresis compared with those treated with immunosuppression alone; however, the number of patients studied is still small. From the random data available to us from individual patients at many centers (patients not treated in a uniform manner), benefits are suggested. In patients with only mild-to-moderate renal damage, only 20% who were untreated retained adequate renal function to support life without dialysis. About 40% of those treated with steroids and immunosuppressive agents alone and 70% of those treated with combined steroids, immunosuppression, and plasma exchange therapy had initial improvement with maintenance of adequate renal function. We do not yet know how many of these with initial improvement will eventually deteriorate and lose renal function but some do so in a matter of months (Johnson *et al.*, 1978; Finch *et al.*, 1979).

Often, patients with anti-GBM antibody disease lose renal function and are considered for renal transplantation. As noted earlier, one of the most convincing pieces of evidence demonstrating the nephrotoxicity of human anti-GBM antibodies was the observation of recurrent GN in kidneys transplanted into patients while circulating anti-GBM antibodies were present (Lerner *et al.*, 1967; Wilson and Dixon, 1973). If transplantation is postponed until anti-GBM antibody has largely disappeared from the circulation, patients do not usually develop clinically severe recurrences when heavily immunosuppressed for transplant management. Whether the patient's ability to produce autoimmune anti-GBM antibody responses has disappeared, or whether this function is simply blunted by the immunosuppressive regimen, remains to be evaluated fully. This question could be answered recently in a woman who had classic anti-GBM antibody-induced Goodpasture's syndrome (Almkuist *et al.*, 1981). Circulating anti-GBM antibody had disappeared after nephrectomy and remained absent over a 2-year period of follow-up. The patient was then transplanted with an identical twin kidney, without the usual transplant immunosuppression. She soon redeveloped circulating anti-GBM antibody and had clinical and immunopathologic evidence of recurrent anti-GBM antibody-induced GN. Subsequently, immunosuppression and plasma exchange terminated the antibody response, and graft function was preserved. The initial nonimmunosuppressed course allowed redevelopment of the anti-GBM antibody response, apparently stimulated by antigens in the identical twin kidney.

We have been interested recently in the differences in nephritogenic basement membrane antigens between individuals as another potential inducer of anti-basement membrane antibody responses in the renal transplant population (Wilson, 1980a). There are strain and individual differences in basement membrane antigens in animals and in man. For example, the brown Norway rat contains a nephritogenic TBM antigen that the Lewis rat lacks (Lehman *et al.*, 1974a). Anti-TBM antibodies can be induced in a Lewis rat by transplanting it with a TBM antigen-positive kidney from a brown Norway × Lewis F_1 hybrid (Lehman *et al.*, 1974b). We have seen one similar example in a man who lacked the usual nephritogenic TBM antigens in his own kidneys, and who, upon receiving two separate kidney grafts, each with the normal TBM antigens, developed anti-TBM antibodies both times (Wilson *et al.*, 1974b).

Some kindreds of individuals with the hereditary kidney disease termed Alport's syndrome lack the usual nephritogenic GBM antigens (McCoy *et al.*, 1976). One individual with Alport's syndrome who lacked the nephritogenic GBM antigens in his own kidney developed anti-GBM antibodies when transplanted with a normal kidney (Wilson, 1980a). Researchers in England recently found that patients with anti-GBM antibody-induced Goodpasture's syndrome had a high frequency of DRW2 alloantigen (Rees *et al.*, 1978). Whether such a genetic distribution, if confirmed, relates to the antibody response or to the distribution of GBM antigens remains to be determined.

2. *Other Nephritogenic Glomerular Capillary Wall Antigens*

These newly recognized nephritogenic immune systems differ from the classical GBM antigenic mechanisms described previously only in the nature of the antigens involved (Table 1). We sometimes elute antibody from human GN kidneys that appears to react with antigens like those from the animal models to be discussed, suggesting that human counterparts of these models will be identified.

2.1. Structural Glomerular Antigens

By immunofluorescence study, 30–40% of older New Zealand white rabbits have evidence of GN (Verroust *et al.*, 1974). Their glomerular disease is characterized by irregular, granular deposits of immunoglobulin and complement in the glomerular wall which are suggestive of those seen in IC types of GN. By electron microscopy, irregular, nearly continuous electron-dense deposits are seen along the subepithelial aspect of the GBM. The electron-dense deposits are not as distinct and circumscribed as deposits usually associated with IC GN. The immunoglobulin eluted from these kidneys reacts with the glomerular capillary wall of normal rabbits (by indirect immunofluorescence) (Woodroffe *et al.*, 1978). The reaction of the eluate is somewhat irregular, with reactive sites appearing to extend away from the epithelial aspect of the GBM. When the fixation of the eluted antibody was evaluated at the ultrastructural level with immunoperoxidase techniques, binding was detected in the areas where the epithelial cell foot processes attach to the GBM (Neale and Wilson, 1978). This, then, is an example of a nonclassic GBM glomerular capillary wall antigen that is involved in spontaneous GN. The physicochemical nature of this new nephritogenic antigen remains to be defined. A radioimmunoassay is being developed to detect the antibody in rabbits and in turn may prove useful in extending our understanding of similar systems to man.

Another GN that seems to involve the direct reaction of antibody with glomerular capillary wall antigens is the model developed by Heymann and colleagues in the late 1950s, employing rats immunized with rat kidney suspensions in adjuvant (Heymann *et al.*, 1959). By immunofluorescence, rats with Heymann's nephritis have granular immunoglobulin and complement deposits along the GBM, and by electron microscopy, electron dense deposits are present on the subepithelial aspect of the GBM. The immunofluorescence deposits are not as round and circumscribed as those usually associated with circulating IC deposits, but are rather more geographic in nature, suggesting that they may outline structures within the glomerular capillary wall. In 1967, it was found that eluates from these kidneys reacted with renal tubular brush border antigens of the proximal renal convoluted tubule, leading to the postulate that this disease was an autologous IC disease involving formation and glomerular deposition of antibody and renal tubular brush border antigen (Edgington *et al.*, 1967, 1968). A crude extract of renal tubules (termed Fx1A) was found which induced the lesion, and a 28 S lipoprotein purified from the Fx1A (termed RTE-α-5) could induce the illness when given in very small quantities (Edgington *et al.*, 1968). In the mid-1970s, a model with similar immunopathologic findings was induced using heterologous anti-Fx1A antibodies (Barabas and Lannigan, 1974; Feenstra *et al.*, 1975). Recent studies indicate that the glomerular binding of the heterologous anti-Fx1A antibodies proceeds slowly over several days (Salant *et al.*, 1980). In 1978, *in vivo* and *in vitro* studies using perfused kidneys suggested that the heterologous anti-Fx1A antibodies bound to antigen already present in the glomerulus (Couser *et al.*, 1978; Van Damme *et al.*, 1978). The antibody was infused in such a way as to exclude the presence of circulating antigen and subsequent IC formation.

A question then arose regarding the nature of reactivity in the active Heymann's nephritis model. We found that eluates of kidneys from rats with Heymann's nephritis contained antibody that could bind to an antigen(s) present within normal rat glomerular capillary walls (Neale and Wilson, 1979). The antibodies binding to the glomerular capillary wall were present in lower dilutions than those also present that bound to the renal tubular brush border antigens, as had been observed earlier by Edgington *et al.* (1967, 1968). By using an immunoperoxidase electron microscopic method, it was possible to localize the reactive antigen in the glomerular wall in a scattered granular distribution concentrated along the subepithelial aspect of the GBM (Neale and Wilson, 1979). Similar eluates bind to glomeruli when passed through the isolated perfused kidney described previously under circumstances in which IC formation is excluded. This process shows that the eluted antibody can bind directly to the glomerulus (T. J. Neale, W. G. Couser, and C. B. Wilson, unpublished observations). These studies, however, neither exclude an additional role of tubular antigen-antibody IC in this model, as postulated by Edgington *et al.* (1967), nor do they provide information regarding a separation, if any, between glomerular and tubular antigens and the antibody reactivities to them.

Based on the rabbit and rat models, the concept of direct antibody attack against glomerular antigens can be expanded to include not only the GBM but at least two other glomerular capillary wall antigens. These antigens are concentrated around the epithelial cell foot processes in the rabbit model and are present as scattered granular accumulations along the subepithelial aspect of the GBM in the Heymann's nephritis model.

2.2. *Planted Glomerular Antigens*

Materials normally exogenous to the glomerulus may become trapped or planted within the glomerular capillary wall for subsequent nephritogenic immune reaction. As mentioned earlier, heterologous anti-GBM antibody in the autologous phase of experimental anti-GBM antibody-induced GN is a classic example of a planted nephritogenic antigen. In IC-induced GN, the IC becomes a source of planted antigen (or antibody) for continued interaction of antibody (or antigen) from the circulation. In experimental situations, it is possible to show that antibody or antigen alone can bind to the IC deposits. Once an IC lesion starts, it can in theory be perpetuated by interactions of either antigen or antibody alone from the circulation, as they react with previously planted IC. The most convincing evidence that materials from the circulation interact with planted IC in the serum sickness models is the situation in which extreme antigen excess is created purposely; just as IC are dissolved *in vitro* by such a manipulation, they are removed quantitatively from the glomerulus (Wilson and Dixon, 1971). As a result, the rabbit with chronic serum sickness GN recovers completely if treatment begins before irreversible damage is done (Wilson, 1974). Extreme antigen excess treatment also rapidly terminates specific antibody production, providing another therapeutic benefit.

Other planted antigens are known or have been discussed. Material taken up in the mesangium can react with antibody and in turn can cause GN (Mauer *et al.*, 1973). It has also been suggested that DNA may combine with the GBM for subsequent IC formation *in situ* when anti-DNA antibody is present (Izui *et al.*, 1976, 1977). If so, this mechanism could play a part in some of the autoimmune anti-DNA diseases that are inducible with bacterial lipopolysaccharide or parasites.

Just as antigen and antibody can combine with deposited IC *in situ*, other antibodies formed by the host to components of the IC deposit, for example, anti-idiotypic antibody, rheumatoid factor, or potentially immunoconglutinins, might add to the deposit and thus increase phlogogenicity. Once a nidus of planted antigen is present, continuing development of the inflammatory lesion is possible.

We were interested to see if material that binds to the glomerular capillary wall for physicochemical reasons could serve as a nephritogenic planted antigen. We used the lectin concanavalin A (Con A), which binds to carbohydrate in the glomerular capillary wall (Golbus and Wilson, 1979). Con A infused into the renal artery of a rat binds to the glomerular capillary wall in a pattern determined by how much is given and the time sequence of sampling; the localization is rather linear early and becomes more irregular and scattered later. Passively administered antibody reacts with the planted Con A-incited GN (Golbus and Wilson, 1979). In quantitative terms, when sufficient Con A is infused to plant 75 μg/g of kidney, glomerular injury occurs when about 70 μg/g of the administered anti-Con A antibody binds. As mentioned earlier, it takes a similar amount (about 75 μg) of anti-GBM antibody per gram of kidney to induce immediate phase anti-GBM antibody injury in the rat (Unanue and Dixon, 1965a). Con A planted in the kidney of a rat previously immunized to Con A also incites glomerular injury by interaction of the autologously formed antibody. This lectin model clearly establishes the nephritogenic potential of antigens fixing to the glomerular capillary wall for any of a variety of physicochemical reasons, including charge characteristics of the polyanionic glomerular capillary wall by attracting cationic substances such as protamine, ruthenium red, and other cationic dyes (Farquhar, 1978). Some infectious organisms pathogenic for man have materials with lectinlike properties, suggesting similar potentials. Occasionally, patients have bacterial antigen localized within the glomeruli, but little or no immunoglobulin, suggesting the possibility that bacterial antigens bind directly to the glomerulus (Treser *et al.*, 1969; Hyman *et al.*, 1975; Pertschuk *et al.*, 1976), in turn serving as planted antigens for *in situ* IC formation within the glomerular capillary wall.

3. Conclusion

In conclusion, the nephritogenic immune reactions involving tissue-fixed antigens, either structural components of the kidney or foreign materials trapped there, have been reviewed. Our current understanding of anti-GBM antibody disease has been outlined. The spontaneous or induced models of nonclassic GBM or planted glomerular capillary wall antigens in nephritogenic immune reactions with the potential human counterparts have been summarized. Research in the area of nephritogenic immune reactions involving tissue-fixed antigens must progress on several interrelated fronts in both man and experimental systems. We need to improve methods of identification to understand incidence, clinical pathologic correlates, and natural history. The role of nephritogenic reactions involving nonclassic GBM and planted antigens in human GN must be determined. The physicochemical nature of the nephritogenic antigens, their physiology, metabolism, and genetic determinants need to be understood. The factors that lead to the induction of the nephritogenic "autoimmune" antibody responses must be explored through basic immunology and clinical observations. Additional information on humoral and cellular mediation systems, and in particular factors influencing progression of immune renal injury, is needed. Manipulation of these factors may provide therapeutic benefit. The therapeutic efforts currently being tried need to be evaluated in large and well-controlled trials to judge their real value. Attempts to develop immunologically specific interruption of the nephritogenic immune reactions should be the goal for effective and lasting management. This is an exciting area and one in which meaningful progress can be expected. This progress will in turn decrease the number of individuals facing the expensive and less than satisfactory management of end-stage renal failure.

References

Almkuist, R. D., Buckalew, V. M., Hirszel, P., Maher, J. F., James, P. M., and Wilson, C. B., 1981, Recurrence of anti-glomerular basement membrane antibody mediated glomerulonephritis in an isograft, *Clin. Immunol. Immunopathol.* **18:**54.

Andres, G. A., and McCluskey, R. T., 1975, Tubular and interstitial renal disease due to immunologic mechanisms, *Kidney Int.* **7:**271.

Barabas, A. Z., and Lannigan, R., 1974, Induction of an autologous immune complex glomerulonephritis in the rat by intravenous injection of heterologous anti-rat kidney tubular antibody. I. Production of chronic progressive immune-complex glomerulonephritis, *Br. J. Exp. Pathol.* **55:**47.

Beirne, G. J., and Brennan, J. T., 1972, Glomerulonephritis associated with hydrocarbon solvents: Mediated by antiglomerular basement membrane antibody, *Arch. Environ. Health* **25:**365.

Beirne, G. J., Wagnild, J. P., Zimmerman, S. W., Macken, P. D., and Burkholder, P. M., 1977, Idiopathic crescentic glomerulonephritis, *Medicine* **56:**349.

Border, W. A., Lehman, D. H., Egan, J. D., Sass, H. J., Glode, J. E., and Wilson, C. B., 1974, Antitubular basement-membrane antibodies in methicillin-associated interstitial nephritis, *N. Engl. J. Med.* **291**:381.

Clagett, J. A., Wilson, C. B., and Weigle, W. O., 1974, Interstitial immune complex thyroiditis in mice. The role of autoantibody to thyroglobulin, *J. Exp. Med.* **140**:1439.

Cochrane, C. G., 1978, Mediating systems in inflammatory disease, *J. Invest. Dermatol.* **71**:40.

Cochrane, C. G., and Janoff, A., 1974, The Arthus reaction: A model of neutrophil and complement-mediated injury, in: *The Inflammatory Process,* 2nd ed., Volume III (B. W. Zweifach, L. Grant, and R. T. McCluskey, eds.), Academic Press, New York, pp. 85–162.

Couser, W. G., and Salant, D. J., 1980, *In situ* immune complex formation and glomerular injury, Editorial, *Kidney Int.* **17**:1.

Couser, W. G., Steinmuller, D. R., Stilmant, M M., Salant, D. J., and Lowenstein, L. M., 1978, Experimental glomerulonephritis in the isolated perfused rat kidney, *J. Clin. Invest.* **62**:1275.

Dahlberg, P. J., Kurtz, S. B., Donadio, J. V., Jr., Holley, K. E., Velosa, J. A., Williams, D. E., and Wilson, C. B., 1978, Recurrent Goodpasture's syndrome, *Mayo Clin. Proc.* **53**:533.

Edgington, T. S., Glassock, R. J., and Dixon, F. J., 1967, Autologous immune complex pathogenesis of experimental allergic glomerulonephritis, *Science* **155**:1432.

Edgington, T. S., Glassock, R. J., and Dixon, F. J., 1968, Autologous immune complex nephritis induced with renal tubular antigen. I. Identification and isolation of the pathogenetic antigen, *J. Exp. Med.* **127**:555.

Farquhar, M. G., 1978, Structure and function in glomerular capillaries: Role of the basement membrane in glomerular filtration, in: *Biology and Chemistry of Basement Membranes* (N. A. Kefalides, ed.), Academic Press, New York, p. 43.

Feenstra, K., Lee, R.vd, Greben, H. A., Arends, A., and Hoedemaeker, P. J., 1975, Experimental glomerulonephritis in the rat induced by antibodies directed against tubular antigens. I. The natural history: A histologic and immunohistologic study at the light microscopic and the ultrastructural level, *Lab. Invest.* **32**:235.

Finch, R. A., Rutsky, E. A., McGowan, E., and Wilson, C. B., 1979, Treatment of Goodpasture's syndrome with immunosuppression and plasmapheresis, *South. Med. J.* **72**:1288.

Golbus, S. M., and Wilson, C. B., 1979, Experimental glomerulonephritis induced by *in situ* formation of immune complexes in glomerular capillary wall, *Kidney Int.* **16**:148.

Heymann, W., Hackel, D. B., Harwood, S., Wilson, S. G. F., and Hunter, J. L. P., 1959, Production of nephrotic syndrome in rats by Freund's adjuvants and rat kidney suspensions, *Proc. Soc. Exp. Biol. Med.* **100**:660.

Holdsworth, S. R., Golbus, S. M., and Wilson, C. B., 1979, Characterization of collagenase solubilized human glomerular basement membrane antigens reacting with human antibodies, *Kidney Int.* **16**:797 (abstr.)

Holdsworth, S. R., Neale, T. J., and Wilson, C. B., 1981, Abrogation of macrophage-dependent injury in experimental glomerulonephritis in the rabbit: Use of an antimacrophage serum, *J. Clin. Invest.* **68**:686.

Hoyer, J. R., 1980, Tubulointerstitial immune complex nephritis in rats immunized with Tamm-Horsfall protein, *Kidney Int.* **17**:284.

Hyman, L. R., Jenis, E. H., Hill, G. S., Zimmerman, S. W., and Burkholder, P. M., 1975, Alternate C3 pathway activation in pneumococcal glomerulonephritis, *Am. J. Med.* **58**:810.

Izui, S., Lambert, P. H., and Miescher, P. A., 1976, *In vitro* demonstration of a particular affinity of glomerular basement membrane and collagen for DNA. A possible basis for a local formation of DNA-anti-DNA complexes in systemic lupus erythematosus, *J. Exp. Med.* **144**:428.

Izui, S., Lambert, P. H., Fournie, G. J., Türler, H., and Miescher, P. A., 1977, Features of systemic lupus erythematosus in mice injected with bacterial lipopolysaccharides. Identification of circulating DNA and renal localization of DNA-anti-DNA complexes, *J. Exp. Med.* **145**:1115.

Johnson, J. P., Whitman, W., Briggs, W. A., and Wilson, C. B., 1978, Plasmapheresis and immunosuppressive agents in antibasement membrane antibody-induced Goodpasture's syndrome, *Am. J. Med.* **64**:354.

Johnson, J. P., Briggs, W. A., Bohan, L., Lombardo, J. V., and Wilson, C. B., 1979, The role of plasmapheresis in anti-glomerular basement membrane antibody-mediated renal disease, in: *Controversies in Nephrology—1979*, Volume 1 (G. Schreiner, W. Winchester, W. Mattern, and B. Mendelssohn, eds.), Georgetown University, Washington, D.C., pp. 303–312.

Klassen, J., Elwood, C., Grossberg, A. L., Milgrom, F., Montes, M., Sepulveda, M., and Andres, G. A., 1974, Evolution of membranous nephropathy into anti-glomerular-basement-membrane glomerulonephritis, *N. Engl. J. Med.* **290:**1340.

Kleinknecht, D., Morel–Maroger, L., Callard, P., Adhemar, J. P., and Mahieu, P., 1979, Antiglomerular basement membrane (GBM) antibody-induced glomerulonephritis after solvent exposure, *Kidney Int.* **15:**450 (abstr.)

Lehman, D. H., Wilson, C. B., and Dixon, F. J., 1974a, Interstitial nephritis in rats immunized with heterologous tubular basement membrane, *Kidney Int.* **5:**187.

Lehman, D. H., Lee, S., Wilson, C. B., and Dixon, F. J., 1974b, Induction of antitubular basement membrane antibodies in rats by renal transplantation, *Transplantation* **17:**429.

Lehman, D. H., Wilson, C. B., and Dixon, F. J., 1975, Extraglomerular immunoglobulin deposits in human nephritis, *Am. J. Med.* **58:**765.

Lerner, R. A., and Dixon, F. J., 1966, Transfer of ovine experimental allergic glomerulonephritis (EAG) with serum, *J. Exp. Med.* **124:**431.

Lerner, R. A., and Dixon, F. J., 1968, The induction of acute glomerulonephritis in rabbits with soluble antigens isolated from normal homologous and autologous urine, *J. Immunol.* **100:**1277.

Lerner, R. A., Glassock, R. J., and Dixon, F. J., 1967, The role of anti-glomerular basement membrane antibody in the pathogenesis of human glomerulonephritis, *J. Exp. Med.* **126:**989.

Lockwood, C. M., Boulton–Jones, J. M., Lowenthal, R. M., Simpson, I. J., Peters, D. K., and Wilson, C. B., 1975, Recovery from Goodpasture's syndrome after immunosuppressive treatment and plasmapheresis, *Br. Med. J.* **2:**252.

Lockwood, C. M., Pussell, B., Wilson, C. B., and Peters, D. K., 1979, Plasma exchange in nephritis, in: *Advances in Nephrology*, Volume 8 (J. Hamburger, J. Crosnier, J.-P. Grünfeld, and M. H. Maxwell, eds.), Year Book, Chicago, pp. 383–418.

Mauer, S. M., Sutherland, D. E. R., Howard, R. J., Fish, A. J., Najarian, J. S., and Michael, A. F., 1973, The glomerular mesangium: III. Acute immune mesangial injury: A new model of glomerulonephritis, *J. Exp. Med.* **137:**553.

McCoy, R. C., Johnson, H. K., Stone, W. J., and Wilson, C. B., 1976, Variation in glomerular basement membrane antigens in hereditary nephritis, *Lab. Invest.* **34:**325.

McPhaul, J. J., Jr., and Dixon, F. J., 1969, Immunoreactive basement membrane antigens in normal human urine and serum, *J. Exp. Med.* **130:**1395.

McPhaul, J. J., Jr., and Dixon, F. J., 1970, Characterization of human anti-glomerular basement membrane antibodies eluted from glomerulonephritic kidneys. *J. Clin. Invest.* **49:**308.

Neale, T. J., and Wilson, C. B., 1978 Non-GBM glomerular antigen in spontaneous nephritis in rabbits, *Kidney Int.* **14:**715 (abstr.)

Neale, T. J., and Wilson, C. B., 1979, Fixed glomerular antigen in Heymann's nephritis: Eluted antibody reactivity with normal rat glomeruli, *Kidney Int.* **16:**799 (abstr.)

Pertschuk, L. P., Woda, B. A., Vuletin, J. C., Brigati, D. J., Soriano, C. B., and Nicastri, A. D., 1976, Glomerulonephritis due to Staphylococcus aureus antigen, *Am. J. Clin. Pathol.* **65:**301.

Rees, A. J., Lockwood, C. M., and Peters, D. K., 1977, Enhanced allergic tissue injury in Goodpasture's syndrome by intercurrent bacterial infection, *Br. Med. J.* **2:**723.

Rees, A. J., Peters, D. K., Compston, D. A. S., and Batchelor, J. R., 1978, Strong association between HLA-DRW2 and antibody-mediated Goodpasture's syndrome, *Lancet* **1:**966.

Salant, D. J., Darby, C., and Couser, W. G., 1980, Experimental membranous glomerulonephritis in rats. Quantitative studies of glomerular immune deposit formation in isolated glomeruli and whole animals, *J. Clin. Invest.* **66:**71.

Schreiner, G. F., Cotran, R. S., Pardo, V., and Unanue, E. R., 1978, A mononuclear cell component in experimental immunological glomerulonephritis, *J. Exp. Med.* **147:**369.

Steblay, R. W., 1962, Glomerulonephritis induced in sheep by injections of heterologous glomerular basement membrane and Freund's complete adjuvant, *J. Exp. Med.* **116:**253.

Treser, G., Semar, M., McVicar, M., Franklin, M., Ty, A., Sagel, I., and Lange, K., 1969, Antigenic streptococcal components in acute glomerulonephritis, *Science* **163:**676.

Unanue, E. R., and Dixon, F. J., 1965a, Experimental glomerulonephritis. V. Studies on the interaction of nephrotoxic antibodies with tissues of the rat, *J. Exp. Med.* **121:**697.

Unanue, E. R., and Dixon, F. J., 1965b, Experimental glomerulonephritis. VI. The autologous phase of nephrotoxic serum nephritis, *J. Exp. Med.* **121:**715.

Unanue, E. R., and Dixon, F. J., 1967, Experimental glomerulonephritis: Immunological events and pathogenetic mechanisms, *Adv. Immunol.* **6:**1.

Unanue, E. R., Dixon, F. J., and Feldman, J. D., 1967, Experimental allergic glomerulonephritis induced in the rabbit with homologous renal antigens, *J. Exp. Med.* **125:**163.

Van Damme, B. J. C., Fleuren, G. J., Bakker, W. W., Vernier, R. L., and Hoedemaeker, Ph. J., 1978, Experimental glomerulonephritis in the rat induced by antibodies directed against tubular antigens. V. Fixed glomerular antigens in the pathogenesis of heterologous immune complex glomerulonephritis, *Lab. Invest.* **38:**502.

Verroust, P. J., Wilson, C. B., and Dixon, F. J., 1974, Lack of nephritogenicity of systemic activation of the alternate complement pathway, *Kidney Int.* **6:**157.

Willoughby, W. F., and Dixon, F. J., 1970, Experimental hemorrhagic pneumonitis produced by heterologous anti-lung antibody, *J. Immunol.* **104:**28.

Wilson, C. B., 1974, Immune complex glomerulonephritis, in: *Proceedings of the 5th International Congress of Nephrology*, Mexico, 1972, Volume 1, Karger, Basel, pp. 68–74.

Wilson, C. B., 1979, Immune reactions with antigens in or of the glomerulus, in: *Immunopathology* (F. Milgrom and B. Albini, eds.), Karger, Basel, pp. 127–131.

Wilson, C. B., 1980a, Individual and strain differences in renal basement membrane antigens, *Transplant Proc.* **12**(Suppl. 1)**:**69.

Wilson, C. B., 1980b, Radioimmunoassay for anti-glomerular basement membrane antibodies, in: *Manual of Clinical Immunology*, 2nd ed. (N. R. Rose and H. Friedman, eds.), American Society for Microbiology, Washington, D.C., pp. 376–379.

Wilson, C. B., and Dixon, F. J., 1971, Quantitation of acute and chronic serum sickness in the rabbit, *J. Exp. Med.* **134:**7s.

Wilson, C. B., and Dixon, F. J., 1973, Anti-glomerular basement membrane antibody-induced glomerulonephritis, *Kidney Int.* **3:**74.

Wilson, C. B., and Dixon, F. J., 1979, Renal injury from immune reactions involving antigens in or of the kidney, in: *Contemporary Issues in Nephrology*, Volume 3 (C. B. Wilson, B. M. Brenner, and J. H. Stein, eds.), Churchill Livingstone, New York, pp. 35–66.

Wilson, C. B., and Dixon, F. J., 1981, The renal response to immunological injury, in: *The Kidney*, 2nd ed., Volume 1 (B. M. Brenner and F. C. Rector, Jr., eds.), Saunders, Philadelphia, pp. 1237–1350.

Wilson, C. B., Dixon, F. J., Fortner, J. G. and Cerilli, J., 1971, Glomerular basement membrane-reactive antibodies in anti-lymphocyte globulin, *J. Clin. Invest.* **50:**1525.

Wilson, C. B., Marquardt, H., and Dixon, F. J., 1974a, Radioimmunoassay (RIA) for circulating antiglomerular basement membrane (GBM) antibodies, *Kidney Int.* **6:**114a (abstr.)

Wilson, C. B., Lehman, D. H., McCoy, R. C., Gunnels, J. C., Jr., and Stickel, D. L., 1974b, Antitubular basement membrane antibodies after renal transplantation, *Transplantation* **18:**447.

Woodroffe, A. J., Neale, T. J., and Wilson, C. B., 1978, Spontaneous glomerulonephritis (GN) in New Zealand white (NZW) rabbits, VIIth International Congress of Nephrology, Montreal, Canada, June 18–23 (abstr.)

4

Deposition of Circulating Immune Complexes in Glomeruli

Mart Mannik

Experimental and clinical investigations have established the relationship between circulating immune complexes and the deposition of immune complexes in glomeruli. In spontaneous disease models, in models induced by antigen administration, and in human glomerulonephritis the principal locations of immune complexes are in the subendothelial, mesangial, and subepithelial areas. The presence of immune complexes in glomeruli can result from local formation, as reviewed in the paper by Dr. Curtis B. Wilson, or from deposition of these substances from circulation. The purpose of this review is to consider the pertinent information on glomerular deposition of circulating immune complexes.

The known and potential variables related to the mechanisms that lead to glomerular deposition of circulating immune complexes are numerous. The categories of variables include: (1) the characteristics and quantity of circulating complexes and (2) the structural and functional features of the glomerular capillaries.

1. Characteristics of Immune Complexes

The essential features of immune complexes are antigens, antibodies, and the nature of the union between these reactants.

1.1. Antigens

Antigens can range from small molecules (e.g., haptens) to macromolecules, cells, or microbes. A consideration of soluble, circulating immune

Mart Mannik • Division of Rheumatology, Department of Medicine, University of Washington, Seattle, Washington 98195.

complexes and their deposition in glomerular structures excludes the discussion of particulate immune complexes, e.g., antibody-coated red cells or antibody-coated microorganisms. The chemical nature of antigens influences the biologic properties of the formed antigen–antibody complexes. The *valence of antigens*, defined as the number of *antigenic determinants* for a specific antibody, alters the nature of formed complexes. Antigens may range from uni- to multivalent for a given antibody, and they may possess one or many different antigenic determinants. The physical size and charge of antigens influence the biologic properties of formed antigen–antibody complexes. Finally, antigens alone may bind to glomeruli or interact with cell receptors thereby altering the fate of circulating immune complexes.

1.2. Antibodies

Antibodies in immune complexes may belong to the IgG, IgA, IgM, IgD, or IgE classes of immunoglobulins that will dictate the biologic activities of immune complexes, including complement activation and interaction with receptors on phagocytic cells. The valence of IgG, monomeric IgA, IgD, and IgE is 2, whereas the polymeric IgA and IgM have higher valences, depending in part on the physical size of antigens.

1.3. The Lattice of Immune Complexes

Defined as the number of antigens and number of antibody molecules in a given immune complex, the lattice of immune complexes has an important role in the expression of biologic properties of these materials. The valence of antigens dictates the lattice of immune complexes. Monovalent antigens at best can form Ag_2Ab_1 complexes. Large-latticed immune complexes and immune precipitates cannot be generated. Even bivalent antigens do not build a sufficient lattice to form a precipitate. Only multivalent antigens form large-latticed soluble complexes and immune precipitates. The degree of antigen excess in relation to the point of maximal precipitation also alters the lattice of complexes; i.e., in very high degrees of antigen excess only small-latticed complexes are formed (e.g., Ag_1Ab_1, Ag_2Ab_1, or Ag_2Ab_2). Furthermore, low-avidity antibodies tend to form small-latticed complexes, and at very low concentrations of the reactants the formed complexes shift toward formation of small-latticed complexes, even when the antigen–antibody ratio and antigen valence favor formation of large-latticed complexes. Thus, a number of features can alter the lattice of circulating immune complexes.

1.4. Characteristics of Circulating Immune Complexes That Influence Glomerular Deposition

In chronic serum sickness models of glomerulonephritis subendothelial, mesangial, and subepithelial deposits of immune complexes were encountered. In these models it was not possible to distinguish with certainty between local formation of antigen–antibody complexes and deposition of immune complexes from circulation. The injection of characterized, preformed immune complexes into experimental animals has elucidated several variables that influence glomerular deposition of complexes. These studies have focused on the use of antibodies of the IgG class of immunoglobulins with few exceptions. Rifai *et al.* (1979) used mouse plasmacytoma (MOPC-315) as a source of IgA antibodies to the dinitrophenyl (DNP) group to form immune complexes with DNP–BSA conjugates. Upon injection into mice these preformed immune complexes localized principally in the mesangial area. Furthermore, soluble, preformed immune complexes prepared with IgA antibodies and dextrans as antigens, varying in size and in isoelectric point, localized after intravenous injection in the mesangial area, most likely because of rapid removal of these antigens from circulation and formation of large-latticed complexes (Isaacs and Miller, 1983). Aggregated human IgM as a surrogate for immune complexes localized upon injection into rats in the mesangial and subendothelial areas (Kijlstra *et al.*, 1978). All subsequent comments will be confined to immune complexes containing the IgG class of antibodies.

The total load or concentration of immune complexes in circulation influences the extent of their deposition in glomeruli. A relatively small amount of circulating antigen was deposited in glomeruli in acute or chronic serum sickness models (Wilson and Dixon, 1970, 1971). A small fraction of injected, preformed complexes deposited in kidneys (Arend and Mannik, 1971). The concentration of circulating immune complexes is a dynamic balance between the rate of immune complex formation and the rate of immune complex removal. Very little is known about the rate of immune complex formation in spontaneous disease models and human diseases. The hepatic mononuclear phagocyte system (Kupffer cells) plays the key role in removal of soluble circulating immune complexes. Large-latticed immune complexes (defined as containing more than two antibody molecules, i.e., $>Ag_2Ab_2$) were effectively removed from circulation by the Kupffer cells owing to interaction with Fc receptors, whereas small-latticed complexes (Ag_1Ab_1, Ag_2Ab_1, Ag_2Ab_2) persisted longer in circulation than large-latticed complexes (Mannik *et al.*, 1971; Arend and Mannik, 1971; Mannik and Arend, 1971; Haakenstad and Mannik, 1976). The hepatic uptake of immune complexes was saturable and resulted in prolonged circulation and enhanced glomerular deposition of complexes (Haakenstad and Mannik, 1974; Haakenstad *et al.*, 1976). When the mononuclear phagocyte system was activated in mice with *Corynebacterium parvum*, clearance of circulating immune complexes was enhanced and glomerular deposition decreased in comparison to control mice (Barcelli *et al.*, 1981).

The injection of preformed immune complexes into unimmunized animals has shown that circulating immune complexes deposit only in the subendothelial and mesangial areas of glomeruli and not in the subepithelial area, when they were examined both by immunofluorescence and by transmission electron microscopy. These studies were all done in mice, using rabbit antibodies to BSA (Okumura *et al.*, 1971), to HSA (Haakenstad *et al.*, 1976), or to DNP·BSA (Koyama *et al.*, 1978).

Several lines of evidence suggested that only large-latticed immune complexes ($>Ag_2Ab_2$) were deposited from circulation into the subendothelial and mesangial areas. First, when mixtures of large-latticed and small-latticed complexes were administered, deposition in glomeruli progressed only while large-latticed complexes persisted in circulation, and the deposits declined in intensity while small-latticed complexes remained in circulation (Haakenstad *et al.*, 1976). Second, when only small-latticed complexes were administered, achieved by preparing HSA–anti-HSA complexes at 50-fold antigen excess, no glomerular deposition was seen over a 4-day period (Mannik and Haakenstad, 1977; Haakenstad *et al.*, 1982). Third, when preformed large-latticed immune complexes were allowed to deposit in the mesangial and endothelial areas, then the administration of excess antigen resulted in release of all extracellular complexes, by conversion of large-latticed to small-latticed immune complexes (Mannik and Striker, 1980).

The role of antibody avidity in deposition of immune complexes in glomeruli has been examined by several investigators, but only some examples will be considered here. In one study preformed complexes were prepared at 80-fold antigen excess from ovalbumin and rabbit antibodies to ovalbumin, using either high- or low-avidity antibodies (Germuth *et al.*, 1979a,b). The injection of preformed immune complexes made with low-avidity antibodies resulted in epithelial deposits, detected by immunofluorescence microscopy and by electron microscopy. In contrast, when complexes prepared with high-avidity antibodies were injected, the complexes were localized in the mesangial area. The difference was attributed to the variation in antibody avidity. Three points are of note in relation to these experiments. First, free ovalbumin, with a molecular weight of 40,000, persists in circulation of mice for a short time with half of the material removed in less than 10 min. Therefore, the injected 80-fold excess antigen is quickly removed from circulation. Second, the complexes prepared at 80-fold antigen excess most likely were small latticed. Third, the lattice of complexes prepared with low- and high-affinity antibodies would differ mainly in the dissociation into free antigen and free antibody. The most likely explanation for the observed results is that with rapid loss of excess antigen, the complexes with high-avidity antibodies were converted to large-latticed complexes and localized in the mesangial area. On the other hand, with loss of excess antigen, the complexes with low-avidity antibodies dissociated into free antigen and free antibody, thus creating alternating presence of antigen and antibody with repeated injections and resulting in local formation of immune complexes in the subepithelial area, as demonstrated experimentally by Fleuren *et al.* (1980).

The conclusion of Koyama *et al.* (1978) that immune complexes made with high-avidity antibodies and DNP_{29}·BSA localized in the mesangial area and immune complexes made with low-avidity antibodies and DNP_{29}·BSA resulted in no glomerular deposition also is best explained on the basis of the lattice of formed complexes. The former combination of reactants resulted in large-latticed and the latter in small-latticed complexes. The same authors also showed that antigen valence influenced glomerular localization of complexes. Complexes prepared with DNP_{29}·HSA and antibodies with moderate avidity localized in the mesangial area, but complexes with the same antibody and DNP_7·BSA had only minimal deposition in glomeruli. The latter complexes most likely consisted only of small lattices under the conditions used. These observations indicate that the influence of antibody avidity in glomerular localization of complexes is expressed through varying lattice formation and the ability of complexes made with low-avidity antibodies to dissociate into free antigen and free antibody.

Several investigations have explored the interaction between the fixed negative charge on the glomerular capillary wall and variations in the charge of immune complexes. Gallo *et al.* (1981) showed that positively charged immune complexes decorated the fixed negative charges of mouse laminae rarae interna and externa, but the development of immune deposits was not further followed since the observations were only extended to 1 hr after injection of the immune complexes. Gauthier *et al.* (1982) showed that cationized antibodies alone or small-latticed (Ag_2Ab_2, Ag_1Ab_1) immune complexes prepared with these antibodies persisted only for a few hours in glomeruli. In contrast, immune complexes with larger lattices and containing cationized antibodies initially bound to the fixed negative sites in the lamina rara interna and then condensed into extensive, subendothelial deposits in the capillary loops. With passage of time these deposits tended to migrate toward the mesangial area (Gauthier *et al.*, 1982). Immune complexes with cationic antigens have a comparable sequence of deposition. Immune complexes with negatively charged antibodies deposited in the mesangial area, indicating that at least some part of mesangial deposition of immune complexes is not dependent on charge–charge interactions (Gauthier *et al.*, 1984).

The significance of charge–charge interactions in the planting of antigens for *in situ* formation of immune complexes has been examined in detail both with passive models in rats (Oite *et al.*, 1982) and with active models in rats and rabbits (Oite *et al.*, 1983; Border *et al.*, 1982). The conclusion has been reached that cationic molecules with molecular sizes up to and above 400,000 can penetrate the glomerular basement membrane to form immune complexes in the subepithelial area as seen in membranous glomerulonephritis, whereas proteins with molecular weight of 900,000 and above do not penetrate the lamina densa (Vogt *et al.*, 1982). Accordingly, small-latticed immune complexes may reach the subepithelial area if the molecular weight does not exceed 900,000. In one study the conclusion was reached that immune complexes can indeed reach the subepithelial area, using complexes that were covalently cross-linked with a two-stage cross-linking reagent, but the size of the injected complexes was not carefully defined (Caulin-Glaser *et al.*, 1983). Thus, some uncertainty remains with regard to the passage of intact immune complexes through the lamina densa of the glomerular basement membrane. On the other hand, Vogt *et al.* (1982) have suggested that immune complexes localized in the subendothelial area may dissociate, pass through the lamina densa as separate molecules of antigen and antibody, and reform immune complexes in the subepithelial area.

The sequence of deposition of circulating immune complexes in glomerular structures by electron microscopy is of some interest. After the intravenous injection of a single bolus of immune complexes (Haakenstad *et al.*, 1976), electron-dense deposits were first seen in endothelial fenestrae and the subendothelial area, particularly adjacent to the mesangium. This was followed by development of mesangial deposits. When the large-latticed complexes cleared from circulation, then the visible deposits disappeared first from the endothelial fenestrae, then the subendotheial area, and eventually from the mesangial area. The injected immune complexes in these preparations were soluble and ranged up to about 22 S on ultracentrifugation, obviously not approaching the size of deposits visualized by electron microscopy in tissue specimens. Therefore, during the glomerular filtration process at the glomerular capillary wall a rearrangement or condensation of immune complexes must occur to form precipitates that become visible by electron microscopy. During this process the excess antigen must not become concentrated locally since otherwise precipitates would not be achieved. The formation of the precipitates or large aggregates as visible deposits appears to depend on immunospecific reactions since (1) the immune deposits are dissolved by large amounts of excess antigen (Mannik and Striker, 1980); (2) when in mice immune deposits developed simultaneously with ferritin and with fibrinogen as the antigens, the immune deposits were segregated by electron microscopy to those containing ferritin and those containing fibrinogen without mixed deposits (Kubeš, 1977).

Proof for condensation of immune complexes into larger lattices was provided with a system where covalent bonds could be established between the haptenic group and antibody-combining site after complexes with a desired lattice had been formed (Mannik *et al.*, 1983). The complexes that had a fixed lattice and were not able to precipitate initially interacted with glomerular structures to the same extent as complexes that were not covalently cross-linked. With passage of time the cross-linked complexes disappeared from glomeruli in less than 8 hr, whereas the non-cross-linked complexes persisted and evolved into large, electron-dense deposits. The necessity of a precipitating antigen–antibody system for development of electron-dense immune deposits in the subepithelial area was demonstrated by using varying hapten density on a carrier protein (Agodoa *et al.*, 1983). With nonprecipitating antigen–antibody systems and cationic antigens, transient immune deposits were present by immunofluorescence microscopy, and electron-dense deposits did not evolve. When precipitating antigen–antibody systems were used, then the deposits persisted by immunofluorescence microscopy and electron-dense deposits evolved. These series of experiments emphasized the requirement for precipitating antigen–antibody systems for development of persisting glomerular immune deposits.

The preceding discussion of rearrangement of soluble immune complexes into immune precipitates during deposition in glomeruli raises the question of how a variety of protein aggregates form deposits in glomeruli, including aggregated albumin, aggregated IgG, and aggregated IgM (Michael *et al.*, 1967; Kijlstra *et al.*, 1978). The answers to this question are not known. Polymers of IgG, however, are known to undergo nonimmunospecific protein–protein interactions (Nardella and Mannik, 1978) that may explain formation of large deposits, again provided that local concentration increases owing to either filtration process or electrostatic interactions.

The current concepts on the role of the nature of circulating immune complexes on glomerular deposition can be expanded by the study of deposition of a carefully characterized spectrum of antigen–antibody complexes containing varying antibodies and varying antigens. The concepts derived from experimental animals can be applied to the characterization of circulating immune complexes in human diseases.

2. *Structural and Functional Features of Glomerular Capillaries in Relation to Deposition of Circulating Immune Complexes*

The role of the negative charge on the glomerular capillary wall in deposition of circulating immune complexes was considered in the preceding section.

The role of the C3b receptors in localization of circulating immune complexes in glomeruli remains uncertain. These receptors have been identified with certainty only in human and primate glomeruli and were identified only on epithelial cells (Carlo *et al.*, 1981). When preformed immune complexes were injected into mice, mouse C3 accumulated in glomerular deposits with some delay (Haakenstad *et al.*, 1976), indicating that the antigen–antibody deposits formed in glomeruli prior to binding C3. Complement components can solubilize already formed immune complexes (reviewed by Takahashi *et al.*, 1980) or prevent formation of immune deposits (reviewed by Schifferli and Peters, 1983). The tissue deposition of such immune complexes with attached components of complement has not been examined.

The purposeful and known alteration of the glomerular structure or function should help to clarify the mechanisms of glomerular deposition of immune complexes. The bulk of completed work in this area has been directed at the deposition and removal of immune complexes or surrogates of immune complexes in the mesangium. This topic was recently reviewed by Michael *et al.* (1980).

The prior deposition of ferritin–antiferritin complexes in the mesangial areas of rats delayed the egress and appeared to have enhanced the deposition of aggregated human IgG, used as a surrogate for immune complexes (Keane and Raij, 1980). Ford and Kosatka (1980) suggested enhanced deposition of circulating immune complexes in mice when prior immune complexes were formed in the mesangium, but kinetics of deposition were not examined, and the systems used may have caused some of the observed changes. The binding of antibodies to rat glomerular basement membrane (Mauer *et al.*, 1974) and the treatment of rats with aminonucleoside of puromycin (Mauer *et al.*, 1972) enhanced the deposition of aggregated human IgG in the mesangium and probably thereby delayed the egress of this substance from the mesangium. The mechanisms for these alterations in mesangial deposition of the surrogates of immune complexes remain uncertain. Furthermore, the reduction of endothelial fenestrae did not impair the mesangial deposition of the same probe for mesangial function (Keane and Raij, 1981). Bilateral obstruction of ureters resulted in initially decreased and subsequently enhanced accumulation of aggregated human IgG in glomerular mesangium of rats (Raij *et al.*, 1979).

A decrease of mesangial deposition of injected, preformed, immune complexes was observed in rats that had subepithelial deposits of immune complexes as part of the induced autologous immune complex nephritis (Schneeberger *et al.*, 1980). In these experiments some loss of the injected immune complexes occurred in urine as part of the induced proteinuria.

All these experiments collectively show that know alterations of the glomerular structure and function can alter the deposition of immune complexes in glomeruli. The meaning of these observations, however, in relation to the mechanisms of immune complex deposition from circulation remains to be elucidated.

References

Agodoa, L. Y. C., Gauthier, V. J., and Mannik, M., 1983, Precipitating antigen-antibody systems are required for the formation of subepithelial electron dense immune deposits in rat glomeruli, *J. Exp. Med.* **158:**1259.

Arend, W. P., and Mannik, M., 1971, Studies on antigen–antibody complexes. II. Quantification of tissue uptake of soluble complexes in normal and complement-depleted rabbits, *J. Immunol* **107:**63.

Barcelli, U., Rademacher, R., Ooi, Y. M., and Ooi, B. S., 1981, Modification of glomerular immune complex deposition in mice by activation of the reticuloendothelial system, *J. Clin. Invest.* **67:**20.

Border, W. A., Ward, H. J., Kamil, E. S., and Cohen, A. H., 1982, Induction of membranous nephropathy in rabbits by administration of an exogenous cationic antigen, *J. Clin. Invest.* **69:**451.

Carlo, J. R., Ruddy, S., and Conway, A. F., 981, Localization of the receptors for activated complement on the visceral epithelial cells of the human renal glomerulus by immunoenzymatic microscopy, *Am. J. Clin. Pathol.* **75:**23.

Caulin-Glaser, T., Gallo, G. R., and Lamm, M. E., 1983, Nondissociating cationic immune complexes can deposit in glomerular basement membrane, *J. Exp. Med.* **158:**1561.

Ebling, F., and Hahn, B. H., 1980, Restricted subpopulations of DNA antibodies in kidneys of mice with systemic lupus. Comparison of antibodies in serum and renal eluates, *Arthritis Rheum.* **23:**392.

Fleuren, G., Groud, J., and Hoedemaeker, P. J., 1980, *In situ* formation of subepithelial glomerular immune complexes in passive serum sickness, *Kidney Int.* **17:**631.

Ford, P. M., and Kosatka, I., 1980, The effect of *in situ* formation of antigen–antibody complexes in the glomerulus on subsequent glomerular localization of passively administered immune complexes, *Immunology* **39:**337.

Gallo, G. R., Caulin–Glaser, T., and Lamm, M. E., 1981, Charge of circulating immune complexes as a factor in glomerular basement membrane localization in mice. *J. Clin. Invest.* **67:**1305.

Gauthier, V. J., Mannik, M., and Striker, G. E., 1982, Effect of cationized antibodies in preformed immune complexes on deposition and persistence in renal glomeruli, *J. Exp. Med.* **156:**766.

Gauthier, V. J., Striker, G. E., and Mannik, M., 1984, Glomerular localization of immune complexes prepared with anionic antibodies or with cationic antigens, *Lab. Invest.* **50:**636.

Germuth Jr., F. G., Rodriguez, E., Lorelle, C. A., Trump, E. I., Milano, L., and Wise, O'L., 1979a, Passive immune complex glomerulonephritis in mice: Models for various lesions found in human disease. I. High avidity complexes and mesangiopathic glomerulonephritis, *Lab. Invest.* **41:**360.

Germuth Jr., F. G., Rodriguez, E., Lorelle, C. A., Trump, E. I., Milano, L. L., and Wise, O'L., 1979b, Passive immune complex glomerulonephritis in mice: Models for various lesions found in human disease. II. Low avidity complexes and diffuse proliferative glomerulonephritis with subepithelial deposits, *Lab. Invest.* **41:**366.

Haakenstad, A. O., and Mannik, M., 1974, Saturation of the reticuloendothelial system with soluble immune complexes, *J. Immunol.* **112:**1939.

Haakenstad, A. O., and Mannik, M., 1976, The disappearance kinetics of soluble immune complexes prepared with reduced and alkylated antibodies and with intact antibodies in mice, *Lab. Invest.* **35:**283.

Haakenstad, A. O., Striker, G. E., and Mannik, M., 1976, The glomerular deposition of soluble immune complexes prepared with reduced and alkylated antibodies and with intact antibodies in mice, *Lab. Invest.* **35:**293.

Haakenstad, A. O., Striker, G. E., and Mannik, M., 1982, The disappearance kinetics and glomerular deposition of small-latticed soluble immune complexes. *Immunology* **47:**407.

Isaacs, K. L., and Miller, F., 1983, Antigen size and charge in immune complex glomerulonephritis. II. Passive induction of immune deposits with dextran–anti-dextran immune complexes, *Am. J. Pathol.* **111:**298.

Keane, W. F., and Raij, L., 1980, Impaired mesangial clearance of macromolecules in rats with chronic mesangial ferritin-antiferritin immune complex deposition, *Lab. Invest.* **43:**500.

Keane, W. F., and Raij, L., 1981, Determinants of glomerular mesangial localization of immune complexes. Role of endothelial fenestrae, *Lab. Invest.* **45:**366.

Kijlstra, A., van der Lelij, A., Knutson, D. W., Fleuren, G. J., and van Es, L. A., 1978, The influence of phagocyte function on glomerular localization of aggregated IgM in rats, *Clin. Exp. Immunol.* **32:**207.

Koyama, A., Niwa, Y., Shigematsu, H., Taniguchi, M., and Tada, T., 1978, Studies on passive serum sickness. II. Factors determining the localization of antigen–antibody complexes in the murine renal glomerulus, *Lab. Invest.* **38:**253.

Kubeš, L., 1977, Experimental immune complex glomerulonephritis in the mouse with two types of immune complexes, *Virchows Arch. B Cell. Pathol.* **24:**343.

Mannik, M., and Arend, W. P., 1971, Fate of preformed immune complexes in rabbits and rhesus monkeys, *J. Exp. Med.* **134:**19s.

Mannik, M., and Haakenstad, A. O., 1977, Circulation and glomerular deposition of immune complexes, *Arthritis Rheum.* **20:**S148.

Mannik, M., and Striker, G. E., 1980, Removal of glomerular deposits of immune complexes in mice by administration of excess antigen, *Lab. Invest.* **42:**483.

Mannik, M., Arend, W. P., Hall, A. P., and Gilliland, B. C., 1971, Studies on antigen–antibody complexes. I. Elimination of soluble complexes from rabbit circulation, *J. Exp. Med.* **133:**713.

Mannik, M., Agodoa, L. Y. C., and David, K. A., 1983, Rearrangement of immune complexes in glomeruli leads to persistence and development of electron dense deposits. *J. Exp. Med.* **157:**1516.

Mauer, S. M., Fish, A. J., Blau, E. B., and Michael, A. F., 1972, The glomerular mesangium. I., Kinetic studies of macromolecular uptake in normal and nephrotic rats, *J. Clin. Invest.* **51**:1092.

Mauer, S. M., Fish, A. J., Day, N., and Michael, A. F., 1974, The glomerular mesangium. II. Studies of macromolecular uptake in nephrotoxic nephritis rats, *J. Clin. Invest.* **53**:431.

Michael, A. F., Fish, A. J., and Good, R. A., 1967, Glomerular localization and transport of aggregated protein in mice, *Lab. Invest.* **17**:14.

Michael, A. F., Keane, W. F., Raij, L., Vernier, R. L., and Mauer, S. M., 1980, The glomerular mesangium, *Kidney Int.* **17**:141.

Nardella, F. A., and Mannik, M., 1978, Nonimmunospecific protein–protein interactions of IgG: Studies of the binding of IgG to IgG immunoadsorbents, *J. Immunol.* **120**:739.

Oite, T., Batsford, S. R., Mihatsch, M. J., Takamiya, H., and Vogt, A., 1982, Quantitative studies of *in situ* immune complex glomerulonephritis in the rat induced by planted, cationized antigen, *J. Exp. Med.* **155**:460.

Oite, T., Shimizu, F., Kihara, I., Batsford, S. R., and Vogt, A., 1983, An active model of immune complex glomerulonephritis in the rat employing cationized antigen, *Am. J. Pathol.* **112**:185–194.

Okumura, K., Kondo, Y., and Tada, T., 1971, Studies on passive serum sickness. I. The glomerular fine structure of serum sickness nephritis induced by preformed antigen–antibody complexes in the mouse, *Lab. Invest.* **24**:383.

Raij, L., Keane, W. F., Osswald, H., and Michael, A., 1979, Mesangial function in ureteral obstruction in the rat. Blockade of the efferent limb, *J. Clin. Invest.* **64**:1204.

Rifai, A., Small, P. A., Teague, P. O., and Ayoub, E. M., 1979, Experimental IgA nephropathy, *J. Exp. Med.* **150**:1161.

Schifferli, J. A., and Peters, D. K., 1983, Complement, the immune-complex lattice, and the pathophysiology of complement-deficiency syndromes, *Lancet* **2**:957.

Schneeberger, E. E., Collins, A. B., Stavrakis, G., and McCluskey, R. T., 1980, Diminished mesangial accumulation of intravenously injected soluble immune complexes in rats with autologous immune complex nephritis, *Lab. Invest.* **42**:440.

Takahashi, M., Takahashi, S., and Hirose, S., 1980, Solubilization of antigen–antibody complexes: A new function of complement as a regulator of immune reactions, *Prog. Allergy* **27**:134.

Vogt, A., Rohrbach, R., Shimizu, F., Takamiya, H., and Batsford, S., 1982, Interaction of cationized antigen with rat glomerular basement membrane: *In situ* immune complex formation, *Kidney Int.* **22**:27.

Wilson, C. B., and Dixon, F. J., 1970, Antigen quantitation in experimental immune complex glomerulonephritis. I. Acute serum sickness, *J. Immunol.* **105**:279.

Wilson, C. B., and Dixon, F. J., 1971, Quantitation of acute and chronic serum sickness in the rabbit, *J. Exp. Med.* **134**:7s.

Cystic Diseases of the Kidney

5

Renal Cystic Disease as the Target of Research

Kenneth D. Gardner, Jr.

1. Introduction

Cystic diseases account for 10% of all end-stage kidney disease (Cleveland and Fellner, 1979). Through Medicaid and Medicare their treatments cost our society about $200 million annually. Federal support for research into these conditions—their cause(s), prevention, arrest, and detection—approximates $500,000 a year. That is to say, of every federal dollar spent on renal cystic disease, more than 99 cents goes for treatment; less than 1 cent goes for research. This pittance of $500,000 reflects not defective central management but rather a relative lack in the field of interested, qualified investigators who are competitive for federal research dollars.

This section is intended to stimulate, intrigue, and inform the non-cystites among us about where we have been in renal cystic disease and where we might go. Our ultimate goal is the arrest, prevention, or cure of these often lethal, most certainly costly, disorders.

2. Cyst Formation

In his classic essay on adult polycystic kidney disease (APKD), Dalgaard (1957) noted a relatively constant pattern of clinical evolution among hundreds of subjects: pain, then enlargement, and finally failure of kidney function. He postulated that cysts, progressively enlarging, compress otherwise normal adjacent renal tissue until it is unable to function. In brief, in APKD, Dalgaard attributed renal failure to cyst expansion.

Kenneth D. Gardner, Jr. • Department of Medicine, University of New Mexico School of Medicine, Albuquerque, New Mexico 87131.

In the quarter century that has ensued, researchers of cystic kidney disease have sought answers to three questions that are inherent in Dalgaard's postulate: Why do cysts form? Why do they enlarge? Does their enlargement cause renal failure?

In the susceptible kidney, cysts conceivably could form for a variety of reasons. Increased compliance of tubular basement membrane or increased intraluminal pressures—the consequence of obstruction, increased filtration, or decreased net reabsorption of water—could cause tubular walls to blow out. Fibrosis in the interstitium could pull on tubular walls, causing them to pouch out. Tubular cells could grow into the interstitium, undergo central necrosis, and leave a cystic cavity communicating with the nephrons. A tubule could elongate, become redundant, and lose its common wall. Adjacent tubules could coalesce, giving rise to cysts between nephrons.

Three of these possibilities can be laid quickly to rest. Microdissection and microscopic examination of susceptible and developing cystic kidneys do not reveal interstitial fibrosis, evidence of looping, or coalescence of tubules (Baert, 1978). Evidence has accumulated, however, to support both the "blowing out" and the neoplasia hypotheses. Virchow saw solutes plugging tubules in adult polycystic disease and cited obstruction as its cause (Editorial, 1969). Several other European pathologists described cellular proliferation in APKD, sometimes to the point of neoplasia (Nauwerck and Huischmid, 1893).

More recently the "blowing out" and the neoplasia hypotheses have been the subject of both clinical and laboratory investigations. The clinical studies, primarily of APKD, group themselves into three major categories: morphologic studies, inulin and isotope perfusion, and cyst fluid analyses.

Microdissection and reconstruction studies reveal that cysts are focal dilations or appendages of nephrons (Lambert, 1947). In APKD they occur at various sites, most commonly in the loop of Henle and along the collecting tubule and duct.

Inulin perfusion studies have yielded conflicting results. Earlier studies demonstrated that inulin enters and accumulates in cysts in the polycystic kidney (Lambert, 1947; Bricker and Patton, 1955). More recent observations, however, contradict this finding (Muther and Bennett, 1980).

In Sweden, Jacobson and his co-workers (1977) injected tritiated water into cysts *in vivo* and serially sampled the cyst fluid thereafter. The concentrations of tritiated water in cyst fluid fell with time. Turnover rates of cyst fluid were calculated to be as high as 100 ml/day, far in excess of the single-nephron glomerular filtration rate in the human kidney. The question of how such high turnover rates might occur was not answered.

Analyses of cyst fluid have yielded several findings of interest: Cysts contain fluid whose compositions resemble that of proximal or distal tubular fluid (Gardner, 1969; Huseman *et al.*, 1980). Sodium concentrations may range, for example, in a bimodal distribution from highs of 150 to lows of 1 or 2 mEq/liter. In cysts with low sodium concentrations, amino acids reach concentrations of 50 mEq/liter (Gardner, 1969). Cyst fluid osmolality approximates that of plasma. "Hippurates" appear in low concentrations in both proximal and distal cysts (Huseman *et al.*, 1980).

The results of these studies of clinical material have led to conclusions that, in APKD at least, cysts communicate with nephrons, are functional, and do contribute to the formation of urine. They shed little, if any, light on the question of pathogenesis.

During these clinical studies, however, several investigators measured intracystic hydrostatic pressures (Jacobson *et al.*, 1977; Huseman *et al.*, 1980). The findings are surprisingly consistent. The conclusions are not. Hydrostatic pressures are elevated in some cysts, but not all, of virtually all cystic kidneys studied *in vivo*. Do these findings confirm or deny the presence of obstruction? The question is under debate.

Dunnill and co-workers (1977) added a new dimension to our understanding of renal cystic disorders when they described the morphology of *acquired* cystic disease in humans. Noncystic kidneys of patients on chronic hemodialysis may undergo new cell growth and cyst formation. Studies of the composition and dynamics of cyst fluid in these kidneys have not been performed. Nonetheless it now is clear that renal cystic disease in man can be acquired as well as inherited.

Because clinical material is relatively scarce and difficult to study, laboratory models of renal cystic disease have been given increasing attention. They consist, like their human counterparts, of both inherited and acquired disease. The former occurs in rats, cats, pigs, and mice. The latter is produced primarily by the feeding of cystogenic chemicals to rats. Of the two varieties, acquired cystic disease is the more widely studied. It resembles human disease in that cysts form and enlarge in once-normal kidneys.

Structurally, the animal models, too, display new cell growth, primarily along collecting tubules and ducts (Evan *et al.*, 1979). It is visible as hyperplasia and micropolyp formation. It occurs in inherited and in acquired disease. It appears, before cysts form, along collecting tubules in response to the cystogens diphenylamine (Evan *et al.*, 1978) and nordihydroguaiaretic acid (Evan and Gardner, 1979). Sometimes the polyps that develop appear to partially obstruct nephrons.

Functionally, in the chemically induced models intracystic hydrostatic pressures are elevated (Evan *et al.*, 1978) or may rise in response to the introduction by microperfusion of fluid into dilated proximal tubules on the surface of the kidney (Evan and Gardner, 1979). Water filtration and reabsorption rates, as measured by micropuncture techniques, appear to be intact. The excretion of tritrated inulin is delayed from these nephrons. From observations such as these, the conclusion has been drawn that cystic nephrons are partially obstructed (Evan *et al.*, 1979).

A second school of thought about pathogenesis has sprung from the study of another chemical model, that induced in rats by the feeding of diphenylthiazole (DPT) (Carone *et al.*, 1974). In that model fewer than 5% of dilated, cystic nephrons had elevated pressures. To explain cyst formation the concept was invoked that DPT increases the compliance of tubular basement membrane, allowing the normal transmural pressure gradient of some 5 mm Hg to distend the wall. This concept focuses on the prevalence of nephrons with normal pressures rather than on those with elevated pressures. As is the case with human disease, then, the significance of some normal and some elevated hydrostatic pressures in the models has given rise to controversy (Gardner, 1981).

3. Summary

To summarize, I have highlighted evidence that supports roles for neoplasia, disordered cell growth, obstruction, and altered mural compliance in the pathogenesis of renal cysts. The new cell growth that occurs in cystic kidneys both in inherited and in acquired disease, both in human and in animal, implicates neoplasia. The occurrence of polyps across species lines and in pathogenetically dissimilar forms of renal cystic disease strengthens the likelihood that neoplasia plays a role in cyst formation. The facts that polyps may partially occlude lumens, that intracystic pressures are increased, and that the excretion of [^{3}H]inulin is delayed from cystic nephrons, all favor obstruction. Altered mural compliance is suggested by the observation that pressures are not elevated in most tubules of one cystic model (DPT).

Based on occasional publications, three additional, possible contributors to renal cyst formation need to be mentioned: There is a chance that cystic renal disease may result from nonspecific tubular damage. When the papillary region of rabbit kidneys is excised, tubules dilate and corticomedullary cysts form (Cuttino *et al.*, 1977). The renal lesion produced by lead is characterized by cysts late, but by acute tubular necrosis early, in its course (Boyland *et al.*, 1962). Small cysts were noted by Oliver in the kidney from a patient with recurrent episodes of paroxysmal cold hemoglobinuria (Oliver *et al.*, 1951).

It also may be that aging contributes to cyst formation. Simple cysts, at least, increase in frequency with age. Baert and Steg (1977) believe their origin lies in collecting tubular diverticulae, which also become more prevalent as the kidney approaches senesence.

Finally, there is the theme of the cystogenic metabolite, introduced by McGeogh and Darmady (1975) from experience with the chemical cystogens. They were the first to suggest that some product of an inherited defect in metabolism might favor the formation of renal cysts.

Among questions that future research into renal cystic disease might answer are the following:

1. What is a "cyst"? Are morphologists satisfied that dilated tubules are cysts or must cysts be fluid-filled sacs with no, one, or two, but not more, communications with the nephron?
2. Are diverticula forerunners of cysts? What is the difference between them?
3. Could accelerated aging explain the process of cyst formation?

4. In fact, is there a cystogenic metabolite? Need we do other experiments, besides transplanting noncystic kidneys into patients whose native cystic kidneys have failed and then waiting to see if the transplanted organs become cystic?
5. Is tubular wall compliance, normally low, increased in the kidney susceptible to cyst formation?
6. Why is tubular cell growth altered in the several forms of renal cystic disease? Is it response to injury, an inherited defect in tubular cell replication, or what? Is it restricted to only cystic diseases of the kidney?
7. Why do cysts form and enlarge?
8. Does their enlargement lead to progressive renal disease?
9. Could pharmacologic intervention limit cyst growth and thereby slow, arrest, or prevent costly end-stage renal disease?
10. Does water get into cysts and if so, how?

In this section, a group of investigators, whose special interests are directly or indirectly relevant to renal cystic disease, review several aspects of this entity. Drs. Bernstein and Evan review the morphology of inherited and of acquired renal cystic disease in man and animals. Dr. Toback seizes on the proliferative element and reviews the subject of ordered and disordered growth of renal tubular cells. Drs. Grantham and Bennett present the issues surrounding the movement and passage of molecules, including inulin and water, into and out of cysts. Dr. Welling correlates cyst function with cyst wall structure. Dr. Holmes presents studies of early polycystic kidney disease. We seek to answer the most practical question of all: Can we cure renal cystic disease by stopping the growth of cysts?

References

Baert, L., 1978, Hereditary polycystic kidney disease (adult form): A microdissection study of two cases at an early stage of the disease, *Kidney Int.* **13**:519.

Baert, L., and Steg, A., 1977, Is the diverticulum of the distal and collecting tubulus a preliminary stage of the simple cyst in the adult? *J. Urol.* **118**:707.

Boyland, E., Dukes, C. E., Grover, P. L., and Mitchley, B. C. V., 1962, The induction of renal tumors by feeding lead acetate to rats, *Br. J. Cancer* **16**:283.

Bricker, N. S., and Patton, J. F., 1955, Cystic disease of the kidney: Study of dynamics and chemical composition of cyst fluid, *Am. J. Med.* **18**:207.

Carone, F. A., Rowland, R. G., Perlman, S. G., and Ganote, C. E., 1974, The pathogenesis of drug-induced renal cystic disease, *Kidney Int.* **5**:411.

Cleveland, W., and Fellner, S. K., 1979, Hereditary nephropathies as a cause of end-stage renal disease, *Dialysis Transplant* **8**:633.

Cuttino, J. T., Herman, P. G., and Mellins, H. Z., 1977, The renal collecting system after medullary damage, *Investigative Radiol.* **12**:241.

Dalgaard, O. Z., 1957, Bilateral polycystic disease of the kidneys, *Acta Med. Scand.* (*suppl*) **328**:17.

Dunnill, M. S., Millard, P. R., and Oliver, D., 1977, Acquired cystic disease of the kidneys: A hazard of long-term intermittent maintenance hemodialysis, *J. Clin. Pathol.* **30**:868.

Editorial, 1969, The enigma of familial polycystic kidneys, *N. Engl. J. Med.* **281**:1013.

Evan, A. P., and Gardner, K. D., Jr., 1979, Nephron obstruction in nordihydroguaiaretic acid-induced renal cystic disease, *Kidney Int.* **15:**7.

Evan, A. P., Hong, S. K., Gardner, K. D., Jr., Park, Y. S., and Itagaki, R., 1978, Evolution of the collecting tubular lesion in diphenylamine-induced renal disease, *Lab. Invest.* **35:**93.

Evan, A. P., Gardner, K. D., Jr., Bernstein, J., 1979, Polypoid and papillary epithelial hyperplasia: A potential cause of ductal obstruction in adult polycystic disease, *Kidney Int.* **16:**743.

Gardner, K. D., Jr., 1969, Composition of fluid in twelve cysts of a polycystic kidney, *N. Engl. J. Med.* **281:**985.

Gardner, K. D., Jr., 1981, Cyst function in adult polycystic kidney disease, in: *Controversies in Nephrology* (G. Schreiner, ed.), Nephrology Division, University of Georgetown Press, Washington, D.C., pp. 279–285.

Huseman, R., Grady, A., Welling, D., and Grantham, J., 1980, Macropuncture study of polycystic disease in adult human kidneys, *Kidney Int.* **18:**375.

Jacobson, L., Lindquist, B., Michaelson, G., and Bjerle, P., 1977, Fluid turnover in renal cysts, *Acta Med. Scand.* **202:**327.

Lambert, P. P., 1947, Polycystic disease of the kidney: A review, *Arch. Pathol.* **44:**34.

McGeogh, J. E. M., and Darmady, E. M., 1975, Polycystic disease of kidney, liver and pancreas; a possible pathogenesis, *J. Pathol.* **119:**221.

Muther, R. S., and Bennett, W. M., 1980, Cyst fluid antibiotic levels in polycystic kidney disease: Differences in proximal and distal cyst permeability, Abstracts of The American Society of Nephrology, p. 26A.

Nauwerck, C., and Huischmid, K., 1893, Uber das multiloculare adenokystom der niere, *Beitr. Path. Anat.* **12:**1.

Oliver, J., MacDowell, M., and Tracy, A., 1951, Pathogenesis of acute renal failure associated with traumatic and toxic injury. Renal ischemia nephrotoxic damage, and the ischaemic episode, *J. Clin. Invest.* **30:**1305.

6

Morphology of Human Renal Cystic Disease

Jay Bernstein

1. *Introduction*

This chapter contains a discussion of certain morphologic features of autosomal dominant, adult polycystic kidney disease (APKD) in relation to current theories of pathogenesis. The principal theories are (1) obstruction of tubular lumina by epithelial hyperplasia and (2) increased compliance of tubular walls secondary to an abnormality in the tubular basement membrane.

The first of the two hypotheses has old roots and was revived recently by Evan and Gardner (1979), who observed epithelial hyperplasia in experimental cystic disease. The observation was then confirmed in human cystic kidneys by Evan, Gardner, and Bernstein (1979), demonstrating the relevance of the experimental models to the clinical disease. The second hypothesis, suggested on the basis of experimental observations by Carone *et al.* (1974), was supported by Grantham and colleagues (Cuppage *et al.*, 1980; Huseman *et al.*, 1980) in clinical studies of solute concentrations and hydrostatic pressures in human cystic kidneys. Their data indicate that cysts probably occupy relatively short segments of nephrons, and they found the pressures in most cysts to lie within the normal range of transmural tubular pressure. They have interpreted their findings to mean that portions of tubules dilate without increased pressure and, hence, without obstruction, perhaps as the result of increased stretchability of tubular basement membranes.

The morphologic observations provide no insight into the etiology of APKD. They do not serve to differentiate between a developmental abnormality in nephrogenesis leading to malformation and an inherited defect in

---

Jay Bernstein • Department of Anatomic Pathology, William Beaumont Hospital, Royal Oak, Michigan 48072. This work was supported in large part by a grant from The William Beaumont Hospital Research Institute.

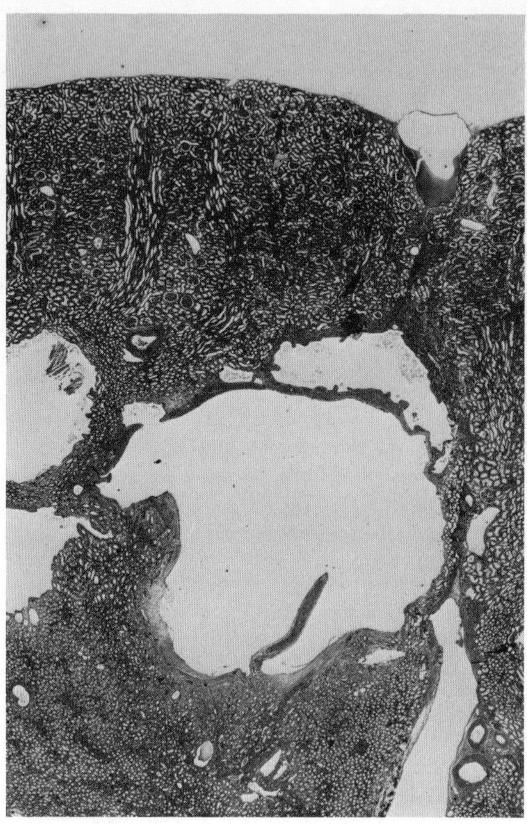

Figure 1. The kidney in an "early" stage of APKD contains numerous cysts with well-preserved intervening parenchyma. The patient was a young adult, asymptomatic for renal disease, who died of a ruptured cerebral aneurysm, and postmortem examination showed renal and hepatic cysts. Hematoxylin and eosin stain, ×10.

metabolism leading to abnormal tubular components. Either could theoretically set the stage for progressive cyst formation, although the distinction does carry implications for potential therapeutic intervention and pharmacologic mediation of the abnormality.

2. *Distribution of Cysts*

Most of us are acquainted with the gross appearance of terminal APKD, in which the kidney is greatly enlarged and in which the parenchyma appears to be replaced entirely by cysts. Cysts in early stages of APKD are restricted and localized in their distribution, which is sometimes disseminated and sometimes segmental, and not all nephrons are affected. Eulderink and Hogewind (1978) have demonstrated focal nephronic involvement of nephrons in young infants with what appears to have been incipient APKD. I have illustrated the point that cysts early in the course of APKD are focally distributed and that the intervening parenchyma is histologically normal (Bernstein, 1979) (Fig. 1). Although I assumed then that APKD progresses

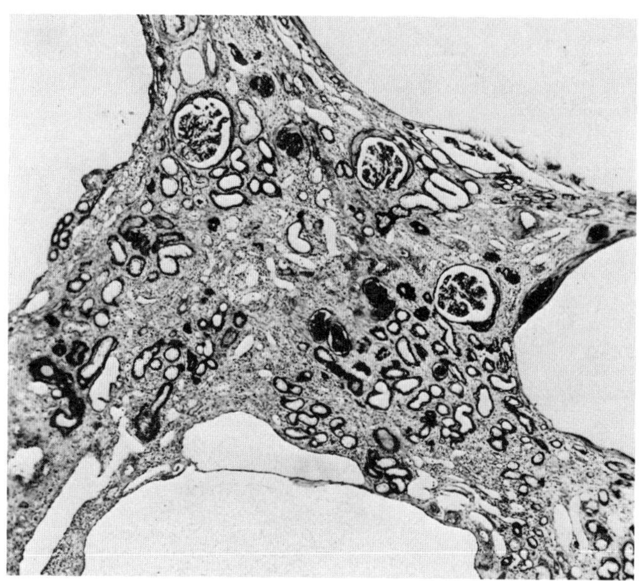

Figure 2. The kidney in a late stage of APKD contains large cysts, and the intervening parenchyma is severely atrophic, with glomerular sclerosis, tubular atrophy, and interstitial fibrosis. Vascular sclerosis is inconsequential. The parenchymal atrophy may have contributed more to renal insufficiency than parenchymal replacement by cysts. Periodic acid–Schiff stain, ×40.

through the involvement of additional nephrons, Huseman *et al.* (1980) have estimated that only a small proportion of the nephrons are likely to be affected. Indeed, microscopic examination of the end-stage lesion shows a surprisingly large amount of solid renal parenchyma, and it appears unlikely from visual impression alone that the disease progresses to renal insufficiency simply because of cystic replacement of the parenchyma. It appears more likely that renal insufficiency results in large part from secondary effects on the adjacent parenchyma. The remaining parenchyma is atrophic and sclerotic (Fig. 2), perhaps from the pressure of enlarging cysts, perhaps from circulatory impairment.

Several earlier morphologic studies have shown, in relation to the observations of Huseman *et al.* (1980) on the functional localization of cysts to segments of nephrons, that cysts do indeed occupy relatively small segments of nephrons. Localized nephronic dilatation was shown by Lambert (1947) in his reconstructions of sectioned kidneys and by Heggö (1966) and Baert (1978) in their microdissections. Baert showed a predilection of the cysts for Henle's loops and the collecting tubules, confirming Heggö's observations, and he showed localized dilatations of proximal and distal convolutions. Incidentally, he found no evidence of abnormal ductal branching or abnormal nephronic attachment to ducts, and he also found the kidneys to contain many normal nephrons. He suggested that the cysts might arise from tubular

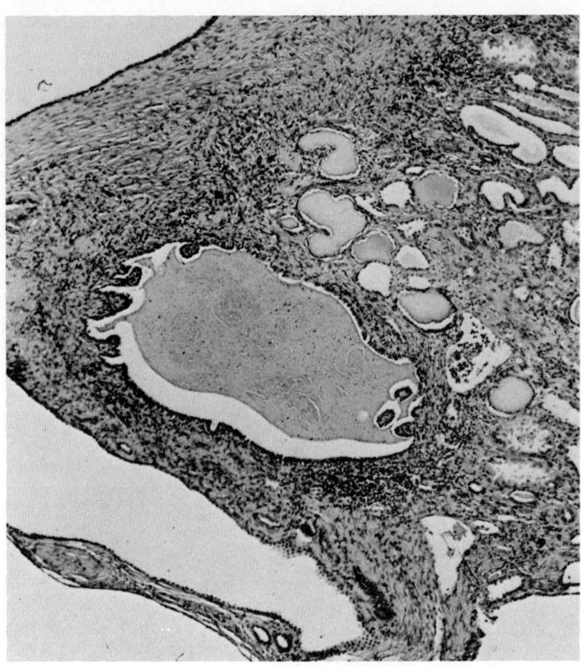

Figure 3. A small cyst is lined with hyperplastic epithelium that is thrown into intracystic polyps and papillae. Note severe fibrosis of the surrounding parenchyma. Hematoxylin and eosin stain, ×50.

diverticula (Baert and Steg, 1977), which increase in number with age, but diverticula are ordinarily restricted to the distal tubule (Darmady and MacIver, 1980).

The occurrence of segmental cyst formation can be interpreted to mean that there are localized points of predilection, i.e., that some segments ordinarily have weaker walls or thinner basement membranes than other segments and dilate preferentially, even were the basement membrane to be diffusely abnormal. It also might mean that any hereditary weakness of the wall must be accompanied by a local factor, such as obstruction, to account for segmental involvement.

3. *Evidence of Local Obstruction*

Our finding of polypoid epithelial hyperplasia within cysts (Fig. 3) was an unexpected observation which assumed immediate significance because of its obvious resemblance to the morphologic findings in experimental cystic disease. Studies carried out by Evan and Gardner (1979) had shown that the dilated ducts in experimental nordihydroguaiaretic acid-induced cystic disease contained epithelial polyps and that luminal obstruction could be

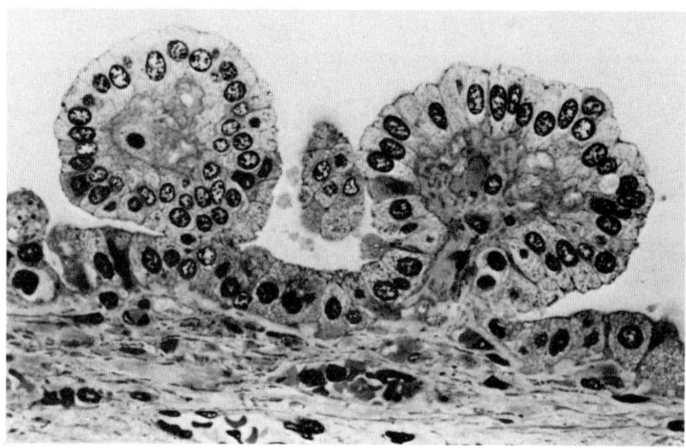

Figure 4. The epithelium lining the cyst is hyperplastic and forms small intracystic polyps with vascular cores. Epon section, Azure II–methylene blue stain, ×400.

inferred from functional studies. The polyps in APKD result from epithelial hyperplasia (Fig. 4), and polyps are sometimes so numerous within individual cysts that they might be regarded as forerunners of neoplasia. Scanning electron microscopy shows the linings of some cysts to be literally studded with polyps, and it shows polyps also to be located at the distal ends of the cysts in position to have occluded the lumens (Evan *et al.*, 1979).

4. Epithelial Hyperplasia in Other Types of Cystic Diseases

The theory according prime importance to luminal obstruction gains support from the presence of epithelial hyperplasia in several other forms of renal cystic disease, both hereditary and acquired. Each of the conditions also postulates a weakness of the tubular basement membrane, but none has been demonstrated. The epithelial hyperplasia, however, is apparent on microscopic examination. For example, in end-stage renal disease, particularly in patients receiving long-term hemodialysis, the kidneys become cystic in association with epithelial hyperplasia (Dunnill *et al.*, 1977; Krempien and Ritz, 1980). Cell proliferation can lead to neoplasia, and the kidneys can become considerably enlarged as the result of disseminated cyst formation.

In localized cystic disease, a form of renal cystic disease that appears to be nonhereditary and nonprogressive (Cho *et al.*, 1979), cyst formation is limited to one portion of one kidney and is accompanied by epithelial polypoid hyperplasia. Cyst formation in tuberous sclerosis and in von Hippel–Lindau disease is associated with epithelial proliferation (Bernstein, 1979), which in von Hippel–Lindau disease places the patient at considerable risk of developing renal cell carcinoma.

In all these conditions cyst formation has been associated with epithelial hyperplasia. Is it necessary also to have increased tubular compliance? Perhaps, but the evidence is lacking.

5. Tubular Enlargment Results from Increased Intratubular Pressure

If cysts enlarge as the result of luminal obstruction, there has to be increased transmural pressure. The studies of cyst pressures in excised kidneys carried out by Huseman and colleagues (1980) failed to demonstrate such increases, but the measurements were carried out on nephrectomized kidneys. Although the statement is unsupported by objective data, I have an impression that excised cystic kidneys are softer and flabbier than the same kidneys *in situ* with intact circulation. Even though the artery and vein of an excised kidney are firmly ligated, considerable fluid is lost through disrupted hilar lymphatics. I assume that pressure is also lost. Others (Bjerle *et al.*, 1971) have found increased pressures.

In the absence of actual measurements and direct evidence, certain circumstantial evidence comes to mind. I indicated earlier that cystic kidneys contain considerable residual parenchyma that has undergone atrophy, with glomerular sclerosis, tubular atrophy, and interstitial fibrosis (Fig. 2). The atrophy and sclerosis are sometimes most marked around cysts or between adjacent ones. The effect appears to have resulted from pressure, although it also could have resulted from ischemia. The arteries in cystic kidneys are not especially or consistently sclerotic, but splaying and stretching could have the same effect as luminal vascular obstruction.

Therefore, it is of some interest to observe that the cysts in APKD are regularly surrounded by layers of smooth muscle cells and that the neighboring interstitium also contains smooth muscle (Bernstein, 1979) (Fig. 5). Whether the cells result from hyperplasia of existing elements or metaplasia of other stromal elements, the phenomenon is present in both early and late specimens. I interpret the muscular hyperplasia to be a response to increased pressure and tension. Precedent for this interpretion lies in studies of arterial muscular hypertrophy in experimental hypertension (Wiener *et al.*, 1977). Smooth muscle increases as a response to increased arterial tension, and I hypothesize that similar changes take place in the stroma surrounding renal cysts. The muscle fibers may differentiate from fibroblasts, as they do in experimentally obstructed kidneys (Nagle *et al.*, 1973), but the fibers in APKD do not have the ultrastructural characteristics of myofibroblasts.

6. Summary

The morphologic features of APKD indicate that cysts arise as localized dilatations of nephrons and ducts as the result of luminal obstruction. The obstruction appears to result from polypoid epithelial hyperplasia. An

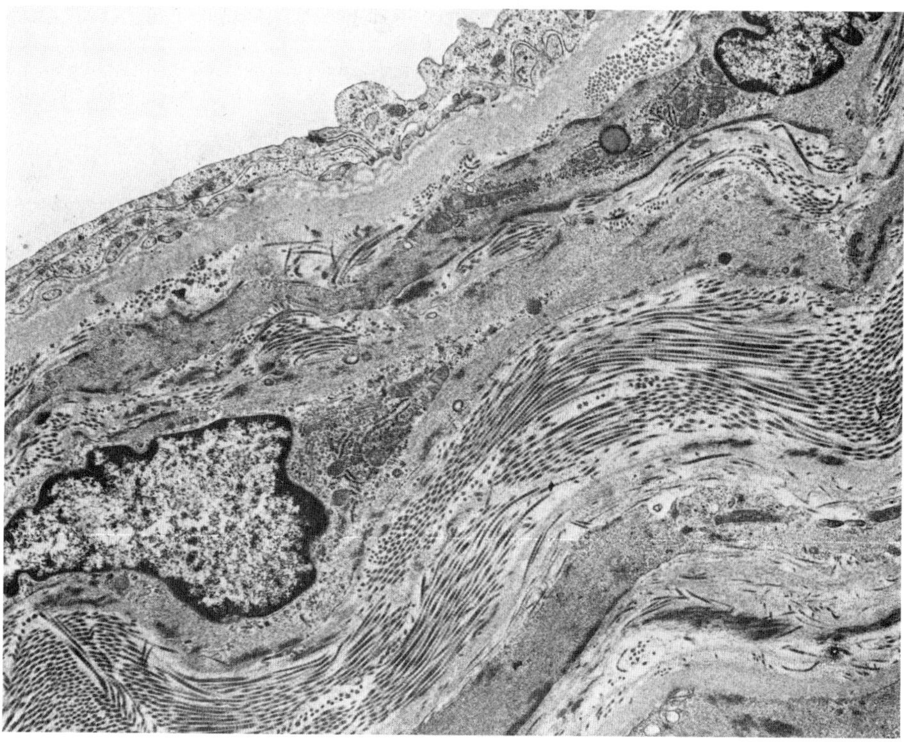

Figure 5. The cyst is lined with flattened epithelium resting on a thickened basement membrane and is surrounded by smooth muscle cells. The smooth muscle fibers are separated by bundles of collagen fibers. Electron micrograph, ×7500.

inherited defect in basement membrane, leading to increased tubular compliance, may be present and may be enhanced by that local obstruction. There are several preferential sites of cyst formation—Henle's loop and the collecting tubule—where there may ordinarily also be inherent weakness of the tubular wall or basement membrane. The morphologic evidence indicates that only a minor proportion of nephrons are involved in the process and that progression of the disease results from atrophy and sclerosis of the remaining parenchyma. Such structural alteration and functional compromise could result from ischemia, but there is also morphologic evidence of increased tubular tension, which may be expected to have compromised the adjacent parenchyma.

References

Baert, L., 1978, Hereditary polycystic kidney disease (adult form): A microdissection study of two cases at an early stage of the disease, *Kidney Int.* **13:**519.

Baert, L., and Steg, A., 1977, Is the diverticulum of the distal and collecting tubules a preliminary stage of the simple cyst in the adult? *J. Urol.* **118**:707.

Bernstein, J., 1979, Hereditary renal disease, in: *Kidney Disease: Present Status*, IAP Monograph No. 20, Chapter 13 (J. Churg, B. H. Spargo, F. K. Mostofi, and M. R. Abell, eds.), Williams & Wilkins, Baltimore.

Bjerle, P., Lindquist, B., and Michaelson, G., 1971, Pressure measurement in renal cysts. *Scand. J. Clin. Lab. Invest.* **27**:135.

Carone, F. A., Rowland, R. G., Perlman, S. G., and Ganote, C. E., 1974, The pathogenesis of drug-induced renal cystic disease, *Kidney Int.* **5**:411.

Cho, K. U., Thornbury, J. R., Bernstein, J., Heidelberger, K. P., and Walter, J. F., 1979, Localized cystic disease of the kidney: Angiographic–pathologic correlation, *AJR* **132**:891.

Cuppage, F. E., Huseman, R. A., Chapman, A., and Grantham, J. J., 1980, Ultrastructure and function of cysts from human adult polycystic kidneys, *Kidney Int.* **17**:372.

Darmady, E. M., and MacIver, A. G., 1980, *Renal Pathology*, Butterworths, London, pp. 57–58.

Dunnill, M. S., Millard, P. R., and Oliver, D., 1977, Acquired cystic disease of the kidneys: A hazard of long-term intermittent maintenance haemodialysis, *J. Clin. Pathol.* **30**:868.

Eulderink, F., and Hogewind, B. L., 1978, Renal cysts in premature children. Occurrence in a family with polycystic kidney disease, *Arch. Pathol. Lab. Med.* **102**:592.

Evan, A. P., and Gardner, K. D., Jr., 1979, Nephron obstruction in nordihydroguaiaretic acid-induced renal cystic disease, *Kidney Int.* **15**:7.

Evan, A. P., Gardner, K. D., Jr., and Bernstein, J., 1979, Polypoid and papillary epithelial hyperplasia: A potential cause of ductal obstruction in adult polycystic disease, *Kidney Int.* **16**:743.

Heggö, O., 1966, A microdissection study of cystic disease of the kidneys in adults. *J. Pathol.* **91**:311.

Huseman, R., Grady, A., Welling, D., and Grantham, J., 1980, Macropuncture study of polycystic disease in adult human kidneys, *Kidney Int.* **18**:375.

Krempien, B., and Ritz, E., 1980, Acquired cystic transformation of the kidneys of haemodialysed patients, *Virchows Arch.* (*Pathol. Anat.*) **386**:189.

Lambert, P. P., 1947, Polycystic disease of the kidney. A review, *Arch. Pathol. Lab. Med.* **44**:34.

Nagle, R. B., Kneiser, M. R., Bulger, R. E., and Benditt, E. P., 1973, Induction of smooth muscle characteristics in renal interstitial fibroblasts during obstructive nephropathy, *Lab. Invest.* **29**:422.

Wiener, J., Loud, A. V., Giacomelli, F., and Anversa, P., 1977, Morphometric analysis of hypertension-induced hypertrophy of rat thoracic aorta, *Am. J. Pathol.* **88**:619.

7

Morphology of Polycystic Kidney Disease in Man and Experimental Models

Andrew P. Evan and Kenneth D. Gardner, Jr.

1. Introduction

Although diagnosis of polycystic kidney disease has been possible for many years, we still have only a limited understanding of the pathogenesis of the disease, partly because of the difficulty in obtaining human cystic kidneys in different stages of cyst formation. At present only a few human kidneys with early-onset polycystic changes have been evaluated for both structural and functional changes (Baert, 1978). Therefore, growing attention has been given to various animal models that possess lesions that mimic human polycystic kidney disease (Goodman *et al.*, 1970; Carone *et al.*, 1974; Gardner *et al.*, 1976; Evan and Gardner, 1976, 1979; Evan *et al.*, 1979). There are presently three types of animal models for experimental polycystic kidney disease: (1) chemically induced, (2) traumatically induced, and (3) genetically transmitted. The chemically induced models have received the most attention in that a large number of compounds have been reported to produce cysts in small laboratory animals. Furthermore, these models allow opportunity to follow the acquisition and sequential growth of cysts. Of the various renal cytogens, three compounds, all of which are antioxidants, have received the greatest attention. These substances are diphenylamine (DPA), nordihydroguaiaretic acid (NDGA), and diphenylthiazole (DPT).

Andrew P. Evan • Department of Anatomy, Indiana University School of Medicine, Indianapolis, Indiana 46223. ***Kenneth D. Gardner, Jr.*** • Department of Medicine, University of New Mexico School of Medicine, Albuquerque, New Mexico 87131.

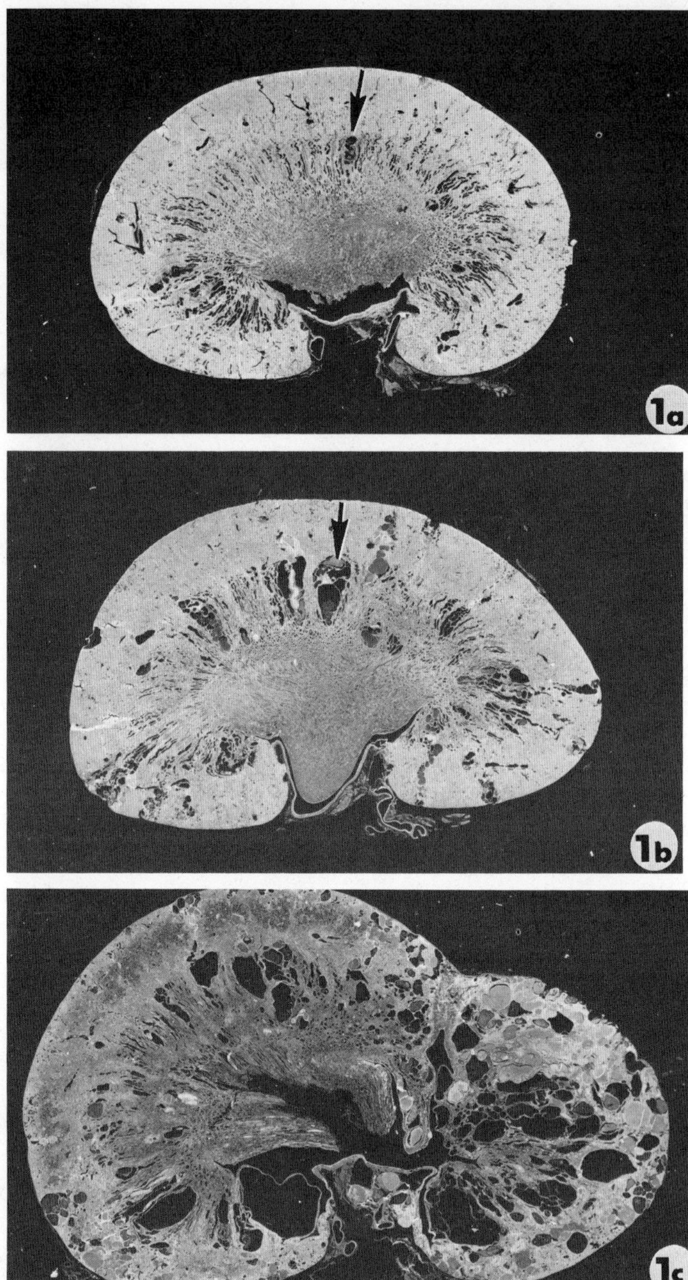

Figure 1. These low-magnification light micrographs show the progression of cystic changes in animals treated with NDGA for 1 week (a), 1 month (b), and 6 months (c). Note the appearance of dilated collecting tubules (arrow) within the cortex and medulla by 1 week. By 1 month both dilated (arrow) and cystic nephrons are clearly seen. The number and size of the cysts appear to increase with time (c). a, ×4; b, ×4; c, ×4 (Reprinted from Gardner and Evan, 1979, with permission.)

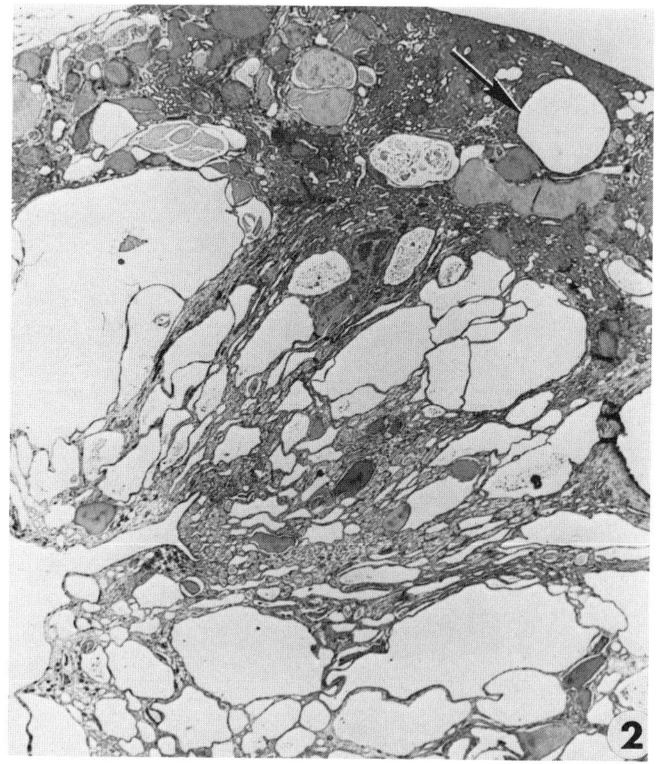

Figure 2. A higher-magnification light micrograph of the cortex from an animal treated with NDGA for 2 months. Numerous cysts of various sizes are found (arrow), some containing cast material. No other changes are noted. ×75.

2. *Chemical Models*

The chemically induced models have several morphologic features that appear to be similar to human polycystic kidney disease. First, cyst formation may be seen throughout the kidney. DPA and NDGA produce cysts that occupy the entire cortex and outer medulla, thus resembling the adult type of human polycystic disease. DPT causes dilation of some collecting tubules which extends from the kidney capsule to the tip of the papilla. These changes mimic the infantile type of human polycystic disease.

Second, the size of the cysts as well as the number appears to increase with time. Figures 1a–c show the progression of cystic changes in animals that have been treated with NDGA for 1 week (Fig. 1a), 1 month (Fig. 1b), and six months (Fig. 1c). It should be noted that at six months not all cysts are of the same size. Figures 1a–c also show an overall increase in kidney size with time.

Third, the cystic changes are induced in kidneys that were once structurally normal. Figure 2 shows the entire length of the cortex from a NDGA-

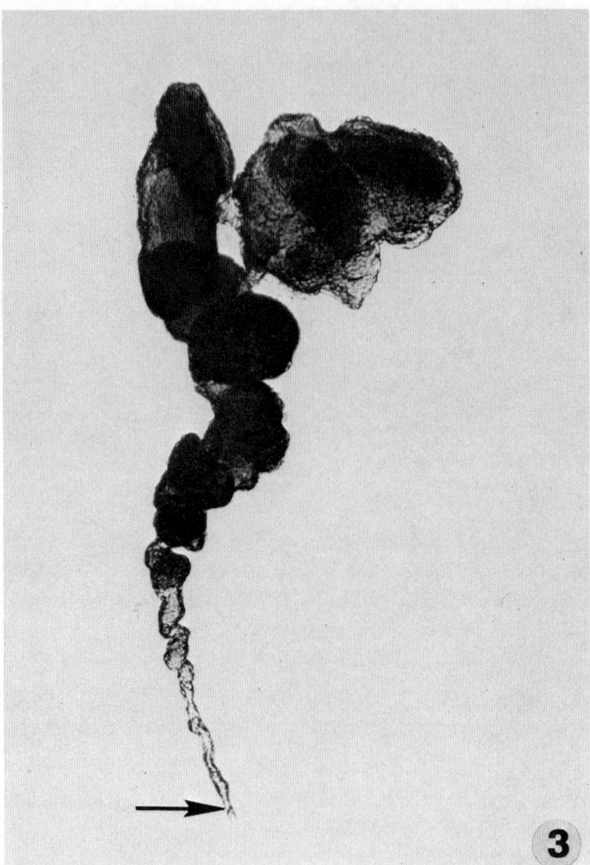

Figure 3. A microdissected collecting tubule from a rat treated for 1 month with NDGA. The lower end (arrow) of the tubule appears normal; however, it slowly dilates and twists upon itself as one progresses up this segment. The upper portion shows frank cysts. ×180. (Reprinted from Evan and Gardner, 1979, with permission.)

treated animal. The only change noted is dilation of portions of the nephron. A this time, no changes are seen in the interstitium as fibrosis, or in the vascular system. This observation has held true for all the chemically induced models in which a thorough morphologic investigation has been performed.

Fourth, microdissection studies reveal the dilated and cystic segments of the nephron to be located initially along the collecting tubules. These observations are in agreement with Potter's work (1972), which shows the collecting duct to be the principal site of involvement in all forms of human polycystic kidney disease. Recently Baert (1978) examined two cases of adult polycystic disease at early onset and found cystic dilations along some proximal and distal tubules, loops of Henle, and collecting tubules. Figure 3 shows a collecting tubule from an animal treated with NDGA for 1 month.

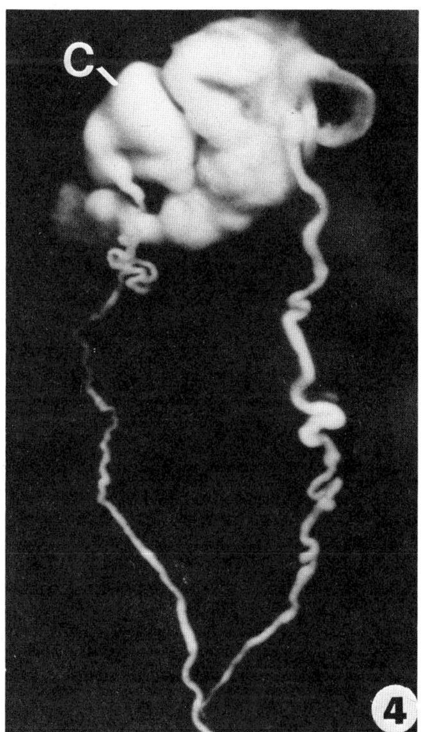

Figure 4. A latex-filled collecting tubule that was microdissected from a rat treated for 6 months with NDGA. A large cyst (c) of the collecting tubule was located just beneath the kidney capsule. The tubule narrows quickly at its outflow end. ×150. (Reprinted from Evan and Gardner, 1979, with permission.)

The lower end of the tubule appears normal. However, as one progresses up the collecting segment, the lumen dilates and the tubular wall twists upon itself, suggesting increased growth. At the upper pole obvious cysts can be seen. Occasionally, we are able to analyze superficially placed cysts by both structural and functional techniques. Figure 4 shows a latex-filled collecting tubule with a larger cyst in contact with the kidney capsule. As one follows this segment, there is an abrupt change in the luminal diameter from dilated to normal size. This kind of observation suggests partial obstruction, while the cyst is obviously continuous with the rest of the nephron.

These last examples resemble those cystic collecting tubules in adult polycystic disease. As mentioned previously, DPT produces a cystic lesion that mimics infantile disease. By microdissection, an entire collecting tubular arcade (Fig. 5) appears dilated beginning at the duct of Bellini.

So far, we have shown that the experimentally induced model of cystic disease in some ways mimics human disease. However, the observations do not shed light on any possible pathogenetic mechanisms of the disease. While examining the renal tissue from an animal that had been exposed to NDGA for 2 weeks, we noted areas of cellular hyperplasia along the walls of some dilated collecting tubules (Fig. 6). By tracing these same tubules through serial sections, we noted an area of obstruction at the outflow end. The tubule appeared to be obstructed by a polyplike growth extending into the

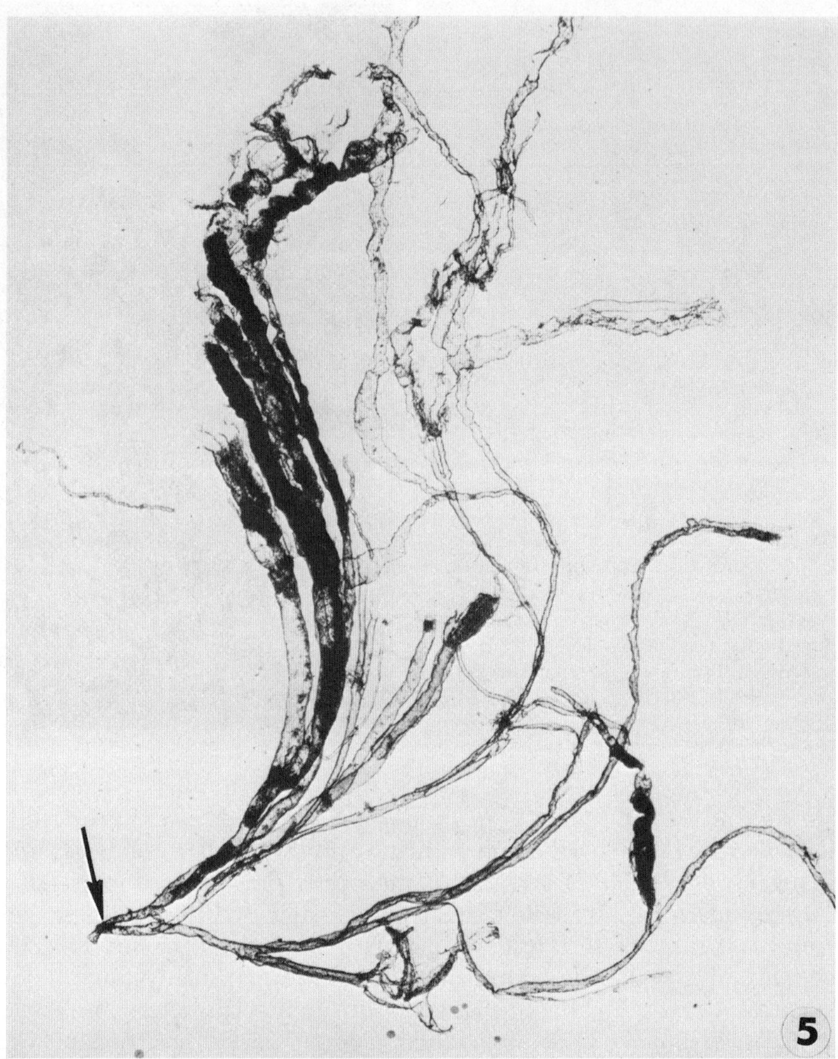

Figure 5. A light micrograph of a collecting duct arcade from an animal treated with DPT for 1 month. Dilation of the tubules begins as early as the duct of Bellini (arrow). The extent of dilation varies between tubules. ×100.

tubular lumen (Fig. 7). By carefully examining numerous light microscopic sections, we were able to find several cysts that were cut longitudinally thereby revealing a polyp at the outflow end of that tubule. In order to examine greater numbers and areas of dilated tubules and to obtain a three-dimensional image of cyst walls, we employed the scanning electron microscope. Figure 8 is a scanning electron microscopic picture (SEM) of a cyst from a NDGA-treated rat. The cyst wall changes from normal to hyperplastic epithelium near the tubular outlet. Associated with the cellular hyperplasia

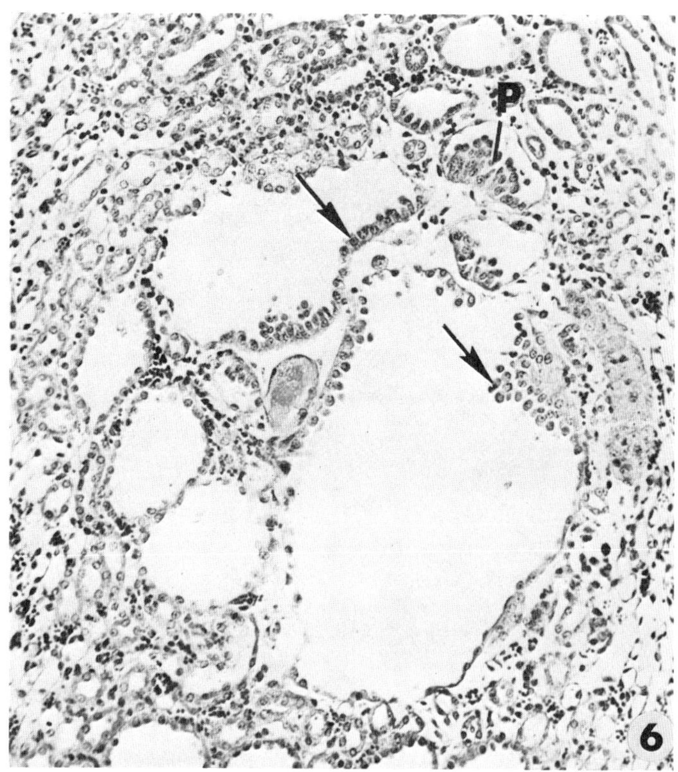

Figure 6. A light micrograph showing several cross sections of dilated collecting tubules from an animal treated with NDGA. Portions of the cyst wall possess hyperplastic cells (arrows). At the exit of one dilated collecting tubule, a polypoid structure (P) is noted partially obstructing this segment. ×170. (Reprinted from Evan and Gardner, 1979, with permission.)

is a polyp positioned at the outflow end of the cyst such that it could partially obstruct the nephron. The hyperplastic cells are irregular in shape (Fig. 9) and often pile upon themselves forming focal polyps (Figs. 9 and 10) along the cyst wall.

Hyperplasia in these models is further identified by doing a tritiated thymidine study or by counting nuclei seen on cross section (Evan *et al.*, 1978; Evan and Gardner, 1979). Although we are clearly showing hyperplasia in our experimental models, this is by no means a new idea related to human polycystic disease. Nauwerck and Huischmid (1893) as early as 1883 showed hyperplasia in the cyst wall in adult polycystic kidney disease. These authors suggested that the proliferating cells were growing away from rather than into the cyst lumen.

The morphologic data mentioned in this chapter in combination with functional observations define conditions that suggest increased resistance to outflow from dilated and cystic nephrons. Findings in the chemically induced models have led us to hypothesize that polypoid hyperplasia partic-

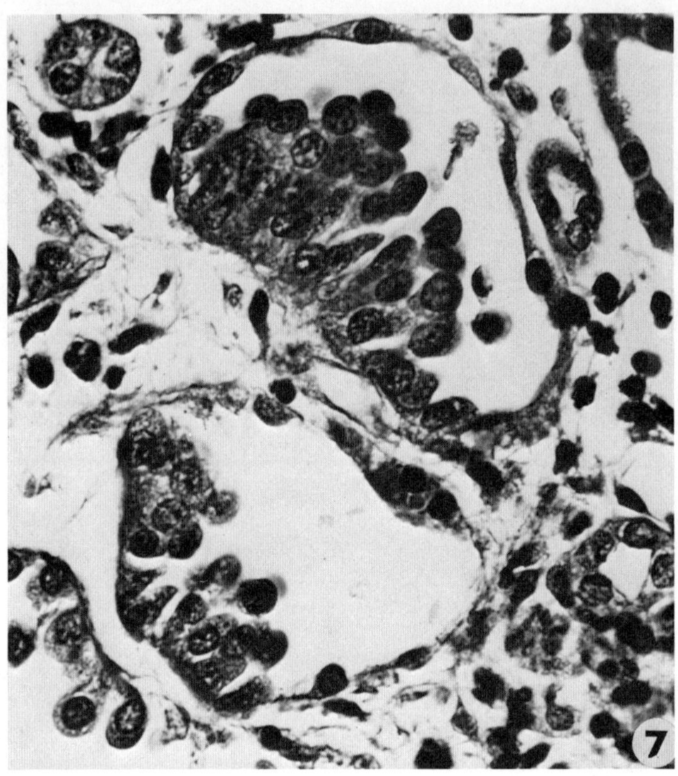

Figure 7. At a higher magnification the polyp is clearly seen. Numerous elongated cells are clustered such that they project into the tubular lumen. ×1300. (Reprinted from Evan and Gardner, 1979, with permission.)

ipates in cyst formation in susceptible kidneys by increasing resistance to the outflow of tubular urine.

To strengthen the hypothesis, we examined several congenital models of polycystic disease (Crowell *et al.*, 1979). By scanning electron microscopy a congenital polycystic kidney from a kitten shows many dilated collecting tubules (Fig. 11). The overall pattern of tubular dilation resembles that of the infantile type of human polycystic disease. As dilated collecting tubules are followed into the inner medulla, areas of hyperplasia and of polyp formation are noted (Fig. 12). Similar changes are seen in the piglet model of congenital polycystic disease.

3. Human Disease

In order to establish the presence, extent, and distribution of cellular hyperplasia and/or of polyp formation in humans, we have examined adult polycystic disease. We established the presence of polypoid hyperplasia in

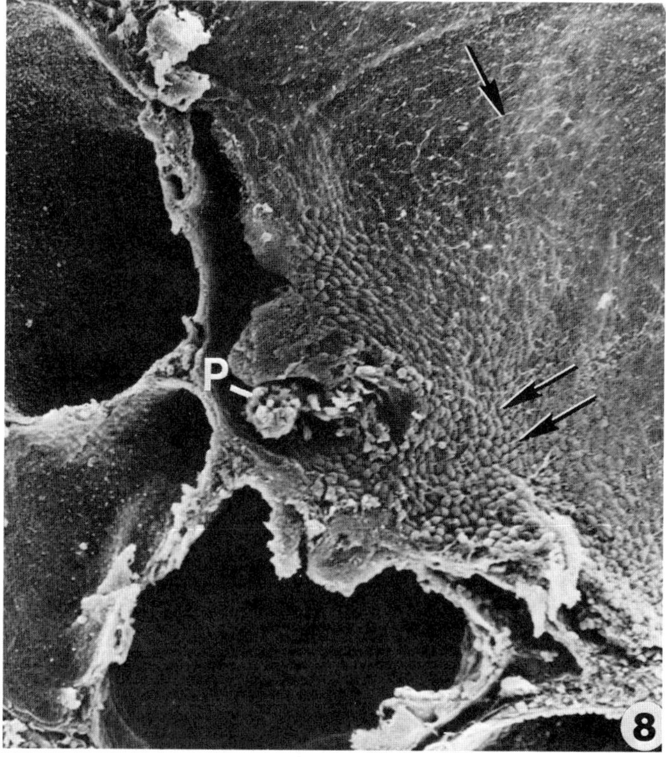

Figure 8. Scanning electron micrograph of a cyst from a NDGA-treated rat. Portions of the wall possess normal cells (arrow); however, as one progresses to the outflow end of the cyst hyperplastic cells are noted (double arrow). Situated within the tubule is a polyp (P) which is partially obstructing the outflow. ×100.

each kidney by light, transmission, and scanning electron microscopy. Figure 13 shows an area of hyperplasia along the cyst wall and the association of numerous focal polyps. A fortuitous fracture of a large cyst is seen in Fig. 14. At the upper end of the cyst. several focal polyps are noted. As one progresses to the outflow end of the cyst a small polyp is found. The polyp is again associated with an area of hyperplasia.

4. *Summary*

In summary, the earliest dilated tubules in models are localized to the collecting tubule. Commonly the wall is characterized by hyperplastic cells. At the outflow end of cysts, one frequently finds polyps that appear to be causing complete, partial, or intermittent obstruction. Distal to the site of polypoid hyperplasia, lumens return to normal diameter. As a possible means of regulating or arresting the development of polycystic kidney disease,

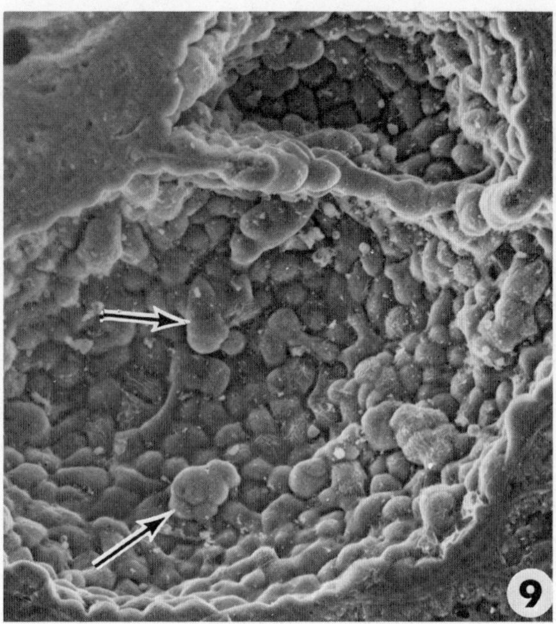

Figure 9. SEM of a cyst wall from a DPT-treated animal. Numerous cells of irregular shape and distribution are noted (arrows). ×650. (Reprinted from Evan and Gardner, 1976, with permission.)

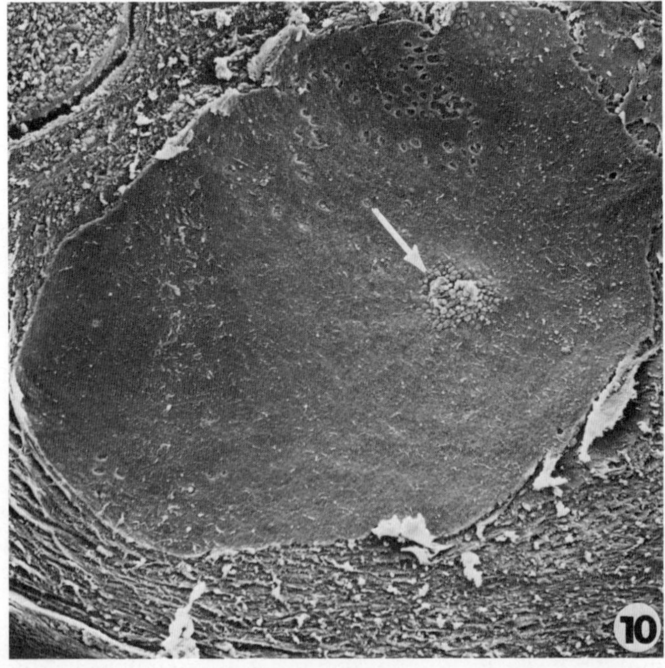

Figure 10. SEM of a cyst from a NDGA-treated animal showing a focal polyp (arrow). ×50.

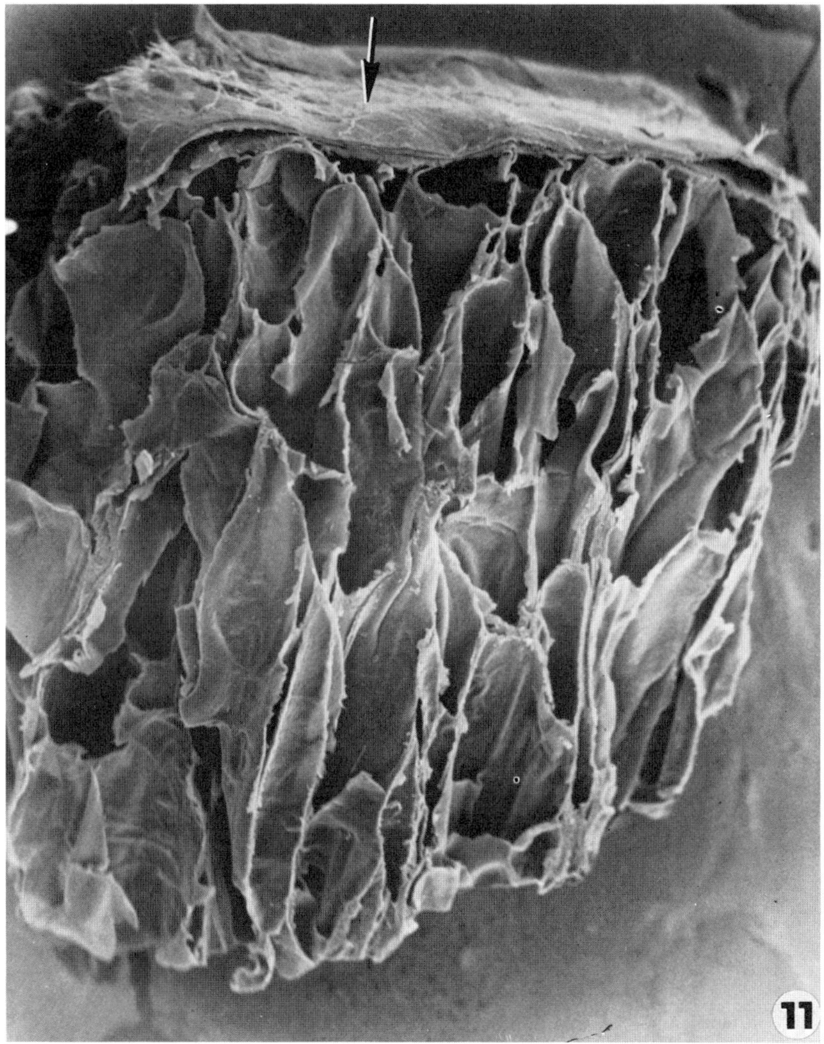

Figure 11. SEM of the cortex from a congenital polycystic kitten. Numerous dilated tubules are noted extending to the kidney capsule (arrow). ×35.

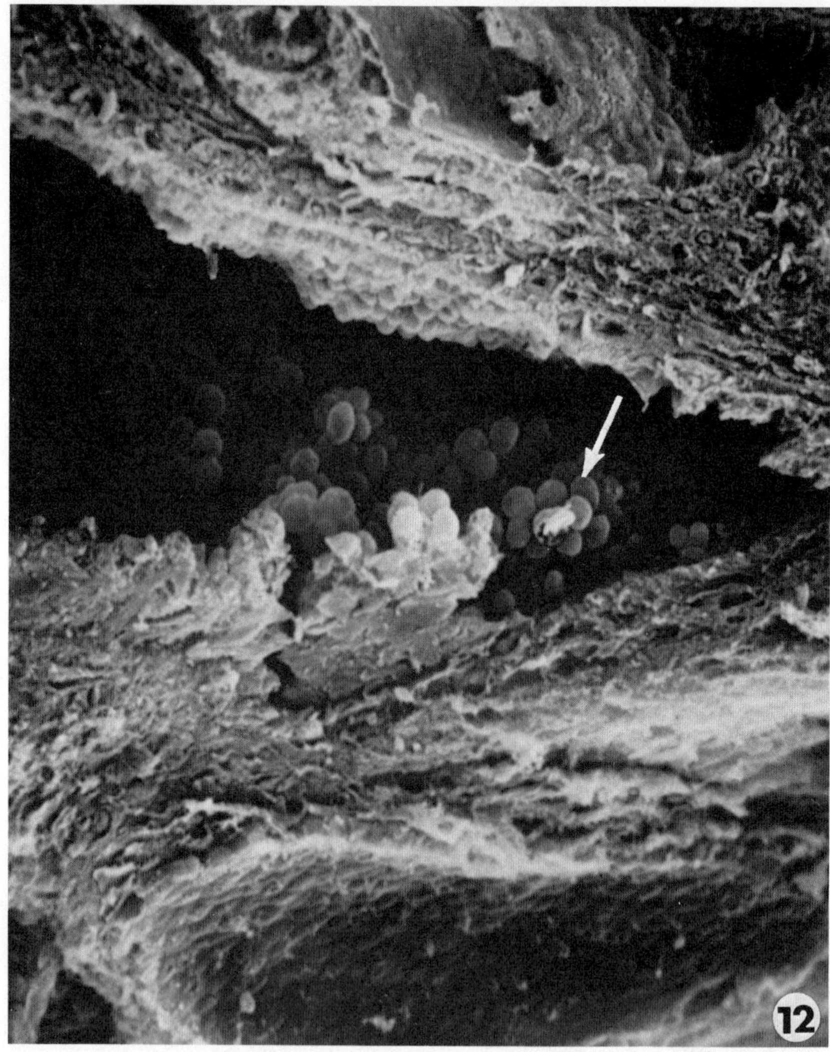

Figure 12. At a higher magnification hyperplasia (arrow) and polypoid formation are noted in the collecting tubules of the inner cortex. ×1500.

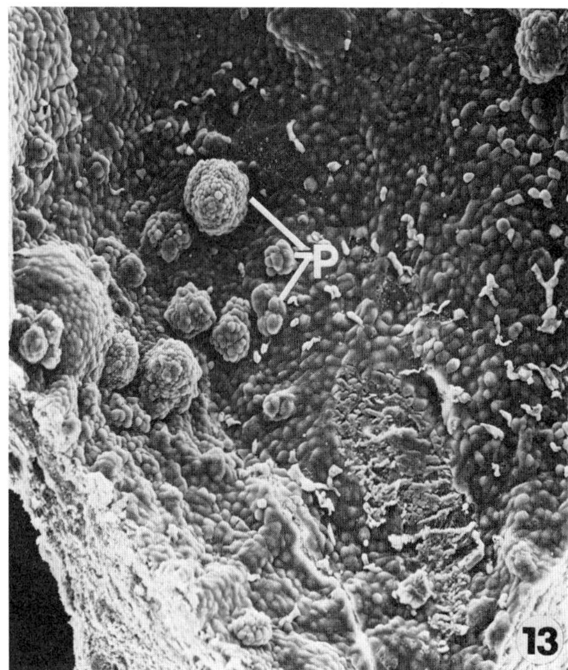

Figure 13. SEM of large cyst from an adult type of human polycystic kidney. The cyst wall is lined by numerous hyperplastic cells as well as several polyps (P). ×180. (Reprinted from Evan *et al.*, 1979, with permission.)

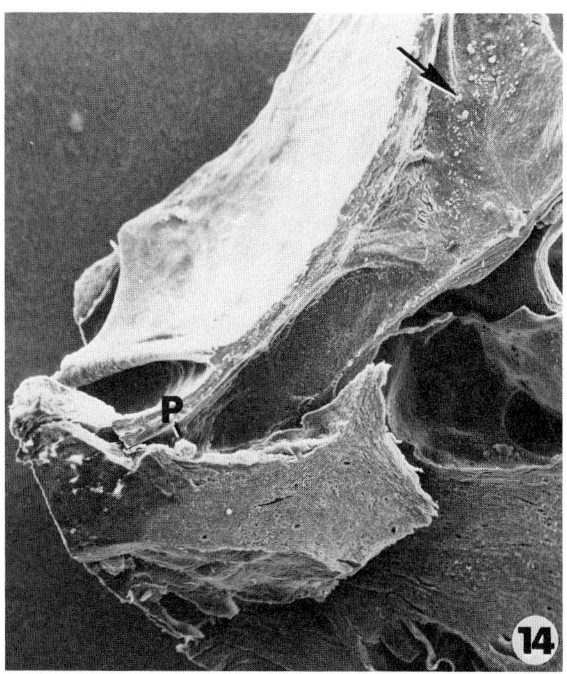

Figure 14. A fortuitous fracture of a large cyst from a human polycystic kidney reveals focal polyps (arrow) and a discrete polyp (P) positioned at the outflow end of the cyst. ×40. (Reprinted from Evan *et al.*, 1979, with permission.)

future studies must explore the mechanisms that control renal cell growth. Particular attention should also be directed toward understanding the mechanisms causing acquired cystic disease of the kidney and the appearance of renal cell carcinoma after long-term hemodialysis (Dunnill *et al.*, 1977).

References

Baert, L., 1978, Hereditary polycystic kidney disease (adult form): A microdissection study of two cases at an early stage of the disease, *Kidney Int.* **13:**519.

Carone, F. A., Rowland, R. G., Perlman, S. G., and Ganote, C. E., 1974, The pathogenesis of drug-induced renal cystic disease, *Kidney Int.* **5:**411.

Crowell, W. A., Hubbell, J. J., and Riley, J. C., 1979, Polycystic renal disease in related cats, *J. Am. Vet. Med. Assoc.* **175:**286.

Dunnill, M. S., Millard, P. R., and Oliver, D., 1977, Acquired cystic disease of the kidneys: A hazard of long-term intermittent maintenance hemodialysis, *J. Clin. Pathol.* **30:**868.

Evan, A. P., and Gardner, K. D., Jr., 1976, Comparison of human polycystic and medullary cystic kidney disease with diphenylamine-induced cystic disease, *Lab. Invest.* **35:**93.

Evan, A. P., and Gardner, K. D., Jr., 1979, Nephron obstruction in nordihydroguaiaretic acid-induced renal cystic disease, *Kidney Int.* **15:**7.

Evan, A. P., Hong, S. K., Gardner, K. D., Jr., Park, Y. S., and Itagaki, R., 1978, Evolution of the collecting tubular lesion in diphenylamine-induced renal disease, *Lab. Invest.* **38:**244.

Evan, A. P., Gardner, K. D., Jr., and Bernstein, J., 1979, Polypoid and papillary epithelial hyperplasia: A potential cause of ductal obstruction in adult polycystic disease, *Kidney Int.* **16:**743.

Gardner, K. D., Jr., Solomon, S., Figzgerrel, W. W., and Evan, A. P., 1976, Function and structure in the diphenylamine-exposed kidney, *J. Clin. Invest.* **57:**796.

Goodman, T., Grice, H. C., Becking, G. C., and Salem, F. A., 1970, A cystic nephropathy induced by nordihydrorguaiaretic acid in the rat: Light and electron microscopic investigations, *Lab. Invest.* **23:**93.

Nauwerck, C., and Huischmid, K., 1893, Über das multiloculare adenokystom der niere, *Beitr. Path. Anat.* **12:**1.

Potter, E. L., 1972, *Normal and Abnormal Development of the Kidney*, Year Book Medical Publishers, Chicago, p. 83.

8

Ordered and Disordered Growth of Renal Cells

F. Gary Toback

1. Cellular Hyperplasia and Renal Cysts

Hyperplasia of tubular cells has been linked to cystic disease of the kidney for more than a century (Sturm, 1875). A sequence of events leading from tubular cell hyperplasia to cyst formation is proposed in Fig. 1. First, there must be an inciting cause of cell proliferation and perhaps a genetic or acquired predisposition to respond to it. Once cell growth is initiated, proliferating epithelial cells pile up on the tubular wall and form adenomatous masses. These masses or polyps are thought to partially obstruct the passage of fluid down the nephron, thereby raising intratubular pressure, dilating the tubule wall, and eventually causing cysts to form.

Evan, Gardner, and colleagues (Evan and Gardner, 1979; Evan *et al.*, 1978; Gardner *et al.*, 1976) obtained physiologic and morphologic support for this sequence by studying the evolution of diphenylamine- and nordihydroguaiaretic acid-induced cysts in rats. They also identified epithelial cell polyps in the kidneys of adults with inherited polycystic kidney disease and suggested that partial tubular obstruction may play a pathogenetic role in this disease in man (Evan *et al.*, 1979). Acquired tubular cell hyperplasia, adenoma, and cyst formation have also been reported in the kidneys of long-term hemodialysis patients whose initial disease was glomerulonephritis (Ishikawa *et al.*, 1980).

These observations support the pathogenetic sequence that links renal cell hyperplasia with cyst formation. This chapter reviews factors involved

F. Gary Toback • Department of Medicine, University of Chicago Pritzker School of Medicine, Chicago, Illinois 60637. This work was supported by USPHS grants AM 18413 and GM 22328 and by the Chicago Heart Association. This chapter was prepared during the author's tenure as an Established Investigator of the American Heart Association.

Proliferative factors ⟶ Tubular cell hyperplasia ⟶ Polyp formation ⟶ Obstruction to fluid flow → Cyst formation

Figure 1. A pathogenetic sequence relating proliferation of renal tubular cells and cyst formation.

in growth control of kidney cells in the rat and in culture. Although cyst formation does not occur in these model systems, increased understanding of the mechanisms that initiate and control cell growth could be of value in defining the pathogenesis of cystic disease of the kidney.

2. *Renal Growth during Potassium Depletion*

In 1937 Schrader, Prickett, and Salmon reported that feeding rats a potassium-deficient diet induced renal growth. Subsequent studies revealed that cellular hyperplasia and hypertrophy occur in the kidneys, whereas overall body growth is retarded (Gustafson *et al.*, 1973; Liebow *et al.*, 1941). In the renal papilla, all cell types become filled with lysosomes which have a multivesicular appearance (Aithal *et al.*, 1977a; Spargo, 1964). In the inner stripe of red medulla, growth is associated with adenomatous hyperplasia in the collecting tubules (Oliver *et al.*, 1957). Scanning electron microscopy (EM) reveals numerous polyplike projections that appear to fill and perhaps obstruct the collecting tubule lumen (Toback *et al.*, 1976). Similar papillary projections have been observed in the kidneys of patients with adult polycystic disease (Evan *et al.*, 1979).

Autoradiography was used to quantify the extent of cell division in the collecting tubules and other cell types in this renal zone (Toback *et al.*, 1979). Rats were given [^{3}H]thymidine intraperitoneally; 1 hr later the kidneys were removed, and slices of inner red medulla were cut and processed for autoradiography. DNA synthesis for new cell growth was estimated by counting labeled nuclei. Figure 2 shows that during potassium depletion the percent of labeled nuclei increased two- to fivefold in the collecting tubules, thick limbs of Henle's loop, and interstitium. Repletion with potassium for 3 days halted cell proliferation and reduced the frequency of labeled nuclei to values that were similar to or less than control.

Membrane metabolism was studied during potassium depletion because organelles, endoplasmic reticulum, and surface structures must be formed in the growing cells. Phospholipid synthesis was measured as a marker of cell growth since cellular membranes are composed largely of phospholipids and proteins. The synthesis of phosphatidylcholine, the major renal phospholipid, occurs primarily via the Kennedy pathway in the kidneys of normal and of potassium-depleted rats (Toback *et al.*, 1977b; Rouser *et al.*, 1969; Kennedy and Weiss, 1956) (Fig. 3). In this pathway, choline is phosphorylated to phosphorylcholine, which then reacts with cytidine triphosphate (CTP) to

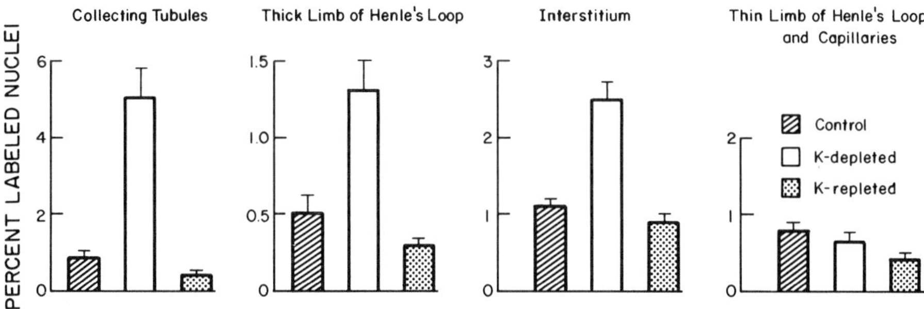

Figure 2. Effect of dietary potassium depletion and repletion on cell proliferation in the inner stripe of kidney red medulla. The percent of labeled nuclei in tissue from rats potassium depleted for 3–4 weeks was higher than in control animals in collecting tubules, thick limbs of Henle's loop, and interstitium. Values in animals potassium repleted for 3 days were lower than in controls in collecting tubules and thin limbs of Henle's loop and capillaries. (Reprinted from Toback *et al.*, 1979, with permission.)

form cytidine diphosphocholine, the immediate precursor of phosphatidylcholine. An increased rate of choline incorporation into membrane phospholipids occurs during the onset of growth and immediately precedes formation of new cellular membranes in the rodent kidney (Toback *et al.*, 1974, 1976, 1977a).

Increased phosphatidylcholine biosynthesis was observed in the papilla as early as 18 hr after rats were fed the potassium-deficient diet and was associated with phospholipid accumulation in the tissue (Toback *et al.*, 1976). In the inner stripe of red medulla and inner cortex an increase in synthesis was observed by 36 hr and persisted for at least 34 days. Thus, enhanced phosphatidylcholine biosynthesis was associated with lysosome biogenesis in papilla, adenomatous hyperplasia in inner stripe of red medulla, and hyperplasia and hypertrophy in cortex.

To define the biochemical mechanism by which potassium depletion stimulates phospholipid synthesis during the initiation of renal growth, precursor uptake and enzyme activities were measured in cortical tissue

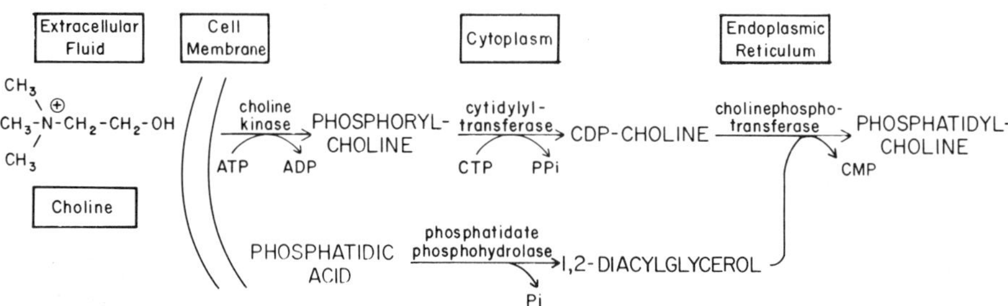

Figure 3. Pathway of phosphatidylcholine biosynthesis. (Reprinted from Toback and Havener, 1979, with permission.)

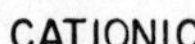

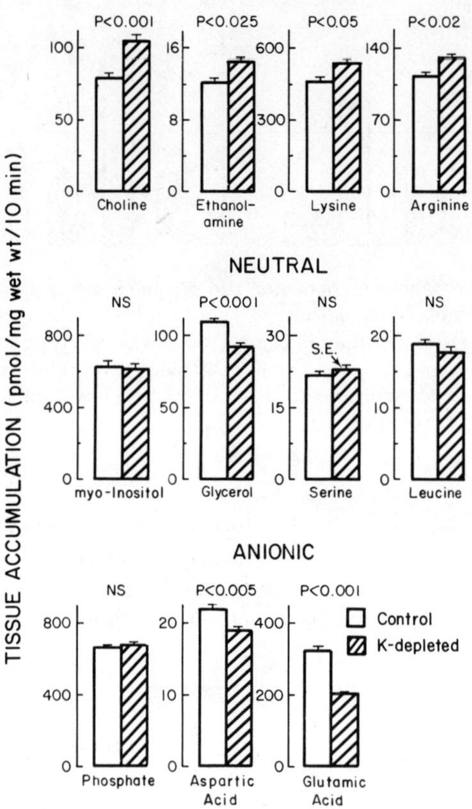

Figure 4. Effect of molecular charge on tissue accumulation. Inner cortical slices from the kidneys of control and potassium-depleted rats were incubated for 10 min and the accumulation of each substrate was determined. (Reprinted from Toback and Havener, 1979, with permission.)

(Toback and Havener, 1979; Toback *et al.*, 1977b). Figure 4 compares tissue accumulation of choline, ethanolamine, lysine, and arginine in renal slices from control and 1-week potassium-depleted rats. The accumulation of each of these cationic phospholipid and protein precursors was enhanced in tissue from potassium-depleted animals. In contrast, the uptake of a variety of anionic and neutral precursors was decreased or unchanged.

The specific activity of CDP-choline: 1,2-diacylglycerol cholinephosphotransferase, the last enzyme in the pathway, was assessed in cortical homogenates. Enzyme activity was up to 33% higher in potassium-depleted animals. Activity was increased further by reducing the medium concentration from 150 mM to 100 mM in the reaction mixture to simulate the observed decrement in intracellular potassium concentration that occurs during potassium depletion. Enzyme activity also was enhanced in microsomal preparations of normal cortical tissue by decreasing the potassium concentration

(Havener and Toback, 1980). Activities of the three other enzymes of the Kennedy pathway, choline kinase, choline phosphate cytidylyltransferase, and phosphatidate phosphohydrolase, were not increased during potassium depletion.

These findings suggested that potassium depletion enhanced renal cortical phosphatidylcholine formation by an effect on two steps of the pathway. Accumulation of the precursor choline was increased as part of a generalized cellular avidity for cations, possibly to maintain electroneutrality during potassium loss. Stimulation of cholinephosphotransferase activity could facilitate utilization of the accumulated phospholipid precursor and thereby increase phosphatidylcholine synthesis for new membrane and organelle biogenesis during the initiation of renal growth.

Cell proliferation during potassium depletion also was associated with increased glycolysis, decreased mitochondrial energy production, and a reduction of the Pasteur effect (Toback *et al.*, 1979; Aithal and Toback, 1978; Aithal *et al.*, 1977b). These aberrations in energy metabolism simulate the bioenergetic pattern observed in cancer cells (Wu and Racker, 1963). Unlike neoplastic cell growth, the biochemical and morphologic changes induced during potassium depletion are reversible. Thus, the return of potassium to the diet leads to regression of hyperplastic cells, correction of bioenergetic defects, and breakdown of accumulated phospholipid (Toback *et al.*, 1979; Ordóñez *et al.*, 1977).

3. *Potassium Depletion and Renal Cyst Formation*

A link between tubular cell proliferation, potassium depletion, and renal cyst formation was suggested by Perey, Herdman, and Good in 1967. These workers found that a single injection of 9-fluoroprednisolone, a long-acting steroid, given to neonatal rabbits induced hypokalemia and cyst formation in cortical collecting tubules. Of interest, was that cyst formation was "almost completely prevented" by daily injections of potassium chloride. These results suggested that a decrease in the serum or tissue potassium concentration, or both, could be important in the pathogenesis of cyst formation. This may be a special case, however, because serum and renal concentrations of potassium are normal in rats with diphenylamine-induced cystic disease. Thus, the exact relationship between steroid administration, potassium depletion, tubular cell hyperplasia, and renal cyst formation remains uncertain.

4. *Renal Growth in Culture*

In renal cells grown in culture several factors have been identified that contribute to growth control. These are hormones and growth factors in normal serum, low-molecular-weight nutrients, and inhibitors produced by the cells (Holley *et al.*, 1977, 1978a,b).

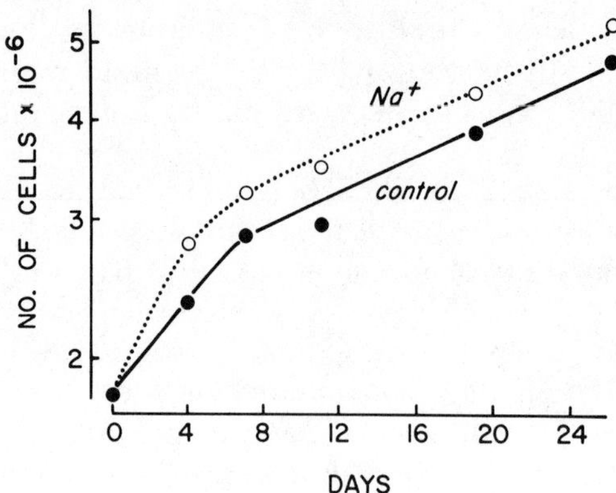

Figure 5. Effect of NaCl on growth of confluent cultures of BSC-1 cells. Cells were plated in Dulbecco-modified Eagle's medium with 1% calf serum and grown to the density shown on day 0 on the graph. Sets of plates were then changed to media containing 0.1% calf serum with (○) or without (●) added NaCl (25 mM). Media were subsequently changed twice a week. (Reprinted from Toback, 1980, with permission.)

Recent studies have suggested that the first event during the onset of cell growth may be a sudden increase in the influx of sodium ions (Koch and Leffert, 1979; Smith and Rozengurt, 1978; Johnson *et al.*, 1976). Na^+ might also play a role during the initiation of kidney growth during potassium depletion. In these animals there is increased uptake of Na^+ in muscle and of cationic amino acids and phospholipid precursors in growing kidney (Toback and Havener, 1979; Heppel, 1940). To test the hypothesis that Na^+ ions mediate the onset of renal growth, NaCl was added to cultures of monkey kidney epithelial cells from the BSC-1 cell line (Toback, 1980). The effect of NaCl was studied in high-density cultures to simulate the low proliferative activity of kidney cells *in vivo*. Figure 5 shows the growth of BSC-1 cells in the presence of added NaCl. On day 0 of the experiment, a solution of NaCl sufficient to raise the medium Na^+ concentration by 25 mM was added to half the cultures. The control cultures were maintained at the normal Na^+ concentration of 155 mM. The results indicate that cell growth occurred at a faster rate at the higher Na^+ concentration. Additional experiments excluded the possibility that this effect was a consequence of an increment in the chloride concentration or osmolality of the medium. Thus, Na^+ appeared to act as a mediator of the molecular events that initiate cell proliferation. *In vivo*, growth factors or hormones in the serum might mediate the increase in Na^+ flux achieved in these experiments by raising the medium Na^+ concentration.

Increasing the availability of a nutrient molecule such as glucose can also induce more renal cells to proliferate. In Fig. 6, the growth of BSC-1 cells at the usual medium glucose concentration of 25 mM is compared to growth in the presence of 100 mM glucose (Holley *et al.*, 1978a). The growth rate was increased about 50% by this fourfold increase in the glucose concentration.

Lithium also was found to induce proliferation of renal cells in culture, as shown in Fig. 7 (Toback, 1980). The addition of sufficient LiCl to raise the medium concentration to 2.5 mM in high-density cultures increased the

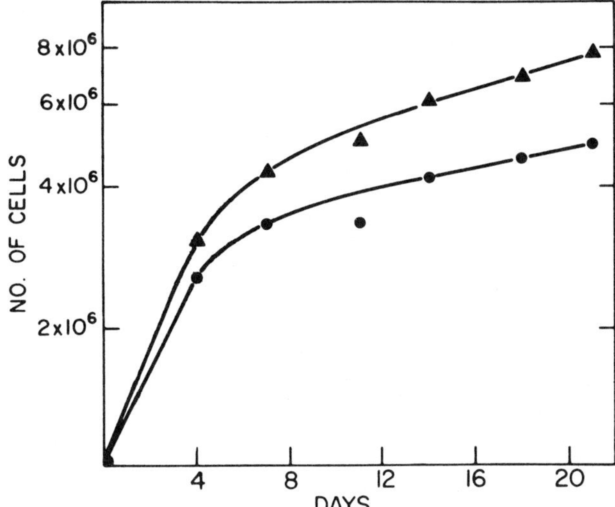

Figure 6. Effect of normal and high concentrations of glucose on growth of confluent cultures of BSC-1 cells. Cells were plated in medium containing 25 mM glucose and 10% serum and grown to the density shown on day 0 on the graph. Sets of plates were then changed to media containing 10% serum with (▲) or without (●) added glucose (100 mM). (Reprinted from Holley *et al.*, 1978a, with permission.)

growth rate for 1 week. However, growth ceased by day 10. Light microscopic examination at that time revealed indistinct plasma membranes and a decrease in cytoplasmic density. Longer exposure to lithium resulted in a decrease in cell number. These observations in cell culture are reminiscent of the toxic effect of lithium on renal tissue in some patients (Burrows *et al.*, 1978). Changes suggestive of tubular necrosis and dilatation of the distal nephron also have been reported in patients and animals after lithium treatment (Lindop and Padfield, 1975; Evan and Ollerich, 1972). Of interest is the

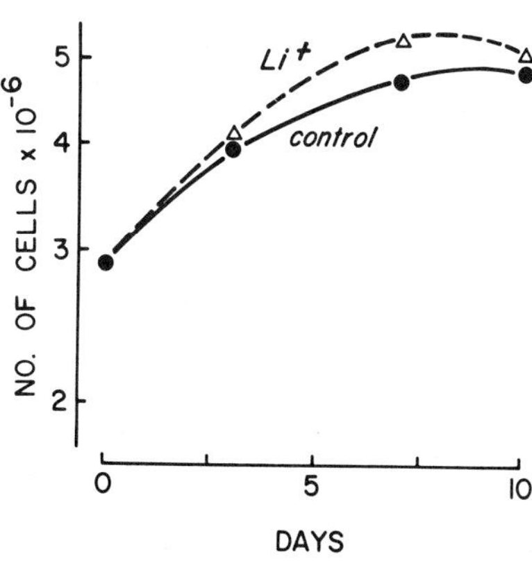

Figure 7. Effect of LiCl on growth of confluent cultures of BSC-1 cells. Cells were plated in medium with 1% calf serum and grown to the density shown on day 0 on the graph. Sets of plates were then changed to media containing 0.5% serum with (△) or without (●) LiCl (2.5 mM). (Reprinted from Toback, 1980, with permission.)

work of Hestbech and co-workers (1977), who described numerous cortical and some medullary cysts in the kidneys of two patients after long-term lithium exposure.

5. Conclusions

A variety of substances appear to play a role in the initiation of renal cell growth. Some of these are sodium chloride (Toback, 1980) and ammonium acetate (Berman *et al.*, 1979), which augment the growth of renal cells in culture, and testosterone (Korenchevsky *et al.*, 1933) and thyroxine (Katz and Lindheimer, 1973), which increase renal mass in rats. Unknown factors in the serum appear to mediate compensatory renal growth after unilateral nephrectomy (Lowenstein and Stern, 1963; Ogawa and Nowinski, 1958). Epidermal growth factor, which is a normal constituent of human blood and urine, stimulates the growth of renal epithelial cells in culture (Carpenter and Cohen, 1979; Holley *et al.*, 1977). It is not yet known if this polypeptide plays a role in the regulation of renal growth in man. Inhibitors of kidney cell growth produced by the cells may also play an important role in the regulation of renal growth *in vivo* (Holley *et al.*, 1978b, 1980; Lozzio *et al.*, 1975).

It seems likely that growth-promoting factors, ions, nutrients, and inhibitors interact with each other so that the initiation of growth may represent a summation of various proliferative and inhibitory influences on the cell (Holley, 1975). Study of the mechanism of action of these diverse substances would provide a fund of knowledge which could form the basis for understanding the causes of renal disease and thereby permit the design of treatments to prevent or to ameliorate it in susceptible or afflicted individuals.

ACKNOWLEDGMENTS. The collaborative efforts of Leah J. Havener, and Drs. H. N. Aithal, Godfrey S. Getz, Nelson Ordóñez, and Benjamin Spargo at the University of Chicago are acknowledged with gratitude. Studies of renal cells in culture were performed in Dr. Robert W. Holley's laboratory at the Salk Institute, San Diego, California, and were supported by a Scholar Grant in Cancer Research from the American Cancer Society.

References

Aithal, H. N., and Toback, F. G., 1978, Defective mitochondrial energy production during potassium depletion nephropathy, *Lab. Invest.* **39:**186.

Aithal, H. N., Toback, F. G., Dube, S., Getz, G. S., and Spargo, B. H., 1977a, Formation of renal medullary lysosomes during potassium depletion nephropathy, *Lab. Invest.* **36:**107.

Aithal, H. N., Toback, F. G., Ordóñez, N. G., and Spargo, B. H., 1977b, Functional defects in mitochondria of renal inner red medulla during potassium depletion nephropathy, *Lab. Invest.* **37:**423.

Berman, J., Perantoni, A., Jackson, H. M., and Kingsbury, E., 1979, Primary epithelial cell culture of adult rat kidney, enhancement of cell growth by ammonium acetate, *Exp. Cell Res.* **121**:47.

Burrows, G. D., Davies, B., and Kincaid-Smith, P., 1978, Unique tubular lesion after lithium, *Lancet* **1**:1310.

Carpenter, G., and Cohen, S., 1979, Epidermal growth factor, *Annu. Rev. Biochem.* **48**:193.

Evan, A. P., and Gardner, K. D., Jr., 1979, Nephron obstruction in nordihydroguaiaretic acid-induced renal cystic disease, *Kidney Int.* **15**:7.

Evan, A. P., and Ollerich, D. A., 1972, The effect of lithium carbonate on the structure of the rat kidney, *Am. J. Anat.* **134**:97.

Evan, A. P., Hong, S. K., Gardner, K., Jr., Park, Y. S., and Itagaki, R., 1978, Evolution of the collecting tubular lesion in diphenylamine-induced renal disease, *Lab. Invest.* **38**:244.

Evan, A. P., Gardner, K. D., Jr., and Bernstein, J., 1979, Polypoid and papillary epithelial hyperplasia: A potential cause of ductal obstruction in adult polycystic disease, *Kidney Int.* **16**:743.

Gardner, K. D., Jr., Solomon, S., Fitzgerrel, W. W., and Evan, A. P., 1976, Function and structure in the diphenylamine-exposed kidney, *J. Clin. Invest.* **57**:796.

Gustafson, A. B., Shear, L., and Gabuzda, G. J., 1973, Protein metabolism *in vivo* in kidney, liver, muscle, and heart of potassium-deficient rats, *J. Lab. Clin. Med.* **82**:287.

Havener, L. J., and Toback, F. G., 1980, Amino acid modulation of renal phosphatidylcholine biosynthesis in the rat, *J. Clin. Invest.* **65**:741.

Heppel, L. A., 1940, The diffusion of radioactive sodium into the muscles of potassium-deprived rats, *Am. J. Physiol.* **128**:449.

Hestbech, J., Hansen, H. E., Amdisen, A., and Olson, S., 1977, Chronic renal lesions following long-term treatment with lithium, *Kidney Int.* **12**:205.

Holley, R. W., 1975, Control of growth of mammalian cells in cell culture, *Nature* **258**:487.

Holley, R. W., Armour, R., Baldwin, J. H., Brown, K. D., and Yeh, Y.-C., 1977, Density-dependent regulation of growth of BSC-1 cells in cell culture: Control of growth by serum factors, *Proc. Natl. Acad. Sci. USA* **74**:5046.

Holley, R. W., Armour, R., and Baldwin, J. H., 1978a, Density-dependent regulation of growth of BSC-1 cells in cell culture: Control of growth by low molecular weight nutrients, *Proc. Natl. Acad. Sci. USA* **75**:339.

Holley, R. W., Armour, R., and Baldwin, J. H., 1978b, Density-dependent regulation of growth of BSC-1 cells in cell culture: Growth inhibitors formed by the cells, *Proc. Natl. Acad. Sci. USA* **75**:1864.

Holley, R. W., Böhlen, P., Fava, R., Baldwin, J. H., Kleeman, G., and Armour, R., 1980, Purification of kidney epithelial cell growth inhibitors, *Proc. Natl. Acad. Sci. USA* **77**:5989.

Ishikawa, I., Saito, Y., Onouchi, Z., Kitada, H., Suzuki, S., Kurihara, S., Yuri, T., and Shinoda, A., 1980, Development of acquired cystic disease and adenocarcinoma of the kidney in glomerulonephritic chronic hemodialysis patients, *Clin. Nephrol.* **14**:1.

Johnson, J. D., Epel, D., and Paul, M., 1976, Intracellular pH and activation of sea urchin eggs after fertilisation, *Nature (London)* **262**:661.

Katz, A. I., and Lindheimer, M. D., 1973, Renal sodium- and potassium-activated adenosine triphosphatase and sodium reabsorption in the hypothyroid rat, *J. Clin. Invest.* **52**:796.

Kennedy, E. P., and Weiss, S. B., 1956, The function of cytidine coenzymes in the biosynthesis of phospholipids, *J. Biol. Chem.* **222**:193.

Liebow, A. A., McFarland, W. J., and Tennant, R., 1941, The effects of potassium deficiency on tumor-bearing mice, *Yale J. Biol. Med.* **13**:523.

Koch, K. S., and Leffert, H. L., 1979, Increased sodium ion influx is necessary to initiate rat hepatocyte proliferation, *Cell* **18**:153.

Korenchevsky, V., Dennison, M., and Kohn-Speyer, A., 1933, Changes produced by testicular hormone in normal and in castrated rats, *Biochem. J.* **27**:557.

Lindop, G. B. M., and Padfield, P. L., 1975, The renal pathology in a case of lithium-induced diabetes insipidus, *J. Clin. Pathol.* **28**:472.

Lowenstein, L. M., and Stern, A., 1963, Serum factor in renal compensatory hyperplasia, *Science* **142:**1479.

Lozzio, B. B., Lozzio, C. B., Bamberger, E. G., and Lair, S. V., 1975, Regulators of cell division: endogenous mitotic inhibitors of mammalian cells, *Int. Rev. Cytol.* **42:**1.

Ogawa, K., and Nowinski, W. W., 1958, Mitosis stimulating factor in serum of unilaterally nephrectomized rats, *Proc. Soc. Exp. Biol. Med.* **99:**350.

Oliver, J., MacDowell, M., Welt, L. G., Holliday, M. A., Hollander, W., Jr., Winters, R. W., Williams, T. F., and Segar, W. E., 1957, The renal lesions of electrolyte imbalance. I. The structural alterations in potassium-depleted rats, *J. Exp. Med.* **106:**563.

Ordóñez, N. G., Toback, F. G., Aithal, H. N., and Spargo, B. H., 1977, Zonal changes in renal structure and phospholipid metabolism during reversal of potassium depletion nephropathy, *Lab. Invest.* **36:**33.

Perey, D. Y. E., Herdman, R. C., and Good, R. A., 1967, Polycystic renal disease: A new experimental model, *Science* **158:**494.

Rouser, G., Simon, G., and Kritchevsky, G., 1969, Species variations in phospholipid class distribution of organs: I. Kidney, liver and spleen, *Lipids* **4:**599.

Schrader, G. A., Prickett, C. O., and Salmon, W. D., 1937, Symptomatology and pathology of potassium and magnesium deficiencies in the rat, *J. Nutr.* **14:**85.

Smith, J. B., and Rozengurt, E., 1978, Serum stimulates the Na^+, K^+ pump in quiescent fibroblasts by increasing Na^+ entry, *Proc. Natl. Acad. Sci. USA* **75:**5560.

Spargo, B., 1954, Kidney changes in hypokalemic alkalosis in the rat, *J. Lab. Clin. Med.* **43:**802.

Sturm, P., 1875, Über das adenom der niere und über die beziehung desselben zu einigen anderen neubildungen der niere, *Arch. Heilk.* **16:**193.

Toback, F. G., 1980, Induction of growth in kidney epithelial cells in culture by Na^+, *Proc. Natl. Acad. Sci. USA* **77:**6654.

Toback, F. G., and Havener, L. J., 1979, Mechanism of enhanced phospholipid formation during potassium depletion nephropathy, *Am. J. Physiol.* **236:**E429.

Toback, F. G., Smith, P. D., and Lowenstein, L. M., 1974, Phospholipid metabolism in the initiation of renal compensatory growth after acute reduction of renal mass, *J. Clin. Invest.* **54:**91.

Toback, F. G., Ordóñez, N. G., Bortz, S. L., and Spargo, B. H., 1976, Zonal changes in renal structure and phospholipid metabolism in potassium-deficient rats, *Lab. Invest.* **34:**115.

Toback, F. G., Havener, L. J., Dodd, R. C., and Spargo, B. H., 1977a, Phospholipid metabolism during renal regeneration after acute tubular necrosis, *Am. J. Physiol.* **232:**E216.

Toback, F. G., Havener, L. J., and Spargo, B. H., 1977b, Stimulation of renal phospholipid formation during potassium depletion, *Am. J. Physiol.* **233:**E212.

Toback, F. G., Aithal, H. N., Ordóñez, N. G., and Spargo, B. H., 1979, Altered bioenergetics in proliferating renal cells during potassium depletion, *Lab. Invest.* **41:**265.

Wu, R., and Racker, E., 1963, Control of rate-limiting factors of glycolysis in tumor cells, in: *Control Mechanisms in Respiration and Fermentation* (B. Wright, ed.), Ronald Press, New York, pp. 265–288.

9

Movements of Salts and Water into Cysts in Polycystic Kidney Disease

Jared Grantham

1. *Cyst Structure and Function in Polycystic Kidney Disease*

The cysts in polycystic kidney disease (PKD) derive from different nephron segments (Potter, 1972; Lambert, 1947; Bricker and Patton, 1955). Recent studies from our laboratory confirmed the earlier study of Gardner (1969) which showed that the cysts are capable of maintaining steep solute concentration gradients between cyst fluid (CF) and plasma (Cuppage *et al.*, 1980; Huseman *et al.*, 1980).

1.1. *Cyst Function*

The cysts can be divided into general groups on the basis of the sodium concentrations: proximal cysts (Na CF/serum $\approx$ 1.0) and distal cysts (Na CF/serum $<$ 0.4) (Fig. 1). Confirmation of the hypothesis that cysts arise from nephrons is obtained when one examines the concentrations in cysts designated as proximal or distal on the basis of the sodium concentration (Figs. 2–5). In proximal cysts the concentrations of K, Cl, H^+, creatinine, and urea are nearly equal to the serum values, whereas the distal cyst values are quite different. In distal cysts the sodium, chloride, and pH values are lower than in serum, whereas the potassium, creatinine, urea, and glucose levels are higher than in serum in both azotemic and nonazotemic patients. The distribution of these solutes conforms to the expectations for fluid in prolonged contact with proximal and distal renal epithelium.

Jared Grantham • Department of Medicine, University of Kansas School of Medicine, Kansas City, Kansas 66103.

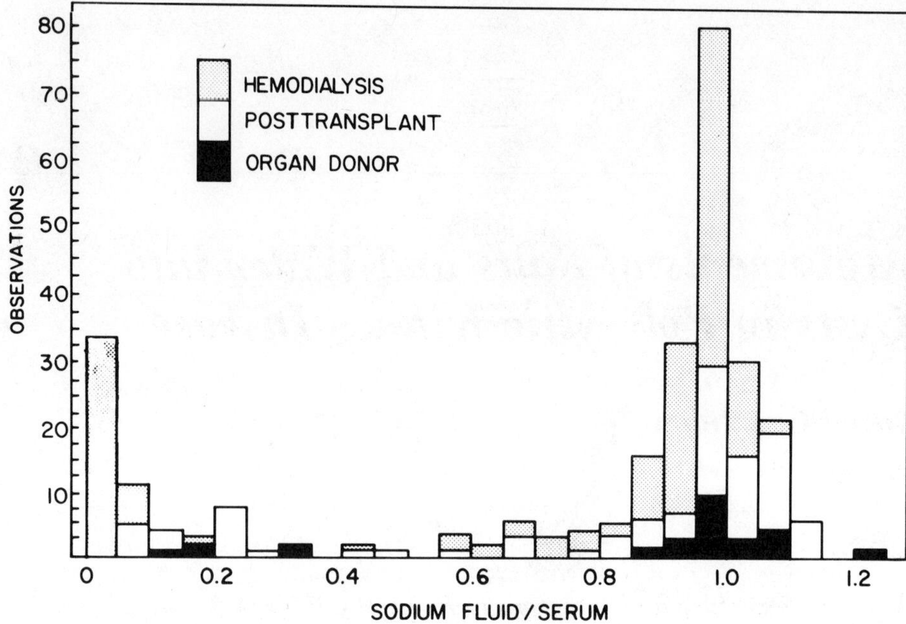

Figure 1. Distribution of cyst fluid sodium concentrations in 271 individual cysts from eight patients. Hemodialysis, five azotemic patients who were nephrectomized prior to renal transplantation. Posttransplant, two nonazotemic patients whose cystic kidneys were removed several weeks after a successful cadaveric allograft. Organ donor, one nonazotemic subject with PKD whose kidneys were donated for renal transplantation. Note the biomodal distribution of sodium concentrations in the cysts. (Reprinted from Huseman *et al.*, 1980, with permission.)

1.2. Cyst Structure

Morphological studies of the walls of cysts show the presence of a single layer of epithelial cells joined at their apices by "tight" or "loose" junctional complexes (Cuppage *et al.*, 1980). Those cysts with "tight" apical junctions had solute concentrations in the fluid typical of distal nephrons, whereas those cysts with "loose" junctions had fluid typical of proximal tubules. The separate analysis of structure and function strongly suggests that the epithelium lining cyst, though dedifferentiated with respect to surface characteristics (e.g., brush borders and basolateral infoldings), functions throughout the life of the patient.

2. Human Findings

Studies in two nonazotemic patients who had their polycystic kidneys removed several weeks after they had received cadaveric renal allografts showed that the solutes in *proximal* cysts had equilibrated with plasma (Figs. 2–5). These serendipitous studies showed that proximal cyst walls are permeable to most endogenous solutes (electrolytes, creatinine, and urea). By

Table 1. Solute Distribution in Distal Cysts of Five Azotemic Patients and in One Patient following Renal Transplantation[a]

		Azotemic patients	Posttransplant patient
Creatinine (mg dl^{-1})	Cyst	49	50
	Serum	12.4	17
	Ratio	3.95	2.94
Urea (mg dl^{-1})	Cyst	92.0	60
	Serum	79.1	113
	Ratio	1.16	0.53

[a] The CF/S ratios of urea ÷ creatinine are reduced from 0.29 in the azotemic to 0.18 in the posttransplant patient.

contrast electrolyte gradients were preserved in distal cysts, although the creatinine and urea levels decreased to a small extent indicating that distal epithelium was slightly permeable to solutes (Table 1). The transplanted patients' cyst values were referenced with the azotemic serum values to permit comparison with the cyst fluids from the azotemic subjects. As shown in Table 1, the distal cyst fluid-to-serum ratios of creatinine and urea were higher in five azotemic patients than in the distal cysts of the nonazotemic patient who had received a successful allograft.

These studies of solute permeability are in agreement with the work of others who showed that tritiated water moved readily across the cyst walls (Jacobsson *et al.*, 1977). Since the cysts are permeable to water, creatinine, and urea, it seems certain that electrolyte gradients in renal cysts are maintained by active cellular transport.

Analysis of hydrostatic pressure differences across the walls of cysts (Fig. 6) shows that the pressures are of a magnitude expected in normal renal tubules.

A recent observation in our laboratory that also bears on the functional significance of renal cysts deserves mention. We removed a polycystic kidney from an azotemic patient who had been given gentamicin and clindamycin for several days prior to nephrectomy. We found that gentamicin levels were higher in proximal than in distal cysts, in keeping with the observations of Muther and Bennett (1980). However, the clindamycin levels were much higher in distal (acidic) than in proximal (normal pH) cysts. Since gentamicin is highly polar and clindamycin is relatively nonpolar and very lipid soluble, we suggest that certain drugs, such as clindamycin, may accumulate preferentially in distal cysts owing to their high permeability through the cyst wall and their propensity to be dissociated and "trapped" in acidic fluid.

In this same patient we learned that the Po_2 of cyst fluid may range from anaerobic (no oxygen) to levels of oxygen equal to that of normally oxygenated blood. Furthermore, some of the so-called "chocolate cysts" (cysts containing heme products) were packed with lipid bodies, i.e., cells that contain polarizing lipid droplets typical of the oval fat bodies seen in the urine of patients with nephrotic syndrome and lipiduria. This latter obser-

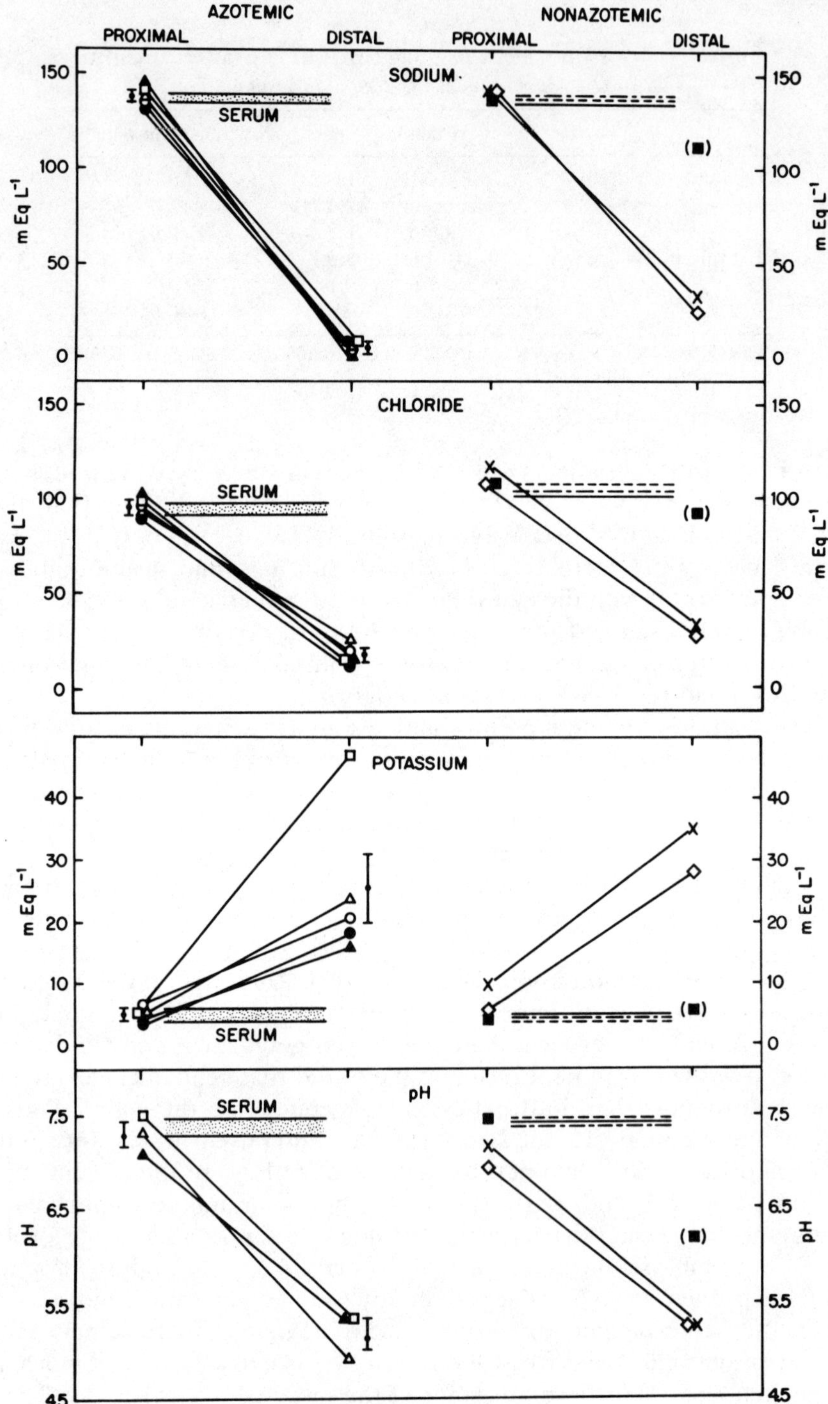

Figures 2–5. Cyst fluid concentrations of solutes. Kidneys from five azotemic and three nonazotemic patients were studied. Range of serum values for nonazotemic patients. (————) Organ donor; (– – – –) transplanted patients; (■) a single "indeterminant" cyst.

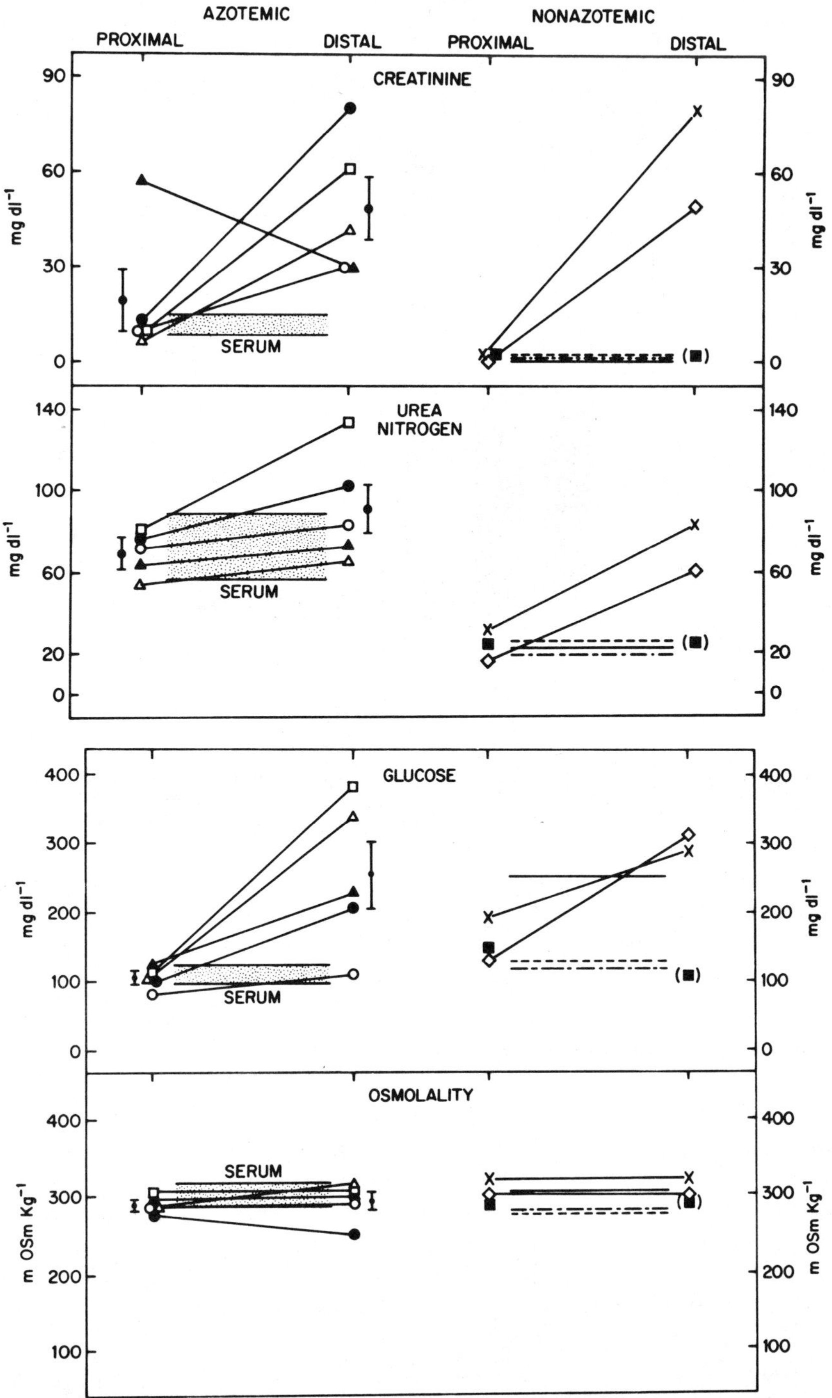

Figures 2–5. *(Continued)*

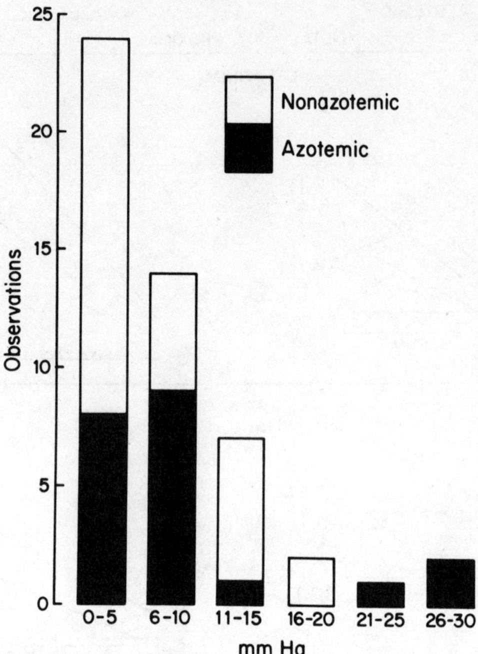

Figure 6. Hydrostatic pressures in cysts.

vation suggests that in some cysts there is considerable "turnover" of cells, since the lipid-laden cells were also found in the epithelium lining the cyst walls.

From the foregoing, it seems reasonable to conclude that cystic nephrons continue to function to some extent throughout the life of the patient. In the remainder of this chapter, I will consider how this information may help us to understand the pathogenesis of cyst formation.

3. Mechanisms of Cyst Formation

A cyst can form in only a limited number of ways in a nephron segment, as shown diagrammatically in Fig. 7. In *normal* nephrons plasma is filtered into the tubules, and about 99% of the water and solutes is reabsorbed. Transtubule pressure measured in laboratory animals shows values ranging from about 11 mm Hg in proximal convoluted to about 5 mm Hg in distal convoluted tubules. In the diagram, the pressure is depicted as coiled springs pushing outward. Fluid movement is shown by the solid arrows.

3.1. Obstruction

If a nephron segment is *obstructed*, either by a cast or by an abnormal growth of cells, the pressure inside the tubule proximal to the obstruction

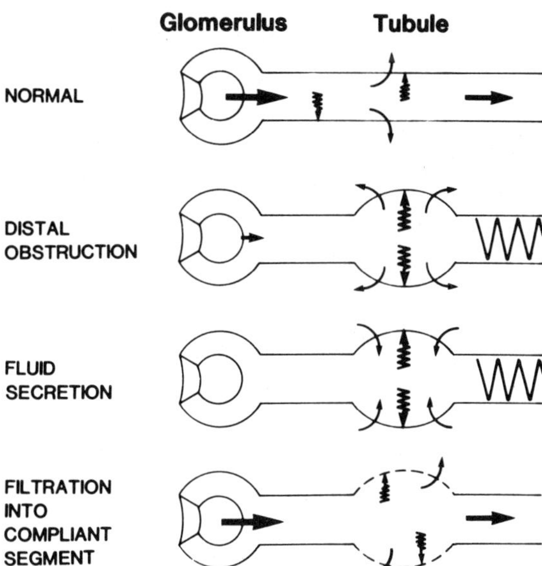

Figure 7. Mechanisms of cyst formation. Solid lines indicate fluid movement. Dashed-coiled lines with arrowheads indicate pressure.

will be increased initially. If the obstruction is total, several studies suggest that the tubular pressure will actually decrease owing to a sharp reduction in glomerular filtration rate (GFR) several hours after the obstruction is placed (Wilson, 1980). Thus, complete obstruction might not cause persistent hypertension in the renal tubule. Alternatively, partial obstruction would permit GFR to continue at some reduced level and would also cause pressure to be chronically increased. In human PKD, we found no evidence for an increase in hydrostatic pressure; rather the pressures were in a range expected for normal nephrons (Fig. 6). Electron microscopy did not show evidence of increased pressure within the cyst, but as Dr. Bernstein has pointed out, one might interpret the atrophy of adjacent noncystic nephrons to reflect some degree of pressure atrophy. If pressure increases by a small magnitude, not detectable by our measurements, and is instrumental in the formation of cysts, we must then explain why the cysts start out as focal dilatations for nephron segments, rather than as a generalized expansion of whole nephrons when the collecting segments are obstructed.

3.2. Secretion

Fluid secretion has been suggested as a possible cause of cyst formation. Secretion is a reasonable mechanism since hippurates have been shown to cause fluid secretion in proximal tubules (Grantham *et al.*, 1973) and the fluid of distal cysts contains unidentified osmotic solutes (probably amino acids) which could cause fluid movement in the cysts (Table 2). A secretion process would require distal obstruction since fluid secreted into the segment would simply drain into the pelvis of a normal nephron. The most damaging

Table 2. Nominal Composition of Cyst Fluids in Azotemic Patients in Steady State

	Proximal (mmoles/liter)	Distal (mmoles/liter)
Na^+	138	4.8
K^+	5.1	25.3
Cl^-	96	18.3
HCO_3^-	25	1.0
PO_4^{3-}	5.0	15.1
Ca^{2+}	3.9	4.0
Glucose	5.8	14.1
Urea	25	32.9
Creatinine	1.7	4.3
Hippurate	2.8	1.4
Total	308.4	121.2
Osmolality	290	301

evidence against fluid secretion is the finding that the creatinine levels are equal to or greater than the plasma creatinine levels in proximal and distal cysts. Secretion of fluid would dilute rather than concentrate the creatinine in the cysts.

3.3. Increased Compliance

The final alternative involves a focal increase in the *compliance* of nephron segments. The tubular basement membrane (TBM) normally determines the distensibility of tubules in response to hydrostatic pressure (Welling and Grantham, 1972). According to this view, the tubular basement membrane is weakened, because of either defective synthesis or abnormal breakdown. This causes the tubular segment to expand to an abnormal degree with normal intratubular pressures. This mechanism does not require distal obstruction, although any factor that would increase intratubular pressure would facilitate the formation of the cyst. In this way cysts would fill with unabsorbed glomerular ultrafiltrate because the resistance to fluid flow into the cysts would be equal to or less than the resistance to flow through the remainder of the nephron and collecting system. The basement membrane "defect" could be due (1) to synthesis of abnormally compliant TBM, or (2) to synthesis of increased amounts of TBM which allows cells to grow in the radial direction. On the one hand, cystic disease may be viewed as a problem of defective synthesis of a supportive framework; on the other hand, the disease may be considered a defect in the growth of tubular epithelium.

3.4. Summation

In summary, we know that in adult PKD the cysts arise from nephrons and collecting segments. The cells dedifferentiate, losing some of the normal surface features, yet they retain their basic solute transport and permeability characteristics.

4. Unresolved Questions

Some unresolved questions are

1. What are the mechanisms of renal insufficiency? Specifically, to what extent do compression, recruitment of new nephrons to form cysts, and/or altered tubuloglomerular feedback contribute to renal failure?
2. Are the lining cells genetically programmed to form cysts, or are the cells passengers hanging onto a superstructure (TBM) that is abnormally compliant?
3. Can advantage be taken of the different electrolyte and solute concentrations in the cysts for diagnostic purposes or for the selective accumulation of drugs in the cysts?

ACKNOWLEDGMENT. The author thanks Janet Rosberg for secretarial assistance.

References

Bricker, N., and Patton, J., 1955, Cystic disease of the kidneys, *Am. J. Med.* **18**:207–219.

Cuppage, F., Huseman, R., Chapman, A., and Grantham, J., 1980, Ultrastructure and function of cysts from human adult polycystic kidneys, *Kidney Int.* **17**:372–381.

Gardner, K., 1969, Composition of fluid in twelve cysts of a polycystic kidney, *N. Engl. J. Med.* **281**:985–988.

Grantham, J., Irwin, R., Qualizza, P., Tucker, D., and Whittier, F., 1973, Fluid secretion in isolated proximal straight renal tubules, *J. Clin. Invest.* **52**(10):2441–2450.

Huseman, R., Grady, A., Welling, D., and Grantham, J., 1980, Macropuncture study of polycystic disease in adult human kidneys, *Kidney Int.* **18**:375–385.

Jacobsson, L., Lindqvist, B., Michaelson, G., and Bjerle, P., 1977, Fluid turnover in renal cysts, *Acta Med. Scand.* **202**:327–329.

Lambert, P., 1947, Polycystic disease of the kidney, *Arch. Path.* **44**:34–58.

Muther, R. S., and Bennett, W. M., 1980, Cyst fluid antibiotic levels in polycystic kidney disease (PCKD): Difference in proximal and distal cyst permeability, American Society of Nephrology 13th Annual Meeting Abstracts, p. 27A.

Potter, E. L., 1972, *Normal and Abnormal Development of the Kidney*, Year Book Medical Publishers, Chicago, pp. 182–208.

Welling, L., and Grantham, J., 1972, Physical properties of isolated perfused renal tubules and tubular basement membranes, *J. Clin. Invest.* **51**(5):1063–1075.

Wilson, D. R., 1980, Pathophysiology of obstructive nephropathy, *Kidney Int.* **18**:281–292.

10

Movement of Organic Molecules into Cysts

William M. Bennett, Curtis G. Wickre, and Richard S. Muther

1. Introduction

Patients with polycystic kidney disease and intercurrent urinary tract infection may develop perinephric abscesses despite prolonged antibiotic treatment directed against susceptible urinary pathogens (Sweet and Keane, 1979). Sweet and Keane (1979), during a 3½-year period of observation, found that 8 of 24 dialysis patients with polycystic kidney disease developed symptomatic urinary infections. Of these, five patients developed perinephric abscesses despite more than 2 weeks of antibiotic treatment. This type of experience suggests that cystic nephrons may not achieve adequate concentrations of antibiotics for sterilization of infected fluid. Poor drainage of cystic nephrons due to outflow obstruction also might contribute to poor therapeutic response.

Impaired renal function in patients with polycystic kidney disease is likely to contribute to poor results by decreased filtration of drugs or by poor diffusion through damaged parenchyma, despite therapeutic antibiotic concentrations in serum. This is analogous to other patients with upper-urinary-tract infection and advanced renal disease, where adequate tissue or urinary antibiotic concentrations are difficult to obtain (Bennett *et al.*, 1977). However, patients with infected simple renal cysts do not respond well to antibiotic therapy (Patel *et al.*, 1978) either. The fact that these patients usually have well-preserved renal function suggests that antibiotic movement

---

William M. Bennett, Curtis G. Wickre, and Richard S. Muther • Division of Nephrology, Department of Medicine, Oregon Health Sciences University, Portland, Oregon 97201. Supported, in part, by Grant RR-00334-14 from the General Clinical Research Centers Branch, Division of Research Resources, National Institutes of Health.

into cystic nephrons may be dependent on mechanisms other than glomerular filtration. This chapter reviews what is currently known about antibiotic movement into cysts. As data have accumulated, it has become evident that such studies provide insight not only into the treatment of infection, but also into cyst physiology and into the transport of other organic molecules by cyst walls.

2. *Simple Cysts*

Simple renal cysts contain fluid that is in equilibrium with extracellular or interstitial fluid. Steg found no penetrance of amoxicillin, minocycline, or rifampicin into simple cysts (Steg, 1976). Other reported cases of infection treated medically have shown poor responses to penicillins (ampicillin, penicillin G, nafcillin) and to streptomycin. In fact, only a solitary patient who was treated with chloramphenicol improved on medical treatment alone (Deliveliotis *et al.*, 1967). Muther and Bennett (1980) recently measured simultaneous levels of gentamicin in urine, serum, and cyst fluid from three patients treated with full therapeutic doses of the antibiotic. Despite creatinine clearances of 40, 52, and 80 ml/min, respectively, only one patient achieved measurable gentamicin in the cyst. In that patient, the concentration was 24% of the serum concentration and 0.6% of that found in urine. An additional patient with a creatinine clearance of 78 ml/min was given trimethoprim-sulfa methoxazole. Neither drug could be detected in the cyst (Deliveliotis *et al.*, 1967). From these data, it would seem that surgical drainage would be preferable to antibiotic therapy for infected simple renal cysts. Changes in permeability due to infection, *per se*, could alter antibiotic penetrance, but this has not been investigated systematically. Patients with solitary cysts might prove to be ideal subjects for studies of transport kinetics of other organic molecules as well as of antibiotics.

3. *Cysts in Patients with Adult Polycystic Kidney Disease*

Few studies have examined penetration of antibiotics into cysts of patients with polycystic kidney disease. We obtained cyst fluid from seven patients with typical adult polycystic kidney disease. All patients had bilaterally enlarged kidneys and positive family histories. Four patients were on maintenance dialysis, and another patient had a creatinine clearance of 15 ml/min. Two patients had normal renal function but came to medical attention because of severe abdominal pain related to massive cyst enlargement. All patients were treated with antibiotics in full therapeutic dosage for 36–48 hr prior to cyst fluid sampling. Simultaneously with aspiration of cyst fluid, serum and urine samples were obtained for antibiotic concentrations. Eighty cysts were sampled, ranging in volume from 1.5 to 967 ml. Of the 80 cysts sampled, 62 were proximal, as classified by the method of Huseman *et al.*

Table 1. Mean Concentration of Antibiotics in Serum, Urine, and Cyst Fluid in Patients with Polycystic Kidney Disease[a]

Drug	No. patients	Serum	Urine	Cyst	Cyst : serum ratio	Cyst : urine ratio
Gentamicin	3	2.3	11	0.59 (33)	0.26	0.05
Tobramycin	2	3.7	28	0 (5)	0	0
Cephapirin	3	46	448	8.8 (43)	0.19	0.02
Ticarcillin	1	400	—	47 (20)	0.12	—
Ampicillin	1	4.7	660	0 (1)	0	0
Erythromycin	1	4.3	32	3.4 (4)	0.79	0.16

[a] All concentrations in μg/ml. Numbers in parentheses indicate number of cysts punctured.

(1980), on the basis of cyst fluid-to-serum sodium ratios of greater than 0.9. Sixteen cysts were of distal nephron origin, as judged by cyst fluid-to-serum sodium ratios of less than 0.2. Two cysts were of indeterminant origin. Three patients had proximal cysts only sampled. The results for the antibiotics studied with simultaneous urine and serum values are shown in Table 1. Table 2 depicts antibiotic concentrations in proximal and distal cysts. In general, all drugs tested penetrate cysts poorly. Proximal cysts seem to achieve higher concentrations for all drugs except cephapirin. However, only one distal cyst was punctured in patients receiving cephapirin, so that firm conclusions are hazardous. Only one patient had infected cysts at the time of these studies. Despite adequate serum levels and sensitive bacteria, sterilization of the cyst was not achieved prior to surgical treatment.

Penicillins and cephalosporins are handled in the normal kidney by the organic acid transport system. Clearances of these drugs exceeded glomerular filtration rates, and proximal tubular secretion has been demonstrated. Thus, since the cysts of patients with polycystic kidney disease presumably arise from single nephrons and have filtration rates of approximately 10^{-8} liters/min (Huseman *et al.*, 1980), drugs transported as organic acids should be transported into cysts better than drugs that depend primarily on glomerular filtration, such as aminoglycosides. The surprising appearance

Table 2. Comparison of Antibiotic Levels between Proximal and Distal Cysts[a]

Drug	No. patients	Serum	Cyst fluid: Proximal	Cyst fluid: Distal
Gentamicin	3	2.3	1.04 (19)	0 (14)
Tobramycin	2	3.7	0 (2)	0 (3)
Cephapirin	3	46	8.1 (42)	38 (1)
Ticarcillin	1	400	135 (7)	0 (13)
Ampicillin	1	4.7	0 (1)	—
Erythromycin	1	4.3	3.4 (4)	—

[a] All concentrations in μg/ml. Numbers in parentheses indicate number of cysts punctured.

Table 3. Mean Cyst Fluid, Serum, and Urine Concentrations of Inulin and PAH following Their Continuous Intravenous Infusion in Two Patients with Normal Renal Function[a]

	Patient 1		Patient 2	
	Inulin	PAH	Inulin	PAH
Serum	0.78	6.30	0.53	3.14
Cyst fluid	0	1.44	0	0
Urine	14	515	2.8	95
Cyst: fluid	0	0.23	0	0

[a] All concentrations in mg/dl. Values in patient 1 are the mean of 13 proximal cysts. Values in patient 2 are from one 250-ml proximal cyst.

of gentamicin in proximal cysts suggests that these cationic drugs may gain access to cysts by a transtubular route. Basolateral transport of aminoglycosides, although quantitatively not important in normal animals, has been implied from renal cortical slice studies (Kluwe and Hook, 1978). Collier *et al.* (1979) showed that only 75% of renal gentamicin uptake could be eliminated by rendering an isolated perfused rat kidney nonfiltering.

In two patients with normal renal function, prolonged infusions of inulin and para-aminohippurate (PAH) were performed. Results are shown in Table 3. In one patient, PAH was detected in proximal cysts in a concentration 23% that of serum values. The other patient, who had only a solitary 250-ml proximal cyst punctured, had no PAH detected. Neither patient achieved measurable inulin concentrations in cysts. Unfortunately, no distal cysts were available from these patients for study. Bricker and Patton (1955) and Lambert (1947) found inulin in cysts shortly after intravenous injection. It is difficult to reconcile these results with the present studies. It is possible that inulin might enter cysts by diffusion across epithelium whose permeability is altered by distention. A similar explanation might be offered for gentamicin entrance into cyst fluid.

It is obvious that further study of organic molecules and their movement into cyst fluid might be fruitful in unraveling mechanisms of cyst growth as well as leading to more rational drug therapy of infected cysts.

References

Bennett, W. M., Hartnett, M. N., Craven, R., Gilbert, D. N., and Porter, G. A., 1977, Gentamicin concentrations in blood, urine and renal tissue of patients with end stage renal disease, *J. Lab. Clin. Med.* **90:**389–393.

Bricker, N. S., and Patton, J. F., 1955, Cystic disease of the kidneys, a study of dynamics and chemical composition of cyst fluid, *Am.J. Med.* **18:**207–219.

Collier, V. V., Leitman, P. S., and Mitch, W. E., 1979, Evidence for luminal uptake of gentamicin in perfused rat kidney, *J. Pharmacol. Exp. Ther.* **210:**247–251.

Deliveliotis, A., Zorgos, S., and Vorkarakis, M., 1967, Suppuration of a solitary cyst of the kidney, *Br. J. Urol.* **39:**472–476.

Huseman, R., Grady, A., Welling, D., and Grantham, J., 1980, Macropuncture study of polycystic kidney disease in adult human kidneys, *Kidney Int.* **18:**375–385.

Kluwe, W. M., and Hook, J. B., 1978, Analysis of gentamicin uptake by rat renal cortical slices, *Toxicol. Appl. Pharmacol.* **45:**531–539.

Lambert, P. P., 1947, Polycystic disease of the kidneys: A review, *Arch. Path.* **44:**34–58.

Muther, R. S., and Bennett, W. M., 1980, Concentration of antibiotics in simple renal cysts, *J. Urol.* **124:**596.

Patel, N. P., Pitts, W. R., and Ward, J. N., 1978, Solitary infected renal cyst: Report of two cases and review of the literature, *Urology* **11:**164–172.

Steg, A., 1976, Renal cysts. II. Chemical and dynamic study of cyst fluid, *Eur. Urol.* **2:**164–170.

Sweet, R., and Keane, W. F., 1979, Perinephric abscess in patients with polycystic kidney disease undergoing hemodialysis, *Nephron* **23:**237–240.

11

Kinetics of Cyst Development in Cystic Renal Disease

Larry W. Welling and Dan J. Welling

1. *Introduction*

The cysts in polycystic renal disease are always filled with fluid. In this chapter we consider the accumulation of that fluid to be a primary event in cyst production, consider the source of that fluid, and then ask whether or not the amount and rate of cyst filling and growth can give us additional information about their cause.

2. *Mass Balance*

Figure 1 shows a hypothetical nephron segment in which a central region is predisposed to cystic dilation by some as-yet-unknown mechanism. Arrows represent volume flows. $J_{V_{in}}$ is the proximal inflow and is equal to the single nephron glomerular filtration rate (GFR) plus or minus any secretory or reabsorptive flux that may have occurred upstream. J_{V_s} is secretory volume flux from peritubular medium to tubule lumen and probably requires an osmotic difference to be effective. $J_{V_{ab}}$ is reabsorptive volume flux from lumen to peritubular medium and may derive from active or passive processes. $J_{V_{out}}$ is the distal outflow and may be influenced by partial or complete distal obstruction. For reference, $J_{V_{in}}$ and $J_{V_{out}}$ are assigned a wide range of normal values to accommodate a variety of species and circumstances. In general, J_{V_s} is small or negligible whereas $J_{V_{ab}}$ may represent a considerable fraction of the $J_{V_{in}}$.

The mass balance equation for this situation is $dV/dt = J_{V_{in}} + J_{V_s} - J_{V_{ab}} - J_{V_{out}}$ in which the rate of volume change, dV/dt, in the segment is seen

---

Larry W. Welling • Veterans Administration Medical Center, Kansas City, Missouri 64128. ***Dan J. Welling*** • Departments of Pathology and Physiology, University of Kansas Medical Center, Kansas City, Kansas 66103.

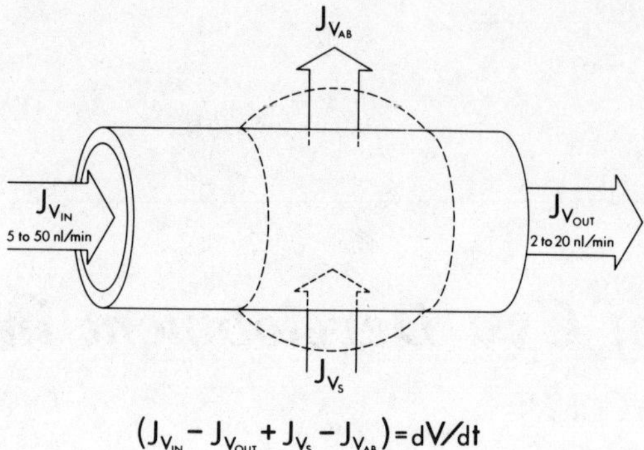

Figure 1. Hypothetical nephron segment predisposed to cystic dilation. Arrows represent volume flows.

to be critically dependent on the four fluid fluxes. In the steady state, dV/dt is zero. In the growing cyst, dV/dt is positive, equal to the net filling rate and thus equal to the rate of cyst growth. Because dV/dt reflects several flows which might vary independently with time, the change in cyst volume with time may have different patterns. Figure 2 shows three possibilities: a linear cyst growth pattern in which dV/dt is constant, a faster-than-linear pattern in which dV/dt is increasing, and an apparently self-limiting growth pattern in which dV/dt gradually decreases to zero.

Because single-nephron GFR, and thus probably $J_{V_{in}}$, is reported to be normal until late in the polycystic kidney disease process, and because J_{V_s} probably remains negligible, these different growth patterns presumably reflect different relative values of the reabsorptive flux, $J_{V_{ab}}$, and the distal outflow, $J_{V_{out}}$. It is interesting to consider the reabsorptive fluxes and outflows in each of the most frequently proposed mechanisms for renal cyst formation, namely, ballooning or blowout, basement membrane defect, and cellular hyperplasia with or without polyp formation.

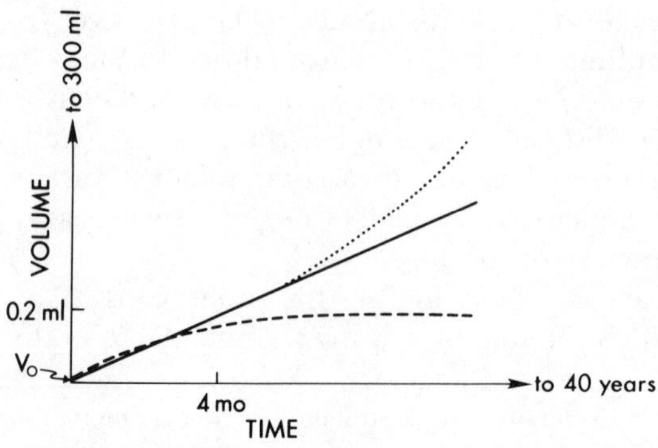

Figure 2. Possible cyst growth patterns.

Table 1. *Linear Cyst Growth*

Cyst volume (ml)	Time *dV/dt*: 5 nl/min	50 nl/min
0.1	14 days	1.4 days
1	140 days	14 days
10	3.8 years	140 days
100	38 years	3.8 years

3. Review of Cyst Models

3.1. Balloon Model

In the balloon theory, partial or complete distal obstruction reduces the $J_{V_{out}}$ such that, in response to continuing proximal filling, $J_{V_{in}}$, there occurs a cystic change analogous to the filling of a stretchable balloon. Historically, it is implied that the cellular and basement membrane mass remains constant and reasonably normal during this dilation process and simply becomes stretched and attenuated to accommodate the increasing surface area of the cyst. In that case, $J_{V_{ab}}$ might conceivably remain constant, and if $J_{V_{out}}$ also were constant though reduced from normal, fairly rapid and linear cyst growth would occur. The mass balance equation then would equal a constant value in the range of 0 to approximately 50 nl/min. The time, t, required to achieve a given cyst volume, V, is given by the equation $t = (V - V_0)/(J_{V_{in}} - J_{V_{out}} + J_{V_s} - J_{V_{ab}})$ in which V_0 is the starting normal volume of about 10^{-5} ml. Listed in Table 1 are representative calculations in which dV/dt has been assigned a reasonable maximum value of 50 nl/min or an arbitrary minimum value of 5 nl/min. It is interesting that the smaller cysts predicted at the earliest times are consistent with those observed experimentally. That is, in rat kidneys made cystic by use of diphenylthiazole, diphenylamine, or nordihydroguaiaretic acid, Carone *et al.* (1974), Gardner *et al.* (1976), and Evan and Gardner (1979) each have reported occasional cysts of 0.2-ml volume at about 35 days and under flow conditions probably not too dissimilar from the 5 nl/min situation. It is possible also that the occasional 100-ml cysts observed in adult polycystic disease may have grown over periods as great as 38 years. However, before this evidence is taken as support for the balloon theory or for the presence of linear growth patterns, additional facts must be considered. First, the larger cysts in the rat models and in human disease are not the general rule but rather are far outnumbered by much smaller cysts. Second, the initial postulate of constant and normally transporting cellular and basement membrane mass in the stretching cyst wall is untenable on geometric grounds. As shown in Table 2, if cell and basement membrane mass did indeed remain constant during cyst growth, the average 7.5-μm cell height and 0.25-μm basement membrane thickness of the parent nephron would become attenuated to 0.25 and 0.01 μm,

Table 2. Attenuation of Constant Cell and Basement Membrane (BM) Mass

Tubule OD (mm)	Cell height (μm)	BM thickness (μm)
0.04	7.5	0.25
1	0.25	0.01
10	0.025	0.001

respectively, in cysts only 1 mm in diameter and to angstrom dimensions in 1-cm cysts. Although some wall thinning is observed in some cystic nephrons, it is not invariable and never is to these predicted extremes, even in very large cysts. Third, Fig. 3 illustrates the relationship between transtubular hydrostatic pressure and the outer diameters of isolated, distally occluded, intact nephron segments or tubule basement membranes from rabbits (Welling and Grantham, 1972). Although all the segments and membranes are seen to be moderately stretchable in the physiologic pressure range of perhaps 5–20 cm H_2O, it is quite apparent that, if the basement membrane is normal in compliance and in quantity, no amount of obstruction or luminal pressure could produce even 1-mm cysts. Finally, if one does not require the maintenance of constant absorptive flux during cyst wall stretching and allows instead a more probably progressive decrease in transport function, zero transport, or even cell death, the result would be, as shown in Fig. 2,

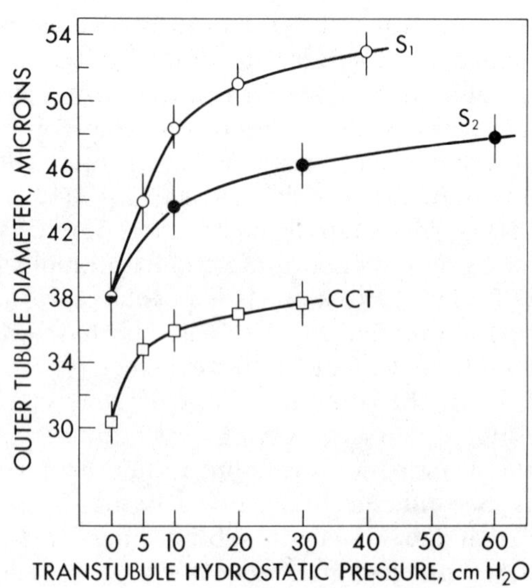

Figure 3. Relationship between transtubular hydrostatic pressure and outer diameters of rabbit proximal S_1 and S_2 segments and cortical collecting tubules (CCT). (Adapted from Welling and Grantham, 1972.)

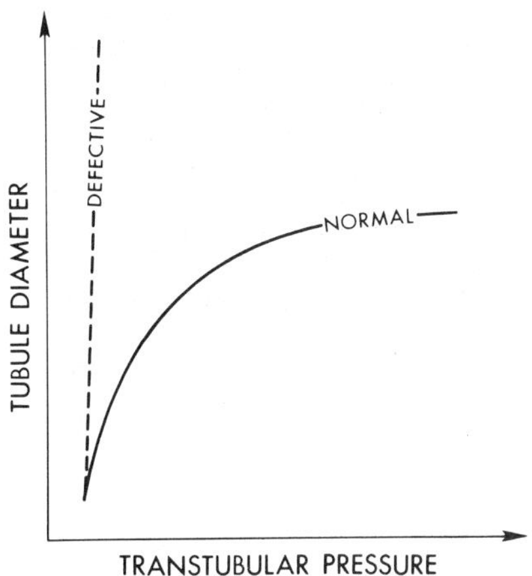

Figure 4. Comparison of compliance curves for normal and hypothetical abnormal tubule basement membrane.

either a faster-than-linear cyst growth pattern or a linear pattern with slope greater than in the original constant flux situation. Then one would predict a larger ratio of large to small cysts and thus a picture even less consistent with the rat model and human disease observations. For all these reasons, our analysis does not support the balloon or blowout theory as presented historically and can accommodate other obstruction theories only if they include the possibility of changing reabsorptive flux and avoid the problems of attenuation and limited tubule distensibility.

3.2. Membrane Defect Model

The second of the most frequently proposed cyst growth mechanisms incorporates a basement membrane defect that might be analogous to the known effects of collagenase on tubule basement membranes. Stated simply, it is proposed that the compliance or stretchability of a presumably defective basement membrane would not decrease with increasing distention as does the normal membrane in Fig. 4. but rather would become effectively infinite (Carone *et al.*, 1974). This in turn would tend to dissipate the proximal to distal pressure gradient in the tubule, decrease the driving force for $J_{V_{out}}$, and allow an accumulation of $J_{V_{in}}$. Large cysts might then develop at normal or even subnormal tubule pressures. It should be noted that the arguments concerning cyst size distribution, cell and basement membrane attenuation, and maintenance of cellular transport capacity used against the balloon model apply here as well. Therefore, unless the membrane defect model is supplemented by the possibility for changing reabsorptive flux and avoidance of attenuation, it cannot be supported by our analysis.

Table 3. Saturation Cyst Growth

$(J_{V_{ab}}/A_0)$ (nl/min · cm)	Volume (diameter)	
	1-cm Cylinders	Spheres
10	3×10^{-4} ml (0.2 mm)	1.4×10^{-3} ml (1.4 mm)
1	3×10^{-2} ml (2 mm)	1.4 ml (14 mm)
0.1	3 ml (20 mm)	1400 ml (140 mm)

3.3. Saturation Filling Model

The third proposed cyst growth mechanism incorporates cellular growth or hyperplasia during cyst growth and proves to be the most interesting for two reasons. First, if the possibility of cellular hyperplasia is added to an obstruction model or to the membrane defect model, both can be made acceptable. Second, concomitant cell growth and cystic dilation can produce the characteristic, self-limiting cyst growth pattern indicated by the lower broken line in Fig. 2, a pattern we shall refer to as saturation filling.

Saturation filling is described by the equation $(J_{V_{in}} - J_{V_{out}} + J_{V_s}) = (J_{V_{ab}}/A_0)A$ and is a situation in which the reabsorption capacity $J_{V_{ab}}$ per unit tubule surface area A_0 is maintained constant and greater than zero during cyst growth and during the enlargment of the cyst wall surface area A. For example, it would occur if growth of absorbing cyst lining cells kept pace with the increasing surface area of the cyst and thereby maintained normal cell spacing and density in a single-layer epithelium. Thus, as the cyst surface area increases so does the total absorptive capacity of the cyst wall. Cyst growth then ceases when that total absorptive capacity comes to equal the algebraic sum of the other volume flows previously available for cyst growth. Using the reference values from Fig. 1, that volume flow would be, maximally, 50 nl/min.

In favor of this viewpoint are the findings of Carone *et al.* (1974), Evan and Gardner (1979), and Cuppage *et al.* (1980) that normal cell size and spacing are indeed found in cyst epithelium. Further support is provided by the sample calculations in Table 3. That is, if saturation filling does occur in human and experimental disease, one might expect to find large populations of cylindrical dilated tubules or spherical cysts of sizes predicted from the reasonable range of absorptive capacities in the left column. It should be noted that the 10 and 1 nl/min·cm absorptive capacities are approximately equivalent to those seen in normal proximal and in distal nephron segments. Although the available observations are few, we do find that the smaller of the calculated cyst sizes are reasonably compatible with the more usual, smaller cysts seen in rat models and human disease and that the larger calculated sizes might correspond to the few larger cysts observed. Further-

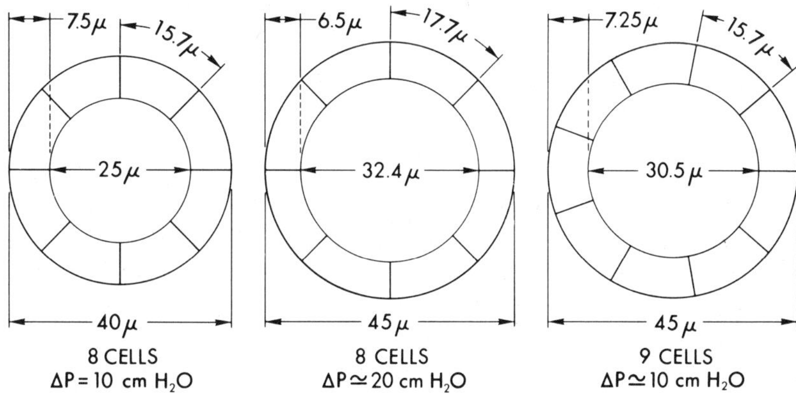

Figure 5. Suggested manner of tubule cell growth induced by tubule dilation.

more, to account for the occasional very large cysts, one can easily accept the possibility of damaged or otherwise poorly functioning cyst epithelium. The calculations using the 0.1 absorption capacity would reflect such a situation. Circumstantial evidence for a poorly functioning epithelium is provided by the several published electron micrographs in which the cyst lining cells are somewhat reduced in height and, more important, lack the complex array of lateral intercellular channels which have been correlated in our laboratory with the cellular capacity for active volume reabsorption (Welling *et al.*, 1978).

4. *Proposed Mechanism*

Having now arrived at our choice of saturation as a reasonable model for cyst growth, two additional points remain for consideration. The first is a reconciliation between the distal obstruction and basement membrane defect models and what might be termed the saturation model. The second is a brief discussion of research procedures that might be used to test the validity of our conclusions.

One overriding consideration in the saturation model is an apparent coordination between cyst growth rate and the rate at which cell growth occurs to maintain an approximately normal reabsorptive capacity per unit surface area. Although the concept of contact inhibition might be involved to assure normal epithelial size and density, one still must find a reasonable initiating stimulus which, in the context of a developing disease state, must presumably be pathologic. We propose two possibilities. First, as illustrated by the difference between the first and the second tubule diagrams in Fig. 5, moderate tubule dilations are possible within the range of physiologic transtubular pressure. Pathologic distal obstruction, possibly by means of the epithelial polyps demonstrated by Evan and Gardner (1979), then could produce moderate cellular stretching and attenuation which, in turn, might trigger cellular hyperplasia sufficient to return cell size to normal, as in the third diagram. Furthermore, if each new cell were allowed to produce its normal allotment of basement membrane, the transtubular pressure could return to normal and thereafter fluctuate between normal and only slight elevation as the cycle is repeated and as the cyst grows and expands progressively. The second possibility is similar to the first but incorporates the basement membrane defect model as proposed by Carone *et al.* (1974). Cellular attenuation and the triggering of hyperplasia then could occur with only trivial elevations of tubular pressure and without the need for significant distal obstruction. Basement membrane attenuation could be prevented if the new cells again were allowed to produce new, but now presumably abnormal, membrane in appropriate quantity.

It should be noted that in both proposed mechanisms the role of transtubular pressure is simply to induce sufficient wall stretching to trigger a single event of cellular hyperplasia. The pressure then could return to normal from which point it might again build up and trigger a second hyperplasia event. Cycles of this type presumably could continue for long periods of time. If the new cells maintain any degree of transport capacity, the cyst eventually would reach a saturation volume at which point no further pressure fluctuations would occur and cyst growth would cease. If the new cells lack or secondarily lose their transport capacity, there would be no saturation volume and cyst growth might continue indefinitely. If a polycystic kidney contained both transporting and nontransporting cysts and if, as supported by the cyst function studies of Gardner (1969) and of Huseman *et al.* (1980), the transporting cysts predominate, one would expect a low ratio of large to small cells, as is in fact observed.

5. *Proposed Experimental Approach*

The conclusions we have reached here have been based on comparisons of predicted events to a very few and often incomplete experimental observations. To continue our approach and to validate our viewpoints, the following experimental procedures will be required. First, to evaluate the possibility of basement membrane defect, attempts should be made to measure the compliance characteristics of cyst walls. Second, it is critically important that we obtain data on cyst growth characteristics and particularly the average, and median sizes and the distribution of sizes of all cysts in samples obtained at numerous time intervals. Third, because of the expected differences between the absorptive capacities of proximal and of distal nephron cysts, careful recording of cyst type must accompany the measurements of cyst growth pattern. Finally, as in the work already begun by Evan and Gardner, careful examination must be made for evidence of cellular hyperplasia and for evidence of obstructive mechanisms.

References

Carone, F. A., Rowland, R. G., Perlman, S. G., and Ganote, C. E., 1974, The pathogenesis of drug-induced renal cystic disease, *Kidney Int.* **5**:411.

Cuppage, F. E., Huseman, R. A., Chapman, A., and Grantham, J. J., 1980, Ultrastructure and function of cysts from human adult polycystic kidneys, *Kidney Int.* **17**:372.

Evan, A. P., and Gardner, K. D., Jr., 1979, Nephron obstruction in nordihydroguaiaretic acid-induced renal cystic disease, *Kidney Int.* **15**:7.

Gardner, K. D., Jr., 1969, Composition of fluid in twelve cysts of a polycystic kidney, *N. Engl. J. Med.* **281**:985.

Gardner, K. D., Jr., Solomon, S., Fitzgerrel, W. W., and Evan, A. P., 1976, Function and structure in the diphenylamine-exposed kidney, *J. Clin. Invest.* **57**:796.

Huseman, R., Grady, A., Welling, D., and Grantham, J., 1980, Macropuncture study of polycystic disease in adult human kidneys, *Kidney Int.* **18**:375.

Welling, D. J., Welling, L. W., and Hill, J. J., 1978, Phenomenological model relating cell shape to water reabsorption in proximal nephron, *Am. J. Physiol.* **234**:F308.

Welling, L. W., and Grantham, J. J., 1972, Physical properties of isolated perfused renal tubules and tubular basement membranes, *J. Clin. Invest.* **51**:1063.

12

Early Polycystic Kidney Disease

Joseph H. Holmes and Patricia Gabow

Over 700 persons either having polycystic kidney disease (PKD) or related to persons having that disease were studied at the University of Colorado Health Science Center for more than 20 years.[1–4] This study was begun in 1960 when it was observed that the ultrasound image of the adult form of PKD was quite distinctive.[4] This distinctive pattern offered a potential for earlier diagnosis of PKD and for more effective family screening without the radiation exposure accompanying the excretory urogram.

The primary goal of the authors was to obtain a clearer picture of the nonazotemic phase of PKD. Not only were the findings useful to facilitate earlier diagnosis, but they also were helpful in genetic counseling of all PKD persons planning to have children. Often PKD is not diagnosed until an affected person has had one or more children. Therefore, if genetic counseling is to be effective, PKD must be diagnosed earlier and family screening must be more effective.

This report presents a number of broad issues which arose from the initial study of this patient group and which could be helpful to the practicing physician/nephrologist for management and treatment of affected persons and their families.

The study group comprised 495 persons having early PKD and their family members. After a positive diagnosis of PKD in a patient, attempts were made to evaluate all other family members. In all persons, blood creatinine was below 3 mg/100 ml.

The protocol, which has been followed with only minor variations throughout the 20-year study period, consisted of a history (including

Joseph H. Holmes • Department of Medicine, University of Colorado School of Medicine, Denver, Colorado 80204. ***Patricia Gabow*** • Department of Medicine, Denver General Hospital, Denver, Colorado 80204. This work was partially supported by Grant HEW RR 0051 to University Colorado CRC, National Foundation Grant 6-105, National Kidney Foundation—Rocky Mountain Chapter, and National Institutes of Health Grant AM 19928. Portions of the data reported herein have previously appeared in ref. 4.

complete questioning about the genitourinary system); a physical examination; and blood sampling for determination of BUN, serum creatinine, uric acid, SGOT, SGPT, and alkaline phosphatase values. Determination of serum sodium and potassium values was included for the last 215 patients seen. Blood calcium and phosphorus determinations were obtained in persons with a history of renal calculi. Hematological studies included hematocrit, hemoglobin, red cell count, white cell count, differential count, red blood cell indices, and platelet counts, which were done on the last 215 patients seen.

Routine urinalysis on a fresh specimen was performed for all patients. In addition, the majority collected 12- (7 P.M. to 7 A.M.) or 24-hr urine specimens for analysis of urea nitrogen, creatinine, uric acid, and, for the last 215 patients, sodium and potassium content also.

Ultrasound examinations were obtained on 451 patients. Intravenous pyelograms were performed in approximately 100 subjects in conjunction with the ultrasound examination.

At least four factors must be considered when classifying cystic disease of the kidney[5–7]: (1) genetic relationship; (2) structural or anatomical aspects; (3) rate of cyst growth; and (4) relation to liver abnormalities (i.e., associated cystic disease or cirrhosis).

In defining the genetic aspects, no method for identifying the gene and assessing its abnormality exists at present. Therefore, in diagnosing the adult form of PKD, a positive genetic history or evidence of polycystic disease in related family members is the most reliable factor.

In 6% of subjects, a positive family history could not be obtained. The accuracy of this figure is difficult to ascertain because of difficulties inherent in obtaining family histories. For example, a patient said to have died of heart disease may have had associated PKD. Consequently, in each patient suspected of having spontaneous mutation (i.e., a negative family history), evaluation of both parents was attempted before a spontaneous mutation was considered.

The advent of new imaging techniques, such as ultrasound, computed tomography (CT), or isotope scanning, has provided a means for more precise definitions and classifications. Study of the rate of cyst growth suggests that when there is no change in the cystic pattern for more than 15 years, the cystic disease may not be genetic in origin because continued cyst growth is assumed to be a characteristic of the adult form of PKD. Finally, if concomitant liver cysts are present, the diagnostic chance of the disease being the adult form of PKD is increased significantly. The literature reports that liver cysts are present in 28–50% of patients with adult PKD.[6,8] This emphasizes the need to examine the liver for cysts in all persons suspected of having PKD.

The diagnosis of PKD was based on one or more of the following criteria: a positive excretory urogram, a positive ultrasound, or direct observation of renal cysts at surgery. CT, isotopic studies, or angiogram were not done routinely in the series but were used only to confirm other studies.

The population was classified as having no evidence of PKD, suspicious for presence of PKD, or definite PKD. The 451 subjects with ultrasound data were classified as follows: without PKD if no cysts were detected; suspicious for PKD if less than a total of five cysts were detectable in both kidneys or cysts were present in only one kidney; definite PKD if cysts were detectable in both kidneys and totaled five or more.

Eighty-one cases were diagnosed as suspicious for PKD. However, experience suggests that this group probably will evolve into two populations: (1) those who develop clear-cut PKD with more and larger cysts; and (2) those in whom the cyst pattern remains unchanged over a period of years. In five patients in the suspicious group, the ultrasound pattern of two or three cysts has remained unchanged over at least 15 years. This means that any patient in the suspicious group must be followed periodically until a final decision can be made.

The PKD group was compared with the 254 uninvolved family members, and any significant difference between the two groups was considered a characteristic of the adult form of PKD. Such comparisons may not take into account unrecognized physical differences between involved families and a corresponding normal group. However, members of PKD families offer an environmental and genetic (unrelated to renal cyst growth) control.

The clinical symptoms that occurred with greater frequency in the positive PKD group were nausea, headache, hematuria, hypertension, infections, back pain, and renal calculi. The physical examination findings occurring with greater frequency in the PKD group were hypertension, systolic murmur, abnormal fundoscopic examination, palpable liver, and peripheral edema.

Hypertension (62%) was of particular interest because it was frequently the presenting symptom, usually discovered during routine physical examination. A blood pressure of greater than 150/90 mm Hg was considered to represent hypertension. The diagnosis of hypertension was based on the history, medical records, and/or measurements during physical examination. In the PKD group, the average age of diagnosis of hypertension was 33 years. Hypertension often was diagnosed before there was overt evidence of cystic disease or of renal enlargement.

The hypertension did not relate to the levels of BUN or serum creatinine. Blood uric acid levels were higher in the PKD group with hypertension. In any unexplained case of hypertension, family history was and should be checked for the possibility of PKD.

Back pain, though present in more than 61% of those having a positive PKD diagnosis, was a difficult symptom to evaluate. In most instances the patient tended to relate the back pain to lifting, unusual work, strain, or trauma. Back pain did not bring the patient in for his initial PKD diagnostic workup. The location of relevant pain varied and could be in the groin, in midabdomen just to the left of the umbilicus, in the lumbar region, or in the flank.

Nineteen percent of the PKD group complained of headaches. Headaches did not correlate significantly with the presence of hypertension.

A few persons in this series with PKD noted intraabdominal pressure, belching, difficulty in eating because of a "full" feeling, constipation or diarrhea, and palpable abdominal masses. Most of the symptoms were vague, but might be explicable on the basis of increased intraabdominal mass. In each of these persons, the serum creatinine concentration was less than 3 mg/100 ml.

In the PKD patients, the most significant findings on physical examination were a higher incidence of palpable kidneys, palpable liver, and abdominal tenderness. A palpable left kidney was noted in 51.2%, a palpable right kidney in 49.4%. Upper abdominal tenderness was present in 19%.

Three other findings were of interest. (1) Abnormal funduscopic changes were noted in 22% of the PKD and correlated with hypertension. (2) It is interesting that a systolic murmur was present in 10.5% of the positive group and did not correlate with hypertension. (3) Edema was noted in 9.3% of the PKD group. The physical findings that appear to be the most significant for early diagnosis are hypertension, palpable kidneys, and palpable liver.

Laboratory tests did not prove very helpful in diagnosis of early PKD. Routine urinalyses done at a time when patients were symptom-free also were not discriminating since abnormal urinalyses occurred with a high frequency in subjects considered to be unaffected family members. Single determinations of serum creatinine and BUN were not useful since most fell within the hospital laboratory's normal range. Blood urea and serum creatinine determinations were most useful in detecting progressive depression of renal function with time. Liver function tests were within normal limits in all groups. These tests were similar in those patients who had hepatic cysts and in those with no hepatic cysts.

Hematuria, occurred in 31% of patients with PKD according to history, is a distinctive symptom, and demands further renal workup. When cystoscope examination was negative, PKD was the most likely diagnosis. In managing hematuria in patients with PKD, the physician should follow a conservative program. Surgery is not indicated except for extreme emergencies. Interestingly, a greater incidence of hematuria was found in PKD patients with hypertension than in those with no hypertension.

Since urinary cultures were done only rarely, the diagnosis of genitourinary or "bladder" infection was made when the referring physician had told the patient that an acute episode of dysuria, hematuria, fever, and back pain that disappeared with antibiotic therapy was a "bladder infection." Only a third of the PKD group had a history of infection. In PKD patients who developed recurrent infections, it was appropriate to treat them vigorously and to follow them periodically. If the infection occured in a cyst, antibiotic therapy was continued for a longer period of time. Vigorous treatment and careful follow-up may prevent future renal damage.

Over the past 20 years, three new imaging techniques have altered significantly the diagnostic approach to PKD. The three techniques are ultrasound, CT scanning, and isotopes scanning.[8–12]

Ultrasonography was more sensitive than excretory urography in detecting PKD and in subjects suspicious for PKD. Routine excretory urograms appeared normal in 5 of 39 subjects with definite PKD diagnosed by ultrasonography. Excretory urography was suspicious in an additional six subjects. Excretory urography with nephrotomography was normal in 2 of 16 subjects and suspicious in an additional subject evaluated with this radiological technique. One subject had a normal ultrasonogram and excretory urogram, but an abnormal arteriogram consistent with PKD.

CT, although effective in demonstrating cysts, has been used most often in this study to determine presence of complications such as cyst hemorrhage or cyst obstruction. CT has not proven useful for screening family members.[11] The problems associated with CT evaluation include patient preparation, contrast administration, radiation exposure, and the difficulties in examination of young children without anesthesia.

Ultrasound has made it possible to achieve an earlier diagnosis of PKD.[1–3,11,12] Its major advantages include noninvasiveness and the ability to demonstrate cysts in both liver and kidney, during the same examination. Recent articles have suggested that ultrasound should be the imaging method of first choice whenever PKD is suspected.[8,9,11,12]

In addition, ultrasound can demonstrate pancreatic and ovarian cysts and cysts in the fetal kidney. This series includes four fetal cystic kidneys demonstrated by ultrasound.

Liver cysts were demonstrated in 38% of the PKD subjects, a figure approximating those in the literature (range 36 to 50%).[6,8] It is likely that as ultrasonic techniques improve, liver cysts will be detected in a higher percentage of PKD patients. Liver cysts have been observed in persons in good health who have no family history of PKD. This might correspond to the presence of one or two renal cysts in individuals in normal populations, especially in many of the older age groups.

The younger age group (under 18) always has presented a difficult diagnostic problem in classification of cystic disease of the kidney.[13] This group can be subdivided into several categories: (1) early appearance of cysts in subjects less than 18 years old with a definite family history of adult PKD; (2) those classified as suspicious, that is, five or fewer cysts; (3) multicystic kidney defined as cysts in only one kidney; (4) infantile PKD; (5) persons referred as having PKD later diagnosed as tuberous sclerosis; and (6) renal cystic disease and portal cirrhosis. Children referred to the University of Colorado group as PKD have had evaluations which reveal this spectrum of diagnoses.

In those with adult PKD, early cyst growth sufficient for diagnosis occurs in about 8.5% before age 18. This finding is in contrast to a general belief that cysts in this disease are not detected until age 20 or 30. An additional

20% were classified as suspicious. In this group it is worthwhile to reexamine the child every 6 months to determine whether more cysts develop or to demonstrate a stable cyst pattern over successive years.

The multicystic group all had a unilateral abdominal mass discovered at birth or shortly thereafter. Surgery was done in five of the six patients, and the cystic kidney was removed since the other kidney was declared normal at surgery. There was no positive family history of PKD. The term "multicystic" as defined by most internists and urologists is restricted to kidneys enlarged unilaterally by cyst growth.[7,14] It is recommended that those patients diagnosed as having multicystic disease shortly after birth be followed conservatively and that greater restraint be exercised in performing surgery.

The diagnosis of infantile PKD often is made by the pathologist. However, there may also be a distinctive X-ray image pattern. When PKD is found in three members of the same generation (as observed in one of the families) one should question whether the diagnosis of infantile PKD is correct.

Two other cases of cystic disease occurred in the under-18 group. One was diagnosed eventually as tuberous sclerosis and the other had renal cystic disease with associated portal cirrhosis. Tuberous sclerosis is occasionally diagnosed as PKD, especially in the younger patient, before other diagnostic characteristics of this disease appear.

With the use of ultrasound, the presence of the cysts in the fetal kidney before birth can be discovered. In three of the four cases discovered *in utero*, there was a family history of the adult form of PKD. All four cases had echo patterns of cystic disease that differed significantly from the pattern of infantile PKD.

Because there are no data to indicate when these children might develop serious uremia, the screening routine has been changed, and young family members are checked with ultrasound in the first decade. If the result is negative, they need not be checked until later, perhaps in their twenties.

One of the most common questions asked by at risk individuals is "What is the likelihood that I have PKD?" At the present time, little more can be offered than an explanation of autosomal dominant inheritance. In trying to detect early PKD in at-risk family members, a history of previous hematuria or hypertension may be helpful although these occur commonly in subjects considered negative. During the physical examination, careful attention should be given to blood pressure and to examination of abdomen. Careful palpation of kidneys and liver should be done. If a systolic murmur or edema is present, further diagnostic evaluation should be carried out. Laboratory studies on a single visit were not helpful in diagnosing or evaluating PKD, but for progressive changes over a period of time, they are clearly useful.

If five or fewer cysts are detected in a person under age 30, it is impossible to make a positive diagnosis on a single visit. Consequently, these patients must be followed, and only when additional cysts appear on subsequent visits can the diagnosis be established. Early in this study it was assumed that whenever two or three cysts were noted in a family member, that person would develop PKD, but this has not always been the case. More difficult diagnostically is the discovery of the first cyst after age 50, when one or two cysts may appear even in normal persons with no history of PKD. Long-term follow-up on this subset of patients is critical in order to develop a predictive index for subjects at risk.

As a result of this study, a logical routine checkup for family members at risk has been devised. It was found that cysts grow slowly in most patients and that an evaluation every 2 or 3 years is probably sufficient. All patients who are planning a family should be checked at that time.

Another question commonly asked by those who have PKD is "When will I require dialysis or renal transplantation and how long can I lead a useful working life? I want to make plans for my family or decide whether to have children or adopt a child." Sufficient longitudinal data have not been obtained on the group with uremia to predict the prognosis on any specific PKD patient. Furthermore, rate of cyst growth may vary considerably.(15) For example, one patient in this series had no evidence of cysts at the age of 17, yet at the age of 18½ had multiple cysts in both kidneys. In contrast, an 82-year-old woman with 55-g cystic kidneys died of pneumonia with a BUN in the normal range.

Patients frequently ask: "Can I alter the course of the disease by a special diet, drinking more fluids, being more active, or by special exercises?" No data regarding such measures have been accumulated in this disorder.

One question often asked by younger subjects is whether they should participate in contact sports. When cysts are large, especially when they occur in the younger age group participating in contact sports like football, there may be merit to a restriction. On the other hand, if cysts are small, perhaps restriction may not be necessary. Three patients in this series suffered complications associated with trauma to the kidney area.

Other important questions are how vigorously the hypertension should be treated in patients with PKD, and how many die of cardiovascular complications. Family histories often reveal a cardiac cause of death in a previous generation. Although the hypertension in PKD may not be severe, proper antihypertensive treatment in these patients is appropriate. However, no longitudinal study has demonstrated the impact of antihypertensive therapy on the natural history of the disease.

Physicians have wondered whether PKD is a disease manifested only by multiple cyst growth in the kidney or whether it represents a systemic disease in which cyst growth in the kidney is only one manifestation. The high incidence of cyst growth in the liver and pancreas in persons with PKD supports the latter concept.(6)

Further evaluation will be needed to assess the pathogenesis of this disease, particularly in relationship to its possible systemic nature.

References

1. Lufkin EG, Alfrey AC, Trucksess ME, Holmes JH: Polycystic kidney disease: Earlier diagnosis using ultrasound. *Urology* 4:5–12, 1974.
2. Holmes JH: Polycystic kidney disease, in: Watanabe, Holmes, Holm, and Goldberg (eds): *Diagnostic Ultrasound in Urology and Nephrology*. Tokyo, Igaku-Shoin, 1981, p 39.
3. Holmes JH: Early application of ultrasound in study of kidney and bladder, in: Watanabe, Holmes, Holm, and Goldberg (eds): *Diagnostic Ultrasound in Urology and Nephrology*. Tokyo, Igaku-Shoin, 1981.
4. Gabow PA, Ikle DW, Holmes JH: Polycystic kidney disease: Prospective analysis of non-azotemic patients and family members. *Ann Intern Med*, 101:238–247, 1984.
5. Grantham JJ: Polycystic renal disease, in: Early LE, Gottschalk CW (eds): *Diseases of the Kidney*. Boston, Little Borwn. 1979, pp 1123–1126.
6. Dalgaard O: Bilateral polycystic disease of the kidney. *Acta Med Scand* (Suppl 328):17–218, 1957.
7. Bernstein J: A classification of renal cyst in cystic disease of the kidney, in: Gardner KD, Jr (ed): *Disease of the Kidney*. New York, Wiley, 1976.
8. Rosenfeld AT, Curtis AM, Putnam CE: Gray scale ultrasonography, computerized tomography, and evaluation of polycystic kidney and liver disease. *Urology* 9:436–438, 1977.
9. Lawson TL, McClennan BL, Shirkhoda A: Adult polycystic kidney disease: Ultrasonographic and compound tomographic appearance. *J Clin Ultrasound* 6:297–302, 1978.
10. Rosenfeld AT, Glickman MG, Hodson J: *Diagnostic Imaging in Renal Disease*. New York, Appleton Century and Crofts, 1979, pp 42–45.
11. Rosenfeld AT, Birdcage AW, Wolf B, *et al*: Ultrasound in the presymptomatic diagnosis of adult dominant polycystic kidney disease, in: White D (ed): *Ultrasound in Medicine*. New York, Plenum Press, 1977, p 143.
12. Kelsey JA, Louey JD: Gray scale ultrasonography in the diagnosis of polycystic kidney disease. *Radiology* 122:791, 1977.
13. Bengtsson J, Hedman L, Svalander C: Adult type of polycystic disease in newborn child. *Acta Med Scand* 197:447–450, 1975.
14. Ambrose SS: Unilateral, mylticystic renal disease in adults. *Birth Defects* 13:349–353, 1979.
15. Trebbin WM, Newhouse JH, Whitmore E: Polycystic kidneys without radiologic enlargement. *Urology* 11:96–98, 1970.

II

RECENT ADVANCES ON SOME COMPLICATIONS OF CHRONIC RENAL FAILURE

Renal Osteodystrophy, Vitamin D Analogues, Parathormone

13

An Overview of Recent Advances in Mineral Metabolism

Saulo Klahr, Eduardo Slatopolsky, and Kevin Martin

1. Introduction

The last decade witnessed a dramatic expansion of knowledge, both fundamental and clinical, about the metabolism of calcium and phosphorus, and about the regulation of bone structure and function in health and disease. Calcium and phosphorus are essential components of the skeleton, which regulate or modulate many biochemical and transport processes. Cystosolic and extracellular fluid concentrations of ionic calcium are maintained within narrow limits despite wide fluctuation in calcium intake. The circulating levels of phosphorus are controlled by many of the same factors responsible for regulating calcium metabolism, though to a less stringent degree.

The regulation of mineral metabolism may be viewed as a coordinated multicomponent system including organs that are directly involved in mineral translocation—the intestine, the bone, and the kidney—and the principal hormones that control these translocations—parathyroid hormone, calcitonin, and vitamin D metabolites. These hormones aid in controlling both the quantity and quality of the skeleton. Chronic progressive renal disease brings about a series of perturbations and distortions in the control systems responsible for mineral homeostasis. Basic advances in the understanding of the synthesis and metabolism of parathyroid hormone, vitamin D, calcium, and phosphorus in health have led to substantial progress in delineating the alterations in bone and the derangements in mineral metabolism brought about by renal disease. These, in turn, have led to significant clinical advances and to a more rational approach to treatment or prevention of these problems.

Saulo Klahr, Eduardo Slatopolsky, and Kevin Martin • Renal Division, Department of Medicine, Washington University School of Medicine, St. Louis, Missouri 63110. Supported by USPHS NIAMDD Grants AM-09976 and AM-07126.

It is impossible within the context of this overview to describe the many advances that have occurred in recent years in understanding of mineral metabolism and its regulation. For an excellent and more comprehensive discussion of the subject, the reader should consult recent texts[1,2] and reviews.[3–8] This overview will be limited to discussion of some topics of current interest in the area of parathyroid hormone and of vitamin D metabolism and their interrelationships.

2. *Parathyroid Hormone*

Parathyroid hormone, an 84-amino-acid peptide, is synthesized in the parathyroid glands from proparathyroid hormone (90 amino acids) and preproparathyroid hormone (115 amino acids).[9] Parathyroid hormone secretion is inhibited by an increase and stimulated by a decrease in serum calcium. This feedback system of regulation involving the parathyroid glands is one of the most important homeostatic mechanisms for the close control of the concentration of calcium in extracellular fluid. Parathyroid hormone is elaborated in response to hypocalcemia, other ionic perturbations, and a variety of humoral stimuli, most notably beta-adrenergic stimulation.[10,11] Its principal effect is to raise circulating levels of ionized calcium by promoting bone resorption, renal tubular calcium reabsorption, and the renal conversion of 25-hydroxy D_3 to 1-α-25-dihydroxy D_3, a potent stimulator of intestinal calcium absorption. In addition, parathyroid hormone promotes the renal excretion of phosphate, an effect that tends to raise serum calcium. The effects of the hormone at the level of kidney and bone seem to be mediated via cyclic AMP.[12]

Substantial evidence also has accumulated which indicates that the release of parathyroid hormone is mediated also by cyclic AMP. The evidence for a role of cyclic AMP in the secretion of parathyroid hormone is derived from several observations: (1) the presence of adenylate cyclase activity in parathyroid tissue; (2) the ability of dibutyryl cyclic AMP, and theophylline, to stimulate hormone secretion; (3) the correlation between *in vitro* cyclic AMP production and hormone release; and (4) the fact that many parathyroid hormone secretagogues (a) stimulate cyclic AMP formation in parathyroid cells and (b) have effects on cyclic AMP and parathyroid hormone secretion that are similar in time course, kinetic characteristics, and dose-response relationships.[13–15] Hypocalcemia, probably due to retention of phosphate and/or to decreased synthesis of 1,25-dihydroxy D_3 by the diseased kidney, is probably the major cause of increased secretion of parathyroid hormone in uremia. The possible contribution of other stimuli (increased beta-adrenergic activity, release of prostaglandins or secretin), which have been shown to augment parathyroid hormone secretion, to the increased release of the hormone observed in uremia has not been adequately explored. However, published data suggest, although not convincingly, that administration of propranolol, a beta-adrenergic blocker, can decrease the levels of parathyroid hormone in uremic subjects.[16] This observation raises the possibility that increased beta-adrenergic activity may be involved, partially in the increased secretion of parathyroid hormone observed in chronic renal disease.

In addition to changes in calcium concentration, it has been postulated that the levels of circulating vitamin D metabolites may play a role in the regulation of parathyroid hormone release. The finding of specific binding sites for vitamin D metabolites within the parathyroid glands has led to the suggestion that these metabolites exert a direct effect on the parathyroid gland which is independent of the levels of serum calcium.[17] Canterbury *et al.*[18] have shown that intravenous administration of 24,25-dihydroxy D_3 in the dog produces an acute suppression of parathyroid hormone (PTH) release in the absence of changes in extracellular fluid calcium. In addition, this same group has found that oral administration of 24,25-dihydroxy D_3 to dogs with chronic renal insufficiency and secondary hyperparathyroidism leads to a progressive decrease in the levels of circulating immunoreactive PTH even in the absence of changes in ionized or total serum calcium.[19] These results suggest a direct effect of some of the vitamin D metabolites on PTH release. It is possible that alterations in the levels of some of these vitamin D metabolites in uremia may be responsible in part for the increased secretion of PTH in patients with chronic renal disease. However, at present the evidence for a direct effect of the vitamin D metabolites on the secretion of PTH is controversial since the results reported by some investigators have not been confirmed by others, and contradictory data have also been reported. Data from our own laboratory indicate that administration of 1,25-dihydroxy D_3 to uremic patients leads to a decrease in the levels of circulating parathyroid hormone only when an elevation in serum calcium occurs. When 1,25-dihydroxy D_3 is administered to uremic subjects but serum calcium levels are not allowed to increase, there is no detectable decrease in the levels of circulating immunoreactive PTH even after 6 months of administration of the D metabolite.

Recent studies have reinvestigated the mechanisms underlying the inability of elevations in serum calcium to turn off PTH secretion in uremic subjects. It has been postulated that the increase in mass (hypertrophy) of the parathyroid glands in chronic renal disease underlies the unresponsiveness of the glands to the normal stimuli capable of "turning off" hormonal secretion. Previous studies in animals with normal parathyroid glands have suggested that a basal secretion of PTH ("calcium unresponsive") may persist even in the presence of marked hypercalcemia. If glandular mass is enlarged, there will be an increase in the basal rate of PTH secretion which may be independent of calcium control and may be sufficient to maintain elevated levels of the hormone even in the presence of hypercalcemia. This will, therefore, mimic the lack of suppression of glandular secretion by an appropriate stimulus (hypercalcemia). On the other hand, it is possible that a "true defect" of the hypertrophic parathyroid glands in uremia may lead to an altered response to the signals that normally "shut off" the secretion of PTH. In an attempt to explore this possibility we have examined the kinetic behavior of the adenylate cyclase (the enzyme responsible for cyclic AMP generation and the release of parathyroid hormone) in membranes obtained from glands of normal animals or animals with experimental renal disease and from glands of normal or uremic individuals.[20] These studies indicate that the kinetic characteristics of the adenylate cyclase from hypertrophic glands are markedly different from those observed in normal glands. Maximal activation of the adenylate cyclase requires lower concentrations of Mg^{2+} in membranes obtained from hypertrophic than in normal glands. This change in the magnesium concentration required for the activation of the adenylate cyclase of hypertrophic glands is reversed by the addition of guanosine triphosphate (GTP) or its analogues to the incubation media. In addition, a similar degree of suppression of adenylate cyclase activity by external calcium requires a greater concentration of the cation in hypertrophic glands than in normal glands. These observations suggest that in addition to an increase in glandular mass, an intrinsic defect in the kinetics of the regulatory enzyme responsible for PTH secretion may underlie the lack of suppression of PTH release in patients with secondary hyperparathyroidism.

It has also become evident in recent years that most of the increased levels of serum immunoreactive PTH observed in uremic subjects is due to accumulation of carboxy terminal fragments of the hormone. Although the gland is capable of secreting both the intact hormone and fragments, a process that may be influenced both quantitatively and qualitatively by the concentrations of serum calcium, it is also clear that peripheral metabolism of the intact hormone contributes to the heterogeneous nature of circulating immunoreactive PTH.[21] Since the major site of catabolism of carboxy terminal PTH fragments is the kidney, via glomerular filtration rate (GFR), a progressive decrease in GFR as it occurs in chronic renal disease will result in accumulation of carboxy terminal fragments. Hence, the markedly elevated levels of PTH seen in chronic renal disease result from a combination of increased secretion of the hormone plus decreased degradation. Several investigators have postulated that these markedly increased levels of circulating immunoreactive PTH may play a role in some of the manifestations of the uremic syndrome. There is no question that elevated levels of PTH contribute to the bone disease and to the electroencephalographic abnormalities seen in many patients with chronic renal disease, but no clear and convincing evidence has been provided for a role of PTH in causing some of the other manifestations of uremia that have been attributed to the hormone (e.g., anemia, carbohydrate intolerance, hyperlipidemia).[22]

It is also clear that the peripheral metabolism of PTH[21] seems to be somewhat selective since certain organs are capable of extracting exclusively intact hormone (liver) and others only the amino terminal fragment (bone), whereas other organs, mainly the kidney, are capable of extracting from blood the intact hormone and both carboxy and amino terminal fragments. In addition, the peripheral metabolism of parathyroid hormone may be

Table 1. Potential Sites at Which Calcium May Influence Calcium Homeostasis

1. The intraglandular synthesis of PTH
2. The rate of release of PTH from the glands
3. The proportion of intact PTH vs. PTH fragments released from the glands
4. The rate of peripheral conversion of intact PTH to fragments in liver and kidney
5. The effects of PTH or its fragments on target organs (bone, kidney)

controlled by the levels of serum calcium since experimental evidence indicates that calcium levels modify the rate of formation of PTH fragments in both liver and kidney.[23,24] The peripheral formation of PTH fragments may be necessary for the expression of the calcemic effect of the hormone. In adult perfused bone, extraction of immunoreactive PTH and a cyclic AMP response can be demonstrated only when the 1-34 biologically active fragment is used, but not when the 1-84 intact hormone is utilized for perfusion. Hence, conversion of the 1-84 intact hormone to fragments may be necessary for the calcemic effect of the hormone. It is also evident that calcium levels may control the physiologic response to the synthetic 1-34 fragment of PTH at the level of both kidney and bone. Hence, calcium levels may exert regulation at multiple sites in the series of events that start with the synthesis of PTH and end with an effect of the hormone at the level of its target organs (see Table 1).

The greater understanding of the mechanisms that control PTH secretion has led to the search for potential means of achieving "medical parathyroidectomy." Certainly, elevations of serum calcium by dietary means or by the use of vitamin D metabolites will, in most instances, decrease the levels of circulating PTH. The demonstration by Canterbury *et al.*[19] that 24,25-dihydroxy D_3 is capable of decreasing circulating levels of PTH in uremic dogs in the absence of elevations of serum calcium suggests that this agent may be of use. The observations of Caro *et al.*[16] suggest that propranolol may be effective in decreasing PTH levels in uremia. In addition, Bourgoignie *et al.*[25] have shown that cimetidine is capable of decreasing the levels of immunoreactive PTH in uremic subjects and animals with experimental renal disease and hyperparathyroidism. Others, however, have not been able to reproduce these results.[26]Severe hypomagnesemia[27] as well as hypermagnesemia[28] of certain degree have also been shown to suppress PTH release.

3. Vitamin D

Substantial evidence has accumulated for a role of the kidney in the conversion of 25-hydroxy D_3, a metabolite formed in the liver by hydroxylation of vitamin D at the 25 position, into 1,25-dihydroxy D_3. Although the measured plasma levels of 1,25-dihydroxy D_3 are normal in patients with chronic renal disease at GFR values above 30 ml/min, a marked decrease in the circulating levels of this vitamin D_3 metabolite are seen in patients with glomerular filtration rates below 25 ml/min.[29] In the presence of decreased renal mass the normal circulating levels of 1,25-dihydroxy D_3 at GFR values of 30 ml/min or above may indicate an increased conversion of $25(OH)D_3$ to $1,25(OH)_2D_3$ per unit of remaining renal mass. This adaptation may be due in part to increased levels of circulating PTH. The fact that a continuous and progressive renal adaptation in $1,25(OH)_2D_3$ production does not occur at GFR values below 25 ml/min may relate to the fact that at this level of GFR the external balance of phosphate is not maintained. At GFR values below 25 ml/min phosphate retention occurs when dietary phosphate intake is not restricted. Since phosphate has been shown to play a key role in the conversion of $25(OH)D_3$ to $1,25(OH)_2D_3$, it is possible that the development of hyperphosphatemia [which will decrease the conversion of $25(OH)D_3$ to $1,25(OH)_2D_3$] is responsible for the lack of a further increase in the renal conversion per unit mass of $25(OH)D_3$ to $1,25(OH)_2D_3$ as renal mass decreases. This may then explain the decrease in the levels of circulating 1,25-dihydroxy D_3 at GFR values of 25 ml/min or below.

It has also become evident in recent years that patients without progressive renal insufficiency but with the nephrotic syndrome may develop bone disease.[30] The sequence of events leading to bone disease in these patients seems to be influenced by the degree of proteinuria and hence the quantitative urinary losses of vitamin D-binding protein. Patients with the nephrotic syndrome have been found to have profoundly decreased levels of 25-hydroxy D_3 and some decrease in 1,25-dihydroxy D_3 levels. However, the major decrease is in the levels of 25-hydroxy D_3, a metabolite whose plasma concentrations are usually normal in patients with end-stage renal disease. The metabolite [$25(OH)D_3$] usually is decreased in states in which the major component of histological bone disease is osteomalacia. The decreased levels of circulating 25-hydroxy D_3 in the nephrotic syndrome may lead to a decreased total and ionized serum calcium and subsequently to elevated levels of immunoreactive PTH. Consequently, the bone disease will be characterized not only by the histological manifestations of osteomalacia but also by those of hyperparathyroidism. It is not known at present whether patients who have had marked proteinuria during the natural history of their renal disease and subsequently develop progressive renal insufficiency have a greater histological component of osteomalacia on bone biopsy when compared to patients who were nonproteinuric during the evolution of their progressive renal disease.

4. Bone

Of recent interest in terms of bone metabolism is the isolation and characterization by Price *et al.*[31–34] of a new bone protein, bone-gla-protein

(BGP). BGP is a 49-amino-acid chain, molecular weight 5800, which contains three residues of the vitamin K-dependent amino acid, gamma-carboxyglutamic acid. This protein is the most abundant noncollagenous protein of mammalian bone and is principally located in the bone extracellular matrix. *In vitro* studies have demonstrated that BGP is probably bound to hydroxyapatite in bone via the association between the carboxyglutamate side chains and the mineral surface. BGP is synthesized in cortical and cancellous bone cultures of calf and is fully gamma-carboxylated and synthesized at a rate of about 1 BGP molecule per molecule of tropocollagen. Although the bone cells that synthesize this protein have not been identified directly, the presence of 4-hydroxy proline at position 9 in the calf BGP sequence indicates that the protein has been modified by prolyl-hydroxylase, an enzyme found in osteoblasts. This indirect evidence suggests that BGP may be synthesized by osteoblasts. A radioimmunoassay against BGP has been recently developed, and it has been reported that BGP can be detected in increased amounts in the blood of individuals with different metabolic bone diseases. Additional work in this area may provide evidence for BGP levels in blood as a new and useful marker of bone disease, particularly of increased bone resorption. Preliminary evidence indicates that the levels of BGP are markedly elevated in the serum of uremic patients. Whether these increased levels are exclusively the result of increased bone resorption or due to a combination of increased bone resorption and decreased excretion of BGP by the kidney remains to be established. BGP may be a better marker of bone disease than alkaline phosphatase since it is not elevated in diseases of organs (i.e., liver) other than bone.

ACKNOWLEDGMENT. The authors would like to thank Mrs. Patricia Verplancke for her help in the preparation of this manuscript.

References

1. Rasmussen H, Bordier, P: *The Physiological and Cellular Basis of Metabolic Bone Disease.* Baltimore, Williams & Wilkins, 1974.
2. Avioli LV, Krane SM (eds): *Metabolic Bone Disease*, Volumes I and II. New York, Academic Press, 1977, 1978.
3. Parfitt AM: The actions of parathyroid hormone on bone: Relation to bone remodeling and turnover, calcium homeostasis, and metabolic bone diseases. I. Mechanisms of calcium transfer between blood and bone and their cellular basis: Morphological and kinetic approaches to bone turnover. *Metabolism* 25:809–844, 1976.
4. Parfitt AM: The actions of parathyroid hormone on bone: Relation to bone remodeling and turnover, calcium homeostasis, and metabolic bone diseases. II. PTH and bone cells; bone turnover and plasma calcium regulation. *Metabolism* 25:909–955, 1976.
5. Parfitt AM: The actions of parathyroid hormone on bone: Relation to bone remodeling and turnover, calcium homeostasis, and metabolic bone diseases. III. PTH and osteoblasts, the relationship between bone turnover and bone loss, and the state of bones in primary hyperparathyroidism. *Metabolism* 25:1033–1069, 1976.
6. Parfitt AM: The actions of parathyroid hormone on bone: Relation to bone remodeling and turnover, calcium homeostasis, and metabolic bone diseases. IV. The state of bones

in uremic hyperparathyroidism—the mechanisms of skeletal resistance to PTH in renal failure and pseudohypoparathyroidism and the role of PTH in osteoporosis, osteopetrosis and osteofluorosis. *Metabolism* 25:1157–1188, 1976.

7. DeLuca HF, Schnoes HK: Metabolism and mechanism of action of vitamin D. *Annu Rev Biochem* 45:631–666, 1976.
8. Hausler MR, McCain TA: Basic and clinical concepts related to vitamin D metabolism and action. *N Engl J Med* 297:974–983, 1977.
9. Habener JF, Potts JT; Parathyroid physiology and primary hyperparathyroidism, in Avioli LV, Krane SM (eds): *Metabolic Bone Disease*, Volume II. New York, Academic Press, 1978, pp. 1–147.
10. Kukreja SC, Hargis GK, Bowser EN, Henderson WJ, Fisherman EW, Williams GA: Role of adrenergic stimuli in parathyroid hormone secretion in man. *J Clin Endocrinol Metab* 40:478–478, 1975.
11. Brown EM, Hurwitz S, Aurbach DG: Beta-adrenergic stimulation of cyclic AMP content and parathyroid hormone release from isolated bovine parathyroid cells. *Endocrinology* 100:1696–1702, 1977.
12. Peck WA, Klahr S: Cyclic nucleotides in bone and mineral metabolism, in Greengard P, Robison GA (eds): *Advances in Cyclic Nucleotide Research*, Volume 11. New York, Raven Press, 1979, pp. 89–130.
13. Brown EM, Carroll RJ, Aurbach GD: Dopaminergic stimulation of cyclic AMP accumulation and parathyroid hormone release from dispersed bovine parathyroid cells. *Proc Natl Acad Sci USA* 74:4210–4213, 1977.
14. Gardner DE, Brown EM, Windeck K, Aurbach GD: Prostaglandin E_2 stimulation of adenosine 3′,5′-monophosphate accumulation and parathyroid hormone release in dispersed bovine parathyroid cells. *Endocrinology* 103:577–582, 1978.
15. Brown EM, Gardner DG, Windeck RA, Aurbach GD: Cholera toxin stimulates 3′,5′-adenosine monophosphate accumulation and parathyroid hormone release from dispersed bovine parathyroid cells. *Endocrinology* 104:218–225, 1979.
16. Caro JF, Burke JF, Besarab A, Glennon JA: A possible role for propranolol in the treatment of renal osteodystrophy. *Lancet* 2:451, 1978.
17. Golden P, Mazey R, Greenwalt A, Martin K, Slatopolsky E: Vitamin D: A direct effect on the parathyroid gland? *J Min Electr Metabol* 2:1–6, 1979 (editorial).
18. Canterbury JM, Lerman S, Claflin AJ, Henry H, Normal A, Reiss E: Inhibition of parathyroid hormone secretion by 1,25-dihydroxycholecalciferol and 24,25-dihydroxycholecalciferol in the dog. *J Clin Invest* 61:1375–1383, 1978.
19. Canterbury JM, Gavellas G, Bourgoignie JJ, Reiss E: Metabolic consequences of oral administration of $24,25(OH)_2D_3$ to uremic dogs. *J Clin Invest* 65:571–576, 1980.
20. Bellorin–Font E, Martin K, Freitag J, Anderson C, Sicard G, Slatopolsky E, Klahr S: Altered adenylate cyclase kinetics in hyperfunctioning parathyroid glands. *J Endocrinol Clin Metab* 52:499–507, 1981.
21. Martin KJ, Hruska KA, Freitag JJ, Klahr S, Slatopolsky D: The peripheral metabolism of parathyroid hormone. *N Engl J Med* 301:1092–1098, 1979.
22. Slatopolsky E, Martin K, Hruska K: Parathyroid hormone metabolism and its potential as a uremic toxin. *Am J Physiol* 239:F1–F12, 1980.
23. Canterbury JM, Bricker LA, Levey JS, Kozlovskis PL, Ruiz E, Zull JE, Reiss E: Metabolism of bovine parathyroid hormone: Immunological and biological characteristics of fragments generated by liver perfusion. *J Clin Invest* 55:1245–1253, 1975.
24. Hruska KA, Martin K, Mennes P, Greenwalt S, Anderson C, Klahr S, Slatopolsky S: Degradation of parathyroid hormone and fragment production by the isolated perfused dog kidney. The effect of glomerular filtration rate and perfusate Ca^{++} concentrations. *J Clin Invest* 60:501–510, 1977.
25. Bourgoignie JJ, Jacob AI, Lanier D Jr, Gavellas G, Canterbury J: Cimetidine (C) inhibition of iPTH in chronic renal disease. Abstracts American Society of Nephrology 12th Annual Meeting, *Kidney Int* 16:918, 1979.

26. Cunningham J, Segre GV, Slatopolsky E, Avioli LV: Effect of histamine H_2-receptor blockade on parathyroid status in normal and uremic man (editorial). *Am J Nephrol* 4:205–207, 1984.
27. Mennes P, Rosenbaum R, Martin K, Slatopolsky E: Hypomagnesemia and impaired parathyroid hormone secretion in chronic renal disease. *Ann Int Med* 88:206, 1978.
28. Massry S, Coburn JW, Kleeman CR: Evidence for suppression of parathyroid gland activity by hypermagnesemia. *J Clin Invest* 49:1619–1629, 1970.
29. Slatopolsky E, Gray R, Adams ND, Lewis J, Hruska K, Martin K, Klahr S, DeLuca H, Lemann J: The pathogenesis of secondary hyperparathyroidism in early renal failure. Fourth International Workshop on Vitamin D, Berlin, 1979.
30. Malluche HH, Goldstein DA, Massry SG: Osteomalacia and hyperparathyroid bone disease in patients with nephrotic syndrome. *J Clin Invest* 63:494–500, 1979.
31. Price PA, Poser JW, Raman N: Primary structure of the γ-carboxyglutamic acid-containing protein from bovine bone. *Proc Natl Acad Sci USA* 73:3374–3375, 1976.
32. Nishimoto SK, Price PA: Proof that the γ-carboxyglutamic acid-containing bone protein is synthesized in calf bone. *J Biol Chem* 254:437–441, 1979.
33. Price PA, Nishimoto S, Parthemore JG, Deftos LJ: A new biochemical marker for bone metabolism. Proceedings of the First Annual Meeting of the American Society for Bone and Mineral Research, Abstract #14A, 1979.
34. Price PA, Epstein DJ, Lothringer JW, Nishimoto SK, Poser JW, Williamson MK: Structure and function of the vitamin K-dependent protein of bone, in Suttie JW (ed): *Vitamin K Metabolism and Vitamin K-Dependent Proteins*. Baltimore, University Park Press, 1979, pp. 219–226.

14

The Pathology of the Uremic Bone Lesion

Steven L. Teitelbaum

1. The Morphological Manifestations of Renal Osteodystrophy

Renal osteodystrophy is a generic term that encompasses the array of biochemical and morphological derangements of bone that attend renal insufficiency. The insights gained into the genesis and, particularly, the natural history of this family of disorders are a reflection of the greater longevity of the uremic patient and, hence, the opportunity for skeletal dysfunctions to become clinically manifest.

Many biochemical and morphological manifestations of renal osteodystrophy occur. Appreciation of the spectrum of these morphological derangements is a result of the development of techniques of performing relatively atraumatic needle bone biopsies under local anesthesia and the ability to prepare well-preserved, nondecalcified histological sections of these biopsy specimens.

When prepared in the routine histology laboratory, hard tissues are invariably decalcified prior to section preparation. This process prevents distinction between bony matrix which was nonmineralized *in vivo* (osteoid) from that which was calcified and thereby renders impossible the histological diagnoses of most disorders of mineralization. A growing number of centers have now established techniques whereby nondecalcified histological sections of bone are prepared. These techniques permit precise identification of the bone lesion in each uremic patient and are essential for the careful management of renal osteodystrophy.

The histological features of renal osteodystrophy consist of innumerable combinations of osteitis fibrosa and osteomalacia associated with either

---

Steven L. Teitelbaum • Division of Bone and Mineral Metabolism, and Department of Pathology and Laboratory Medicine, The Jewish Hospital of St. Louis, Washington University School of Medicine, St. Louis, Missouri 63110. Supported in part by NIH Grant AM-11674.

osteosclerosis or osteopenia. Uremic osteitis fibrosa is the skeletal manifestation of hyperparathyroidism. As parathyroid hormone is a general activator of bone cell proliferation, the lesion is characterized by abundant osteoblasts and osteoclasts (Fig. 1). Osteoid is also in excess, and the presence of peritrabecular marrow fibrosis probably reflects activation of fibroblastlike osteoblast precursor cells. Osteomalacia, on the other hand, is the histological manifestation of abnormal mineralization and is also characterized by abundant osteoid, but associated with a paucity of osteoblasts and osteoclasts and an absence of marrow fibrosis (Fig. 2). Although "pure" examples of osteitis fibrosa and osteomalacia do exist in uremia, a combination of these lesions within a given bone biopsy is the rule.

Alterations of bone mass generally occur with progressive renal failure. The most common such change is an increase in the quantity of bone matrix per unit volume of marrow space (osteosclerosis). There is, in fact, an inverse correlation between glomerular function and the magnitude of osteosclerosis.[(1)] However, the increased skeletal radioopacity that occurs in many patients with end-stage renal disease is a manifestation of trabecular change. In fact, the cortical bone of uremic patients with osteosclerosis typically becomes more porous, resulting in loss of distinction between cortex and trabeculum. Abundant osteoid always accompanies the increase in the mineralized mass of trabecular bone,[(2)] indicating that osteomalacia and osteitis fibrosa may exist in radiodense bone.

The major application of the use of nondecalcified, histological sections of bone is the ability to identify those osteopenias with excess osteoid. Osteoporosis is a histological entity defined as a decreased mass of normally mineralized bone and therefore exhibits a normal quantity of osteoid. As the skeletons of uremic patients almost invariably contain excess osteoid, osteoporosis is a most unusual manifestation of renal failure.

Despite the virtual universality of excess osteoid in renal osteodystrophy, this accumulation of unmineralized bone matrix may reflect two distinctly different kinetic phenomena, namely: (1) a decreased rate of osteoid mineralization, i.e., osteomalacia, or (2) an absolute increase in the rate of organic matrix synthesis. Although standard histological features of uremic bone, such as the paucity or abundance of osteoblasts, are suggestive of defective mineralization or accelerated matrix synthesis, respectively, these kinetic disorders must ultimately by diagnosed by kinetic means.

The autofluorescent properties of tetracyclines have placed the skeleton in the unique position of being the organ system in man whose rate of turnover may be morphometrically measured in a single biopsy specimen.[(3)] These antibiotics bind stoichiometrically to divalent cations of newly formed, relatively acrystalline hydroxyapatite.[(4–7)] If the antibiotic is administered a short time prior to bone biopsy, it appears as a fluroescent line at the site of mineral deposition (calcification front), namely, the interface of osteoid and mineralized bone. Osteomalacia is reflected by a decreased rate of hydroxyapatite deposition at the osteoid–mineralized bone interface and conse-

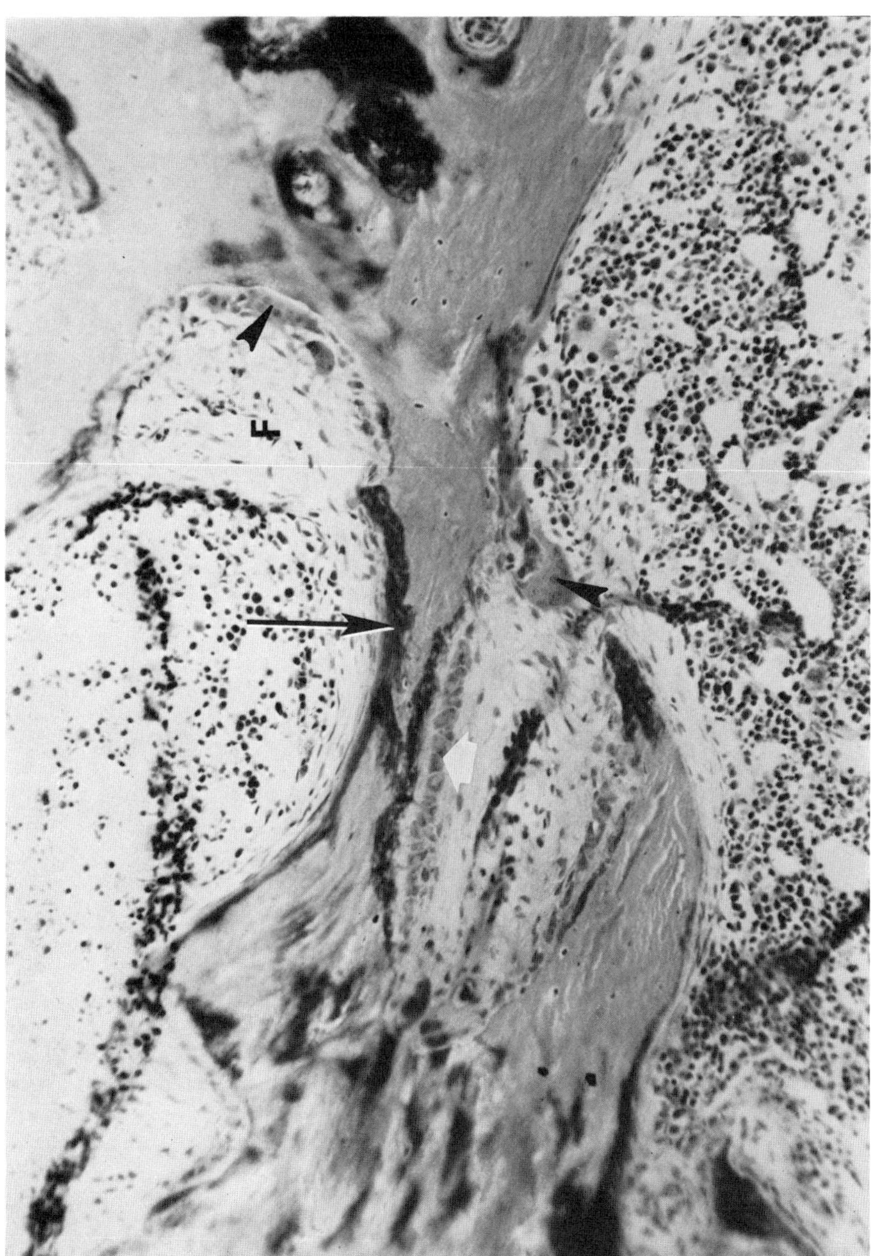

Figure 1. Renal osteitis fibrosa characterized by excess osteoid (black arrow), peritrabecular marrow fibrosis (F), and numerous osteoclasts (arrowheads) and osteoblasts (white arrow). Undecalcified, Goldner, ×200.

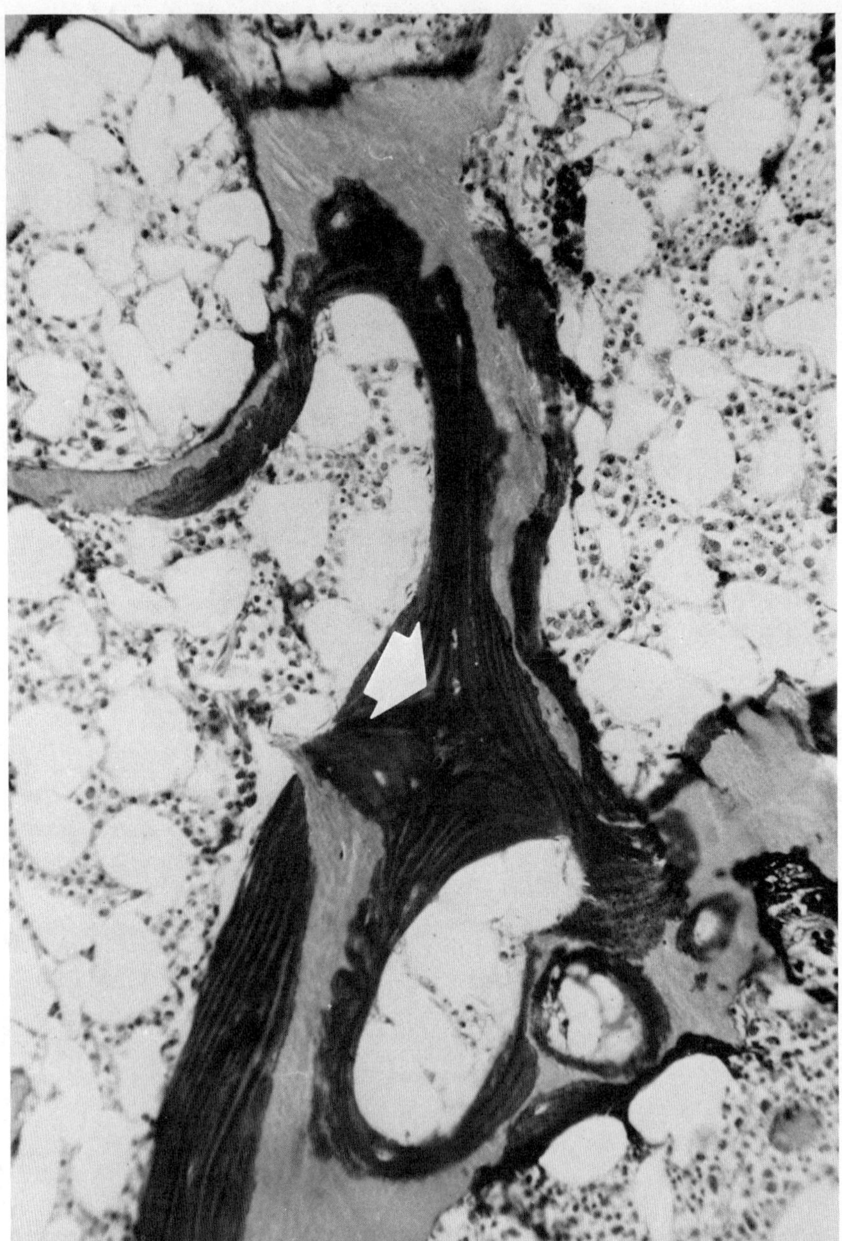

Figure 2. Renal osteomalacia characterized by excess osteoid (arrow), a paucity of osteoblasts and osteoclasts, and an absence of peritrabecular marrow fibrosis. Undecalcified, Goldner, ×200.

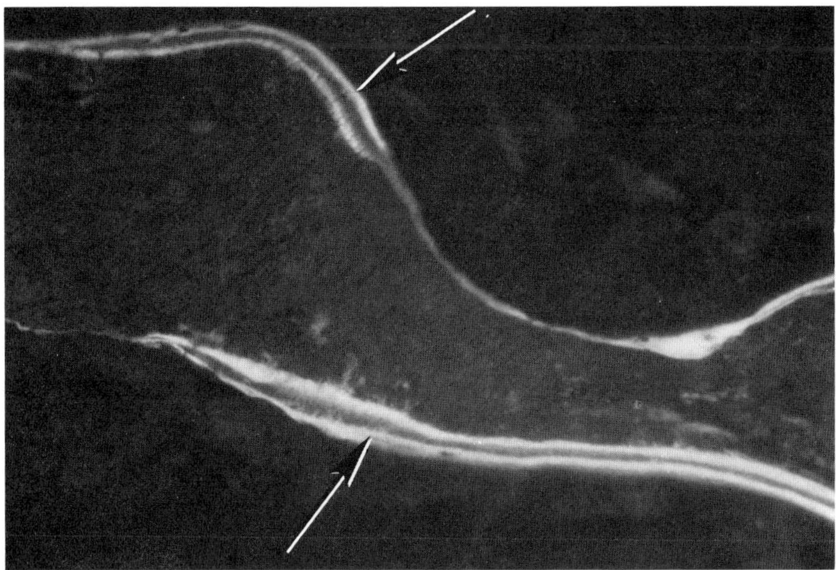

Figure 3. Parallel fluorescent lines in normal bone representing two courses of tetracycline administered 14 days apart. The label (arrows) located at the interface of osteoid and mineralized bone represents the second course of the antibiotic and identifies the calcification front. Undecalcified, unstained, fluorescent micrograph, ×250.

quently insufficient calcium to bind tetracycline in adequate quantities to produce fluorescence.(3) The consequence of this phenomenon is the absence of fluorescence at most osteoid–mineralized bone interfaces.(3)

At those sites where tetracycline deposition does occur, the fluorescent line is buried deeper in the bone as new mineral is appositionally deposited. Consequently, one may determine the actual rate of bone mineralization by administering two time-spaced courses of the antibiotic and micromorphometrically determining the mean distance between the two resulting, parallel fluorescent bands (Fig. 3). Division of that distance by the interdose duration yields the *cellular rate of mineralization* or the appositional rate of osteoid mineralization of the average bone-forming unit. For example, if the mean distance between labels is 14 μm and the interdose duration 14 days, the average bone-forming unit is appositionally mineralizing bone at the rate of 1 μm/day. Determination of the cellular rate of mineralization is particularly important in evaluating conditions of excess osteoid (hyperosteoidosis). Those hyperosteoidoses due to osteomalacia are characterized by a decreased cellular rate of mineralization, whereas excess osteoid due to accelerated organic matrix synthesis is associated with a cellular rate of mineralization that is at least normal.(8)

The two tetracycline-based morphological abnormalities of the osteomalacic skeleton described previously, namely diminished calcification front formation and decreased cellular rate of mineralization, reflect a defective

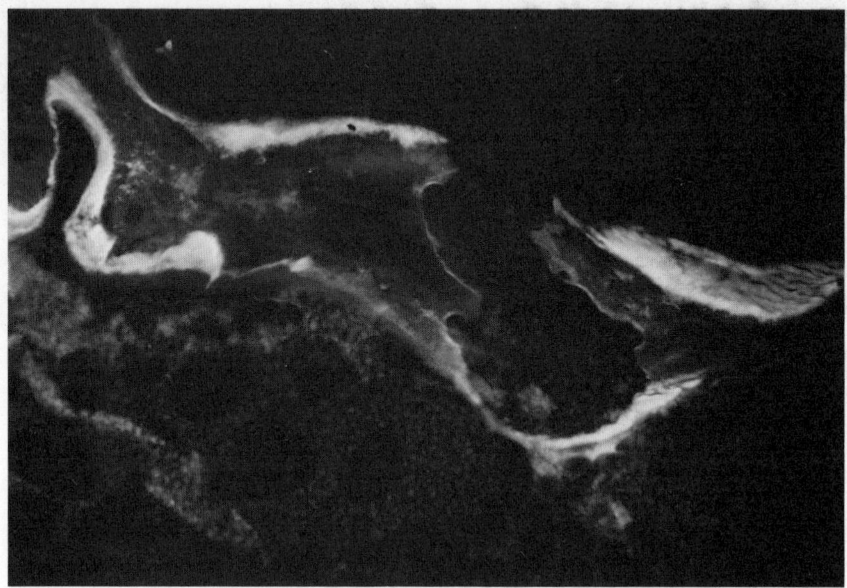

Figure 4. Wide and diffuse tetracycline labeling in bone of a patient with end-stage renal disease following a single course of tetracycline. Compare to normal calcification front in Fig. 3. Undecalcified, unstained, fluorescent micrograph, ×250.

rate of mineral deposition. However, another form of osteomalacia, namely, abnormal bone mineral maturation, may also be recognized by tetracycline fluorescence.

Normally, newly deposited bone mineral "matures" in a given period of time to a more perfectly crystalline form which is incapable of binding tetracycline in sufficient quantities to produce fluorescence.[9] The uremic skeleton, however, is characterized by delayed mineral maturation and hence an accumulation of immature hydroxyapatite capable of tetracycline fluorescence.[10,11] The morphological consequence of this mineral maturational defect is the presence of wide and irregular fluorescent labels (Fig. 4). It should be pointed out that the uremic skeleton generally develops a variety of combinations of tetracycline-based abnormalities.[12]

Organic matrix deposition is also abnormal in renal bone disease. Biochemically, this defect is manifest by a paucity of collagen cross-links.[13] It is unresolved if this abnormality is related to one of the earliest morphological alterations to occur in uremic bone, namely, the deposition of immature, woven, rather than mature, lamellar collagen (Figs. 5a,b). Woven collagen is, however, characterized by diffuse tetracycline fluorescence indicating an associated immaturity of its mineral content (Fig. 6).

2. The Genesis of Renal Osteodystrophy

The genesis of renal osteodystrophy initially lies in circulating abnormalities which in turn affect bone cell function resulting in derangements of

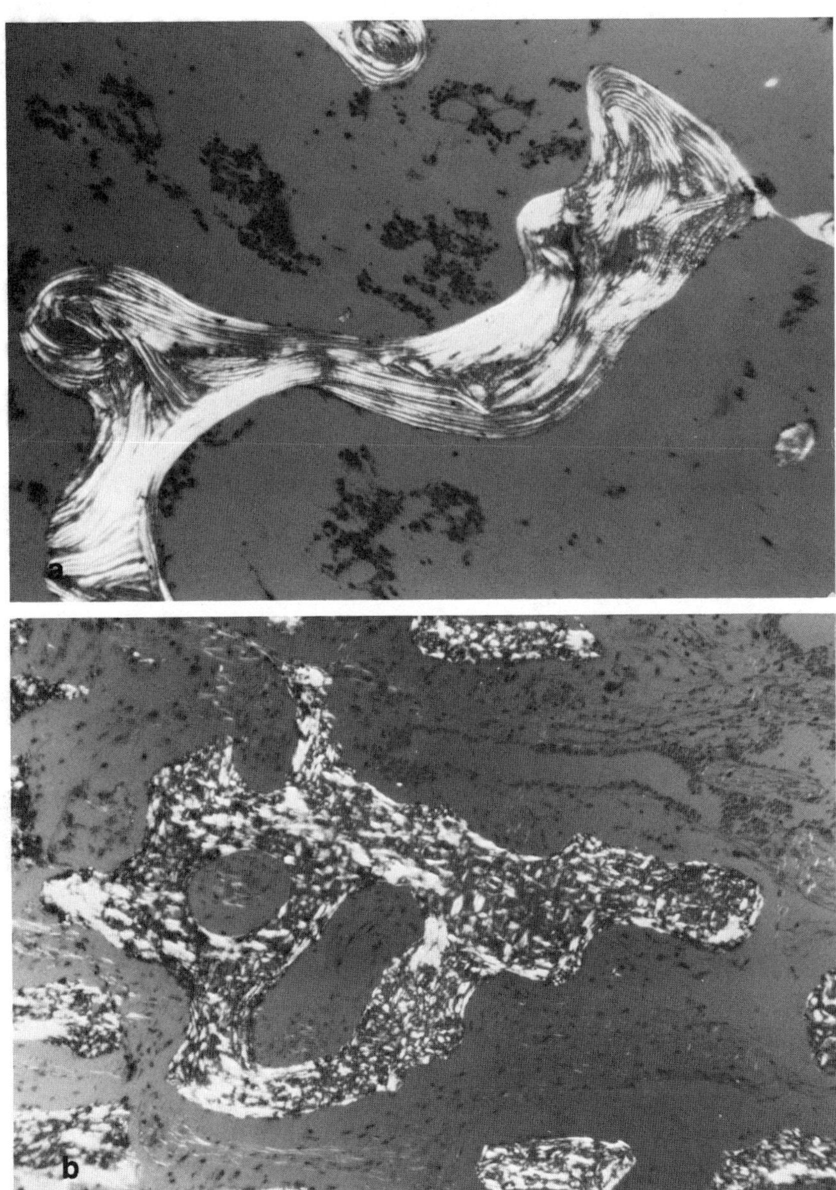

Figure 5. (a) "Mature" lamellar bone collagen as viewed by polarizing microscopy. Hematoxylin–eosin, ×100. (b) "Immature" woven bone collagen as viewed by polarizing microscopy. Hematoxylin–eosin, ×100.

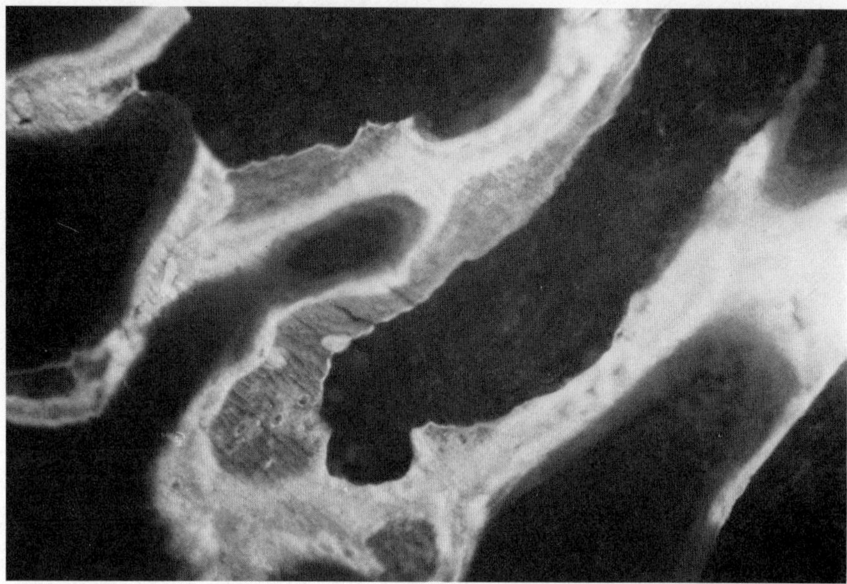

Figure 6. Diffuse fluorescence of woven bone following a single course of tetracycline. Compare to lamellar bone fluorescence in Fig. 3. Undecalcified, unstained, fluorescent micrograph, ×250.

matrix production and mobilization. There are undoubtedly consequences of renal failure whose profound effects on bone are yet to be discovered. However, the most readily appreciated circulating abnormalities of renal failure which dramatically influence bone are those of parathyroid hormone, vitamin D, and inorganic phosphorus.

There is little question that the progressive hyperparathyroidism which parallels declining renal function has profound skeletal manifestations. It is well known that most patients with end-stage renal disease have some degree of osteitis fibrosa. What is less commonly appreciated, however, is that patients with relatively mild renal insufficiency also have skeletal changes reflecting hyperparathyroidism.[1] For example, woven bone formation occurs when glomerular filtration rate falls beneath 80 cc/min per 1.73 m^2.[1] Excessive osteoid also accumulates under these circumstances. However, as most osteoid seams exhibit calcification front formation, osteomalacia is generally not a component of early renal failure.[1]

It should also be appreciated that although severe uremic hyperparathyroidism has detrimental skeletal effects, hypoparathyroidism results in perhaps the most crippling form of renal osteodystrophy. Totally parathyroidectomized patients with end-stage renal disease develop severe osteomalacia which is resistant to treatment with vitamin D metabolites.[14] As most circulating immunoreactive parathyroid hormone in end-stage renal disease is biologically inactive,[15,16] it is probable that some patients with relatively mild excesses of the immunologically determined hormone are indeed functionally hypoparathyroid. Moreover, hyperparathyroidism, either directly or indirectly, appears to retard the development of osteomalacia in uremia. Not only is calcification front formation directly related to the log of circulating immunoreactive parathyroid hormone levels, but the cellular rate of mineralization is markedly increased in those patients whose bone biopsies exhibit a predominance of osteitis fibrosa.(14)

Abnormal vitamin D metabolism undoubtedly contributes to the development of end-stage renal osteodystrophy. However, investigators have recently noted normal circulating levels of 1,25-dihydroxyvitamin D [1,25$(OH)_2$D] in early and moderate renal failure (R. W. Chesney, personal communication; E. Slatopolsky, personal communication). Consequently, the contribution which defective vitamin D metabolism makes to incipient renal bone disease is controversial. Furthermore, blood 25-hydroxyvitamin D (25-OHD) levels have been noted to be decreased,(17) normal,(18) or elevated (19) in patients with advanced renal insufficiency, and the contributions that deficiencies of this metabolite may make to the development of renal osteodystrophy have not been identified.

On the other hand, there is abundant evidence that administration of pharmacological doses of vitamin D or its 25-(20) or 1-α-hydroxylated metabolites(21) is generally strikingly beneficial to the uremic skeleton. It should be mentioned, however, that there is as yet no convincing evidence that these different compounds have distinct effects on renal osteodystrophy.

Those patients who respond most dramatically to treatment with vitamin D or its metabolites have bone lesions that exhibit a predominance of osteitis fibrosa. Concomitant with a fall in the level of circulating immunoreactive parathyroid hormone, osteoblasts and osteoclasts decrease in number, woven bone and marrow fibrosis usually become scarce and often disappear, and the volume of osteoid diminishes.(20) The responsivity of the predominantly osteomalacic skeleton is, however, more inconsistent (22) (*vide infra*).

Although conclusive evidence of a direct enhancement of vitamin D on bone mineralization is not available, circumstantial data suggest such a phenomenon occurs in uremia. For example, we have demonstrated improvement of mineral maturation by both biochemical and histological methods in uremic patients treated with either 25-OHD or the parent compound.(12,20,26) The histological evidence rests on the observation that the wide and irregular fluorescent calcification fronts that characterize osteomalacia are partially normalized by vitamin D.(12) On the other hand, it has been shown that merely increasing the Ca $\times$ P product in renal osteomalacia augments the mass of mineralized bone but does not improve calcification front formation.

Abnormalities of circulating phosphorus are closely linked to the hyperparathyroidism of renal failure, and it is apparent that those patients with the highest blood phosphorus levels also have the most severe hyperparathyroidism.(25) Because of concomitant hyperparathyroidism, the contribution that hyperphosphatemia *per se* makes to the development of renal osteodystrophy is not clear. It is unlikely, however, that the acceleration of bone formation in uremia is a direct effect of excess parathyroid hormone. For example, the cellular rate of mineralization is diminished in primary hyperparathyroidism,[26] a state that differs from renal hyperparathyroidism, at least in part, by changes in circulating phosphorus. Although the factor(s) responsible for enhanced skeletal synthesis in uremia is yet to be identified, the preceding observation suggests phosphorus may be extremely important. Moreover, phosphorus administration to man promotes bone formation,[29,30] and renal osteomalacia, which is generally characterized by relatively low circulating phosphorus levels, is associated with striking serum elevations of this anion when successfully treated with 25-OHD.[22]

3. *The Role of the Bone Biopsy in the Management of Renal Osteodystrophy*

A number of studies have demonstrated that bone histology is essential for optimal management of renal osteodystrophy. The necessity of the bone biopsy reflects the heterogeneity of uremic skeletal lesions and the relative inability to predict the response of these lesions to treatment. Prior to therapy, there are, however, noninvasive tests which are often indicative of the histology of the uremic skeleton. We and others have found that circulating immunoreactive parathyroid hormone levels,[25] and, to a lesser extent, alkaline phosphatase,[21,25,29,30,31] are generally predictive of the magnitude of osteitis fibrosa. Similarly, the radiographic appearance of subperiosteal resorption and osteosclerosis reflect the skeletal manifestations of excess parathyroid hormone.[25,31] On the other hand, in the absence of pseudofractures, there are no nonhistological methods which predict the degree of osteomalacia.[25,31]

After therapy, noninvasive techniques are often of limited value in predicting the skeletal response. For example, although circulating immunoreactive parathyroid hormone levels may decline after treatment with vitamin D analogues, the bone biopsy may, on occasion, demonstrate accentuation of the features of osteitis fibrosa. Although yet unproven, this phenomenon may reflect enhanced skeletal responsivity to parathyroid hormone. In addition, one of the hallmarks of successful treatment of renal osteodystrophy is reduction in osteoid volume, a histological feature that is unpredictable by nonhistological methods.[25,31]

It is apparent that the ultimate resolution of the uremic bone syndrome rests in identification and correction of biochemical derangements of the skeleton. Consequently, interest has recently turned toward gaining insight into the morphological manifestations of these derangements. It has been shown, for example, that the volume of osteoid reflects the excess quantities of magnesium that accumulate in uremic bone.[35] This is of interest as magnesium is a potent inhibitor of mineral maturation.[34] Similarly, aluminum accumulation in bone is associated with osteomalacia.[34] Such coupling of bone biochemistry and morphology cannot help but yield greater insight into the uremic bone syndrome.

Note added in proof: Since preparation of this chapter, it has become apparent that aluminum toxicity is the major cause of uremic osteomalacia and plays the major role in clinically significant renal osteodystrophy.

References

1. Malluche HH, Ritz E, Lange HP, Kutschera J, Hodgson M, Seiffert, U, Schoeppe W: Bone histology in incipient and advanced renal failure. *Kidney Int* 9:355, 1976.
2. Cohen MEL, Cohen GF, Ahad V, Kaye M: Renal osteodystrophy in patients on chronic haemodialysis. A radiological study. *Clin Radiol* 21:124, 1970.
3. Frost HM: Tetracycline-based histological analysis of bone remodeling. *Calc Tiss Res* 3:211, 1969.
4. Milch RA, Rall DP, Tobie JE: Fluorescence of tetracycline antibiotics in bone. *J Bone Joint Surg (AM)* 40:897, 1958.
5. Urist MR, Ibsen KH: Chemical reactivity of mineralized tissue with oxytetracycline. *Arch Pathol* 76:28, 1963.
6. Harris WH, Jackson RJ, Jowsey J: The *in vivo* distribution of tetracycline in canine bone. *J Bone Joint Surg (AM)* 44:1308, 1962.
7. Tam CS Reed R, Cruickshand B: Bone growth kinetics: I. Modifications of the tetracycline labeling technique. *J Pathol* 113:27, 1973.
8. Meunier P, Edouard C, Richard D, Laurent D: Histomorphometry of osteoid tissue. The hyperosteoidoses, in Meunier PJ (ed): *Bone Histomorphometry*. Toulouse, France, Sociétaé de la Nouvelle Imprimerie Fournié, 1977.
9. Termine JD: Mineral chemistry and skeletal biology. *Clin Orthop* 85:207, 1972.
10. Burnell JM, Teubner E, Wergedal JE, Sherrard DJ: Bone crystal maturation in renal osteodystrophy in humans. *J Clin Invest* 53:52, 1974.
11. Russell JE, Termine JD, Avioli LV: Abnormal bone mineral maturation in the chronic uremic state. *J Clin Invest* 52:2848, 1973.
12. Teitelbaum SL, Hruska KA, Shieber W, Debnam JW, Nichols SH: Tetracycline fluorescence in uremic and primary hyperparathyroid bone. *Kidney Int* 12:366, 1977.
13. Russell JE, Avioli LV, Mechanic G: The nature of the collagen cross-links in bone in the chronic uraemic state. *Biochem J* 145:119, 1975.
14. Teitelbaum SL, Bergfeld MA, Freitag J, Hruska KA: Accelerated bone formation in end stage renal disease, in Norman AW, Schaefer K, von Herrath D, Grigoleit H-G, Coburn JW, DeLuca HF, Mawer EB, Suda T (eds): *Vitamin D: Basic Research and Its Clinical Application*. Berlin, Water de Gruyter, 1979, p. 373.
15. Canterbury JM, Reiss E: Multiple immunoreactive molecular forms of parathyroid hormone in human serum. *Proc Soc Exp Biol Med* 140:1393, 1972.
16. Canterbury JM, Levey GS, Reiss E: Activation of renal cortical adenylate cyclase by circulating immunoreactive parathyroid hormone fragments. *J Clin Invest* 52:524, 1973.
17. Eastwood JB, Stamp TCB, Harris E, De Wardener HE: Vitamin-D deficiency in the osteomalacia of chronic renal failure. *Lancet* 2:7997, 1976.
18. Goldstein DA, Oda Y, Kurokawa K, Massry SG: Blood levels of 25-hydroxyvitamin D in nephrotic syndrome. Studies in 26 patients. *Ann Intern Med* 87:664, 1977.
19. Shen F, Baylink DJ, Sherrard DJ, Shen L, Maloney NA, Wergedal JE: Serum immunoreactive parathyroid hormone and 25-hydroxyvitamin D in patients with uremic bone disease. *J Clin Endocrinol Metab* 40:1009, 1975.
20. Teitelbaum SL, Bone JM, Stein PM, Gilden JJ, Bates M, Boisseau VC, Avioli LV: Calcifediol in chronic renal insufficiency. Skeletal response. *JAMA* 235:164, 1976.
21. Pierides AM, Skillen AW, Ellis HA: Serum alkaline phosphatase in azotemic and hemodialysis osteodystrophy: A study of isoenzyme patterns, their correlation with bone histology,

and their changes in response to treatment with 1αOHD$_3$ and 1,25(OH)$_2$D$_3$. *J Lab Clin Med* 93:899, 1979.

22. Frost HM, Griffith DL, Jee WSS, Kimmel D, McCandlis RP Teitelbaum SL: Histomorphometric changes in trabecular bone of renal failure patients treated with calcifediol. *Metabol Bone Dis Rel Res* 2:285, 1981.
23. Russell JE, Roberts ML, Teitelbaum SL, Stein PM, Avioli LV: The therapeutic effects of 25-hydroxyvitamin D$_3$ on renal osteodystrophy. Biochemical and morphometric analyses. *Min Electrolyte Metab* 1:129, 1978.
24. Eastwood JB, Bordier PJ, Clarkson EM, Tun Chot S, De Wardener HE: The contrasting effects on bone histology of vitamin D and of calcium carbonate in the osteomalacia of chronic renal failure. *Clin Sci Mol Med* 47:23, 1974.
25. Hruska KA, Teitelbaum SL, Kopelman R, Richardson CA, Miller P, Debnam J, Martin K, Slatopolsky E: The predictability of the histological features of uremic bone disease by non-invasive techniques. *Metabol Bone Dis Rel Res* 1:39, 1978.
26. Mosekilde L, Melsen F: A tetracycline-based histomorphometric evaluation of bone resorption and bone turnover in hyperthyroidism and hyperparathyroidism. *Acta Med Scand* 204:97, 1978.
27. Goldsmith RS: Discussion. *Fed Proc* 29:1198, 1970.
28. Goldsmith RS, Woodhouse CF, Ingbar SH, Segal D: Effect of phosphate supplements in patients with fractures. *Lancet* 1:7492, 1967.
29. Duursma SA, Visser WJ, Dorhout Mees EJ, Njio L: Serum calcium, phosphate and alkaline phosphatase and morphometric bone examinations in 30 patients with renal insufficiency. *Calc Tiss Res* 16:129, 1974.
30. Sherrard DJ, Baylink DJ, Wergedal JE, Maloney NA: Quantitative histological studies on the pathogenesis of uremic bone disease. *J Clin Endocrinol Metab* 39:119, 1974.
31. Debnam JW, Bates ML, Kopelman RC, Teitelbaum SL: Radiological/pathological correlations in uremic bone disease. *Radiology* 125:653, 1977.
32. Teitelbaum SL, Russell JE, Bone JM, Gilden JJ, Avioli LV: The relationship of biochemical and histometric determinants of uremic bone. *Arch Pathol Lab Med* 103:228, 1979.
33. Boskey AL, Posner AS: Magnesium stabilization of amorphous calcium phosphate: A kinetic study. *Mat Res Bull* 9:907, 1974.
34. Ellis HA, McCarthy JH, Herrington J: Bone aluminum in haemodialyzed patients and in rats injected with aluminum chloride: Relationship to impaired bone mineralisation. *J Clin Pathol* 32:832, 1979.

15

Vitamin D Metabolism in Chronic Renal Disease

Jacob Lemann, Jr., Richard W. Gray, and Nancy D. Adams

This chapter provides a summary of current knowledge of vitamin D metabolism and abnormalities of vitamin D nutrition and metabolism among patients with chronic kidney disease.

1. Vitamin D Metabolism

The scheme in Fig. 1 provides an overview of present knowledge regarding vitamin D metabolism. Pre-vitamin D_3 is synthesized in the skin from 7-dehydrocholesterol under the influence of ultraviolet light and is then thermally converted to vitamin D_3.[1] Vitamin D_3, cholecalciferol, is also obtained from the diet principally from milk, eggs, liver, some fish, and fish oils.[2] Some foods, especially milk and dry cereals, in the United States are fortified with vitamin D_3 or with vitamin D_2, ergocalciferol, derived from irradiated plant sterols. Vitamin D is then transported to the liver and undergoes hydroxylation at carbon atom 25 to form 25-OH-D, calcifidiol, the principal circulating metabolite of the vitamin.[3] The liver appears to be the major site of 25-hydroxylation although it may occur in other tissues in some species.[4] 25-OH-D appears to undergo an enterohepatic circulation.[5] There appears to be only partial feedback regulation by 25-OH-D of the hepatic hydroxylation of vitamin D since administration of large quantities

Jacob Lemann, Jr., and Richard W. Gray • Departments of Medicine and Biochemistry and the Clinical Research Center, Medical College of Wisconsin and Milwaukee County Medical Complex, Milwaukee, Wisconsin 53226. ***Nancy D. Adams*** • Division of Nephrology, University of Connecticut School of Medicine, Farmington, Connecticut 06032. Work supported in part by USPHS Grants RR-00058, AM-15089, and AM-22014.

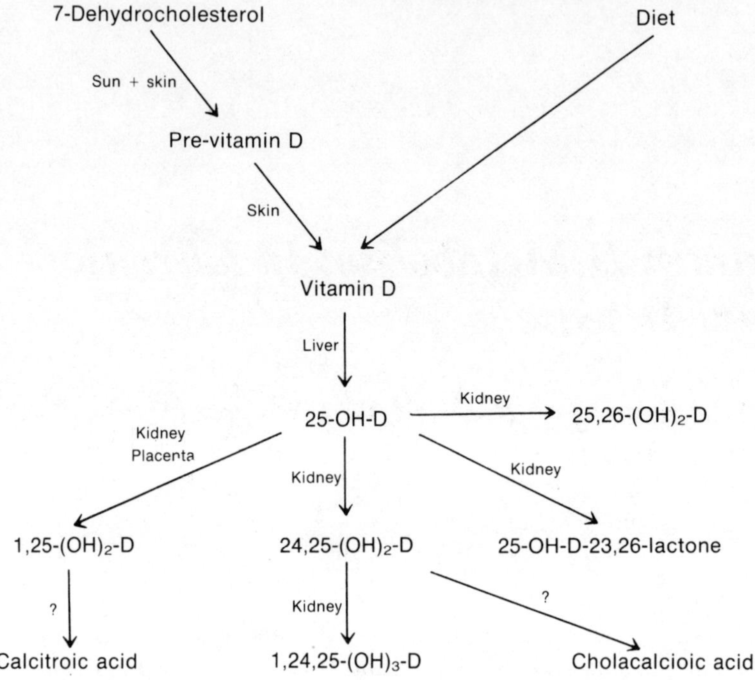

Figure 1. Schematic representation of present knowledge regarding vitamin D metabolism.

of vitamin D result in marked elevations of plasma 25-OH-D concentrations.[(6,7)] 25-OH-D currently appears to be the precursor for all other known vitamin D metabolites. 25-OH-D is converted by the kidney to several other compounds. One-α-hydroxylation results in the formation of 1,25-$(OH)_2$-D, calcitriol, which is the most potent biologically active vitamin D metabolite[(3,8)] but which probably does not account for all the biological actions of vitamin D,[(9,10)] an issue that is considered in further detail in a subsequent section of this chapter. Recent studies have shown that 1,25-$(OH)_2$-D may also be synthesized in the placenta of rats.[(11)] The synthesis of 1,25-$(OH)_2$-D by the kidney is independent of precursor 25-OH-D and is stimulated by parathyroid hormone,[(12–14)] by phosphate deficiency,[(15,16)] and perhaps directly by calcium deficiency.[(17)] The other major metabolite of 25-OH-D that is produced in the kidney is 24,25-$(OH)_2$-D.[(18)] The renal synthesis of 24,25-$(OH)_2$-D appears to depend largely on the availability of precursor 25-OH-D[(19,20)] but also may be regulated by other factors. The kidney, and perhaps other tissues, also produce 25,26-$(OH)_2$-D[(21)] and 25-OH-D-23,26-lactone.[(22)] 1,25-$(OH)_2$-D and 24,25-$(OH)_2$-D can be converted to more polar metabolites including 1,24,25-$(OH)_3$-D[(23)] and the recently discovered calcitroic and cholacalcioic acids.[(24)] 1,24,25-$(OH)_3$-D appears to be relatively inactive,[(25)] and the regulation of its synthesis as well as the synthesis and possible actions of the acid metabolites is not yet known.

Table 1. Effects of Vitamin D and Its Metabolites

Metabolite	Site of synthesis	Function
Vitamin D	Skin	Precursor of other metabolites ?Direct effects
25-OH-D	Liver ?Other tissues	Precursor of other metabolites Bone formation ?Renal Ca and P reabsorption
1,25-$(OH)_2$-D	Kidney	Intestinal Ca absorption ?Intestinal P reabsorption Bone resorption Renal P excretion
24,25-$(OH)_2$-D	Kidney	Bone formation ?Intestinal Ca absorption

2. The Function of Vitamin D

Table 1 outlines the currently known functions of vitamin D and its metabolites. Vitamin D serves as the precursor for subsequent metabolites. It is unlikely that vitamin D itself has any direct effects since 25-OH-D does not stimulate intestinal calcium transport in anephric animals[(26)] nor does vitamin D stimulate bone resorption *in vitro* even in pharmacological doses.[(27)] 25-OH-D serves as a precursor for subsequent vitamin D metabolites. In addition, 25-OH-D may also be required for normal bone formation[(9,10)]and has been shown to stimulate renal tubular calcium and phosphate reabsorption in dogs and rats.[(28,29)] 1,25-$(OH)_2$-D appears to be the principal determinant of intestinal Ca transport in humans.[(30–32)] It also appears to slightly augment intestinal phosphate absorption[(33)] although intestinal phosphate absorption in anephric humans, who cannot synthesize 1,25-$(OH)_2$-D, is not markedly impaired.[(31)] 1,25-$(OH)_2$-D is also capable of stimulating calcium mobilization from bone both *in vivo*[(26)] and *in vitro*.[(34)] Whether it has a direct effect on bone formation remains controversial. 1,25-$(OH)_2$-D does not appear to alter renal calcium transport[(35)] but has been observed to inhibit renal tubular phosphate reabsorption[(36)] in rats. 24,25-$(OH)_2$-D may increase intestinal calcium absorption and retention of calcium in the body[(37)] and appears to participate in normal bone formation.[(9,10)]

3. Plasma Levels of Vitamin D Metabolites in Health

Over the past several years, appropriate techniques for the extraction, chromatographic separation, and measurement of vitamin D and its metabolites have been developed. Table 2 presents the average plasma concentrations of vitamin D and its metabolites in healthy adults.[(19,20,38–41)] 25-OH-D is the major form of vitamin D in plasma having a mean concentration of

Table 2. Average Plasma Vitamin D Metabolite Concentrations in Health

	SI units	Mass units	Half-life
Vitamin D	8 nmoles/liter	4 ng/ml	<1 day
25-OH-D	60 nmoles/liter	25 ng/ml	25 days
1,25-$(OH)_2$-D	80 pmoles/liter	33 pg/ml	<1 day
24,25-$(OH)_2$-D	4 nmoles/liter	2 ng/ml	Probably >7 days

about 60 nmoles/liter or 25 ng/ml. The concentrations of vitamin D itself and 24,25-$(OH)_2$-D are approximately tenfold lower whereas the concentration of 1,25-$(OH)_2$-D is almost 1000-fold lower than that of 25-OH-D. The half-life of vitamin D in plasma based on the disappearance of ^{3}H-vitamin D_3 is about 1 day[(42)] since vitamin D is rapidly converted to 25-OH-D by the liver. The half-life of 25-OH-D in plasma is about 3 weeks based both on the disappearance of injected tracer doses of ^{3}H-25-OH-D_3[(43)] and on the fall in plasma 25-OH-D levels after administration of pharmacological doses of 25-OH-D_3.[(44)] Thus plasma levels of 25-OH-D appear to provide the best assessment of body stores of vitamin D. The plasma half-life of 1,25-$(OH)_2$-D_3 is very short. Injected ^{3}H-1,25-$(OH)_2$-D_3 in quantities approaching those of a tracer disappear from the plasma with a half-time of less than 10 min[(45)] whereas the half-time of decline of plasma 1,25-$(OH)_2$-D after its oral administration is about 6 hr in both healthy adults[(46)] and anephric patients (R. W. Gray, N. D. Adams, and J. Lemann, Jr., unpublished). The plasma half-life of 24,25-$(OH)_2$-D is probably more than 1 week.

4. *Abnormalities of Vitamin D in Kidney Disease*

Vitamin D deficiency results in rickets in children and osteomalacia in adults and is associated with impaired intestinal calcium absorption. Some patients with chronic renal disease, especially children, have rickets in the face of apparently normal sun exposure and normal dietary vitamin D intake. Bone biopsy in patients with chronic renal disease and bone disease, termed renal osteodystrophy, often shows variable degrees of osteomalacia in addition to the changes resulting from secondary hyperparathyroidism.[(47)] It has also long been known and repetitively documented that patients with chronic renal disease exhibit impaired intestinal calcium absorption.[(48–50)] Liu and Chu,[(48)] 40 years ago, demonstrated that net intestinal calcium absorption among five patients with renal osteodystrophy averaged only 1.8 mmoles/day or 7% of dietary calcium intake as compared to about 8.1 mmoles/day or 28% of dietary calcium intake in seven healthy subjects[(51)] when both groups were eating diets providing about 27 mmoles of calcium per day. Moreover, Liu and Chu observed that abnormally low rates of intestinal calcium absorption in their patients with renal osteodystrophy were not improved by physiological

Table 3. Plasma 25-OH-Vitamin D Levels in Patients with Chronic Renal Failure

		Healthy subjects		Patients with chronic renal disease		
Location	Reference	No.	25-OH-D (nmoles/liter)	No.	Creatinine (mg/100 ml)	25-OH-D (nmoles/liter)
Toulouse, France	Bayard *et al.*, 1972, 1973[55,56]	18	38 ± 10[a]	22	9.4 ± 6.4	23 ± 12
Berlin, Germany	Offerman *et al.*, 1974[57]	20	71 ± 35	27	~7.0	38 ± 18
New York, U.S.A.	Letteri *et al.*, 1975[58]	41	75 ± 21	44	6.7 ± 6.0	54 ± 38
Newcastle, U.K.	Cook *et al.*, 1977[59]	44	50 ± 20	13	—	20 ± 8
Katowice, Poland	Pietrek and Kokot, 1977[60]	25	41 ± 17	13	—	29 ± 6
London, U.K.	Eastwood *et al.*, 1979[61]	40	46 ± 20	19	~12.0	27 ± 20

[a] Standard deviation.

doses of vitamin D that caused healing of rickets in patients with vitamin D deficiency.[48]

5. Vitamin D Nutrition in Chronic Renal Disease

In health, available ultraviolet radiation from the sun appears to be the principal determinant of body stores of vitamin D as reflected by the plasma concentrations of 25-OH-D. Observations in the United Kingdom have shown that plasma 25-OH-D levels in healthy individuals are highest in midsummer, somewhat after the summer solstice, and lowest in the late winter, a month or so after the winter solstice.[52] Similar data have been obtained in Kalamazoo, Michigan.[53] Moreover, plasma 25-OH-D concentrations have been observed to increase by about 40% after only 2 weeks of increased sun exposure whereas plasma 1,25-$(OH)_2$-D levels are unaffected by sunlight.[54]

Table 3 summarizes some reported measurements of plasma 25-OH-D concentrations in patients with chronic renal disease, not yet on dialysis, in comparison to measurements in healthy subjects in several areas of Europe, the United Kingdom, and the United States. In each report, plasma levels of 25-OH-D were found to be lower among the patients with renal disease, averaging only about 60% of the values in healthy individuals.[55–61] Moreover, Offerman and associates[57] have observed that plasma 25-OH-D levels decrease as serum creatinine concentrations rise from the range of 1.2–4.0 mg/100 ml to the range of 8–12 mg/100 ml among patients with chronic renal disesae. Although these data suggest that body stores of vitamin D are reduced as renal failure advances, other investigators in Denmark[62] and in

Los Angeles[63] have not observed low plasma 25-OH-D concentrations among patients with chronic renal disease. Nevertheless, since the majority of reports do indicate that plasma 25-OH-D levels may be reduced among patients with chronic renal failure, possible explanations of such observations must be considered.

First, many of the reports of such lower values come from latitudes where there is a pronounced seasonal effect of the sun on plasma 25-OH-D levels, and some of the reports do not specify that samples from normal subjects and from patients with renal disease were drawn at the same time of year. Thus, it is conceivable, although unlikely, that many of the measurements in normals were made in summer and those in renal patients during the winter.

Second, it is possible, although not proven, that patients with advanced renal failure may be less active and thus may not be exposed to the sun as much as healthy individuals—especially during the summer in extreme northern or southern climates where sun exposure appears to be the principal determinant of body stores of vitamin D.[52,53]

Third, it is conceivable that production of vitamin D in the skin from 7-dehydrocholesterol may be impaired in patients with chronic renal disease despite adequate sun exposure. There are, however, no data supporting such a possibility.

Fourth, it is common practice to prescribe a restricted dietary protein intake for patients with chronic renal failure. To the extent that limitations are placed on eggs, milk (even milk that is not fortified with vitamin D), cheese, and fish, the foods that normally contain significant quantities of vitamin D,[2] the dietary intake of vitamin D would be reduced. Careful dietary histories have not been reported for the patients in whom low 25-OH-D levels were observed so that the relative contribution of reduced dietary vitamin D intake to low plasma 25-OH-D levels cannot be evaluated. It is possible that the use of foods fortified with vitamin D and the use of vitamin supplements containing vitamin D account for the normal plasma 25-OH-D levels in patients with chronic renal disease in Copenhagen and Los Angeles.[62,63]

Fifth, heavy proteinuria may account for reduced plasma 25-OH-D levels among some patients with chronic renal disease since plasma levels of 25-OH-D have been observed to fall both as the magnitude of proteinuria increases and as serum albumin levels fall among patients with the nephrotic syndrome.[60,63] Haddad and Walgate[64] reported that serum vitamin D-binding protein concentrations were low among patients with hypoproteinemia,[63] and since presumably some of their hypoproteinemic patients were nephrotic, it is likely that the vitamin D-binding protein and 25-OH-D can thus be lost into the urine. Although some of the reports of low plasma 25-OH-D concentrations in patients with chronic renal disease do not provide measurements of urinary protein excretion, thereby evaluating the possible contribution of heavy proteinuria, some reports indicate that plasma 25-OH-D levels may be reduced even among patients without the nephrotic syndrome.[60] Thus, it would appear that additional data are needed to document the relative importance of proteinuria in reducing plasma 25-OH-D levels in patients with chronic renal disease.

Sixth, it is possible that hepatic conversion of vitamin D to 25-OH-D may be impaired among patients with chronic renal failure. This possibility has been evaluated by Avioli and associates,[42] who studied the metabolism of orally administered ^{3}H-vitamin D_3 in patients with renal disease in comparison with healthy subjects. Intestinal absorption of the radiolabeled vitamin was similar in the two groups, but 2 days after dosing the percentage of serum radioactivity as ^{3}H-25-OH-D_3 was increased among the patients with renal disease. Moreover, the serum half-life of ^{3}H-D_3 was shorter among the patients with renal disease. These results imply more-rapid-than-normal, not impaired, hepatic synthesis of 25-OH-D from precursor vitamin D in patients with chronic renal disease. More recently, Farrington and associates have provided confirmation of these data by showing that plasma levels of 25-OH-D following intramuscular injection of 600,000 units of vitamin D_2 increased to a greater extent among patients with chronic renal disease than among normal subjects.[65]

Finally, the possibility that patients with chronic renal disease have low plasma 25-OH-D levels as a result of accelerated degradation of 25-OH-D has been suggested.[47] To our knowledge, this possibility has not been studied.

6. *Vitamin D Nutrition in Dialysis Patients*

Table 4 summarizes measurements made in several locations of plasma 25-OH-D concentrations in patients on hemodialysis in comparison to levels in healthy subjects.[43,55–57,59,60,66] In contrast to the low plasma 25-OH-D concentrations among patients with kidney disease who have not yet reached end-stage renal failure (Table 3), patients on dialysis appear to have normal plasma 25-OH-D concentrations. In fact, in three of the reported series (Table 3), plasma 25-OH-D levels were, on the average, higher among dialysis patients than in normal subjects.

Possible explanations for the normal or even somewhat elevated average plasma 25-OH-D levels among dialysis patients require consideration. First, these patients may well feel better, resume more normal activities, and thus be exposed to the sun to a greater extent than patients with chronic renal disease. Second, neither cutaneous synthesis of vitamin D nor hepatic conversion of vitamin D to 25-OH-D appears to be impaired among dialysis patients since Pietrek and Kokot in Poland have observed that plasma levels of 25-OH-D are higher in August than in March among dialysis patients.[60] Third, plasma 25-OH-D levels may be higher among dialysis patients because dietary protein intake is less limited and thus dietary vitamin D intake is improved. Dialysis patients also customarily are given a multiple-vitamin capsule daily to replace dialyzable water-soluble vitamins, and these prepa-

Table 4. *Plasma 25-OH-Vitamin D Levels in Hemodialysis Patients*

Location	Reference	Healthy subjects No.	Healthy subjects 25-OH-D (nmoles/liter)	Dialysis patients No.	Dialysis patients 25-OH-D (nmoles/liter)
Toulouse, France	Bayard *et al.*, 1972, 1973[55,56]	18	38 ± 10[a]	22	32 ± 22
Berlin, Germany	Offerman *et al.*, 1974[57]	20	71 ± 35	20	99 ± 66
Milwaukee, U.S.A.	Gray *et al.*, 1974[43]	8	68 ± 21	10	50 ± 16
Seattle, U.S.A.	Shen *et al.*, 1975[66]	20	65 ± 10	20	88 ± 29
Newcastle, U.K.	Cook *et al.*, 1977[59]	44	50 ± 25	14	46 ± 22
Katowice, Poland	Pietrek and Kokot, 1977[60]	25	41 ± 17	15	51 ± 20

[a] Standard deviation.

rations generally also provide 400–1000 units (10–25 μg) of vitamin D. In addition, urinary losses of protein, and thus presumably losses of vitamin D-binding protein, wane as glomerular filtration falls to minimal levels even among previously nephrotic patients. Finally, the metabolic clearance of 25-OH-D is apparently slowed among dialysis patients. We have observed that the plasma half-life of ^{3}H-25-OH-D_3 averages 44 ± 9 days among anephric dialysis patients as compared to only 23 ± 3 days in healthy adults.[43] Thus, greater sun exposure, better diet, vitamin D supplements, reduced urinary 25-OH-D losses, and slowed extrarenal degradation of 25-OH-D may all contribute to the higher plasma 25-OH-D concentrations among dialysis patients.

7. *24,25-(OH)$_2$-D in Chronic Renal Disease*

Haddad and associates reported that plasma levels of 24,25-$(OH)_2$-D were normal in anephric patients.[67] On the other hand, plasma 24,25-$(OH)_2$-D levels have been observed to decline with progressive degrees of renal insufficiency among both adults[20] and children[68] and that has been our own experience in adults (unpublished). Taylor and associates in the United Kingdom have observed that plasma 24,-25-$(OH)_2$-D levels are undetectable in anephric patients (20) and have presented evidence indicating that 25,26-$(OH)_2$-D_2 comigrates with 24,25-$(OH)_2$-D_3 during the chromatographic separation of vitamin D metabolites (69). It was thus suggested that 25,26-$(OH)_2$-D_2 derived from vitamin D_2 supplements accounted for the measurement of 24,25-$(OH)_2$-D among anephric patients in the United States.[67] Recently, Dr. Ronald Horst of the National Animal Disease Center,

Ames, Iowa, has kindly measured plasma levels of vitamin D_2 and vitamin D_3 and their hydroxylated metabolites in seven anephric patients under our care in Milwaukee. Additional high-pressure chromatographic techniques were required to separate the metabolites. All seven samples were obtained in July and August 1979, and total 25-OH-D_3 plus 25-OH-D_2 levels averaged 79 ± 26 nmoles/liter of which about half represented 25-OH-D_2 since each patient was taking a vitamin supplement containing vitamin D_2. Nevertheless, 24,25-$(OH)_2$-D_3 was undetectable in the sera of all seven patients, and only very small amounts of 24,25-$(OH)_2$-D_2 were detectable in two of the seven anephric sera. These data thus effectively confirm the observations of Taylor and associates[20,69] indicating that serum 24,25-$(OH)_2$-D is virtually absent in anephric humans. However, 25-26-$(OH)_2$-D_2 was also undetectable in our patients so the latter compound cannot account for the apparent normal 24,25-$(OH)_2$-D levels previously reported in anephrics in the United States.[67]

8. 1,25-$(OH)_2$-D in Chronic Renal Disease

Plasma 1,25-$(OH)_2$-D levels in healthy adults exhibit a broad range averaging 82 ± 27 pmoles/liter or 34 ± 11 pg/ml[19] and have been repeatedly found to be undetectable in anephric patients.[8,16,40] More recently, Slatopolsky and associates have reported measurements of plasma 1,25-$(OH)_2$-D levels among adults with chronic renal disease and varying degrees of renal failure.[70] Plasma 1,25-$(OH)_2$-D levels were clearly normal or even slightly above normal at 106 ± 31 pmoles/liter in 12 subjects with moderate renal insufficiency [glomerular filtration rate (GFR) 50 ± 13 ml/min]. Plasma 1,25-$(OH)_2$-D levels only fell below normal among eight patients with far-advanced renal failure (GFR 16 ± 6 ml/min) averaging 46 ± 14 pmoles/liter. Similar observations have now been made in children with chronic renal disease[71] although these measurements suggest that the levels may fall below normal earlier in the course of renal failure in children. Most of the children studied thus far have had primary tubulointerstitial renal diseases whereas the adults have principally had glomerular diseases. Whether the type of renal disease is an important determinant of the capacity of the remaining renal tissue to synthesize 1,25-$(OH)_2$-D will require additional study. The availability of 1,25-$(OH)_2$-D appears to be the principal determinant of intestinal calcium absorption when dietary calcium intake is normal since net intestinal calcium absorption is, on the average, indistinguishable from zero when plasma 1,25-$(OH)_2$-D levels are unmeasurably low and net intestinal calcium absorption rises proportionally as plasma 1,25-$(OH)_2$-D levels increase.[31] Systematic studies of intestinal calcium absorption, utilizing isotopic calcium, among patients with varying degrees of chronic renal insufficiency have shown that calcium absorption is generally within the range of normal until GFR declines to levels below 50 ml/min.[72] These data taken together with the roughly similar relationship for the decline in plasma 1,25-$(OH)_2$-D levels as GFR falls[70] imply that limitation of renal 1,25-$(OH)_2$-D synthesis is responsible for the progressive decline of intestinal calcium absorption as renal failure advances. Obviously, paired measurements of plasma 1,25-$(OH)_2$-D concentrations and intestinal calcium absorption will be required to determine whether there are exceptions to this relationship.

Brickman and associates[(73)] have clearly documented that oral 1,25-$(OH)_2$-D_3 therapy in patients with chronic renal disease can augment intestinal calcium absorption in a dose-related manner. Approximately 1.6 nmol or 0.68 μg/day of 1,25-$(OH)_2$-D_3 increased rates of intestinal calcium absorption to rates observed in healthy subjects.[(74)] However, despite normalization of intestinal calcium absorption by 1,25-$(OH)_2$-D therapy, with elevation of serum calcium concentration, a fall in serum iPTH and alkaline phosphatase levels, and a decline in osteoclastic bone resorption among patients with renal osteodystrophy, more recent observations by Coburn and associates have indicated that 1,25-$(OH)_2$-D therapy alone may fail to produce healing of the osteomalacic component of renal osteodystrophy.[(74)] Among patients with renal osteodystrophy whose bone biopsies showed principally osteomalacia, 1,25-$(OH)_2$-D_3 therapy resulted in the rapid development of hypercalcemia and failed to reduce the severity of skeletal osteomalacia. Since osteomalacia is classically the skeletal hallmark of vitamin D deficiency, these observations raise the possibility that there may be additional abnormalities of vitamin D metabolism that contribute to the pathogenesis of bone disease in uremia other than simply the progressive failure of renal 1,25-$(OH)_2$-D synthesis.

Evidence in support of the view that 1,25-$(OH)_2$-D does not account for all the biological actions of the vitamin D endocrine system has recently become available from observations in patients with nutritional vitamin D deficiency. Measurements of plasma vitamin D metabolites in three such patients with osteomalacia proven by bone biopsy have demonstrated that plasma 1,25-$(OH)_2$-D levels are normal despite undetectable or very low plasma levels of both 25-OH-D and 24,25-$(OH)_2$-D.[(75)] These data provide indirect evidence that 25-OH-D itself or 24,25-$(OH)_2$-D may play a critical role in the pathogenesis of osteomalacia. More direct evidence in support of this view has been provided by studies of the histological effects on bone produced by treatment of vitamin D deficiency and osteomalacia with vitamin D and its metabolites.[(9)] Treatment with either vitamin D_3 or 25-OH-D_3 for 8 weeks restored the mineralization front and markedly reduced osteoid volume whereas neither treatment with 1,25-$(OH)_2$-D_3 alone or 24,25-$(OH)_2$-D_3 alone caused any evidence of healing of osteomalacia. Combination therapy employing 1,25-$(OH)_2$-D_3 and 24,25-$(OH)_2$-D_3 did, however, improve the mineralization front and reduce osteoid volume (9). These studies therefore strongly suggest that 25-OH-D itself, or more likely 24,25-$(OH)_2$-D, may play an important role in normal bone formation and remodeling.

Studies of patients with chronic renal disease also provide data in support of an important role for 25-OH-D and/or 24,25-$(OH)_2$-D in the pathogenesis of the osteomalacic component of renal osteodystrophy since the extent of osteomalacia seen in bone biopsies from such patients has been observed to increase as plasma 25-OH-D levels fall.[76] This relationship could reflect reduced availability of 25-OH-D itself in these patients who were studied in the United Kingdom. It seems more likely, however, that reduced availability of 24,25-$(OH)_2$-D may be important since studies of patients with comparable degrees of renal failure and osteomalacia in Denmark showed both normal plasma 25-OH-D levels and a lack of correlation between plasma 25-OH-D concentrations and the severity of osteomalacia.[77]

In summary, several abnormalities of vitamin D metabolism have been identified among patients with chronic renal disease. First, plasma 25-OH-D levels may be low or normal depending on (1) sun exposure and cutaneous vitamin D synthesis, (2) urinary losses of 25-OH-D among patients with primary glomerular diseases and heavy proteinuria, and (3) speculatively, accelerated extrarenal catabolism of 25-OH-D. Second, plasma 1,25-$(OH)_2$-D levels fall as functioning kidney mass is reduced to one half or less as renal disease progresses and the resulting deficiency of 1,25-$(OH)_2$-D causes progressive impairment of intestinal calcium absorption when dietary calcium intake is normal. Moreover, the resulting tendency toward hypocalcemia further aggrevates preexisting secondary hyperparathyroidism and skeletal osteitis fibrosa. Plasma 24,25-$(OH)_2$-D levels also appear to fall as renal failure advances because of reduced availability of precursor 25-OH-D in some patients and, ultimately and probably more importantly, failure of renal synthesis in most patients. The low plasma 24,25-$(OH)_2$-D levels thus appear to contribute to the osteomalacic component of renal osteodystrophy. Therapeutic trials of 24,25-$(OH)_2$-D_3 together with 1,25-$(OH)_2$-D_3 are clearly needed to clarify the importance of 24,25-$(OH)_2$-D in the pathogenesis of renal osteodystrophy. The effects, if any, of the other vitamin D metabolites also remain to be evaluated.

References

1. Holick MF, Richtand NM, McNeill SC, Holick SA, Frommer JE, Henley JW, Potts JT Jr: Isolation and identification of previtamin D_3 from the skin of rats exposed to ultraviolet irradiation. *Biochemistry* 18:1003, 1979.
2. Paul AA, Southgate DAT: *McCance and Widdowson's The Composition of Foods*, 4th ed. Elsevier/North-Holland Biomedical Press, 1978.
3. DeLuca HF: Recent advances in our understanding of the vitamin D endocrine system. *J Lab Clin Med* 87:7, 1976.
4. Tucker G III; Gagnon RE, Haussler MR: Vitamin D_3-25 hydroxylase: Tissue occurrence and apparent lack of regulation. *Arch Biochem Biophys* 155:47, 1973.
5. Arnaud SN, Goldsmith RS, Lambert, PW, Go VLW: 25-Hydroxy-vitamin D_3: Evidence of an enterohepatic circulation in man. *Proc Soc Exp Biol Med* 149:570, 1975.
6. Stamp TCB, Haddad JG, Twigg CA: Comparison of oral 25-hydroxycholecalciferol, vitamin D and ultraviolet light as determinants of circulating 25-hydroxyvitamin D. *Lancet* 1:1341, 1977.
7. Hughes MR, Baylink DJ, Jones PG, Haussler, MR: Radioligand receptor assay for 25-hydroxyvitamin D_2/D_3 and 1α,25-dihydroxy-vitamin D_2/D_3. Applications to hypervitaminosis D. *J Clin Invest* 58:61, 1976.

8. Haussler MR, McCain TA: Vitamin D metabolism and action. *N Engl J Med* 297:974, 1041, 1977
9. Bordier P., Rasmussen H., Marie P., Miravet L., Gueris J, Ryckwaert, A: Vitamin D metabolism and bone mineralization in man. *J Clin Endocrinol Metab* 46:284, 1978.
10. Queille ML, Miravet L, Bordier P, Redel J: The action of vitamin D metabolites [25-OH-D_3, 1,25-$(OH)_2$-D_3, 24,25-$(OH)_2$-D_3, 25,26-$(OH)_2$-D_3] on vitamin D deficient rats. *Biomedicine* 28:237, 1978.
11. Tanaka Y., Halloran B, Schnoes HK, DeLuca HF: *In vitro* production of 1,25-dihydroxyvitamin D_3 by rat placental tissue. *Proc Natl Acad Sci USA* 76:5033, 1979.
12. Bilezikian JP, Canfield RE, Jacobs TP, Polay JS, D'Adamo AP, Eisman JA, DeLuca HF: Response of 1α,25-dihydroxyvitamin D_3 to hypocalcemia in human subjects. *N Eng J Med* 299:437, 1978.
13. Adams ND, Gray RW, Lemann J Jr: The effects of oral $CaCO_3$ loading and dietary calcium deprivation on plasma 1,25-dihydroxyvitamin D concentrations in healthy adults. *J Clin Endocrinol Metab* 48:1008, 1979.
14. Trechsel U, Bonjour J–P, Fleish, H: Regulation of the metabolism of 25-hydroxyvitamin D_3 in primary cultures of chick kidney cells. *J Clin Invest* 64:206, 1979.
15. Hughes MR, Brumbaugh PF, Haussler MR, Wergedal JE, Baylink DT. Regulation of serum 1α,25-dihydroxyvitamin D_3 by calcium and phosphate in the rat. *Science* 190:578, 1975.
16. Gray RW, Wilz DR, Caldas AE, Lemann J Jr: The importance of phosphate in regulating plasma 1,25-$(OH)_2$-vitamin D levels in humans: Studies in healthy subjects, in calcium-stone formers and in patients with primary hyperparathyroidism. *J Clin Endocrinol Metab* 45:299, 1977.
17. Trechsel U, Eisman JA, Bonjour J–P, Fleish, H: Evidence for a calcium-dependent, PTH-independent regulation of plasma 1,25-dihydroxy-vitamin D in rats, in Norman AW, Schaefer K, von Herrath D, Grigoleit H-G, Coburn JW, DeLuca HF, Mawer EB, Suda T (eds): *Vitamin D. Basic Research and Its Clinical Application.* Proc. IVth Vitamin D Workshop, Berlin, Walter deGruyter, 1979, p 511.
18. Holick MF, Schnoes HK, DeLuca HF, Gray RW, Boyle I, Suda, T: Isolation and Identification of 24,25-dihydroxycholecalciferol, a metabolite of vitamin D_3 made in the kidney. *Biochemistry* 11:4251, 1972.
19. Caldas AE, Gray RW, Lemann J Jr: The simultaneous measurement of vitamin D metabolites in plasma: studies in healthy adults and in patients with calcium nephrolithiasis. *J Lab Clin Med* 91:840, 1978.
20. Taylor CM, Mawer EB, Wallace JE, St. John J, Cochran M, Russell, RGG, Kanis JA: The absence of 24,25-dihydroxycholecalciferol in anephric patients. *Clin Sci Mol Med* 55:541, 1978.
21. Tanaka Y, Shepard RM, DeLuca HF: The 26-hydroxylation of 25-hydroxyvitamin D_3 *in vitro* by chick renal homogenates. *Biochem Biophys Res Commun* 83:7, 1978.
22. Horst RL: 25-OH-D_3-26,23-lactone: a metabolite of vitamin D_3 that is 5 times more potent than 25-OH-D_3 in the rat plasma competitive protein binding assay. *Biochem Biophys Res Commun* 89:286, 1979.
23. Holick MF, Kleiner–Bossaler A, Schnoes HK, Kasten PM, Boyle IT, DeLuca, HF: 1,24,25-trihydroxyvitamin D_3. A metabolite of vitamin D_3 effective on intestine. *J Biol Chem* 248:6691, 1973.
24. DeLuca HF, Schnoes HK. Recent developments in the metabolism of vitamin D, in Norman AW, Schaefer K, von Herrath D, Grigoleit H-G, Coburn JW, DeLuca HF, Mawer EB, Suda T (eds): *Vitamin D. Basic Research and Its Clinical Application.* Proc. IVth Vitamin D Workshop, Berlin, Walter deGruyter, 1979, p 445.
25. Cundy T, Kanis JA, Paton S, Smith R, Warner GT, Bartlett M, Russell RGG. The biological effects of 1,24,25-trihydroxyvitamin D_3 in man. *Metab Bone Dis Rel Res* 1:293, 1979.
26. Holick MF, Garabedian M, DeLuca, HF: 1,25-Dihydroxycholecalciferol. A metabolite of vitamin D_3 active on bone in anephric rats. *Science* 176:1146, 1972.

27. Trummel CL, Raisz LG, Blunt JW, DeLuca HF: 25-Hydroxycholecalciferol: Stimulation of bone resorption in tissue culture. *Science* 163:1450, 1969.
28. Puschett JB, Moranz J, Kurnick WS: Evidence for a direct action of cholecalciferol and 25-hydroxycholecalciferol on the renal transport of phosphate, sodium and calcium. *J Clin Invest* 51:373, 1972.
29. Popovtzer MM, Robinette JB, DeLuca HF, Holick MF. The acute effect of 25-hydroxycholecalciferol on renal handling of phosphorus. Evidence for a parathyroid hormone-dependent mechanism. *J Clin Invest* 53:913, 1974.
30. Kaplan RA, Haussler MR, Deftos LJ, Bone H, Pak CYC. The role of 1α,25-dihydroxyvitamin D in the mediation of intestinal hyperabsorption of calcium in primary hyperparathyroidism and absorptive hypercalciuria. *J Clin Invest* 59:756, 1977.
31. Wilz DR, Gray RW, Dominguez JH, Lemann J Jr: Plasma 1,25-$(OH)_2$-vitamin D concentrations and net intestinal calcium, phosphate and magnesium absorption in humans. *Am J Clin Nutr* 32:2052, 1979.
32. Gallagher JC, Riggs BL, Eisman J, Hamstra A, Arnaud SB, DeLuca HF: Intestinal calcium absorption and serum vitamin D metabolites in normal subjects and osteoporotic patients. *J Clin Invest* 64:729, 1979.
33. Brickman AS, Hartenbower DL, Norman AW, Coburn, JW: Actions of 1α-hydroxyvitamin D_3 and 1,25-dihydroxyvitamin D_3 on mineral metabolism in men. I. Effects on net absorption of phosphorus. *Am J Clin Nutr* 30:1064, 1977.
34. Raisz LG, Trummel CL, Holick MF, DeLuca HF: 1,25-Dihydroxycholecalciferol: a potent stimulator of bone resorption in tissue culture. *Science* 175:768, 1972.
35. Hugi K, Bonjour J–P, Fleisch H: Renal handling of calcium: Influence of parathyroid hormone and 1,25-dihydroxyvitamin D_3. *Am J Physiol* 236:F349, 1979.
36. Bonjour J–P, Preston C, Fleisch H: Effect of 1,25-dihydroxy-vitamin D on the renal handling of P_i in thyroparathyroidectomized rats. *J Clin Invest* 60:1419, 1977.
37. Kanis JA, Cundy T, Bartlett M, Smith R, Heynen G, Warner GT, Russell RGG: Is 24,25-dihydroxycholecalciferol a calcium-regulating hormone in man? *Br Med J* 1:1382, 1978.
38. Haddad JG, Chyu KJ: Competitive protein-binding radioassay for 25-hydroxycholecalciferol. *J Clin Endocrinol Metab* 33:992, 1971.
39. Brumbaugh PF, Haussler HD, Bursac KM, Haussler MR. Filter assay for 1α25-dihydroxyvitamin D_3. Utilization of the hormone's target tissue chromatin receptor. *Biochemistry* 13:4091, 1974.
40. Eisman JA, Hamstra AF, Kream BE, DeLuca HF. 1,25-Dihydroxy-vitamin D in biological fluids: a simplified and sensitive assay. *Science* 193:1031, 1976.
41. Lambert PW, Syverson BF, Arnaud CD, Spelbery TC: Isolation and quantitation of endogenous vitamin D and its physiologically important metabolite in human plasma by high pressure liquid chromatography. *J Steroid Biochem* 8:929, 1977.
42. Avioli LV, Birge S, Lee SW, Slatopolsky E. The metabolic fate of vitamin D_3-^3H in chronic renal failure. *J Clin Invest* 47:2239, 1968.
43. Gray RW, Weber HP, Dominguez JH, Lemann, J Jr: The metabolism of vitamin D_3 and 25-hydroxyvitamin D_3 in normal and anephric humans. *J Clin Endocrinol Metab* 39:1045, 1974.
44. Haddad JG, Rojanasathit S: Acute administration of 25-hydroxycholecalciferol in man. *J Clin Endocrinol Metab* 42:284, 1976.
45. Gray RW, Caldas AE, Wilz DR, Lemann J Jr, Smith GA, DeLuca HF: Metabolism and excretion of ^3H-1,25-$(OH)_2$-vitamin D_3 in healthy adults. *J Clin Endocrinol Metab* 46:756, 1978.
46. Bell NH, Schaefer PC, Goldsmith R: Effects of pharmacologic doses of 1,25-dihydroxyvitamin D_3 on serum calcium, parathyroid hormone and 1,25-dihydroxyvitamin D_3 in man. American Society for Bone and Mineral Research, 1979, p. 29A.
47. Avioli LV, Teitelbaum SL: Renal osteodystrophy, in Earley LE, Gottschalk CW (eds): *Strauss and Welt's Diseases of the Kidney*, Volume 1. Boston, Little, Brown 1979, Chapter 9, p 307.
48. Liu SH, Chu HI: Studies of calcium and phosphorus metabolism with special reference to pathogenesis and effects of dihydrotachysterol (A.T.10) and iron. *Medicine* 22:103, 1943.

49. Stanbury SW, Lumb GA: Metabolic studies of renal osteodystrophy. I. Calcium, phosphorus and nitrogen metabolism in rickets, osteomalacia and hyperparathyroidism complicating chronic uremia and in the osteomalacia of the adult Fanconi syndrome. *Medicine* 41:1, 1962.
50. Coburn JW, Koppel MH, Brickman AS, Massry SG: Study of intestinal absorption of calcium in patients with renal failure. *Kidney Int* 3:264, 1973.
51. Chu HI, Liu SH, Hsu HC, Chuo HC, Cheu SH: Calcium, phosphorus, nitrogen and magnesium metabolism in normal young Chinese adults. *Chinese Med J* 59:1, 1941.
52. Poskitt EME, Cale TJ, Lawson DEM. Diet, sunlight and 25-hydroxyvitamin D in healthy children and adults. *Br Med J* 1:331, 1979.
53. Stryd RP, Gilbertson TJ, Brunden MN: A seasonal variations study of 25-hydroxyvitamin D_3 serum levels in normal humans. *J Clin Endocrinol Metab* 48:771, 1979.
54. Morita R, Dokoh S, Fukunaga M, Yamamoto I, Torizuka K: Effects of sunlight exposure on blood concentration of vitamin D derivatives in healthy Japanese adults, in Norman AW, Schaefer K, von Herrath D, Grigoleit H-G, Coburn JW, DeLuca HF, Mawer EB, Suda T (eds): *Vitamin D. Basic Research and Its Clinical Application*. Proc. IVth Vitamin D Workshop, Berlin, Walter deGruyter, 1979, p 165.
55. Bayard F, Bec PH, Lounet JP: Measurement of plasma 25-hydroxycholecalciferol in man. *Eur J Clin Invest* 2:195, 1972.
56. Bayard F, Bec PH, Tonthat H, Lounet JP: Plasma 25-hydroxycholecalciferol in chronic renal failure. *Eur J Clin Invest* 3:447, 1973.
57. Offerman G, vonHerrath D, Schaffer K. Serum 25-hydroxycholecalciferol in uremia. *Nephron* 13:260, 1974.
58. Litteri J, Roginsky M, Moo F, Scipione R, Ellis K, Cohn S. The relationship between calcified tissue mass and plasma 25-hydroxycholecalciferol in chronic renal failure, in Norman AW, Schaefer K, von Herrath D, Grigoleit H-G, Coburn JW, DeLuca HF, Mawer EB, Suda T (eds): *Vitamin D and Problems Related to Uremic Bone Disease*, Berlin, Walter deGruyter, 1975, p 303.
59. Cook DB, Pierides AM, Shannon G: Seasonal variations of serum 25-hydroxyvitamin D in patients with chronic renal failure treated by regular haemodialysis. *Clin Chem Acta* 76:251, 1977.
60. Pietrek J, Kokot F: Serum 25-hydroxyvitamin D in patients with chronic renal disease. *Eur J Clin Invest* 7:283, 1977.
61. Eastwood JB, Daly A, Carter GD, Alaghband–Zadeh J, DeWardener HE: Plasma 25-hydroxyvitamin D in normal subjects and patients with terminal renal failure on maintenance haemodialysis and after transplantation. *Clin Sci* 57:473, 1979.
62. Nielsen SP, Sørensen OH, Lund B, Bärenholdt O, Munck O, Pedersen K: Calcium metabolism in patients with chronic non-dialytic renal disease. *Calcif Tissue Res* 21:202, 1976.
63. Goldstein DA, Yoshitaka O, Kurokawa K, Massry SG: Blood levels of 25-hydroxyvitamin D in nephrotic syndrome, studies in 26 patients. *Ann Int Med* 87:664, 1977.
64. Haddad JG Jr, Walgate J: 25-Hydroxyvitamin D transport in human plasma. Isolation and partial characterization of calcifiediol-binding proteins. *J Biol Chem* 251:4803, 1976.
65. Farrington K, Skinner RK, Varghese Z, Morehead JF: Hepatic metabolism of vitamin D in chronic renal failure. *Lancet* 1:321, 1979.
66. Shen FH, Baylink DJ, Sherrard DJ, Shen L, Maloney NA, Wergedal JE: Serum immunoreactive parathyroid hormone and 25-hydroxy-vitamin D in patients with uremic bone disease. *J Clin Endocrinol Metab* 40:1009, 1975.
67. Haddad JG, Min C, Mendelsohn M, Slatopolsky E, Hahn TJ: Competitive protein-binding radioassay of 24,25-dihydroxyvitamin D in sera from normal and anephric subjects. *Arch Biochem Biophys* 182:390, 1977.
68. Weisman Y, Lum GM, Reiter EO, Gilboa N, Knox GF, Root AW: Serum concentrations of 24,25-$(OH)_2$-D in uremic children: A reflection of renal function. *J Pediatr* 94:190, 1979.
69. Taylor CM: 24,25-Dihydroxyvitamin D in human serum, in Norman AW, Schaefer K, von Herrath D, Grigoleit H-G, Coburn JW, DeLuca HF, Mawer EB, Suda T (eds): *Vitamin D.*

Basic Research and Its Clinical Application. Proc. IVth Vitamin D Workshop, Berlin, Walter deGruyter, 1979, p 197.

70. Slatopolsky E, Gray RW, Adams ND, Lewis J, Hruska K, Martin K, Klahr S, DeLuca HF, Lemann J Jr: Low serum levels of 1,25-$(OH)_2$-D are not responsible for the development of secondary hyperparathyroidism in early renal failure. *Kidney Int* 14:733, 1978.
71. Portale AA, Booth BE, Tsai HC, Morris RC Jr: Reduced plasma 1,25-$(OH)_2$-D concentrations in children with moderate renal insufficiency. *Kidney Int* 16:922, 1979.
72. Mulluche HH, Werner E, Ritz E: Intestinal absorption of calcium and whole-body calcium retention in incipient and advanced renal failure. *Mineral Electrolyte Metab* 1:263, 1978.
73. Brickman AS, Coburn JW, Friedman GR, Okamura WH, Massry SG, Norman AW: Comparison of effects of 1α-hydroxyvitamin D_3 and 1,25-dihydroxyvitamin D_3 on mineral metabolism in man. *J Clin Invest* 57:1540, 1976.
74. Coburn JW, Sherrard DJ, Brickman AS, Wong EGC, Norman AW, Singer FR: A skeletal mineralizing defect in dialysis patients: A syndrome resembling osteomalacia but unrelated to vitamin D, in: *Contributions in Nephrology*, Volume 18. Berlin, Karger, 1980, p 172.
75. Eastwood JB, DeWardener HE, Gray RW, Lemann J Jr: Normal plasma 1,25-$(OH)_2$-vitamin D concentrations in nutritional osteomalacia. *Lancet* 1:1377, 1979.
76. Eastwood JB, Stamp TCB, Harris E, DeWardener HE: Vitamin D deficiency in the osteomalacia of chronic renal failure. *Lancet* 2:1209, 1976.
77. Nielsen HE, Melson F, Lund B, Sorenson OH, Christiansen, MS: Serum 25-hydroxycholecalciferol and renal osteodystrophy. *Lancet* 1:754, 1977.

16

Metabolism of Parathyroid Hormone and Interpretation of Radioimmunoassays for PTH

Eduardo Slatopolsky, Kevin Martin, Keith Hruska, and Saulo Klahr

1. Introduction

With the development of radioimmunoassays that are specific for certain regions of the parathyroid hormone (PTH) molecule, the fate of PTH that is secreted into the circulating blood has been partially clarified.

PTH, a single-chain polypeptide containing 84 amino acids, is synthesized within the parathyroid gland from a biosynthetic precursor, a prohormone known as pro-PTH.[1–3] Pro-PTH has six additional amino acids attached to the NH_2 terminus of the PTH 1-84 molecule. Pro-PTH is synthesized in the rough endoplasmic reticulum of the chief cells in the parathyroid glands and converted to PTH by proteolytic cleavage in the Golgi apparatus.[4] So far there is no convincing evidence that pro-PTH is secreted into the circulation. The storage form of PTH 1-84 is packaged in secretory granules that take several hours to mature.

A precursor of pro-PTH called prepro-PTH consisting of a 25-amino-acid sequence covalently linked to the amino-terminal portion of pro-PTH has been demonstrated.[5,6] Thus, prepro-PTH has 115 amino acids, pro-PTH 90, and PTH 84.

A controversial issue in the understanding of the metabolism of PTH has been the interpretation of the finding of fragments of PTH in the

---

Eduardo Slatopolsky, Kevin Martin, and Saulo Klahr • Renal Division, Department of Medicine, Washington University School of Medicine, St. Louis, Missouri 63110. ***Keith Hruska*** • Renal Division, Jewish Hospital of St. Louis, St. Louis, Missouri 63110. Work supported by USPHS NIAMdd Grants AM-09976 and AM-07126 and by NIH Grant RR-00036.

peripheral blood. Early studies[7,8] with radioimmunoassay gave variable results in patients with primary hyperparathyroidism. It was thought that the radioimmunoassay for PTH was measuring in blood the peptide secreted by the parathyroid glands. However, Berson and Yalow[9] demonstrated that PTH in plasma of patients was heterogeneous and differed immunologically from the hormone extracted from parathyroid glands of humans. Using different antisera they clearly demonstrated the presence of fragments with very short half-lives, so that some fragments rapidly became undetectable after parathyroidectomy whereas other fragments had prolonged half-lives in the circulation. They also demonstrated that the half-life of immunoreactive PTH was markedly prolonged in patients with uremia. Studies from several laboratories showed that the predominant circulating species of i-PTH had a molecular weight smaller than that of native hormone (i.e., mol. wt. approximately 7000 versus 9500 daltons). Moreover, Canterbury, Levey, and Reiss,[10] employing gel filtration of concentrated serum samples from patients with hyperparathyroidism, demonstrated the presence of three separate forms of PTH. The first, called peak 1, was consistent with the native PTH; peak 2, the main component, was found to be a biologically inactive form that represents fragments of the carboxyl portion of the molecule; and peak 3, with a mol. wt. around 4000, was shown to have biological activity in the adenylate cyclase system of rat renal cortical membranes. There is evidence that PTH fragments are produced in the peripheral circulation, particularly by the liver and kidney,[11–13] and are also directly secreted by the parathyroid glands.[14]

2. *Role of the Kidney in PTH Metabolism*

The kidney accounts for approximately 60% of the total metabolic clearance rate of the carboxy-terminal fragments of i-PTH with an arteriovenous extraction of 20%.[15] After the injection of the synthetic amino-terminal fragment of bovine PTH (syn b-PTH 1-34), the renal extraction of this peptide accounted for 45% of the total metabolic clearance rate from plasma. After a single injection of purified bovine PTH 1-84 (the native hormone), the circulating species of iPTH changes first from predominantly intact hormone to a mixture of intact hormone and carboxy- and amino-terminal hormone fragments and finally to carboxy-terminal fragments alone. Studies using the isolated perfused canine kidney demonstrated that the uptake of i-PTH by the kidney resulted in the production of circulating PTH fragments.

Specifically, it appeared that the kidney could remove from the circulation both intact PTH and also carboxy-terminal PTH fragments which are thought to be biologically inactive. Recently, Martin *et al.*[16] examined the mechanisms of i-PTH uptake by the kidney. The proposed mechanisms of the renal uptake of PTH and its fragments are illustrated in Fig. 1. The biologically active forms of PTH (both intact hormone and amino-terminal

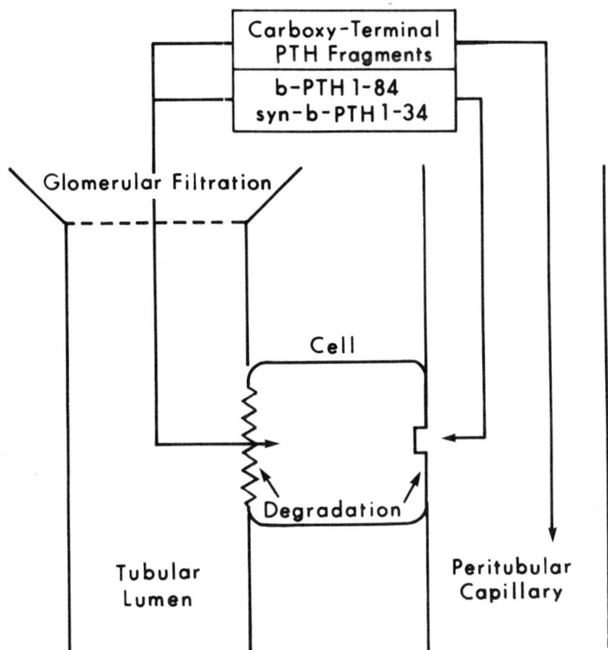

Figure 1. Schematic representation of the renal mechanisms of PTH uptake. (Reprinted from ref. 16, with permission.)

fragments) are removed by both peritubular uptake and glomerular filtration, whereas the biologically inactive forms of i-PTH (carboxy-terminal fragments) depend exclusively on glomerular filtration and tubular reabsorption for their catabolism. The clinical applications of these physiological observations have been demonstrated in studies by Freitag *et al.*,[17] who examined the time course of the changes in the plasma levels of carboxy-terminal i-PTH in patients with chronic renal failure after a successful renal transplantation. There is a marked accumulation of carboxy-terminal PTH fragments in peripheral plasma of patients with chronic renal failure, as would be predicted by the dependence of these fragments on glomerular filtration for their removal from the circulation. However, after renal transplantation from living related donors, plasma i-PTH decreased rapidly to 20% of the preoperative value within 24 hr.

3. Role of the Liver in PTH Metabolism

Barrett *et al.*[18] have recently reviewed the effects of PTH on the liver: Early studies using ^{123}I-labeled hormone did not reveal impressive uptake of radioactivity by the liver.[19] However, the radioactive PTH used was biologically inactive because of oxidation of methionine residues by the chloramine T method used for labeling. Oxidized PTH does not bind specifically to membranes *in vitro*.[20–22] Using radioimmunoassay techniques, Fang and Tashjian[23] demonstrated that partial hepatectomy significantly prolonged the plasma disappearance of i-PTH, thereby demonstrating a role of the liver in PTH metabolism. Subsequent studies have shown that this organ is a major site of PTH metabolism. Canterbury *et al.*, using an isolated perfused rat liver preparation, demonstrated that b-PTH was cleaved by the perfused liver resulting in PTH fragments similar by gel filtration to those found in the peripheral circulation.[11]

Martin *et al.*[13] examined the uptake of PTH by the liver *in vivo*; dogs with indwelling hepatic venous catheters were studied after either single injections or constant infusions of b-PTH 1-84 and syn b-PTH 1-34. These studies suggest that the uptake of i-PTH by the liver is selective for the intact hormone and indicate that the liver does not remove either amino-terminal or carboxy-terminal fragments from the circulation. On the other hand, this organ is a source of carboxy-terminal i-PTH fragments found in the circulation. Since the liver did not extract synthetic b-PTH 1-34 from the circulation and the kidney accounted for only 45% of the metabolic clearance rate of this PTH fragment, this suggests that some other organ or organs are involved in the peripheral metabolism of the amino terminal portion (1-34) of PTH.

4. *Role of Bone in PTH Metabolism*

Parsons and Robinson[24] demonstrated that the injection of b-PTH 1-84 into a cat whose isolated tibia was being perfused with blood from the whole animal caused a rapid release of calcium from the perfused bone. On the other hand, no effect was seen when intact b-PTH 1-84 was added directly to the blood supplying the bone; the latter procedure did not allow the hormone to enter the whole animal. These studies suggested that intact PTH must undergo some alteration in the intact animal before it could exert its effect on bone.

Recently, Martin *et al.*[25] have reexamined and extended these findings utilizing an isolated, perfused canine tibia preparation. During the infusion of syn b-PTH 1-34, there was a 36% arteriovenous difference in the level of amino-terminal i-PTH across the perfused bone. However, there was no significant uptake of i-PTH during the infusion of intact b-PTH 1-84. These findings were correlated with a biological effect by the demonstration of a marked rise in the production of cyclic AMP by the perfused bone during the infusion of syn b-PTH 1-34, whereas perfusion with high concentrations of b-PTH 1-84 resulted in only a minimal increase in the production of cyclic AMP. These studies indicate that there is selective uptake of syn b-PTH 1-34 by the bone, a feature different from that seen with the kidney or liver.

The differences in the uptake of PTH by liver, kidney, and bone are illustrated in Fig. 2. The upper panel shows the arteriovenous difference

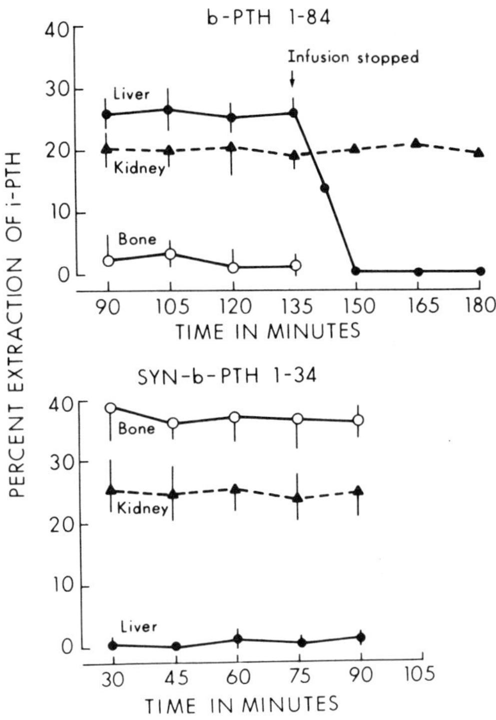

Figure 2. Extraction of i-PTH by liver (●), kidney (▲), and bone (○) during constant infusion of b-PTH (upper panel) and syn b-PTH 1-34 (lower panel). (Reprinted from ref. 30, with permission.)

for i-PTH across these organs during the constant infusion of b-PTH 1-84. The difference between the hepatic and renal uptake of i-PTH becomes apparent when the infusion of b-PTH 1-84 is discontinued. As the intact hormone disappeared from the circulation the hepatic arteriovenous difference rapidly fell, whereas a significant arteriovenous difference persisted across the kidney as long as i-PTH fragments remained in the circulation. The lower panel depicts the arteriovenous difference for i-PTH across the bone, kidney, and liver during the infusion of syn b-PTH 1-34. Both kidney and bone showed considerable extraction of this amino-terminal fragment, but liver did not.

5. *Radioimmunoassay for PTH*

In patients with hypercalcemia, the most direct method for verification of the diagnosis of hyperparathyroidism is the PTH radioimmunoassay (RIA). Over the past several years the heterogenous nature of PTH in the circulation has been elucidated. With this knowledge the binding specificities

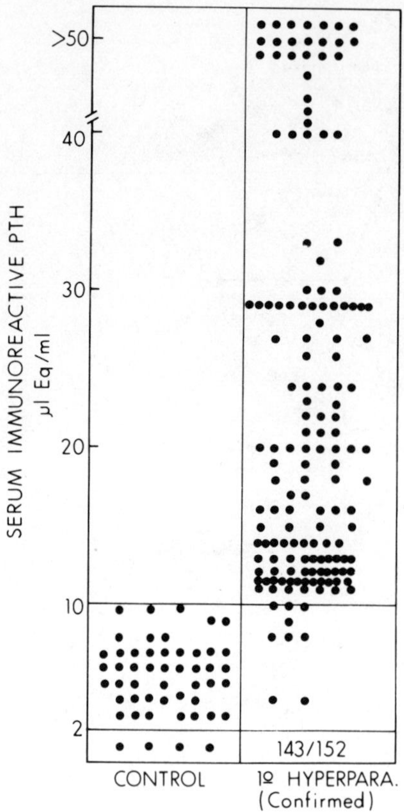

Figure 3. Results for serum i-PTH obtained in 152 patients with surgically confirmed hyperparathyroidism. Using CH9 antibody, a predominantly C-terminal antibody, elevated levels were found in 96% of the patients. (Reprinted from ref. 31.)

of the polyvalent antisera in widespread use can be characterized as that portion of the PTH molecule against which a particular antiserum is chiefly directed. Since both intact PTH and amino-terminal fragments have short half-lives in the circulation (circa 5 min), and carboxyl-terminal fragments have much longer half-lives, it is the latter peptides that comprise the bulk of the circulating hormone. In addition, recent data suggest that primary hyperparathyroidism is characterized by the secretion of COOH-terminal fragments of PTH from the parathyroid gland. Thus, antisera with binding specificities for the carboxy-terminal portion of the molecule bind the greatest fraction of circulating PTH (intact hormone and carboxy-terminal fragments), and these antisera display greater sensitivity in separating normal individuals from those with hyperparathyroidism. When carboxy-terminal-specific antisera are used, abnormal PTH levels have been reported in 90% of patients with primary hyperparathyroidism.[26] The experience of our laboratory with the use of carboxy-terminal anti-serum (CH9) is portrayed in Fig. 3. Ninety-six percent of patients with surgically proven hyperparathyroidism had high PTH levels utilizing this RIA. On the other hand, PTH immunoassays that utilize antisera directed toward the amino-terminal portion of the molecule generally display a 50–70% ability to separate patients with primary hyperparathyroidism from normal.[26]

Recent studies have documented the major role of glomerular filtration in the clearance of carboxy-terminal fragments of PTH from the circulation.[16] Thus, in all hyperparathyroid states associated with renal failure, the half-life of carboxy-terminal fragments in the circulation is markedly prolonged; for example, studies utilizing a carboxy-terminal antiserum show a very slow disappearance of i-PTH from the circulation after parathyroidectomy in dialysis patients.[17] In this situation, PTH assays utilizing antisera with amino-terminal binding specificities may be more useful in the determination of acute variations in PTH secretion, for instance, during a calcium infusion. However, over long follow-up periods carboxy-terminal assays of PTH in patients with renal failure do correlate with the manifestations of parathyroid activity on the bone.[27–29]

In summary, radioimmunoassays of PTH utilizing C-terminal antibodies usually detect high i-PTH in 90–95% of patients with primary hyperparathyroidism. In uremia, although the levels of i-PTH are influenced by the decrease in GFR, they correlate well with bone histology, and if samples are obtained on a monthly basis, they are a good "index" of the degree of secondary hyperparathyroidism.

ACKNOWLEDGMENT. Ms. Sandra Maul assisted in the preparation of the manuscript.

References

1. Cohn DV, MacGregor RR, Chu LLH, Kimmel JR, Hamilton JW: Calcemic fraction-A: Biosynthesis peptide precursor of parathyroid hormone. *Proc Natl Acad Sci USA* 69:1521, 1972.
2. Habener JR, Kemper B, Potts JT, Rich A: Proparathyroid hormone: Biosynthesis by human parathyroid adenomas. *Science* 178:680, 1972.
3. Hamilton JW, Niall HD, Jacobs HW, Keutmann HT, Potts JT Jr, Cohn DV: The N-terminal amino acid sequence of bovine pro-parathyroid hormone. *Proc Natl Acad Sci USA* 71:653, 1974.
4. Kemper B, Habener JF, Potts JT Jr, Rich A: Pro-parathyroid hormone: Identification of a biosynthetic precursor to parathyroid hormone. *Proc Natl Acad Sci USA* 69:643, 1972.
5. Kemper B, Habener JF, Ernst MD, Potts JT Jr, Rich A: Preproparathyroid hormone: Analysis of radioactive tryptic peptides and amino acid sequence. *Biochemistry* 15:15, 1976.
6. Habener JF, Potts JT Jr, Rich A: Pre-proparathyroid hormone. *J Biol Chem* 251:3893, 1976.
7. Berson SA, Yalow RS: Parathyroid hormone in plasma in adenomatous hyperparathyroidism, uremia and bronchogenic carcinoma. *Science* 154:907, 1966.
8. Reiss E, Canterbury JM: A radioimmunoassay for parathyroid hormone in man. *Proc Soc Exp Biol* 128:501, 1968.
9. Berson SA, Yalow RS: Immunochemical heterogeneity of parathyroid hormone in plasma. *J Clin Endocrinol Metab* 28:1037, 1968.
10. Canterbury JM, Levey GS, Reiss E: Activation of renal cortical adenylate cyclase by circulating immunoreactive parathyroid fragments. *J Clin Invest* 52:524, 1973.

11. Canterbury JM, Bricker LA, Levey GS, Kozlovskis PL, Ruiz E, Zull JE, Reiss E: Metabolism of bovine parathyroid hormone. Immunological and biological characteristics of fragments generated by liver perfusion. *J Clin Invest* 55:1245, 1975.
12. Hruska KA, Martin K, Mennes P, Greenwalt A, Anderson C, Klahr S, Slatopolsky E: Degradation of parathyroid hormone and fragment production by the isolated perfused dog kidney. The effect of glomerular filtration rate and perfusate Ca^{++} concentrations. *J Clin Invest* 60:501, 1977.
13. Martin K, Hruska K, Greenwalt A, Slatopolsky E: Selective uptake of intact parathyroid hormone by the liver. Differences between hepatic and renal uptake. *J Clin Invest* 58:781, 1976.
14. Flueck JA, DiBella FP, Edis AJ, Kehrwald JM, Arnaud CD: Immunoheterogeneity of parathyroid hormone in venous effluent serum from hyperfunctioning parathyroid glands. *J Clin Invest* 60:1367, 1977.
15. Hruska KA, Kopelman R, Rutherford WE, Klahr S, Slatopolsky E: Metabolism of immunoreactive parathyroid hormone in the dog. The role of the kidney and the effects of chronic renal disease. *J Clin Invest* 56:39, 1975.
16. Martin KJ, Hruska KA, Lewis J, Anderson C, Slatopolsky E: The renal handling of parathyroid hormone. Role of peritubular uptake and glomerular filtration. *J Clin Invest* 60:808, 1977.
17. Freitag J, Martin KJ, Hruska KA, Anderson C, Conrades M, Ladenson J, Klahr S, Slatopolsky E: Impaired parathyroid hormone metabolism in patients with chronic renal failure. *N Engl J Med* 298:29, 1978.
18. Barrett PQ, Teitelbaum S, Neuman WF, Neuman MW: The role of the liver in the peripheral metabolism of parathyroid hormone, in Copp DH, Talmage RV (eds): *Edocrinology of Calcium Metabolism.* Amsterdam, Excerpta Medica, 1978, p 324.
19. DeLuise M, Martin TJ, Melick RA: Tissue distribution of calcitonin in the rat: Comparison with parathyroid hormone. *J Endocrinol* 48:173, 1970.
20. Sutcliffe HS, Martin TJ, Eisman JA, Pilczyk R: Binding of parathyroid hormone to bovine kidney cortex plasma membrane. *Biochem J* 134:913, 1973.
21. Malbon CC, Zull JE: Interactions of parathyroid hormone and plasma membranes from rat kidney. *Biochem Biophys Res Commun* 56:952, 1974.
22. McIntosh CHS, Hesch RD: Characterization of the parathyrin receptor in renal plasma membranes by labeled hormone and labeled antibody binding techniques. *Biochem Biophys Acta* 426:535, 1976.
23. Fang VS, Tashjian AH: Studies on the role of the liver in the metabolism of parathyroid hormone. I. Effects of partial hepatectomy and incubation of the hormone with tissue homogenates. *Endocrinology* 90:1177, 1972.
24. Parsons JA, Robinson CJ: A rapid indirect hypercalcemic action of parathyroid hormone demonstrated in isolated perfused bone in Talmage RV, Belanger LF (eds): *Parathyroid Hormone and Thyrocalcitonin (Calcitonin).* Amsterdam, Excerpta Medica, 1968, p 329.
25. Martin KJ, Freitag JJ, Conrades M, Hruska KA, Klahr S, Slatopolsky E: Selective uptake of the synthetic amino terminal fragment of bovine parathyroid hormone by isolated perfused bone. *J Clin Invest* 62:256, 1978.
26. Arnaud CD, Goldsmith RS, Bordier PJ, Sizemore GW: Influence of immunoheterogeneity of circulating parathyroid hormone on results of radioimmunoassays of serum in man. *Am J Med* 56:785, 1974.
27. Bordier P, Marie P, Arnaud CD: Evolution of renal osteodystrophy: Correlation of bone histomorphometry and serum mineral and immunoreactive parathyroid hormone values before and after treatment with calcium carbonate or 25-hydroxycholecalciferol. *Kidney Int* 7:S102, 1975.
28. Rutherford WE, Bordier P, Marie P, Hruska K, Harter H, Greenwalt A, Blondin J, Haddad J, Bricker N, Slatopolsky E: Phosphate control and 25-hydroxycholecalciferol administration in preventing experimental renal osteodystrophy in the dog. *J Clin Invest* 60:332, 1977.
29. Hruska KA, Teitalbaum SL, Kopelman R, Richardson CA, Miller P, Depmen J, Martin K, Slatopolsky E: The predictability of the histologic features of uremic bone disease by non-invasive techniques. *Metab Bone Dis Rel Res* 1:39, 1978.

30. Martin KJ, Hruska KA, Freitag JJ, Klahr S, Slatopolsky E: The peripheral metabolism of parathyroid hormone. *N Engl J Med* 301:1092, 1979.
31. Slatopolsky E, Hruska K, Martin K, Freitag J: Physiologic and metabolic effects of parathyroid hormone, in Brenner B, Stein J (eds): *Hormonal Function and the Kidney*. New York, Churchill Livingstone, 1979, pp 169–193.

17

Collagen Metabolism in Uremia

Stephen M. Krane

Collagens are among the most abundant structural proteins of the extracellular matrix and are important components of basement membranes. Although many tissue collagens under normal circumstances have slow turnover rates (e.g., in dermis), other collagens are degraded and new collagens synthesized in the course of tissue remodeling (e.g., in bone). In chronic renal failure abnormalities occur in bone remodeling as well as lesions in dermis and subcutaneous tissue (necrosis) and tendons (spontaneous rupture). These changes should be interpreted with respect to our current knowledge of collagen metabolism.

1. Collagen Structure and Biosynthesis

The term *collagens* refers to a class of proteins characterized by their amino acid composition and the structural organization of the component polypeptide chains.[1–6] Most tissue collagens have regions containing a specific collagen triple helix, the structure of which is determined by the presence of a glycyl residue in every third position. The collagen helix is stabilized by certain posttranslational modifications, particularly hydroxylation of specific prolyl residues. Although many other proteins undergo posttranslational modifications of their component amino acids, collagen has a greater abundance and variety of structural modifications than most proteins in the animal kingdom. The noncollagenous regions of collagen molecules, which do not contain the glycine in every third position, may be integral parts of the molecular structure or may be present only during intermediate stages of biosynthesis and removed prior to deposition of the

---

Stephen M. Krane • Department of Medicine, Harvard Medical School, and Medical Services (Arthritis Unit), Massachusetts General Hospital, Boston, Massachusetts 02114. This is publication No. 803 of the Robert W. Lovett Memorial Group for the Study of Diseases Causing Deformities.

finished product. Procollagens refer to the completed precursor molecule stripped from the polyribosome and assembled intracellularly. The collagen molecule refers to the completely processed procollagen molecule from which the extensions at either end have been removed, although some noncollagenous sequences are retained at both ends. The collagen fiber is a higher-order structure that is formed by the specific alignment of the collagen molecules and eventually interactions with noncollagenous components of the specific tissue. Many tissues contain different kinds of collagens, each of which has a different primary structure determined by a different gene. In addition, collagens with the same primary structure present in different tissues may have distinctive and characteristic posttranslational modifications. In most tissues, the collagens can be considered as containing molecules which may be visualized as long, rigid rods with dimensions of approximately 300×1.5 nm. Each of these molecules is comprised of three polypeptide chains, all of which have the unique collagen helical structure. The helical structure is determined by the amino acid sequence. In addition to glycine at every third residue, other abundant amino acids include alanine and proline. Collagens contain little tyrosine and phenylalanine and no tryptophan and, with the exception of type III collagen, usually lack cysteine in the body of the helical portion. The most abundant posttranslational modification involves hydroxylation of prolyl residues in the 4 position, but in addition, there are small amounts of 3-hydroxyproline. Certain lysyl residues are also hydroxylated in the 5 position to form hydroxylysine. Some of the ϵ-amino groups are lysines as well as hydroxylysines and are also oxidized to their respective aldehydes, forming derivatives termed *allysine* and *hydroxyallysine*, respectively. The hydroxylysine residues within the helical portion of the molecule may also be glycosylated, again in a unique way, by the addition of galactose residues, and in some instances glucose residues are added to the galactose residues. The hydroxylysines, lysines, and aldehydes of these amino acids are involved in cross-links from one collagen chain to another, through their side-chain groups. In tissues, the collagen molecules are aggregated in a specific manner with respect to their long axis and are usually staggered at a distance of approximately one quarter the length of the molecule. This pattern results in interactions of the side chains, producing a predictable distribution of charge densities which in turn form the basis for the unique banding pattern observed by electron microscopy in many collagens. In the most common collagens, for example, those from bone and skin, these interactions produce a pattern of banding with major periods of approximately 64–70 nm. The manner in which the collagen molecules are aggregated also produces regions in which the molecules overlap and others in which there is no overlap. The latter results in voids or holes which are probably the predominant location of deposition of the mineral phase of bone.

It has also been appreciated over the last several years that different tissues contain either a unique type of collagen or mixtures of collagens,

Table 1. Sequence of Cellular Collagen Biosynthesis

1. Amino acid entry
2. Utilization of particular species of tRNA
3. Initiation of polypeptide α chains by formation of hydrophobic amino terminal leader sequence followed by assembly of proregion and helix
4. Hydroxylation of prolyl residues begins on nascent chains
5. Hydroxylation of lysyl residues
6. Glycosylation of hydroxylysyl residues
7. Formation of —S—S— bonds at carboxyterminal extension
8. Formation of triple helix
9. Packaging for secretion
10. Amino-terminal extension cleavage
11. Carboxy-terminal extension cleavage
12. Formation of microfibril
13. Lysyl and hydroxylysyl oxidation
14. Formation of reducible cross-links
15. Maturation and growth
16. Further cross-linking and interaction with other components

each of which has the same basic amino acid composition and higher-order structure.

The most common type of collagen is found in skin and bone and is comprised of so-called type I molecules, which are composed of two α1 chains (type I) and one α2 chain. Three identical polypeptide chains ($\alpha 1[II]_3$) comprise the collagens of cartilage. In addition, blood vessels, parenchymal organs, and skin contain a collagen which is the product of yet another gene, so-called type III collagen ($\alpha 1[III]_3$). Small amounts of type I trimer ($\alpha I[I]_3$) have also been identified in certain tissue culture systems and probably *in vivo* as well. Basement membranes contain collagens with a primary structure (type IV) different from those just described, and even other types have been identified in tissues such as muscle and placenta (type A and B).

The synthesis, secretion, and deposition of such complicated macromolecules have been examined in many systems, and considerable information is available concerning the steps of biosynthesis. These are summarized in Table 1. The amounts and the properties of the collagens thus produced are controlled by cells in several different ways. In some instances, controls exist at the level of the gene. Under certain circumstances, for example, it can be shown in cultured chondrocytes that a shift in ambient calcium concentrations causes a switch from one type of collagen to another. Increases in calcium content of the incubation medium are associated with decreased synthesis of type II collagen and augmented synthesis of type I collagen.[7] Control of structure and function is also exerted by hormones and metabolites at multiple steps in the posttranslational modification and processing of the molecules from the beginning of synthesis to the formation of the finished product. For example, ascorbic acid deficiency affects collagen synthesis since ascorbic acid is one substrate of prolyl hydroxylase. When prolyl hydroxylation is deficient, and formation of 4-hydroxyproline decreased, the triple helical structure is unstable, and collagen molecules synthesized intracellularly are degraded and not secreted. Substances known as lathyrogens (e.g., β-aminopropionitrile) interfere with cross-linking by inhibiting the enzyme lysyl oxidase and blocking the formation of the aldehyde derivatives of lysine and hydroxylysine. Penicillamine forms complexes with aldehydic groups on collagens and prevents their interaction with side-chain groups on other chains and also prevents cross-linking.

2. *Collagen Degradation*

Some collagens undergo turnover in the tissues. This turnover involves resorption of molecules in the collagen fiber and deposition of new molecules. Current evidence suggests that collagenolysis in animal tissues is carried out by the action of specific enzymes, collagenases, which have a number of properties in common.[1,8–10] These collagenases are metalloenzymes operating at neutral pH which catalyze the cleavage of collagens at specific sites in the polypeptide chains. This site is usually between a glycine and a leucine or isoleucine residue at a distance ¾ from the amino terminus. In general, undenatured collagen molecules, collagen fibrils, and fibers are refractory to cleavage by proteolytic enzymes other than collagenases at temperatures below denaturation. The collagenases appear to preferentially attack the native structure, probably cleaving molecules at the surface of the fibril, causing them to be solubilized. The fragments in solution, once denatured, may then be cleaved by other proteases. It is likely that most collagenases are secreted by cells in a latent, or inactive, form and interact with a variety of inhibitors present in many tissues. Some mechanism therefore must exist for the activation of these latent collagenases. It is probable that such collagenases are also operative in the resorption of bone collagen, but in bone there is an additional problem since mineralized collagen cannot be attacked by any proteases. It is obvious, therefore, that some mechanism must be operative for removal of the mineral phase prior to proteolytic attack. The resorptive function is carried out by cells such as osteoclasts, but the exact mechanism for removal of the mineral phase prior to collagenolysis is not known.

3. *Collagen Metabolism in Chronic Renal Failure*

In experimental chronic renal failure and in end-stage human renal disease, alterations in bone collagen and mineral "maturation" have been documented which have been assumed to reflect abnormal bone remodeling. Many of these observations have been based on analyses of mineralized bone powder, fractionated by density gradient centrifugation in bromoform toluene. It had been shown that the more recently formed bone containing newly synthesized collagen is of the lowest mineral density, whereas more mature bone containing older collagen molecules is of higher mineral density. In uremic animals, there is a shift in the distribution of collagens from fractions of high mineral density to those of low mineral density.[11] Such abnormalities have also been seen in chronic renal failure in humans.[12] In experimental animals, when reducible cross-links have been examined using tritiated sodium borohydride, an increase has been found in the ratio of the reducible cross-links dihydroxylysinonorleucine to hydroxylysinonorleucine in uremic animals compared to pair-fed controls.[13] In normal animals with advancing age (maturity) this ratio of these two reducible cross-links tends to fall. The results of these studies have been interpreted as indicating a specific molecular defect in the collagenous protein of the organic matrix of bone in uremia, perhaps owing to some toxic factor analogous to the lathyrogens. However, a similar pattern of abnormal reducible cross-links has been described in vitamin D deficiency.[14] Indeed, in human chronic renal failure, administration of therapeutic doses of 25-hydroxy vitamin D_3 has resulted in alteration of the bone powder density pattern toward normal ("more mature").[12] Other observations are also pertinent to interpreting the data in uremic animals and in man.

The collagen of bone in experimental vitamin D-deficient rickets is type I, as in normal bone, and rachitic epiphyseal cartilage contains predominantly type II collagen, as does normal cartilage.[15] There is an increased content of hydroxylysine in rachitic bone collagen, which is not found in the skin from rachitic animals.[15,16] It was initially suggested by Toole *et al.*[15] that increased glycosylation of these hydroxylysine residues could interfere with mineralization if the carbohydrate residues were located in the hole region of the fiber where most of the mineral is normally deposited. However, it was subsequently found that there is only a small increase in the glycosylation of rachitic collagen and no alteration in its pattern of glycosylation.[17] It has also been shown that the increased hydroxylysine content of bone—but not skin—collagen can be reproduced by dietary calcium deficiency or parathyroidectomy, but also by vitamin D- and phosphate-deficient states.[16] Purified lysyl hydroxylase, the enzyme involved in the posttranslational modification of specific lysyl residues, is inhibited by several divalent cations (calcium, zinc, copper), but the concentration of calcium ions that produces 50% inhibition of activity is quite high (15 mM).[18] Inhibition of lysyl hydroxylase by calcium ions would not in itself explain the observations described since skin collagen hydroxylation is not altered under conditions where bone collagen hydroxylation is. It is possible, however, that there are multiple forms of lysyl hydroxylases which could have different tissue distribution, different kinetics, and different metabolic regulation.

Increased lysyl hydroxylation observed in calcium deprivation and vitamin D deficiency could also explain the abnormal pattern of reducible cross-links observed in uremic animals as determined by tritiated sodium borohydride reduction (relative increase of the dihydroxylated derivative). The increased bone collagen lysine hydroxylation might also account for observations on the effects of vitamin D deficiency on a stable, *nonreducible* cross-link recently identified in collagens of mature animals. The compound, pyridinoline, first described in bovine Achilles tendon collagen,[19] is probably derived from two hydroxyallysine residues and one hydroxylysine residue. In immature bone (from chicks 6 weeks of age), the content of pyridinoline is low (~ 5–10 mmoles/100 moles hydroxyproline), but the levels are 40–50 mmoles in bone from older animals.[20] When the young chicks are made vitamin D deficient, the content of bone collagen pyridinoline is high (30–40 mmoles/100 moles hydroxyproline). The demineralized bone collagen is also less susceptible to proteolysis with pepsin or papain consistent with the *increased* cross-linking. By these criteria, rachitic bone collagen is *more* mature. Whether a similar pattern is present in uremic bone remains to be demonstrated. We are not sure why increased collagen hydroxylation *per se* would have such striking effects on the function of the structural protein, unless critical cross-links are affected as discussed previously. In actuality, the most profound alterations in collagen are seen when hydroxylysine content is deficient as observed in genetic disorders of lysyl hydroxylase.[21,22] However, a lethal recessive form of osteogenesis imperfecta has been described in which the hydroxylysine content of bone collagen is also increased.[23] Unfortunately, no information is available with respect to extracellular fluid concentrations of mineral ions. Hypocalcemia or vitamin D deficiency *in utero* could account for the increased lysyl hydroxylation.

Bone resorption is a feature of the osteodystrophy of chronic renal failure.[24] It is obvious that matrix (collagen) degradation is characteristic of this resorption. Secondary hyperparathyroidism must have an important role, perhaps mediated through stimulation or activation of specific collagenases. In severe uremia other data are consistent with increased collagen degradation.[24,25] Since investigators have shown that there is no increase in excretion of peptide-bound hydroxyproline, although excretion of free hydroxyproline may be increased, probably owing to decreased renal excretory function, the increased excretion of free hydroxyproline and high circulatory levels in human chronic renal failure and in experimental renal disease may be accounted for by impairment of hepatic hydroxyproline oxidase which accompanies the uremia. Normally, only small amounts of free hydroxyproline are found in plasma or urine even in states of increased collagen catabolism.[25] Since the hydroxyproline released from its peptides is rapidly degraded by the hepatic oxidase, the effects on the enzyme in uremia are probably not accounted for by the metabolic acidosis.

Several hormones and metabolites can alter collagen metabolism through effects on collagen synthesis and degradation. Parathyroid hormone increases bone degradation but also inhibits collagen synthesis in responsive cells and tissues,[26,27] although the net effects of excessive parathyroid hormone *in vivo* may be seen as increased synthesis in bone.[28] The latter may be the result of the well-known coupling between bone resorption and formation (? mediator) which may overcome inhibitory effects of parathyroid hormone on bone formation. Calcitonin inhibits resorption but may have effects on

Table 2. Hormones and Metabolites That Affect Collagen Synthesis

Agent	Effect
Ascorbic acid	Substrate for prolyl and lysyl hydroxylation (deficiency inhibits hydroxylation)
Iron	Substrate for prolyl and lysyl hydroxylation (desferrioxamine and αα′dipyridyl inhibit)
O_2	Substrate for prolyl and lysyl hydroxylation (N_2 inhibits)
Superoxide	Stimulates hydroxylation
Parathyroid hormone	Decreases synthesis
β-Adrenergic agonists	Inhibit collagen synthesis
β-Adrenergic antagonists	Stimulate collagen synthesis
Somatomedins	Stimulate collagen synthesis
Insulin	Stimulates collagen synthesis
Glucocorticoids	Inhibit collagen synthesis
Prostaglandin E	Inhibits collagen synthesis
Monocyte–lymphocyte products	Stimulate or inhibit collagen synthesis
Procollagen peptides	Inhibit collagen synthesis
Copper deficiency	Decreased lysyl oxidase
β-Aminopropionitrile	Inhibits lysyl oxidase
Cysteine, penicillamine	Bind to aldehydes
Vitamin D deficiency	Increased lysyl hydroxylation
Ca deficiency	Increased lysyl hydroxylation

formation (osteoblast function) particularly in uremia.[29] Other agents that have been shown to alter collagen synthesis in different systems[5] are listed in Table 2. Whether any of these has a role in the collagen turnover in uremia, particularly in uremic bone, remains to be demonstrated. At the present time it is probable that the changes observed in chronic renal failure are due predominatly to aberrations in vitamin D metabolism, excessive circulatory levels of parathyroid hormone, and abnormal concentration of mineral ions in the extracellular fluid. Whether factors other than these are operative to influence collagen metabolism in uremia remains a possibility since potent effects of a number of substances have been demonstrated.

Note added in proof: The reader should refer to recent reviews on collagen metabolism, such as ref. 30.

References

1. Gross J: Collagen biology: Structure, degradation and disease. *Harvey Lect* 68:351–432, 1974.
2. Fietzek PP, Kühn K: The primary structure of collagen. *Int Rev Connect Tis Res* 7:1–60, 1976.
3. Miller EJ: Biochemical characteristics and biological significance of the genetically-distinct collagens. *Mol Cell Biochem* 13:165–192, 1976.
4. Gay S, Miller EJ: *Collagen in the Physiology and Pathology of Connective Tissue*. Stuttgart, Gustav Fischer Verlag, 1978, pp 1–110.

5. Prockop DJ, Kivirikko KI, Tuderman L, Guzman NA: The biosynthesis of collagen and its disorders. *N Engl J Med* 301:13–23, 77–85, 1979.
6. Rojkind M: Chemistry and biosynthesis of collagen. *Bull Rheum Dis* 30:1006–1011, 1980.
7. Deshmukh K, Kline WG, Sawyer BD: Role of calcium in the phenotypic expression of rabbit articular chondrocytes in culture. *FEBS Lett* 67:48–51, 1976.
8. Harris ED Jr, Krane SM: Collagenases. *N Engl J Med* 291:557–563, 605–609, 652–661, 1974.
9. Weiss JB: Enzymatic degradation of collagen. *Int Rev Connect Tis Res* 7:101–157, 1976.
10. Woolley DE, Evanson JM (ed): *Collagenase in Normal and Pathological Connective Tissues.* London, Wiley, 1980.
11. Russell JE, Avioli LV: Effect of experimental chronic renal insufficiency on bone mineral and collagen maturation. *J Clin Invest* 51:3072–3079, 1972.
12. Russell JE, Roberts ML, Teitelbaum S, Stein PM, Avioli LV: Therapeutic effects of 25-hydroxy vitamin D_3 on renal osteodystrophy. *Mineral Electrolyte Metab* 1:129–138, 1978.
13. Russell JE, Avioli LV, Mechanic G: The nature of the collagen cross-links in bone in the chronic uremic state. *Biochem J* 145:119–120, 1975.
14. Mechanic GL, Toverud SU, Ramp WK: Quantitative changes of bone collagen crosslinks and precursors in vitamin D deficiency. *Biochem Biophys Res Commun* 47:760–765, 1972.
15. Toole BP, Kang AH, Trelstad RL, Gross J: Collagen heterogeneity within different growth regions of long bones of rachitic and non-rachitic chicks. *Biochem J* 127:715–720, 1972.
16. Barnes MJ, Constable BJ, Morton LF, Kodicek E: The influence of dietary calcium deficiency on bone collagen structure. *Biochim Biophys Acta* 328:373–382, 1973.
17. Royce PM, Barnes MJ: Comparative studies on collagen glycosylation in chick skin and bone. *Biochim Biophys Acta* 498:132–142, 1977.
18. Ryhänen L: Lysyl hydroxylase. Further purification and characterization of the enzyme from chick embryos and chick embryo cartilage. *Biochim Biophys Acta* 438:71–89, 1976.
19. Fujimoto D, Akiba K–Y, Nakamura N: Isolation and characterization of a fluorescent material in bovine Achilles tendon collagen. *Biochem Biophys Res Commun* 76:1124–1129, 1977.
20. Fujimoto D, Fujie M, Abe E, Suda T: Effect of vitamin D on the content of the stable crosslink, pyridinoline, in chick bone collagen. *Biochem Biophys Res Commun* 91:24–28, 1979.
21. Pinnell SR, Krane SM, Kenzora JE, Glimcher MJ: A heritable disorder of connective tissue: hydroxylysine-deficient collagen disease. *N Engl J Med* 286:1013–1020, 1972.
22. Krane SM, Pinnell SR, Erbe RW: Lysyl protocollagen hydroxylase deficiency in fibroblasts from siblings with hydroxylysine-deficient collagen. *Proc Natl Acad Sci USA* 69:2899–2903, 1973.
23. Trelstad RL, Rubin D, Gross J: Osteogenesis imperfecta congenita: evidence for a generalized molecular disorder of collagen. *Lab Invest* 36:1501–1508, 1977.
24. Avioli LV: Renal osteodystrophy in Avioli LV, Krane SM (eds): *Metabolic Bone Disease.* New York, Academic Press, 1978, pp 149–215.
25. Kivirikko KI: Urinary excretion of hydroxyproline in health and disease. *Int Rev Connect Tis Res* 5:93–163, 1970.
26. Raisz LG, Kream BE, Canalis EM: Regulation of the synthesis of bone matrix in organ culture, in Horton JE, Tarpley TM, Davis WF (eds): *Mechanisms of Localized Bone Loss.* Washington, DC, Information Retrieval Inc., 1977, pp 39–45.
27. Wong GL, Cohn DV: The effect of parathyroid hormone on the synthesis of collagenous matrix by isolated bone cells, in Horton JE, Tarpley TM, Davis WF (eds): *Mechanisms of Localized Bone Loss.* Washington DC, Information Retrieval Inc., 1977, pp 47–59.
28. Parsons JA: Physiology of parathyroid hormone, in DeGroot LJ (ed): *Endocrinology,* Volume 2. New York, Grune & Stratton, 1979, pp 621–629.
29. Kanis JA, Earnshaw M, Heynen G, Ledingham JGG, Oliver DO, Russell RGG, Woods CG, Franchimont P, Gaspar S: Changes in histologic and biochemical indexes of bone turnover after bilateral nephrectomy in patients on hemodialysis. *N Engl J Med* 296:1073–1079, 1977.
30. Piez KA, Redd AH (eds): *Extracellular Matrix Biochemistry.* New York, Elsevier, 1984.

Neurologic Complications of Renal Failure

18

Neurologic Complications of Renal Failure

The State of the Art

Allen I. Arieff

In the patient with renal failure, the nervous system is the primary barometer of patient well-being. Whereas other manifestations of the uremic state such as anemia, heart failure, bone pain, muscle dysfunction, and skin rashes are evaluated by the physician, it is via the nervous system that patients with renal failure perceive that which is abnormal.[1]

1. Uremic Encephalopathy

An encephalopathy associated with uremia may have among its early manisfestations clouding of the sensorium and decreased mental alertness.[2] Patients are easily fatigued, become apathetic, and are unable to concentrate appropriately; their recent memory is impaired. As the uremia becomes more advanced, attention span may diminish, the patients may have perceptual errors which include misidentification of people and objects, and there may be illusions and hallucinations and tremors of the hand. With the widespread use of dialysis and renal transplantation to treat patients with end-stage renal disease, the more advanced manifestations of uremia are seldom seen. The latter may consist of asterixis and myoclonus; tetany may be apparent. There may be abnormalities of gait and reflexes, such as snouting, rooting, and grasping reflexes. Seizures, either focal or grand mal, may occur.[3]

Allen I. Arieff • Nephrology Service, Department of Medicine, Veterans Administration Medical Center, and University of California School of Medicine, San Francisco, California 94121.

It is probably a safe statement that the pathogenesis of any of the aforementioned manifestations of uremic encephalopathy is not known. There is very little data either on patients or on laboratory animals that reveal the biochemical or pathological abnormalities that may lead to uremic encephalopathy. However, there have been some intriguing biochemical and pathological observations. Prior to the early 1970s, there had been only a few studies on the brain in laboratory animals with renal failure.[4,5] These have revealed that there is increased entry into the uremic brain of ^{14}C-labeled sucrose and ^{42}K. There is delayed entry of [^{24}Na]- and [^{14}C]penicillin, with no apparent effect on the entry of [^{35}S]sulfate and [^{14}C]dimethadione. There is probably a decrease in brain levels of Na–K ATPase. In rats with acute renal failure, van den Nort and associates[5] have studied brain energy metabolism. They found that total brain adenine nucleotides were normal but that there was a decrease of both metabolic rate and lactate formation. Glucose concentration was increased and high-energy phosphate utilization was abnormally low, suggesting the decreased brain metabolic rate.

Histological studies of the brain in renal failure have not been rewarding.[6,7] Studies in patients dying with renal failure have shown a small incidence of subdural hemorrhages, some intracerebral hemorrhage, and generalized neuronal degeneration. There are some necrotic foci and focal glial proliferation. However, all these changes are not specific and do not serve to differentiate uremia from other encephalopathies.

Since neither biochemical nor pathological studies have yet revealed the origin of uremic encephalopathy, investigators have next turned to toxins. More than 50 substances have been described as being "uremic toxins."[8–10] At our present level of knowledge, none of these so-called uremic toxins has been validated experimentally in either patients or laboratory animals.

More recent studies have concentrated on abnormalities of water, electrolyte, and acid–base metabolism in the nervous system. Studies in both patients and laboratory animals with acute renal failure have revealed that brain water is normal as are brain content of K^+ and Mg^{2+}, whereas brain Na^+ is low.[3,11] In patients who have chronic renal failure, brain Na^+ content is normal. Some investigators had suggested that intracellular pH (pHi) in brain might be abnormal in patients with uremia, thus accounting for some of the mental abnormalities associated with the uremic state. Studies in both patients and laboratory animals have not revealed this to be the case. In animals with acute renal failure, despite an acidotic pH of blood, pH is normal in CSF and pHi is normal in both brain and skeletal muscle[12] (Fig. 1). Despite an extracellular acidosis, pHi is normal in muscle, whole body, and white blood cells of patients who have chronic renal failure. Preliminary data suggest that despite the presence of an extracellular acidosis, pHi is not abnormal in liver, brain, or skeletal muscle of animals with chronic renal failure.[13] Brain water is not abnormal in either patients or experimental animals with either acute or chronic renal failure.[3,11–13]

From a biochemical standpoint, one of the first abnormalities reported in uremic brain was the significantly elevated brain (cerebral cortex) Ca^{2+}

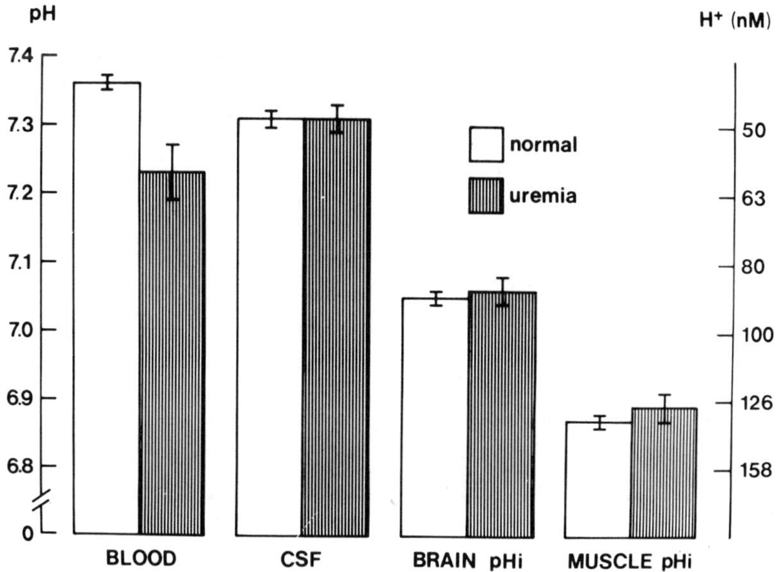

Figure 1. The intracellular pH (pHi) in brain (cerebral cortex) and skeletal muscle of dogs with acute renal failure. Despite an extracellular acidosis, pHi is normal. (Reprinted from ref. 12.)

found in laboratory animals with acute renal failure.[14] These findings have been confirmed in brain (post mortem) of humans with acute renal failure, where brain Ca^{2+} (cerebral cortex) is approximately twice the normal value.[11] The observed elevation in brain Ca^{2+} brings to the forefront the problem of what might have caused this to occur. An increase in the plasma calcium–phosphate product could account for an increased brain Ca^{2+}. However, studies in both humans and animals with acute renal failure reveal no correlation between brain Ca^{2+} content and plasma calcium–phosphate product.[11,14] Another factor that might have caused brain Ca^{2+} to be elevated is parathyroid hormone. Parathyroid hormone is elevated in patients with chronic renal failure. Although they are somewhat nonspecific, symptoms of primary hyperparathyroidism overlap substantially with those of renal failure.[15] In particular, patients with hyperparathyroidism may have impaired recent memory, depression, increased fatigue, impaired mental alertness, and impaired ability to concentrate. Mallette and associates[15] found that mental abnormalities such as weakness, easy fatigability, and various mental disturbances were among the major manifestations of primary hyperparathyroidism. In a recent study on primary hyperparathyroidism by Heath and associates,[16] it was found that of 51 patients with this disorder, 20% had emotional disorders. This was a higher percentage of patients than those presenting with either renal stones, bone disease, or diminished renal function. We thus decided to look at the effects of parathyroid hormone on both brain Ca^{2+} and neuropsychological status. In laboratory animals, it is

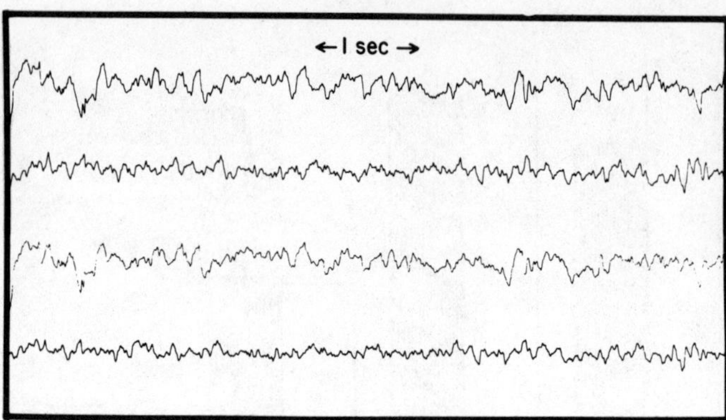

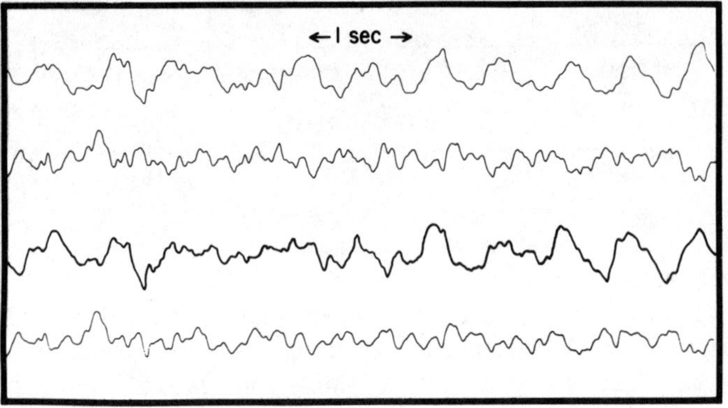

Figure 2. The EEG in a normal subject compared to that of a patient with acute renal failure for 18 hr. The EEG in the patient with renal failure consists almost entirely of abnormal slow waves, despite the fact that the BUN, arterial pH, and plasma concentrations of creatinine, Na^+, K^+, and Cl^- were in the normal range. (Data from ref. 11.)

difficult to conduct any sort of mental status examination, so we did electroencephalograms (EEG). In both patients and laboratory animals who had either uremia or hyperparathyroidism without uremia, it was found that the presence or absence of excess levels of parathyroid hormone in plasma was the main contributor to an abnormal EEG.[3,14,17] In particular, we found that uremic dogs who had previously been parathyroidectomized had near-normal EEGs, whereas normal dogs infused for 3½ days with parathyroid hormone had uremic EEGs.[14] Figure 2 shows the EEG of a patient with acute renal failure. Although the EEG is grossly abnormal, this patient had a BUN below 30 mg/dl, a creatinine below 1.2 mg/dl, and normal pH and K^+ in blood. However, his plasma level of parathyroid hormone was four times the normal value after only 18 hr of acute renal failure. In a dozen patients who had acute renal failure from various causes, we found that the mean Ca^{2+} was only 7.6 mg/dl, and parathyroid hormone was approximately four times the normal value after only 1½ days.[11] Looking at serial EEGs in the same patients at the time of diagnosis, it was found that they were grossly abnormal.[11] After 2–6 weeks of dialysis, there was no change whatsoever in the EEG of patients who had stable chemistries. However, within 24 hr of the onset of the diuretic phase of acute renal failure, the EGGs were not significantly different from normal. At a 3-month follow-up of the same patients, the EEGs were still normal. Among patients who did not survive, it was found that brain Ca^{2+} was increased by approximately 30–50% in patients who had chronic renal failure not treated with dialysis[14,17] (Fig. 2). However, among patients with chronic renal failure treated with dialysis for at least 2 years, both the brain Ca^{2+} and the EEG were not abnormal.[14,17]

We then conducted psychological evaluations of patients who had either primary hyperparathyroidism or uremia with secondary hyperparathyroidism. These patients were evaluated both before and after parathyroidectomy. The controls were patients who underwent major neck surgery for reasons other than parathyroid disease. The EEGs of patients with hyperparathyroidism were abnormal in several different parameters. Both the mean EEG frequency and the percent of frequencies less than 7 hertz were abnormal in patients with either primary or secondary hyperparathyroidism. The percent EEG power less than 5 hertz was abnormal only in patients with secondary hyperparathyroidism. After neck surgery, the EEGs improved toward normal in patients with either primary or secondary hyperparathyroidism, particularly the percent EEG frequencies less than 7 hertz (Fig. 3). Significant improvements toward normal were noted in patients with primary or secondary hyperparathyroidism. Psychological testing was repeated after parathyroidectomy. The patients who had primary hyperparathyroidism showed essentially no change when compared to controls. However, patients with secondary hyperparathyroidism showed improvement in at least four different parameters of psychological function: Raven's progressive matrices, several visual motor items, the trailmaking test, and the profile of moods fatigue scale. Thus, in patients with hyperparathyroidism, the EEGs are abnormal and are improved by parathyroidectomy; certain tests of psychological function improve in patients with secondary hyperparathyroidism after parathyroidectomy; and brain Ca^{2+} in patients with chronic renal failure and secondary hyperparathyroidism is elevated. It may be that the elevated brain Ca^{2+} relates to the EEG and psychological abnormalities (Fig. 4). These studies complete this brief review of the literature on uremic encephalopathy.

2. *Uremic Neuropathy*

Early uremic neuropathy is characterized by periodic numbness and tingling of feet and hands with mild leg weakness. There may be restless leg

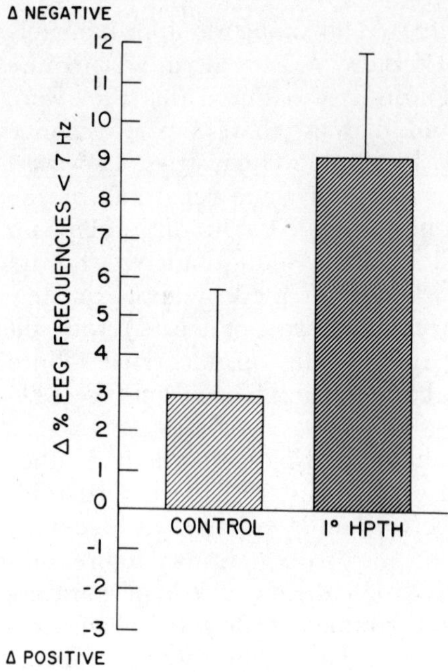

Figure 3. The change (postoperative–preoperative) in the percentage of the EEG occupied by the frequences <7 hertz is shown. Means ± SE are illustrated. There is significant improvement for the patients with primary hyperparathyroidism in this frequency class without a significant change for the control subjects. (Reprinted from ref. 17.)

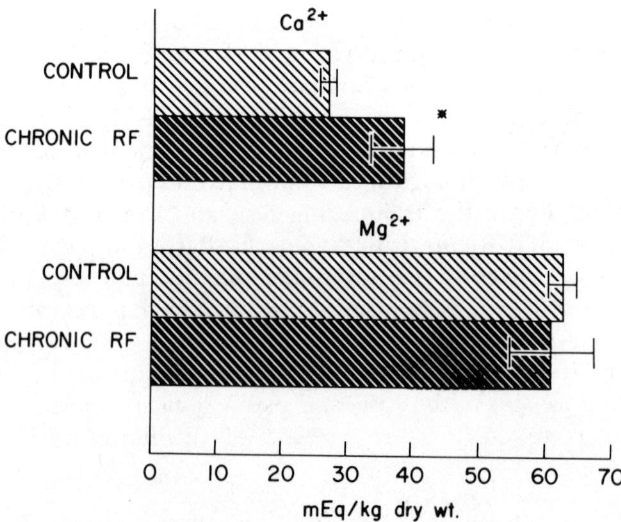

Figure 4. The postmortem calcium and magnesium contents in brain tissue from normal control subjects and from patients with chronic renal failure and secondary hyperparathyroidism are shown. Means ± SE are illustrated, with significance ($p < 0.05$, unpaired t test) denoted by a *. A significant increase in cerebral cortical calcium, but not magnesium, is found in the brains of patients with secondary hyperparathyroidism. (Reprinted from ref. 17.)

syndrome or an unsteady gait. As uremic neuropathy becomes more severe, there may be reduced tendon reflexes and loss of vibration sense. There is impairment of the patient's ability to perceive pain, light touch, or temperature. Typically, the distribution in the legs is that of a stocking glove. Functionally, with very severe uremic neuropathy, the patient may notice persistent numbness and tingling of the extremities, difficulty with walking, and clumsiness with fine movements of the hands, such as problems with writing and buttoning clothes. There may be also associated muscle wasting with weakness.[(18)] It is often overlooked, but uremic neuropathy also may affect the autonomic nervous system. This may be manifested by absence of sweating, impotence, and abnormal Valsalva maneuver, and perhaps by hypotension associated with hemodialysis.

Pathologically, studies on sural nerve of patients who have uremic neuropathy reveal that there is axonal degeneration along with demyelination.[(19)] The demyelination is thought to be a secondary phenomenon.[(19)] Histologically, this is characterized by less fiber density and a decreased thickness of those fibers which are present, along with a loss of myelin on fibers.[(20)] It is not generally appreciated, but as shown by Asbury and associates,[(19)] uremic neuropathy may also effect the spinal cord. There may be pallor of the posterior columns in the spinal cord as well as chromatolysis of the anterior horn cells. In the anterior horn cells at the lower lumbar segments, there often is a characteristic axonal reaction.

Many so-called uremic toxins have been suggested to be important in the pathogenesis of uremic neuropathy.[(2,8–10)] Such so-called toxins include parathyroid hormone, third factor, middle molecules, and several trace metals such as lead, tin, cadmium, zinc, and mercury. However, Nielsen[(18)] showed that if one attempts to correlate a reduction in motor nerve conduction velocity (MNCV) with glomerular filtration rate (GFR), as assessed by several different means, there is a correlation coefficient of 0.68 to 0.84. Neilsen suggested that for any substance to be a uremic toxin, it would therefore have to have a better correlation with MNCV than does GFR. At this time, no "toxin" has been able to fulfill these criteria.[(10)] In human studies, various authors have measured the correlation between MNCV and blood levels of parathyroid hormone, urea, creatinine, myoinositol, and several other substances (Table 1). The correlation coefficients with these substances range from 0.09 to 0.67, none of them being as high as is the correlation with GFR. In addition, it must be pointed out that if one correlates two things that are by definition unrelated, i.e., random numbers, one obtains a correlation coefficient of 0.28 when matching 80 pairs of random numbers. This is significant at the 0.01 level, thus showing that the correlation coefficients in no way show causality.

Another way of looking at neurotoxicity is to study MNCV in animals or patients with acute renal failure. If there is a uremic toxin present in blood, there should be reductions in MNCV in the early phases of renal failure. Preliminary studies in our laboratory show that with acute renal failure for a period of 3½ days to 6 months in the dog, there is no

Table 1. Correlation (r Value) between Motor Nerve Conduction Velocity (MNCV) and Various "Uremic Toxins"[a]

Author	"Uremic toxin"	r	Other
Giulio *et al.*	PTH	0.09	—
Avram *et al.*	PTH	0.45	—
Nielsen	Urea	0.41	—
Blagg *et al.*	Urea	0.51	—
Nielsen	Creatinine	0.51	—
Blagg *et al.*	Creatinine	0.57	—
Blumberg *et al.*	Myoinositol	0.03	—
Reznek *et al.*	Myoinositol	0.67	—
Nielsen	GFR	0.68–0.84	—
Man *et al.*	Middle molecules	Not available	No *in vivo* evidence of peripheral nerve function impairment in patients or animals with renal failure
Scribner *et al.*	Middle molecules		
Kjellstrand *et al.*	Middle molecules		
Giovannetti *et al.*	Methylguanidine	Not available	Chronic injection depresses MNCV in dogs after 10 days
Sterzel *et al.*	Transketolase deficiency	Not available	Deficiency related to impaired MNCV in patients
Lonergan *et al.*	Transketolase deficiency		

[a] From ref. 23; references refer to citations in that reference.

alteration of MNCV.[13] Similarly, studies in 33 patients with acute renal failure demonstrate that MNCV is normal in patients with acute renal failure and is affected neither by dialysis nor by the diuretic phase of acute renal failure; at 3 months' follow-up, MNCV remains normal.[11] Studies by Giulio and associates[21] on uremic patients undergoing hemodialysis have shed some light on the possible role of parathyroid hormone in the pathogenesis of uremic neuropathy. They did MNCV studies on 35 patients before and up to 1 year after parathyroidectomy. The MNCV did not change as a result of the parathyroidectomy. There have been some suggestions that parathyroid hormone might impair MNCV secondary to a deposition of Ca^{2+} in uremic nerve. However, preliminary studies in our laboratory show that in dogs with renal failure for periods of 3½ days to 6 months, there is not a significant increase in nerve Ca^{2+} content.[13] In summary, if one evaluates the role of parathyroid hormone in the pathogenesis of uremic neuropathy in patients, MNCV is normal before and after parathyroidectomy in patients with primary hyperthroidism, MNCV is normal before and after treatment for secondary hyperparathyroidism not due to renal failure, and MNCV is not affected acutely by fourfold elevations in plasma parathyroid hormone in patients with acute renal failure.[10]

Another way of looking at uremic neuropathy is to study the effects of renal transplantation on nerve function. It is the general rule that following renal transplantation, MNCV improves toward normal, but usually not for several months.[18] However, this has not been a universal experience. Ibrahim and associates[22] studied a number of patients with chronic renal failure. They found that after renal transplantation, although some patients did have a return toward normal of MNCV, in other patients, this did not occur even after periods of up to 8 months.

In summary, at this time the etiology of uremic neuropathy must be regarded as complex and unknown. It is probably due to multiple factors and is related to anatomical nerve damage.

References

1. Teschan PE, Ginn HE: The nervous system, in Massry SG, Sellers AL (eds): *Clinical Aspects of Uremia and Dialysis*. Springfield, Illinois, Charles C Thomas, 1976, pp 3–33.
2. Raskin NH, Fishman RA: Neurologic disorders in renal failure. *N Engl J Med* 294:143–148, 204–210, 1976.
3. Arieff AI, Schmidt RW: Fluid and electrolyte disorders and the central nervous system, in Maxwell MH, Kleeman CR (eds): *Clinical Disorders of Fluid and Electrolyte Metabolism*. New York, McGraw–Hill, 1979, pp 1409–1480.
4. Fishman RA: Permeability changes in experimental uremic encephalopathy. *Arch Int Med* 126:835–837, 1970.
5. van den Nort S, Eckel RE, Brine KL, Hrdlicka J: Brain metabolism in experimental uremia. *Arch Int Med* 126:831–834, 1970.
6. Olsen S: The brain in uremia. *Acta Psychiat Scand* 36(Suppl 156):1–128, 1961.
7. Burks JS, Alfrey AC, Huddlestone J, Norenberg MD, Lewin E: A fatal encephalopathy in chronic hemodialysis patients. *Lancet* 1:764–7689, 1976.
8. Massry SG: Is parathyroid hormone a uremic toxin? *Nephron* 19:125–130, 1977.
9. Black DAK: A perspective on uremic toxins. *Arch Int Med* 126:906–909, 1970.
10. Arieff AI, Armstrong DK: Parathyroid hormone and uremic neurotoxicity: An unproven association. *Contr Nephr* 20:56–66, 1980.
11. Cooper JD, Lazarowitz VC, Arieff AI: Neurodiagnostic abnormalities in patients with acute renal failure: Evidence for neurotoxicity of parathyroid hormone. *J Clin Invest* 61:1448–1455, 1978.
12. Arieff AI, Guisado R, Massry SG, Lazarowitz VC: Central nervous system pH in uremia and the effects of hemodialysis. *J Clin Invest* 58:306–311, 1976.
13. Mahoney C, Arieff AI: Central and peripheral nervous system effects of chronic renal failure. *Kidney Int* 24:170–177, 1983.
14. Guisado R, Arieff AI, Massry SG, Lazarowitz VC, Kerian A: Changes in the electroencephalogram in acute uremia: Effects of parathyroid hormone and brain electrolytes. *J Clin Invest* 55:738–745, 1975.
15. Mallette LE, Bilezikian JP, Heath DA, Aurbach GD: Primary hyperparathyroidism: Clinical and biochemical features. *Medicine* 53:127–146, 1974.
16. Heath H, Hodgson SF, Kennedy MA: Primary hyperparathyroidism. *N Engl J Med* 302:189–193, 1980.

17. Cogan M, Covey CM, Arieff AI, Wisniewski A, Clark O, Lazarowitz VC, Leach WJ: Central nervous system manifestations of hyperparathyroidism. *Am J Med* 65:963–970, 1978.
18. Nielsen VK: The peripheral nerve function in chronic renal failure: A survey. *Acta Med Scand* 573(Suppl):7–32, 1974.
19. Asbury AK, Victor M, Adams RD: Uremic polyneuropathy. *Arch Neurol* 8:413–428, 1963.
20. Thomas PK, Hollinrake K, Lascelles RG, O'Sullivan DJ, Baillod RA, Moorhead JF, Mackenzie JC: The polyneuropathy of chronic renal failure. *Brain* 94:761–780, 1971.
21. Giulio SD, Chkoff N, Lhoste F, Zingraff J, Drueke T: Parathormone as a nerve poison in uremia. *N Engl J Med* 299:1134–1135, 1978.
22. Ibrahim MM, Barnes AD, Crosland JM, Edwards PD, Honigsberger L, Newman CE, Robinson BHB: Effect of renal transplantation on uraemic neuropathy. *Lancet* 2:739–742, 1974.
23. Arieff AI: Neurological complications of uremia, in Brenner BM, Rector FC (eds): *The Kidney*, Philadelphia, WB Saunders, 2nd ed, 1981, pp 2306–2343.

19

Dialysis Encephalopathy

Questions and Answers

D. N. S. Kerr, M. K. Ward, and I. S. Parkinson

In this chapter we address ourselves to the questions in Table 1, as a means of reviewing the current state of knowledge about dialysis encephalopathy and of suggesting areas for further research.

1. Is It a Distinct Clinical Syndrome?

The original description by Alfrey *et al.*[1] suggests a distinct entity. However, some investigators remain skeptical, believing that the term embraces a medley of neurological insults inflicted on dialysis patients by such factors as hypertension, atheroma, underdialysis, disequilibrium, hypoxia, hypotension, and drug therapy. A strong argument against this view was the distribution of epidemics; they were often confined to one of several linked dialysis centers where they affected patients without regard for age, blood pressure, adequacy of dialysis, drug therapy, or evidence of arterial disease (Table 2). We were particularly struck by the relative freedom of our patients from cerebral atheroma at autopsy.

There have now been several full descriptions of the disease,[1–11] which are summarized in Table 3 and in Section 2. There is a subclinical prodromal period, during which intellectual impairment can be detected by psychometric tests such as the performance intelligence quotient (IQ)[12] or by formal speech assessment.[13] Often the next phase is recognized only in retrospect; there is a subtle change in personality which earns the patient the reputation

D. N. S. Kerr • Royal Postgraduate Medical School, Hammersmith Hospital, London W12 OHS, England. ***M. K. Ward*** • Department of Medicine, Royal Victoria Infirmary, Newcastle upon Tyne NE1 4LP, England. ***I. S. Parkinson*** • Department of Clinical Biochemistry, Royal Victoria Infirmary, Newcastle upon Tyne NE1 4LP, England.

Table 1. Questions and Answers about Dialysis Encephalopathy

Question	Suggested answer
1. Is it a distinct clinical syndrome?	Yes
2. Are there specific confirmatory investigations?	No, but the EEG is helpful
3. Has it a specific pathology?	Probably yes, but unpublished
4. Is aluminum intoxication the cause?	Yes
5. What is the usual source of the aluminum?	The dialysate, from tap water
6. Can aluminum be removed reliably from tap water?	Yes, but water supplies are idiosyncratic
7. Are aluminum-containing gels a cause of raised serum aluminum?	Yes, but a much less powerful influence than the dialysate
8. Do aluminum gels cause encephalopathy?	Uncertain: very rare if it happens
9. Is the syndrome reversible	
a. by transplantation?	Yes, if carried out early
b. by exclusion of aluminum during dialysis?	Yes, if carried out early and thoroughly
10. How does aluminum damage the brain?	Your guess is as good as ours
11. Does hyperparathyroidism predispose to encephalopathy?	Doubtful, more work needed
12. How is the uptake of dialysate aluminum affected by other solutes?	Critically, but there is a lot to learn

of being obstinate, truculent, or difficult and which led to the breakdown of home dialysis in three of our patients before the disease was diagnosed. The feature that commonly leads to diagnosis is speech impairment. It is usually described as dysphasia, but there is an element of dysarthria. It often appears first during dialysis and may be precipitated by fluid depletion. However, it soon affects the patient at any time, and eventually he may be reduced to permanent aphasia.

Myoclonic jerks are a common early feature and may be accompanied by facial grimacing. These can reach disabling proportions, interfering with swallowing and eventually causing aspiration pneumonia. At an early stage

Table 2. Potentially Etiological Features in Which Newcastle Encephalopathy Patients Did Not Differ Significantly from Others on the Same Dialysis Unit

Age and sex
Blood pressure—present and past
Predialysis creatinine
Drug therapy (other than phosphate binders)
Other evidence of atheroma
History of dialysis complications

Table 3. Clinical Features of Dialysis Encephalopathy

Prodromal
Impaired performance IQ
Reduced fluency in speech tests
Change in personality
Marital and dialysis difficulties
EEG: slow wave activity
Clinically manifest
Dysphasia and dysarthria: dialysis related → intermittent → continuous
Myoclonic jerks
Facial grimacing
Dyspraxia
Ataxia
Grand mal seizures
EEG: slow wave activity, biphasic and triphasic spikes
Terminal
Dementia
Dysphagia → aspiration
Extreme ataxia—inability to feed or clothe
Associated features
Osteomalacia, Myopathy: Common, not invariable
Anemia, Vomiting, Malaise: Described by some authors
Weight loss

the grimacing and dysphagia are often relieved by an injection of diazepam or clonazepam; this is one of several features that led Alfrey *et al.*[1] and later Nadel and Wilson[9] to describe dialysis encephalopathy as a seizure disorder. Grand mal fits are common and affected nearly half our patients. The gait is unsteady and on a wide base. Dyspraxia affects all activities and eventually prevents the patient from feeding himself; it is often detectable first in the handwriting, which deteriorates rapidly with the effort of writing a few lines. Intellectual deterioration is rapid, but insight appears to be retained longer than in most forms of dementia. The patients weep easily, and it appears that two patients who had become aphasic were trying to let us know that they would like to die in peace.

2. *Are There Specific Confirmatory Investigations?*

The clinical picture of advanced dialysis encephalopathy is readily recognized, but early diagnosis is more difficult and is necessary if possible preventive measures such as renal transplantation are to be undertaken. The electroencephalogram (EEG) shows a characteristic, though nonspecific, combination of abnormalities—slow wave activity at 1–4 waves/sec and biphasic or triphasic spike waves, spread uniformly over the leads. No other laboratory test is of much value. Cerebrospinal fluid pressure is normal, and the concentrations of protein, dextrose, and chloride are also normal. The isotope brain scan shows minor or no abnormalities and the CAT scan may reveal slight ventricular enlargement.[8]

3. Has It a Specific Pathology?

Remarkably little has been found on postmortem examination of the brain. Burks *et al.*[4] described slight loss of Purkinje cells in the cerebellum and gliosis, in one of their patients, and these were more striking features of our own cases.[11] Chokroverty *et al.*[5] found only a few nonspecific lacunar infarcts. Galle *et al.*[11a] have published electron micrographs depicting a unique lesion—deposition of uniform crystals of aluminum phosphate in the lysosomes of brain cells. The lack of specific abnormalities on electron microscopy may relate to the fact that autolysis of the brain is extensive within 24 hr and the brain is rarely available for study in less than that interval.

4. Is Aluminum Intoxication the Cause?

We have recently reviewed the evidence,[6,10] which we find convincing. Alfrey *et al.*[14] showed that the aluminum content of brain, bone, and muscle was substantially raised in patients with encephalopathy. This has been confirmed for brain by workers in Britain,[15] France,[16] and the Netherlands.[17] Flendrig *et al.*[17] also showed aluminum overload in several other tissues. However, several investigations have not confirmed the rise in brain aluminum. Platts and Hislop[18] found only a modest increase, and Pascoe and Gregory[19] found none. Others have shown that aluminum in brain is similar in patients with chronic renal failure with or without dialysis dementia. The weight of evidence is strongly in favour of aluminum overload being a constant feature of the disease.

The epidemiological evidence is also compelling. In our study of British dialysis centers, encephalopathy was almost unknown if the tap water aluminum was below 50 μg/liter; the association between encephalopathy and exposure to aluminum was so high as to suggest that there were no obvious other factors of major importance involved in the disease.[20]

Some support to the aluminum theory is lent by the close association between encephalopathy and fracturing, osteomalacic osteodystrophy,[11,17,20–23] which is also a disease associated with increased solutes in the dialysis fluid.[24,25] There is growing evidence from bone biopsy[26,27] and from experimental studies in rats[28] that aluminum is the solute in question.

Serum aluminum in dialyzed patients reflects the aluminum content of the dialysate to which they have been recently exposed,[24] so it is not a reliable guide to body burden. However, if the dialysate has been kept constant, it may better reflect aluminum exposure over the whole dialysis experience.[16,19,29]

5. What Is the Usual Source of the Aluminum?

Flendrig *et al.*[17] gave the first convincing evidence that dialysis fluid could be an important source of aluminum. One of two dialysis centers in Eindhoven, using the same city water supply, suffered an outbreak of encephalopathy while the other was immune. City water had a low aluminum content but the affected center had aluminum anticorrosion devices (anodes) in the water supply; these dissolved, releasing aluminum into the dialysate. Almost all subsequent studies have shown the dialysate to be the most important source. In the EDTA European survey,[30] there was no association between encephalopathy and consumption of aluminum gels, but there was a relationship to the use of untreated water. Our British survey[20] showed a clear-cut relationship to water aluminum level, and a similar relationship has been found in many single-center or local surveys.[3,8,16,18,23,29,31–34] There is one puzzling exception; at Nashville 5% of the patients developed dementia in spite of a water aluminum well below 50 μg/liter.[35] The aluminum content of municipal water supplies often fluctuates considerably from day to day; outbreaks of encephalopathy have followed a change in flocculation procedure at a waterworks[8] or the malfunction of a deionizer,[31] but these possibilities seem to have been ruled out at Nashville. Further information on this interesting epidemic is eagerly awaited, but the overwhelming evidence is that dialysate aluminum is the most important source of intoxication.

Uptake from the dialysate into the patient, against a concentration gradient since plasma aluminum is largely protein bound, was shown by Kaehny *et al.*[36] and confirmed by others,[16,37,38] though some of the studies are difficult to interpret; e.g., Salvadeo *et al.*[38] found uptake from the dialysate but no rise in plasma level. Our studies (unpublished) are in broad agreement with those of Kaehny *et al.*[36] Aluminum is taken up, and serum aluminum rises, unless dialysate is reduced to a very low level (circa 10 μg/liter) when changes in serum aluminum can be explained on hemoconcentration alone. Graf *et al.*,[39] using very pure water to prepare dialysate, were able to remove some aluminum from their patients. More work is needed in this field; some of the anomalies may be explained by differences in dialysate pH, which has a profound effect on aluminum transfer.[40]

6. *Can Aluminum Be Removed Reliably from Tap Water?*

In a preliminary study[41] we showed that water softeners were unreliable and, on some supplies, almost completely ineffective, despite the strong affinity of ionized aluminum for cation-exchange resins. This phenomenon deserves more study than it has received, but it seems likely that it depends on water pH. Aluminum has a U-shaped solubility curve, its nadir being close to the pH we seek in our water supplies (around 7.4). At this pH most of the aluminum in water is in colloidal form and probably unreactive with resins; a small shift in pH results in a big change in ionization.

Deionizers are much more effective; presumably the changes in water pH that occur during the passage through a deionizer ensure that much of the aluminum is ionized at some stage. However, we have monitored the effluent from a deionizer attached to the Newcastle water supply, and regenerated regularly, and have found peaks of aluminum in the "deionized" water into the danger range over 50 μg/liter. Two reverse osmosis systems—one hollow fiber and one spirally wound—have consistently produced water with an aluminum content below 20 μg/liter.

7. *Are Aluminum-Containing Gels a Cause of Raised Serum Aluminum?*

Kaehny *et al.*[42] detected a small rise in serum aluminum when they gave aluminum hydroxide and other antacids to normal subjects; there was also a fourfold increase in urinary aluminum. Dialysis patients are denied this excretory pathway, so one would expect them to show a greater rise in serum aluminum for a give intake. Our own studies[43] showed a modest rise in serum aluminum in chronic renal failure, in the absence of dialysis of aluminum gel ingestion, but a much more substantial rise when aluminum gels were ingested. Similar results were obtained by others[44,45] except that Zumkley *et al.*[45] found no elevation of serum aluminum in nondialyzed patients taking no gels. All are agreed that phosphate binders elevate serum aluminum in renal failure.

8. *Do Aluminum Gels Cause Encephalopathy?*

The elevated serum levels found in patients taking aluminum gels are usually well below those found in centers with epidemic encephalopathy. There are a few exceptions; two of our patients have had persistently elevated serum levels of >200 μg/liter when taking aluminium hydroxide at the predialysis clinic. Both have stable chronic renal failure with a plasma creatinine around 600 μmole/liter, and one has taken the medicine for more than 3 and the other for more than 14 years; neither shows signs of dementia, and the latter has retained his job as chairman of a large company. It may be that orally administered aluminum is less damaging than rapid infusions during dialysis. In dogs, the infusion of aluminum causes retention of more than half the aluminum in body pools even if renal function is normal.[46] The enormous quantities of aluminum-containing medicines given to patients in renal failure worldwide, with so little proven harm, encourage us to go on using this invaluable weapon against hyperparathyroidism. However, we suggest that patients taking large doses should have regular checks on serum aluminum, and alternatives such as parathyroidectomy should be considered if the level climbs above, say, 100 μg/liter. At least seven patients have now been described who appeared to develop dialysis encephalopathy without dialysis.[10,47] Our own patient has been described only in brief outline. She was a 63-year-old woman with stable chronic renal failure, with plasma creatinine around 1000 μmoles/liter for more than 3 years. During this period she had persistent hyperphosphataemia for which she took, conscientiously, increasing doses of aluminium hydroxide gel BP eventually rising to 80 ml/day. Her total ingestion remained well below that achieved by many of our other patients with a longer duration of treatment. After 3 years, she developed progressive dementia but without the typical speech disturbance of dialysis encephalopathy. She died of a myocardial infarction and at autopsy had very severe osteomalacia of the type seen with dialysis encephalopathy, and her bone aluminum was the highest recorded in a nondialyzed patient in the study of Ellis *et al.*[28]

Several other patients have been described whose encephalopathy was attributed to ingestion of aluminum though, as they were on dialysis, it is difficult to exclude the possibility that some of their overload came from that source.[48,49] Eade's patient had a relapse when aluminum gel was readministered and a further remission when it was withdrawn.[49]

Much more information is needed, but at the moment it appears that encephalopathy due to aluminum ingestion alone is a very rare but probably real phenomenon. We need to know how to limit aluminum absorption by choice of preparation, timing of dose, and other means.

9. *Is the Syndrome Reversible?*

The results of transplantation in our own patients are shown in Table 4. They are in line with other reports[50,51] which show that transplantation performed early in the course of the disease arrests its progress whereas patients with advanced disease continue to deteriorate and die. However, it is no easy decision to transplant. Residual intellectual loss can be considerable. One of our "successes" was an accountant before he developed encephalopathy; he now upholsters chairs under supervision. Speech often improves but dysphasia recurs when the patient is agitated; bone disease slowly heals.

Transfer to a purer water supply, and restriction of oral aluminum, has arrested the disease in four of our patients. They have not returned to normal, perhaps because the deionized water was not sufficiently free of

Table 4. Attempts to Reverse Encephalopathy at Newcastle

Cadaver transplantation	
Transplanted early in the disease: neurological status stabilized	5
Dementia progressed in spite of functioning graft (performed late in two cases)	3
Graft failed: patient returned to dialysis with high dialysate aluminum; dementia progressed to death	3
Transferred to purer dialysate (made with distilled or deionized water, 3; transferred to Sunderland, 1)	
Encephalopathy stabilized	4

aluminum. Others have reported more impressive clinical improvement and substantial change in the EEG[48,52–54] in striking contrast to the rapid downhill course of those whose water supply is unchanged.[55]

10. How Does Aluminum Damage the Brain?

There is a little speculation in the literature but almost no fact.

11. Does Hyperparathyroidism Predispose to Encephalopathy?

Mayor and his group have adduced considerable evidence for this hypothesis, in the rat[56–59]; aluminum is better absorbed if parathyroid hormone (PTH) is given, its migration into the brain is enhanced, and the learning behavior of rats is impaired. Subtotal parathyroidectomy appeared to benefit one patient.[60] However, the clinical evidence is not impressive; the fracturing osteodystrophy that often accompanies encephalopathy is characterized by a normal or minimally elevated serum alkaline phosphatase, a slightly elevated serum PTH, and little evidence of osteitis fibrosa. It may be that this is the end result, after aluminum poisoning enhanced by previous hyperparathyroidism, but our case records do not suggest it.

12. How Is the Uptake of Dialysate Aluminum Affected by Other Solutes?

We return to the dialysate, possibly the main cause of encephalopathy, to emphasize in closing how little we know about the chemistry of aluminum in tap water. Does the fluoride, added by our water board in the interests of dental health, form stable compounds with aluminum, and if so, are these protected from removal during water purification? How rapidly does colloidal aluminum redissolve in a deionizer or a dialysis bath? To these and many other questions we need answers that must come from research workers with a more appropriate background than clinical nephrology.

13. Addendum

Since this chapter was first written, dialysis encephalopathy has been universally accepted as a distinct entity, though it must still be distinguished from the other neurological syndromes occurring in renal failure.[61] A recently described encephalopathy of infants in chronic renal failure[62] has occurred in children who had never taken aluminum or been exposed to dialysis. It is characterized by delayed head growth, seizures, dyskinesia, hypotonia, and developmental delay. Although there are some resemblances to dialysis encephalopathy, and aluminum may be incriminated in some children, it seems likely that it is a distinct manifestation of uremic damage to the growing brain.[61]

The association of dialysis encephalopathy and vitamin D-resistant osteomalacia and iron-unresponsive microcytic anemia has been confirmed.[63,64] Little has been added to the clinical description of the encephalopathy, and laboratory investigations, other than the EEG, remain unhelpful. Some further information has emerged in response to Questions 4–7 and 9–12.

4. Is Aluminum Intoxication the Cause?

The epidemiological evidence is now overwhelming and has led to almost universal acceptance of a cause-and-effect relationship. There have been further reports of epidemics in which the occurrence of encephalopathy was closely related to the presence of high aluminum concentrations in water used to make dialysis fluid and improvement in the condition followed effective water treatment.[65–68] No good animal model of the disease has been devised; infusion or ingestion of aluminum causes reduced bone formation, sometimes osteomalacia, damage to hepatocytes, and occasionally renal failure[69–73] but does not produce dialysis encephalopathy. Possibly the right experimental conditions have not been found.

5. What Is the Usual Source of the Aluminum?

It remains true that epidemics of encephalopathy have been almost confined to centers with high dialysis fluid aluminum. There has been no published equivalent of the Nashville epidemic described previously.[35] However, further information about that outbreak has been published[74,75]; the evidence that it was caused by gastrointestinal absorption of aluminum is hard to contravert; five patients improved when aluminum-containing phosphate binders were withdrawn or replaced by magnesium hydroxide. We conclude that most epidemics are caused by contaminated dialysis fluid, usually as a result of inadequate treatment of the water supply, but occasional epidemics and a growing number of sporadic cases have been caused by oral absorption of aluminum.

6. Can Aluminum Be Removed Reliably from Tap Water?

There is now plentiful evidence that tap water aluminum can be reduced to almost undetectable levels (less than 5 μg/liter) by sequential softening, reverse osmosis, and deionization. However, the cost of treating water with this thoroughness is high, expecially in home hemodialysis. A recent British paper suggests that a lower standard (up to 27 μg/liter) is an acceptable compromise.[76] We disagree; the standard commercial concentrate in the United Kingdom contributes about 10 μg/liter to the final concentration, and a dialysate of 37 μg/liter will cause substantial uptake by all but the most heavily overloaded patients. Deionization alone will reduce water aluminum to less than 27 μg/liter consistently in some water supplies[76] but not in others.[63] One reason for the difference is the pH of water; at a pH of 6, most of the aluminum in Newcastle water is in colloidal form, which passes through mixed-bed deionizers largely unchanged.[63]

7. Are Aluminum-Containing Gels a Cause of Raised Serum Aluminum?

The answer is now an emphatic "yes," but the patients vary widely in serum aluminum on a given prescribed dose. Some authors have attributed this largely to differences in compliance,[77] but others have not found this an adequate explanation. We observed a wide range in rise of serum aluminum when a standard dose of aluminum hydroxide was given to a group of well-motivated patients whose compliance was checked by weekly measurements of serum phosphate.[78] It now seems likely that some patients are "hyperabsorbers" of aluminum who can produce dangerous levels of serum aluminum; at Nashville levels greater than 600 μg/liter were recorded, and a number of similar reports are in press in the proceedings of a conference at Antwerp in 1983. Although encephalopathy from this cause is rare, osteomalacia is not, and it is clear that aluminum-containing phosphate binders will have to be used with much more caution. Fortunately they can sometimes be replaced by oral calcium carbonate[79] and a synthetic aluminum-free phosphate binder is performing well in premarketing trials in Germany.[80]

9. Is the Syndrome Reversible?

Further reports of the results of renal transplantation bear out what was stated previously; operation late in the disease is not helpful, but in the early stages it may effect a partial or complete cure, often preceded by an exacerbation in the early postoperative period.[68,81,82] Although water treatment and withdrawal of aluminum-containing medications is often followed by improvement, it is not easy to remove aluminum by hemodialysis. Protein binding of aluminum has been found by several authors to be in the range 60–90%, so a very low dialysis fluid level is needed to prevent uptake during dialysis if the patient's serum aluminum is below 100 μg/liter. Graf and colleagues[83,84] achieved a fall in serum aluminum during dialysis in all their patients with a dialysate of 3–8 μg/liter, but Fleming and his colleagues[77] could not achieve this with a dialysis fluid consistently below 10 μg/liter.

The outlook for patients was changed by the introduction of desferrioxamine as a chelating agent.[85] Subsequent reports have confirmed the substantial improvement that takes place within weeks in dialysis encephalopathy,[86–88] and many more reports attest the value of desferrioxamine in treating bone disease and anemia. It is given in a dose of 2–4 g as a slow infusion toward the end of one dialysis; mobilization of aluminum from tissues is maximum at about 48 hr, in good time for the next dialysis. The Al–desferrioxamine complex is better removed by high-permeability membranes, or hemoperfusion, than by conventional dialysis, but improvement occurs with any of these techniques. There have been occasional reports of visual disturbance from high doses of desferrioxamine, and there is sometimes a transient exacerbation of symptoms after the first few doses, so it is wise to start with a dose no greater than 2 g.

10. *How Does Aluminum Damage the Brain?*

Aluminum has been shown to induce neurofibrillary tangles,[89,90] inhibit various brain enzymes,[91,92] increase blood–brain permeability,[93] and bind with calmodulin,[94,95] but whether any of these effects explains its action in dialysis encephalopathy remains uncertain.

11. *Does Hyperparathyroidism Predispose to Encephalopathy?*

The evidence that PTH increases transport of aluminum into and out of the rat brain is impressive,[96] but its effect on aluminum absorption from the gut is more controversial. There is little clinical evidence that hyperparathyroidism predisposes to any form of aluminum toxicity.

On the other hand, there is increasing evidence that aluminum intoxication suppresses the parathyroids. It prevents secretion of PTH from isolated parathyroids,[97] suppresses PTH in intact rats,[98] and prevents a normal rise in serum PTH in response to hypocalcemia in dialysis patients.[99,100]

12. *How Is the Uptake of Dialysate Aluminum Affected by Other Solutes?*

Our ignorance of this topic is still profound. It is clear that aluminum reacts with many compounds in tap water, forming monomeric compounds with hydroxyl and fluoride ions, polynuclear compounds, and associations with organic materials such as humic acids in tap water.[101] It moves readily from colloidal to ionized form as water pH changes or dialysate concentrate is added.[63] An *in vitro* study showed that aluminum transfer across a dialysis membrane fell almost to zero if the dialysate pH was kept in the range 6.3–7.7.[40] We think this is unlikely to be true *in vivo* since this is the pH range that dialysis centers seek to achieve, and we have confirmed that it is consistently achieved in two dialysis units (Newcastle and Sunderland) in which serum aluminum rises rapidly when the dialysis fluid is made from base-softened water.[(63)]

The earlier models of the Redy dialysate regeneration cartridge leaked aluminum, particularly into bicarbonate-containing solutions.[(102,103)] A new cartridge has been produced (D-3160) from which most of the aluminum content has been eliminated; preliminary studies with this system suggest that aluminum release is no longer a serious problem.[(104)]

References

1. Alfrey AC, Mishell JM, Burks J, Contiguglia SR, Rudolph H, Lewin E, Holmes JH: Syndrome of dyspraxia and multifocal seizures associated with chronic hemodialysis. Transactions. *Am Soc Artif Intern Organs* 18:257–261, 1972.
2. Barratt LJ, Lawrence JR: Dialysis-associated dementia. *Aust New Zeal J Med* 5:62–65, 1975.
3. Bone I: Progressive dialysis encephalopathy: "Dialysis dementia," in Davison AM (ed): *Dialysis Review*. Tunbridge Wells, Pitman, 1978, pp 216–229.
4. Burks JS, Alfrey AC, Huddlestone J, Norenberg MD, Lewin E: A fatal encephalopathy in chronic haemodialysis patients. *Lancet* 1:764–768, 1976.
5. Chokroverty S, Bruetman ME, Berger V, Reyes, MG: Progressive dialytic encephalopathy. *J Neurol Neurosurg Psychiatr* 39:411–419, 1976.
6. Kerr DNS: Clinical and pathologic changes in patients on chronic dialysis: The central nervous system, in Hamburger J, Crosnier J, Grünefeld J-P, Maxwell MH (eds): *Advances in Nephrology*, Vol 9. Chicago, Year Book, 1980, pp 109–132.
7. Mahurkar SD, Dhar SK, Salta R, Meyers L, Smith EC, Dunea G: Dialysis dementia. *Lancet* 1:1412–1415, 1973.
8. Mahurkar SD, Smith EC, Mamdani BH, Dunea G: Dialysis dementia—the Chicago experience. *J Dialysis* 2:447–458, 1978.
9. Nadel AM, Wilson WP: Dialysis encephalopathy: A possible seizure disorder. *Neurology* 26:1130–1134, 1976.
10. Ward MK, Feest TG: Dialysis encephalopathy, in Anderton JL, Parsons FM, Jones DE: *Living with Renal Failure*. Lancaster, MTP Press, 1978, pp 123–133.
11. Ward MK, Pierides AM, Fawcett P, Shaw DA, Perry RH, Tomlinson BE, Kerr DNS: Dialysis encephalopathy syndrome. *Proc Eur Dial Transpl Assoc* 13:348–354, 1976.
11a. Galle P, Chatel M, Berry JP, Menault F: Encephalopathie progressive des dialysés: Preésence d'aluminium en forte concentration dans les lysosomes des cellules cérébrales. *Nouv Presse Med* 8:4091–4094, 1979.
12. English A, Savage RD, Britton PG, Ward MK, Kerr DNS: Intellectual impairment in chronic renal failure. *Br Med J* 1:880–890, 1978.
13. Ackrill P, Barron J, Whiteley S, Horn AC, Ralston AJ: A new approach to the early detection of dialysis encephalopathy. *Proc Eur Dial Transpl Assoc* 16:659–660, 1979.
14. Alfrey AC, LeGendre GR, Kaehny WD: The dialysis encephalopathy syndrome. Possible aluminium intoxication. *N Engl J Med* 294:184–188, 1976.
15. McDermott JR, Smith AI, Ward MK, Parkinson IS, Kerr DNS: Brain-aluminium concentration in dialysis encephalopathy. *Lancet* 1:901–904, 1978.
16. Cartier F, Allain P, Gary J, Chatel M, Menault F, Pecker S: Encéphalopathie myoctonique progressive des dialysés. Rôle de l'eau utilisée pour l'hémodialyse. *Nouv Presse Méd* 7:97–102, 1978.
17. Flendrig JA, Kruis HK, Das HA: Aluminium intoxication: The cause of dialysis dementia? *Proc Eur Dialy Transpl Assoc* 13:355–361, 1976.
18. Platts MM, Hislop JS: Aluminium and dialysis encephalopathy. *Lancet* 2:98, 1976.

19. Pascoe MD, Gregory MC: Dialysis encelphalopathy: Aluminum concentration in dialysate and brain. *Kidney Int* 16:90, 1979.
20. Parkinson IS, Ward MK, Feest TG, Fawcett RWP, Kerr DNS: Fracturing dialysis osteodystrophy and dialysis encephalopathy: An epidemiological survey. *Lancet* 1:406–409, 1979.
21. Platts MM, Moorhead PJ, Grech P: Dialysis dementia. *Lancet* 2:159, 1973.
22. Platts MM, Goode GC, Hislop JS: Composition of the domestic water supply and the incidence of fractures and encephalopathy in patients on home dialysis. *Br Med J* 2:657–660, 1977.
23. Masramon J, Ricart MJ, Caralps A, Lloveras J, Andreu J, Brulles A, Solá R: Dialysis encephalopathy. *Lancet* 1:1370, 1978.
24. Ward MK, Feest TG, Ellis HA, Parkinson IS, Kerr DNS, Herrington J, Goode GL: Osteomalacic dialysis osteodystrophy: Evidence for a water-borne aetiological agent, probably aluminium. *Lancet* 1:841–845, 1978.
25. Hudson G, Milne J, Reis P, Meyer AM, Hayward A: Renal osteodystrophy in regular hemodialysis patients using softened or deionized water. *Kidney Int* 16:87, 1979.
26. Alfrey AC, Hegg A, Miller N, Berl T, Berns A: Interrelationship between calcium and aluminium metabolism in dialyzed uremic patients. *Mineral Electrolyte Metab* 2:81–87, 1979.
27. Cournot–Witner G, Zingraff J, Bourdon R, Drueke T, Balsan S: Aluminium and dialysis bone disease. *Lancet* 2:795–796, 1979.
28. Ellis HA, McCarthy JH, Herrington J: Bone aluminium in haemodialysed patients and in rats injected with aluminium chloride: Relationship to impaired bone mineralisation. *J Clin Pathol* 32:832–844, 1979.
29. Elluott HL, Dryburgh F, Fell GS, Sabet S, MacDougall AI: Aluminium toxicity during regular haemodialysis. *Br Med J* 1:1101–1103, 1978.
30. Jacobs C, Brunner FP, Chantler C, Donckerwolcke RA, Gurland HJ, Hathway RA, Selwood NH, Wing AJ: Combined report on regular dialysis and transplantation in Europe VII, 1976. *Proc Eur Dial Transpl Assoc* 14:3–67, 1977.
31. Berkseth R, Mahowald M, Anderson D, Shapiro F: Dialysis encephalopathy: Diagnostic criteria and epidemiology of 39 patients. *Kidney Int* 14:670, 1978.
32. Rozas VV, Port FK, Easterling RD: An outbreak of dialysis dementia due to aluminium in the dialysate. *J Dialysis* 2:459–470, 1978.
33. Rozas VV, Port FK, Rutt WM: Progressive dialysis encephalopathy from dialysate aluminum. *Arch Intern Med* 138:1375–1377, 1978.
34. Schreeder MT: Dialysis encephalopathy. *Arch Intern Med* 139:510–511, 1979.
35. McKinney TD, Dewberry FL, Stone WJ, Alfrey AC: Dialysis dementia at the Nashville Veterans Administration Hospital. *Kidney Int* 14:680, 1978.
36. Kaehny WD, Alfrey AC, Holman RD, Shorr WJ: Aluminum transfer during hemodialysis. *Kidney Int* 12:361–365, 1977.
37. Allain P, Thebaud HE, Dupouet L, Coville P, Pissant M, Spiesser J, Alquier P: Étude des taux sanguins de quelques métaux (Al, Mn, Cd, Pb, Cu, Zn) chez les hémodialysés chroniques avant et aprés dialyse. *Nouv Presse Méd* 7:92–96, 1978.
38. Salvadeo A, Minoia C, Segnagni S, Villa G: Trace metal changes in dialysis fluid and blood of patients on hemodialysis. *Int J Artificial Organs* 2:17–21, 1979.
39. Graf H, Stummvoll HK, Meisinger V, Kovarik J, Wolf A, Pingerra WF: Aluminium in haemodialysis. *Lancet* 1:379, 1979.
40. Gacek EM, Babb AL, Uvelli DA, Fry DL, Scribner BH: Dialysis dementia: The role of dialysate pH in altering the dialyzability of aluminum. *Trans Am Soc Artif Intern Organs*, 25:409–415, 1979.
41. Parkinson IS, Beckett A, Ward MK, Feest TG, Hoenich N, Strong A, Kerr DNS: Aluminium: Removal from water supplies. *Proc Eur Dial Transpl Assoc* 15:586–587, 1978.
42. Kaehny WD, Hegg AP, Alfrey AC: Gastrointestinal absorption of aluminum from aluminum-containing antacids. *N Engl J Med* 296:1389–1390, 1977.

43. Marsden SNE, Parkinson IS, Ward MK, Ellis HA, Kerr DNS: Evidence of aluminium accumulation in renal failure. *Proc Eur Dial Transpl Assoc* 16:588–594, 1979.
44. Boukari M, Rottembourg J, Jaudon MC, Clavel JP, Legrain M, Galli A: Influence de la prise prolongée de gels d'alumine sur les tauz sériques d'aluminium chez les patients atteints d'insufficance rénale chronique. *Nouv Presse Méd* 7:85–88, 1978.
45. Zumkley H, Bertram HP, Lison A, Knoll O, Losse H: Aluminium, zinc and copper concentrations in plasma in chronic renal insufficiency. *Clin Nephrol* 12:18–21, 1979.
46. Kovalchik MT, Kaehny WD, Hegg AP, Jackson JT, Alfrey AC: Aluminum kinetics during hemodialysis. *J Lab Clin Med* 92:712–720, 1978.
47. Mehta RP: Encephalopathy in chronic renal failure appearing before the start of dialysis. *Can Med Assoc J* 120:1112–1114, 1979.
48. Buge A, Poisson M, Masson S, Bleibel JM, Mashaly R, Jaudon MC, Lafforgue B, Lebkin B, Raymond P: Encephalopathie réversible des dialysés après arrêt de l'apport d'aluminium. *Nouv Presse Méd* 8:2729–2733, 1979.
49. Eade OA, Krawitt EL, Grice D, Wright R, Trowell J: Reversible dialysis encephalopathy: Role for aluminium-containing gels. *Lancet* 2:1386–1387, 1978.
50. Silke B, Fitzgerald GGR, Hanson S, Carmody M, O'Dwyer, WF: Dialysis dementia and renal transplantation. *Dialysis Transplant* 7:486–487, 1978.
51. Sullivan PA, Murnaghan DJ, Callaghan N: Dialysis dementia: Recovery after renal transplantation. *Br Med J* 2:740–741, 1977.
52. Pierides AM: Dialysis dementia, osteomalacic fractures and myopathy: A syndrome due to chronic aluminum intoxication. *Int J Artificial Organs* 1:206–208, 1978.
53. Pierides AM, Edwards W, Cullum U, Ellis HA: An epidemic of the haemodialysis encephalopathy, myopathy and fracture syndrome in Columbia, SC, USA, in *Abstracts 7th International Congress of Nephrology*, Montreal, ISN, 1978, p S-13.
54. Poisson M, Mashaly R, Lebkiri B: Dialysis encephalopathy: Recovery after interruption of aluminium intake. *Br Med J* 2:1610–1611, 1978.
55. Berkseth RO, Anderson DC, Mahowald MW, Shapiro F: Dialysis encephalopathy: Effects of continued aluminum exposure and clonazepam on prognosis. *Kidney Int* 14:670, 1978.
56. Mayor GH, Keiser JA, Makdani D, Ku PK: Aluminum absorption and distribution: Effect of parathyroid hormone. *Science* 197:1187–1189, 1977.
57. Mayor GH, Kesier JA, Sanchez TV, Sprague SM, Hook JB: Factors affecting tissue aluminum concentration. *J Dialysis* 2:471–481, 1978.
58. Noordewier B, Commissaris RL, Cordon J, Keiser JA, Mayor GH, Rech RH: Effect of chronic oral aluminium administration on shuttlebox avoidance behavior in rats. *Kidney Int* 14:682, 1978.
59. Sprague SM, Sanchez TV, Hourani MR, Keiser JA, Mayor GH: Egress of aluminum from rat brain following withdrawal of parathyroid hormone, in *Abstracts 7th International Congress of Nephrology*, Montreal, ISN, 1978, p S-18.
60. Ball JH, Butkus DE, Madison DS: Effect of subtotal parathyroidectomy on dialysis dementia. *Nephron* 18:151–155, 1975.
61. Mahoney CA, Arieff AI: Uremic encephalopathies: Clinical, biochemical and experimental features. *Am J Kidney Dis* 2:324–336, 1982.
62. Rotundo A, Nevins TE, Lipton M, Lockman LA, Mauer SM, Michael AF: Progressive encephalopathy in children with chronic renal insufficiency in infancy. *Kidney Int* 21:486–491, 1982.
63. Parkinson IS, Ward MK, Kerr DNS: Dialysis encephalopathy, bone disease and anaemia: The aluminium intoxication syndrome during regular haemodialysis. *J Clin Pathol* 34:1285–1294, 1981.
64. Wills MR, Savory J: Aluminium poisoning: Dialysis encephalopathy, osteomalacia, and anaemia. *Lancet* 2:29–34, 1983.
65. Leather HM, Lewin IG, Calder E, Braybrooke J, Cox RR: Effect of water deionisers on "fracturing osteodystrophy" and dialysis encephalopathy in Plymouth. *Nephron* 29:80–84, 1981.

66. Davison AM, Walker GS, Oli H, Lewins AM: Water supply aluminium concentration, dialysis dementia and effect of reverse-osmosis water treatment. *Lancet* 2:785–787, 1982.
67. Martin de Francisco AL, Fernandez MD, Ordoñez R, Alvarez C, Cotorruelo JG, Arias M, Sousa F, Llamarares y C: El aluminio en la insuficiencia renal crónica, hemodialysis y trasplante renal. *Nefrologia* 3:95–107, 1983.
68. Platts MM, Anastassiades E: Dialysis encephalopathy; Precipitating factors and improvement in prognosis. *Clin Nephrol* 15:223–228, 1981.
69. Galle P, Giudicelli CP: Toxicité de l'aluminium pour l'hépatocyte. Localisation ultrastructurale et micro-analyse des dépôts. *Nouv Presse Med* 11:1123–1125, 1982.
70. Henry DA, Nudelman RK, Didomenico NC, Stanley TM, Alfrey AC, Goodman WG, Slatopolsky E, Coburn JW: Metabolic and toxic effects of aluminum in the dog. *Kidney Int* 21:229, 1982. (abstr).
71. Chan Y–L, Alfrey AC, Posen S, Lissner D, Hills E, Dunstan CR, Evans RA: Effect of aluminium on normal and uremic rats: Tissue distribution, Vitamin D metabolites, and quantitative bone histology. *Calcif Tissue Int* 35:344–351, 1983.
72. Robertson JA, Felsenfeld AJ, Haywood CC, Wilson P, Clarke C, LLach F: Animal model of aluminum-induced osteomalacia: Role of chronic renal failure. *Kidney Int* 23:327–335, 1983.
73. Goodman WG, Gilligan J, Horst R: Short-term aluminum administration in the rat. Effects on bone formation and relationship to renal osteomalacia. *J Clin Invest* 73:171–181, 1984.
74. Dewberry FL, McKinney TD, Stone WJ: The dialysis dementia syndrome: report of fourteen cases and review of the literature. *Asaio J* 3:102–108, 1980.
75. McKinney TD, Basinger M, Dawson E, Jones MM: Serum aluminum levels in dialysis dementia. *Nephron* 32:53–56, 1982.
76. Platts MM, Owen G, Smith S: Water purification and the incidence of fractures in patients receiving home haemodialysis supervised by a single centre; evidence for "safe" upper limit of aluminum in water. *Br Med J* 288:969–972, 1984.
77. Fleming LW, Stewart WK, Fell GS, Halls DJ: The effect of oral aluminium therapy on plasma aluminium levels in patients with chronic renal failure in an area with low water aluminium. *Clin Nephrol* 17:222–227, 1982.
78. Biswas CK, Arze RS, Ramos JM, Ward MK, Dewar JH, Kerr DNS, Kenward DH: Effect of aluminium hydroxide on serum ionised calcium, immunoreactive parathyroid hormone, and aluminium in chronic renal failure. *Br Med J* 284:776–778, 1982.
79. Moriniere Ph, Roussel A, Tahiri Y, de Fremont JF, Maurel G, Jaudon MC, Gueris J, Fournier A: Substitution of aluminium hydroxide by high doses of calcium carbonate in patients on chronic haemodialysis: Disappearance of hyperaluminaemia and equal control of hyperparathyroidism. *Proc. Eur Dial Transpl Assoc* 19:784–787, 1982.
80. Schneider H, Kulbe KD, Weber H, Streicher E: High-effective aluminium free phosphate binder. *In vitro* and *in vivo* studies. *Proc. Eur Dial Transpl Assoc* 20:725–729, 1983.
81. Mittal VK, Sharma MJ, Toledo–Pereyra LH, Baskin S, McNichol LJ: Complete recovery from dialysis dementia following kidney transplantation. *Dial Transpl* 10(No 1):41–42, 1981.
82. O'Hare JA, Callaghan NM, Murnaghan DJ: Dialysis encephalopathy. Clinical, electroencephalographic and interventional aspects. *Medicine* 62:129–141, 1983.
83. Graf H, Stummvoll HK, Meisinger V, Kovarik J, Wolf A, Pingerra WF: Aluminum removal by hemodialysis. *Kidney Int* 19:587–592, 1981.
84. Graf H, Stummvoll HK, Meisinger V: Desferrioxamine-induced changes of aluminium kinetics during haemodialysis. *Proc Eur Dial Transpl Assoc* 18:674–680, 1981.
85. Ackrill P, Ralston AJ, Day JP, Hodge KC: Successful removal of aluminium from patient with dialysis encephalopathy. *Lancet* 2:692–693, 1980.
86. Arze RS, Parkinson IS, Cartlidge NEF, Britton P, Ward MK: Reversal of aluminium dialysis encephalopathy after desferrioxamine treatment. *Lancet* 2:1116, 1981.
87. Pogglitsch H, Petek W, Wawschinek O, Holzer W: Treatment of early stages of dialysis encephalopathy by aluminium depletion. *Lancet* 2:1344–1355, 1981.

88. Milne FJ, Sharf B, Bell P, Meyers AM: The effect of low aluminum water and desferrioxamine on the outcome of dialysis encephalopathy. *Clin Nephrol* 20:202–207, 1983.
89. Bugiani O, Bernardino G: Progressing encephalomyelopathy with muscular atrophy, induced by aluminum powder. *Neurobiol Aging* 3:209–222, 1982.
90. Wisniewski HM, Sturman JA, Shek JW: Chronic model of neurofibrillary changes induced in mature rabbits by metallic aluminum. *Neurobiol Aging* 3:11–22, 1982.
91. Crapper McLachlan DR, Dam T–V, Farnell BJ, Lewis PN: Aluminum inhibition of ADP-ribosylation *in vivo* and *in vitro. Neurobehav Toxicol Teratol* 5:645–647, 1983.
92. Lai JCK, Blass JP: Inhibition of brain glycolysis by aluminum. *J Neurochem* 42:438–446, 1984.
93. Banks WA, Kastin AJ: Aluminium increases permeability of the blood-brain barrier to labelled DSIP and B-endorphin: Possible implications for senile and dialysis dementia. *Lancet* 2:1227–1229, 1983.
94. Siegel N, Suhayda C, Haug A: Aluminum changes the conformation of calmodulin. *Physiol Chem Phys* 14:165–167, 1982.
95. Siegel N, Haug A, Aluminum interaction with calmodulin. Evidence for altered structure and function from optical and enzymatic studies. *Biochim Biophys Acta* 744:36–45, 1983.
96. Mayor GH, Sprague SM, Sanchez TV: Determinants of tissue aluminum concentration. *Am J Kidney Dis* 1:141–145, 1981.
97. Morrissey J, Rothstein M, Mayor G, Slatopolsky E: Suppression of parathyroid secretion by aluminum. *Kidney Int* 23:699–704, 1983.
98. Robertson JA, Felsenfeld AJ, Haygood CC, Wilson P, Clarke C, Llach F: Animal model of aluminum-induced osteomalacia; Role of chronic renal failure. *Kidney Int* 23:327–335, 1983.
99. Andress D, Felsenfeld AJ, Voigts A, Llach F: Parathyroid hormone response to hypocalcemia in hemodialysis patients with osteomalacia. *Kidney Int* 24:364–370, 1983.
100. Kraut JA, Shinaberger JH, Singer FR, Sherrard DJ, Saxton J, Miller JH, Kurokawa K, Coburn JW: Parathyroid gland unresponsiveness to acute hypocalcemia in dialysis osteomalacia. *Kidney Int* 23:725–733, 1983.
101. Campbell PGC, Bisson M, Bougie R, Tessier A, Villeneuve J–P: Speciation of aluminum in acidic freshwater. *Anal Chem* 55:2246–2252, 1983.
102. Pierides AM, Frohnert PP, Sharbrough FW: Release of aluminum by the Redy dialysis cartridge. Osteomalacia and dialysis encaphalopathy after prolonged usage. *Blood Purification* 1:145–153, 1983.
103. Shapiro WB, Schilb TP, Waltrous CL, Levy SR, Porush JG: Aluminum leakage from REDY sorbent cartridge. *Kidney Int* 23:536–539, 1983.
104. Odell RA, Yang J, George CR, Farrell PC: Aluminum kinetics during sorbent (Redy) dialysis. *Contemporary Dialysis*, pp 57–62, July 1982.

20

Uremic Neuropathy

Viggo Kamp Nielsen

1. Introduction

Uremic neuropathy was fully recognized in the 19th century, and detailed descriptions of its clinical picture and pathology were given by, among others, Kussmaul.[59] Lanceraux[60] was the first to apply the modern term *polynévrite urémique,* in his thesis of 1887, "Troubles nerveux de l'urémie." By the end of the century, uremic polyneuropathy had entered medical textbooks, but only to disappear again after 1909.[81] During the following five decades, it was apparently forgotten by nephrologists and neurologists. In 1963, uremic neuropathy was rediscovered by Asbury *et al.*[2] This was at a time when long-term intermittent dialysis treatment was newly invented in the management of terminal chronic renal failure. The "new" neuropathy aroused a deep concern in dialysis centers all over the world, being regarded as a *complication* to the dialysis procedure as such. The general experience was that of a patient, otherwise well adapted to dialysis, who suddenly developed the picture of progressive sensorimotor polyneuropathy, which might eventually lead to complete physical incapacity. During the subsequent decade intensive research was initiated, and clinical, pathological, and electrophysiological features of the neuropathy were outlined in great detail. As a result, uremic neuropathy was reinstated as an integral part of the uremic syndrome, since evidence of peripheral nerve dysfunction could be demonstrated in most patients with end-stage chronic renal failure *before* regular dialysis was instituted. The pathogenesis of the neuropathy was firmly linked to the deteriorating kidney function, and this relationship was strongly supported by the dramatic recovery observed after a successful renal transplantation.

Viggo Kamp Nielsen · Neuromuscular Laboratory, Department of Neurology, University of Pittsburgh, School of Medicine, Pittsburgh, Pennsylvania 15261.

In recent years, technical advances in dialysis procedures and large-scale renal transplant programs have resulted in a marked decrease in the number of new cases with clinically overt neuropathy. Thus, in 1977 the Annual Report to the European Dialysis and Transplant Association[25] does not even mention uremic neuropathy in its analysis of the rehabilitation of more than 60,000 patients on regular dialysis treatment or in transplant programs. (A special section was devoted to uremic encephalopathy.[103])

Several reviews on uremic neuropathy have appeared in the literature.[3,74,75,85,100,103] This chapter focuses on the pathophysiology and pathogenesis of the neuropathy from clinical, electrophysiological, and experimental studies.

2. *Clinical Features*

Uremic neuropathy can be defined as a distal, symmetrical, mixed sensorimotor polyneuropathy of subacute onset, which develops during the uremic phase of chronic renal failure of any etiology. Most patients present with distal sensory symptoms in the usual stocking–glove distribution, but in a small group of patients rapidly progressive motor symptoms predominate, eventually resulting in a paraplegiclike condition. Uremic neuropathy does not present any distinctive features from other metabolic neuropathies,[3,74] and the diagnosis should be applied only in patients with true irreversible uremia in order to exclude neuropathies due to pharmacologic or environmental neurotoxins[3] or focal peripheral nerve lesions.[46,101]

It was claimed that neuropathy might be prevented by a strict low-protein diet,[7,40] but this has not been confirmed by others. Once established, the only measure to prevent progression seems to be regular dialysis treatment, which should be instituted even if the residual kidney function is capable of sustaining life. Signs of rapid progression, especially with motor pareses, are an urgent indication for renal transplantation.

2.1. *Dialysis*

Early after the invention of regular dialysis treatment it was suggested that the prevention of neuropathy should be the criterion for "adequate" dialysis.[53] However, the relevant parameter for the control of the nerve function in patients on long-term dialysis is a matter of dispute. Measurements of motor nerve condition velocity have been the method most commonly employed. However, there are important objections: Conduction velocities do not correlate well with the clinical picture.[71] Even when the influence of methodological variability is limited by repeated measurements,[62] it is still a major objection that the changes in conduction velocity take place so slowly (over months) that the clinical usefulness of the method is minimal.[56,71] Many authors have advocated that regular determination of the vibratory perception threshold offers a better clinical guidance,[28,36,74] but a controlled study of several clinical and electrophysiological variables reached the negative conclusion that none of them gave an adequate prediction of changes in the neurological state that could be useful for the adjustment of the intensity of dialysis.[34]

Reports on the effectiveness of regular dialysis in the management of already established neuropathy are also conflicting. Caccia *et al.*[16] found that the course of the neuropathy could not be favorably influenced by hemodialysis for up to 6 years, and Thomas,[101] updating 10 years of experience in 139 patients, found no conspicuous changes in the incidence or distribution of neurological findings, except that paresthesias tended to disappear early after onset of dialysis. On the other hand, Cadilhac *et al.*[17] reported that mild deterioration of nerve conduction proved to be reversible on intensified dialysis, and that even severe neuropathies with inexcitable nerves showed improvement over several years of dialysis. In controlled prospective clinical studies, the appearance of neurological signs including slowed nerve conduction could be reversed by an improved dialytic clearance of "middle molecules"[67] or by increasing the weekly dialysis time.[34]

The acute effect of a single dialysis on the nerve function is of special pathophysiological interest. A single dialysis does not induce any acute change in the nerve conduction velocity, but a significant increase in the amplitude of sensory and mixed nerve potentials and muscle action potentials have been reported.[61,94] It has also been shown that the vibratory perception threshold is significantly reduced within 36 hr after a dialysis.[28,36] These observations both suggest that dialysis may induce a temporary improvement of the axon membrane function. This is in keeping with the study by Cotton *et al.*,[26] showing that the resting transmembrane potential difference in skeletal muscle cells and the intracellular Na^+, K^+, and Cl^- concentrations could be normalized after a short period of dialysis.

2.2. *Transplantation*

Successful renal transplantation usually leads to a dramatic recovery even of severe uremic neuropathy.[12,38,48,72,80] Early studies[72] of the conduction velocity, evoked muscle and nerve potential amplitudes, and vibratory perception thresholds in individual patients showed that the remission followed a *biphasic* course with an early rapid improvement, followed by a considerably more protracted restoration of the nerve function to normal. It is noteworthy that the rapid improvement is a general effect, manifested by a parallel increase in conduction velocity in different nerves and nerve segments, in upper and lower extremities, and in mildly and severely affected nerves. Even nerves with conduction velocities in the lower range of normal variation may show improvement that exceeds the expected intraindividual variation.[72] The initial rapid improvement has been confirmed in later studies,[48,80] and it is of particular pathophysiological interest that Oh *et al.*[80] could demonstrate a significant increase in conduction velocity as early as a few days after transplantation. This could not possibly represent structural regeneration of nerve fibers; rather it favors the concept that substances depressing the axon membrane function in uremia are degraded or excreted in the polyuric phase immediately after transplantation.[72]

It is usually assumed that a precondition for remission of uremic neuropathy is the return of a normal renal excretory function, with a high creatinine clearance of the kidney graft. However, considerable neurological improvement has been observed in patients even before the graft started functioning or still showed severe functional impairment.[5,48,79] These observations suggest that normal kidney tissue in a well-vascularized graft may exert an endogenous degradation of neurotoxic substances or elaborate an endocrine substance supportive of neural function. This could be the key to the well-known fact that patients with acute renal failure (shock kidney) never show signs of uremic neuropathy.

3. Pathology

Available data in the literature on the pathology of uremic nerves are relatively small in number, comprising less than 50 patients with terminal chronic renal failure of whom only two thirds presented evidence of clinical neuropathy. Moreover, the pathological material is very selected. Most studies are confined to the pathology of a single distal nerve in the leg, sural, or posterior tibial; nerves in the upper extremity have been studied in only four patients at autopsy. Light-microscopical post-mortem studies[2] showed that pathological findings were practically absent in proximal nerve segments and in nerves of the upper extremity. Teased nerve fiber studies in the sural nerve showed varying degrees of abnormalities from mild paranodal to severe segmental demyelination, which was often unrelated to clinical or electrophysiological findings.[1,29,32,51] Dyck *et al.* [33] and Thomas *et al.*[102] opposed the prevailing hypothesis that findings in teased fibers represented a primary segmental demyelination due to a uremic Schwann cell dysfunction. They advanced the current concept of a primary axonal degeneration with secondary paranodal and segmental demyelination. They emphasized the predominant distal localization[2,33] and that the pathology predominantly affected large-diameter fibers, as evidenced by the extinction of the normal bimodal fiber diameter distribution.[102] The concept of uremic neuropathy as an axonopathy of the "dying-back" type was concordant with that described in certain toxic neuropathies,[92] and the relatively mild slowing of nerve conduction velocity was taken in support of this concept in analogy with findings in acrylamide neuropathy, a prototype of "dying-back" axonopathies.[97]

These arguments do not take into account that slowing of nerve conduction far exceeds the territory of the peripheral nervous system, where pathological abnormalities have been demonstrated. Nor do they rule out alternative mechanisms for slowing of nerve conduction, as for instance biochemical depression of the axon membrane function without underlying morphological abnormalities, in analogy to changes observed during short-lasting ischemia.[77] Albeit distal axonopathy with secondary paranodal and segmental demyelination offers the best description of the pathology of uremic nerves, the concept of a "dying-back" neuropathy, in my opinion, is insufficient to account for electrophysiological and clinical findings in uremic neuropathy.

4. *Pathophysiology*

The conduction velocity is by far the most extensively studied nerve function in chronic renal failure, and slowed velocity has been demonstrated in virtually all peripheral nerves examined, cranial as well as motor and sensory extremity nerves, in distal and proximal segments of the same nerve, and in both large- and small-diameter fibers.[70] Various nerves in the same patient usually show a rather uniform degree of slowing, which in terminal chronic renal failure amounts to an average of 80–85% of the normal mean value.[72] In long-standing cases of neuropathy, during dialysis, nerves in the legs tend to deteriorate more rapidly.

The generalized slowing of nerve conduction that characterizes chronic renal failure led to the suggestion that the average velocity in several nerves in an individual patient might be a more accurate index of the peripheral nervous status.[52,62] However, as already stated, it is questionable whether the conduction velocity is an appropriate index of clinical neuropathy: In addition to objections made previously, it should be noted that although slowing of conduction precedes the development of clinical symptoms and signs, "subclinical neuropathy," clinical signs do not appear at any critical level of slowing. Moreover, the distribution and severity of clinical signs do not parallel the nerve conduction pattern, and during dialysis clinical improvement may take place despite unchanged slowing of nerve conduction.

It was early recognized that impaired nerve conduction also affects *proximal* segments of uremic nerves.[69] This may possibly turn out to be a unique feature in uremic neuropathy. At least, a similarly uniform distribution of conduction abnormalities has not been reported in any other neuropathy. In patients with chronic renal failure prior to the institution of regular dialysis, we found that the sensory conduction velocity was slowed in three consecutive segments of the median nerve: digit–wrist, wrist–elbow, and elbow–axilla. Furthermore, contrary to expectation (from the "dying-back" hypothesis), the digit–wrist segment was in fact the least affected. In a large number of patients ($n = 141$), the relationship between simultaneous measurements of the sensory conduction velocity in the digit–wrist (Y) and the wrist–elbow (X) segments was expressed by $Y = 16.0 + 0.55X$, $r = 0.71$, $p < 0.001$. This indicates that nerve conduction in the wrist–elbow segment was about twice as severely affected as in the digit–wrist segment.[73] In motor fibers of the same nerve, the distal motor latency from wrist to the abductor pollicis brevis muscle was abnormal in only 7 of the 65 nerves with reduced conduction velocity in the elbow–wrist segment.[73]

Subsequent studies, using other techniques, have provided further support for impaired conduction in proximal nerve segments in uremia. The latency of the monosynaptic Hoffmann reflex (H reflex) to the soleus muscle was increased in nearly all of 79 uremic patients,[44] and the conduction velocity in the proximal reflex arch was linearly correlated with the motor velocity in the knee–ankle segment of the peroneal nerve. In fact, Knoll[55] considered the H reflex to be more sensitive than the standard motor conduction velocity in more distal segments, since the H reflex latency in his 64 patients was prolonged earlier in the course of uremia and was abnormal in several patients who had normal distal motor conduction velocities. Others have studied the muscle F response, which is due to recurrent discharges in anterior horn cells when activated by antidromic impulses after peripheral stimulation of motor nerves. In uremic nerves, the proximal conduction velocity (spinal cord–knee) was reduced to the same degree as the motor velocity in the distal knee–ankle segment of the peroneal nerve.[82] Even in patients with normal proximal and distal conduction velocities, the scatter of consecutively recorded F-wave latencies ("F chronodispersion") was greatly increased, suggesting that these seemingly normal nerves contained many abnormal fibers.[83]

The pathological concept of uremic neuropathy as a degenerative distal axonopathy implies that the slowing of nerve conduction is due to conduction block of predominantly large-diameter, fast-conducting fibers. This is not unequivocally supported by electrophysiological data. In addition to the slowing of sensory nerve conduction velocity, the amplitude of the compound nerve action potential commonly shows a significant decrease. This is usually interpreted as indicating a conduction block in a fraction of sensory fibers. In uremic nerves, however, we could show that the amplitude reduction was a simple consequence of a simultaneous and parallel increase in the temporal dispersion of the compound action potential.[70] Hence, the reduction in amplitude did not provide any support for a presumed degeneration of sensory axons. On the other hand, evidence of axonal conduction block in uremic patients has been provided through electromyographic findings in muscles, showing signs of denervation and loss of motor units during volitional contraction.[45,49,70] Electromyographic (EMG) changes appear later than slowing of motor nerve conduction and are usually confined to distal muscles of the leg. Thus, EMG showed signs of moderate-to-severe loss of motor units in the extensor digitorum brevis muscle in 72% of our patients, whereas in hand muscles similar EMG findings were present in only 14%, despite a decrease of the median nerve motor conduction velocity in 58% of these patients. Furthermore, in a single-fiber EMG study the jitter and fiber density was found to be normal in uremic patients with reduced motor conduction velocity.[99] This implies that there was no evidence of reinnervation, which would be expected in case of axonal degeneration. Abnormal

EMG findings are the earliest, and often the only, electrophysiological signs in axonopathies. In uremia, the relationship between EMG and nerve conduction velocity findings is exactly the opposite. This calls for an alternative explanation, as will be discussed at the end of this section.

The *excitability* of uremic nerves was studied by Tackmann *et al.*,[98] using a double stimulation technique. They found an increase of the absolute and relative refractory period in sensory fibers. With an interval between two stimuli shorter than 3 msec, the second "test" response showed a significantly greater increase in latency and a greater reduction in amplitude relative to the first "conditioning" response than were observed in normal controls. They concluded that these findings provided evidence of a change of the axon membrane properties in uremic nerves, characterized by a lowering of the safety factor for impulse propagation. Delbeke *et al.*[31] were unable to reproduce these observations. However, this may be entirely due to the fact that all their patients were on regular dialysis for a protracted period of time, which may have normalized the excitability of nerves.

Uremic nerves exhibit an increased *resistance to acute ischemia.*[19,20,75] Again, this is not a specific feature of uremic neuropathy; the phenomenon is also known in diabetes,[42,95] hyperparathyroidism,[19,43] and chronic hepatic failure.[54,89] Electrophysiologically, during ischemia the evoked nerve action potential is preserved for a longer period of time and the final decline in amplitude is slower than in normal subjects, and this is true also for the decrease in conduction velocity along the ischemic nerve segment.[78] As a result, the perception of sensory stimuli applied to the ischemic limb is abnormally well preserved.[54] This could be shown in our patients on dialysis, where we recorded an average ischemic perception time for vibrations of 25.8 ± 1.1 min, as compared with 17.9 ± 0.5 min in normal controls, $p < 0.001$,[75] indicating that peripheral nerves in uremic patients were abnormally resistant to anoxic depolarization.

However, whether this observation has any implications for the pathophysiology of uremic neuropathy, or is just an epiphenomenon, is still a matter of dispute. The ischemic perception time for vibration shows a positive linear correlation with the serum calcium concentration, being prolonged in patients with primary and secondary hyperparathyroidism and abnormally short in patients with hypoparathyroidism.[43] In both cases, the perception time can be restored to normal after normalization of the serum calcium level. A high extracellular Ca^{2+} concentration stabilizes the nodal axon membrane through a more effective "screening" of the negative surface potential. This raises the threshold for depolarization, equivalent to a hyperpolarization of the membrane,[18,47] which might account for the increased resistance to anoxic depolarization. A similar mechanism may apply to uremic nerves, since uremia is often accompanied by secondary hyperparathyroidism.[93] More data are needed to test this possibility and also to elucidate alternative hypotheses, as discussed in a recent review.[76]

4.1. Cell Membrane Function

The biophysical properties of the cell membrane in uremia have attracted considerable attention during the past decades, and extensive research has been conducted from widely different angles of approach. In the present context, it is of particular interest that a significant reduction of the resting transmembrane potential difference (E_m), often to very low levels, has been demonstrated in patients with terminal uremia by various groups.[11,26,27] A reduction of E_m in muscle cells is not a specific finding in uremia but can also be demonstrated in other patients, "severely ill" for a variety of causes. Nor is a depressed E_m correlated with specific muscular symptoms or signs, except for subjective weakness.[27] Experimental data show that the lowered E_m in uremia is a consequence of a reduced Na^+ efflux with an increase in the intracellular concentration of Na^+ and Cl^- and a decrease in the K^+ concentration. These findings have general application to uremic cells. Of more specific importance to uremic neuropathy and its management are biophysical studies demonstrating that the ouabain-sensitive Na^+–K^+-activated ATPase in cell membranes can be reversibly inhibited by dialyzable substances in uremic plasma. Further experimental studies have shown that the activity of ouabain-sensitive Na^+–K^+-activated ATPase rapidly increases after a successful renal transplantation, with a concomitant reduction of the intracellular sodium concentration.[23,24] The erythrocyte membrane was the preferred model in the earliest and many subsequent studies,[22,58,88,104,105] but concordant results have been obtained in similar studies using other cellular system, such as crab muscle fibers,[8] toad oocytes,[9] frog skin,[14,15] brain cells,[68] leukocytes,[35] and intestinal epithelium.[57]

More recently, these experimental findings have been reproduced in part in clinical studies. Cotton *et al.*[26] directly measured the resting membrane potential *in situ* in the anterior tibial muscle of uremic patients. They confirmed the presence of a reduced E_m and showed that the decrease was linearly correlated with the deterioration in endogenous creatinine clearance below a value of 6.3 ml/min per 1.73 m^2, above which level E_m was consistently normal. (This, incidentally, is the same clearance level, where by regression analysis I found that nerve conduction velocities became abnormally slow in more than 50% of patients.[71] The abnormal E_m and intracellular electrolyte concentrations could be normalized after 7 weeks of hemodialysis. But if the weekly dialysis time then was shortened to a suboptimal level, a secondary drop in E_m developed after a few weeks.

4.2. Summary

All available electrophysiological evidence points to the fact that impulse propagation in uremic nerves is generally impaired. This can be naturally associated with the previously mentioned studies showing that a reversible impairment of the cell membrane function is an integral part of the uremic syndrome. Results from *in vitro* studies in various cell models and the direct demonstration of a lowered E_m in skeletal muscle cells in uremic patients can readily be applied to the nerve axon membrane as well. Slowing of the nerve conduction is a logical consequence of a reduced resting axon membrane potential. The effect of a reduced axon membrane potential difference is a decreased current generation capacity at the node of Ranvier, which will delay the depolarization of the adjacent nodes, and hence the rate of impulse propagation. Admittedly, the same effect might result from paranodal or internodal leakage of current, as seen in advanced demyelinating disorders.[86] But, as emphasized earlier, demyelination of uremic nerves is not prominent and above all not a universal feature. The rapid improvement of nerve conduction after renal transplantation in conjunction with the similarly rapid decrease in the intracellular Na^+ concentration in newly transplanted patients constitutes a strong argument in favor of the membrane dysfunction hypothesis. Incidentally, it is noteworthy that rats with experimental neuropathy demonstrated slowing of the nerve conduction, irrespective of the fact that sophisticated histomorphometric techniques failed to demonstrate any structural abnormalities in the nerve fibers.[90,91]

As a consequence of these considerations, in 1973 we advanced the hypothesis that peripheral neuropathy in chronic renal failure was due to a reversible toxic–metabolic inhibition of the Na^+-K^+-activated ATPase in axon membranes of peripheral nerves, resulting in a depression of the resting membrane potential.[70] This hypothesis was in concordance with the current concept of the uremic syndrome, as a generalized metabolic disorder due to the accumulation of enzymatic inhibitors.[6,48] Moreover, with the aim of documenting the direct relationship between impaired axon membrane function and nerve conduction, we subjected peripheral nerves in normal subjects to short-lasting ischemia.[77] The model employed does not involve any degenerative changes of the nerve, among others evidenced by the restitution of a fully normal nerve function within a few minutes after reestablishment of normal blood flow. One of the major observations in these experiments was that nerve conduction during ischemic became slowed more rapidly in proximal than in distal segments of the same nerve. Hence, the changes in nerve conduction in the course of minutes of ischemia closely mimicked the longitudinal changes over months in uremic neuropathy.[73]

5. *Pathogenesis*

As in most other metabolic neuropathies, the pathogenesis of uremic neuropathy is virtually unknown. The preceding presentation of clinical, pathological, and pathophysiological aspects portrays a neurological picture of such complexity that it seems difficult to encompass all features within one unitary concept. Although the various neurological dysfunctions are present only in advanced chronic renal failure, they still show a statistically significant correlation with the endogeneous creatinine clearance or other measures of renal failure. Evidently, this is an indirect relationship which only reinforces the search for a linking factor, the uremic neurotoxin(s). On the other hand, the strength of this correlation sets a measure for the credibility of an alleged uremic "neurotoxin," which should fullfil the following criteria: (1) It should show a statistically significant correlation with the neurological dysfunction studied, independent of the kidney function. (As an example: A multivariate analysis ruled out an effect of the serum urea or creatinine concentrations on the nerve conduction velocity, independent of the kidney function, although the simple correlation between serum levels and conduction velocities was highly significant.[71]) (2) It should show a neurotoxic effect on normal nerves at clinically relevant concentrations. (3) The substance should be dialyzable, and (4) the neurotoxic effect should be reversible.

Accumulation of myoinositol in uremic serum has been incriminated,[21,30] but there is not sufficient clinical or electrophysiological evidence to show that this is related to the presence of uremic neuropathy,[10,87] and a suspected direct toxic effect on normal nerves[30] has yet to be confirmed.[50] It was suggested that inhibition of transketolase activity in nervous tissue by a dialyzable substance in uremic serum might be responsible for demyelination of nerves,[37,63,96] but a correlation to the presence of neuropathy could not be demonstrated.[85] Recently, it has been claimed that the parathyroid hormone (PTH) was "equal to" the uremic toxin and responsible for neurological disturbances.[41,66] This claim was partly based on a statistically significant covariation between serum levels of PTH and motor nerve conduction velocities in uremic patients.[4] However, the actual correlation coefficient, $r = -0.45$, was much lower than the coefficient for the correlation between nerve conduction and kidney function, $r = 0.68$,[71] suggesting, as was pointed out, that other factors might be involved. In addition, it is known that motor and sensory conduction velocity is normal in patients with primary and secondary hyperparathyroidism.[64,84] Moreover, as discussed earlier, hyperparathyroidal hypercalcemia would rather tend to stabilize the nodal axon membrane potential against toxic–metabolic depolarization[43] and hence theoretically raise the safety factor for impulse propagation. This is exemplified by the increased resistance to ischemia in patients with hyperparathyroidism.[43]

For many years, the possibility has been discussed that an accumulation of "middle molecules" (5000–10,000 daltons) in uremic plasma might be responsible for the development of uremic symptoms, especially relating to the peripheral neuropathy.[67] Man *et al.*[65] recently isolated a substance from the "middle-molecule" plasma fraction with what seems to be promising characteristics. This substance appears to be an acid-polyol with carbohydrate structure. It is excreted in the urine of normal subjects and found in the dialysate from uremic patients treated with hemodialysis. The plasma concentration is greatly increased in patients with uremic neuropathy but can be reduced by hemodialysis, when specially directed against "middle molecules." This is accompanied by improvement of the neurological status. In *in vitro* studies on frog sural nerves,[39] the substance isolated from normal urine causes a decrease in the nerve potential amplitude with a linear correlation to the concentration of the substance. A similar correlation was found with the substance extracted from plasma ultrafiltrate from uremic patients with and without neuropathy. As a control, the same potential amplitude changes were observed when frog nerves were immersed in varying concentrations of xylocaine, which depolarizes the axon membrane.

Further investigations of the biochemistry, physiology, and pathology of nerves to elucidate pathophysiological and pathogenetic aspects of uremic neuropathy would benefit greatly from the access to a suitable animal model for chronic renal failure. A promising model has been suggested by Boudet *et al.*,[13] involving electrocoagulation of the renal cortex in rats. However, it still remains to be seen whether these animals develop neuropathy.

6. Conclusion

Twenty years have passed since the rediscovery of uremic neuropathy. These have been exceedingly productive years, both clinically and scientifically. From its appearance on the scene, uremic neuropathy has passed through several stages. Initially, it was the unknown and feared demon that threatened the success of every dialysis program throughout the world. With time, it became more manageable. Nephrologists recognized the merits of prevention through early institution of regular dialysis. Technical improvements of the dialysis procedures and, equally important, the invention of disposable equipment enabled them to increase the frequency and efficiency of treatment. After 10 years of intensive research, advanced renal transplant programs became available in most centers, by which the seemingly ultimate solution could be offered to intractable cases of neuropathy. Today, uremic neuropathy is still a matter of concern in many dialysis centers, but it certainly plays a far less conspicuous role in the clinical syndrome of uremia. Symptoms and signs are now so widely recognized by the medical profession that there is an impending risk of overdiagnosing the condition, at the expense of other manageable nerve lesions. With prolonged life expectancy and full rehabilitation for uremic patients, more commonplace peripheral nerve syndromes (median, ulnar, peroneal nerve compressions) and other metabolic neuropathies, especially the diabetic, should be considered.

Hardly ever before has so much scientific information been accumulated in such a short span of time within the clinical neurosciences. It is probably no exaggeration that clinical and electrophysiological research has become almost exhausted, and most of this took place within the first 10 years. This can be accredited to certain exceptionally fortunate conditions. Uremic neuropathy offered a hitherto unique opportunity to study the induction, the progression, and, for the first time, the remission of a metabolic neuropathy. The magnitude of the problem and its importance for the outcome of dialysis as a new and lifesaving intervention in uremia were strong incentives for a devoted research effort. Another factor that cannot be overestimated relates to the fact that uremic neuropathy appeared at a time when medical electronics made accessible a growing variety of sophisticated electrophysiological techniques that here found a fruitful area for application, including basic axon membrane research. Uremic neuropathy has contributed to directing the attention of a new group of basic investigators toward the opportunities in applied clinical research. Undoubtedly, this has also fertilized the ground for research in other areas of peripheral neuropathies through new and perhaps provocative concepts regarding the significance of nerve membrane dysfunction. In the field of nephrological research, uremic nerves will remain a useful model, and a suitable animal model for uremia will no doubt become available soon, which may initiate a new boom in joined biochemical and biophysical research with clinical applications.

References

1. Appenzeller O, Kornfeld M, McGee J: Neuropathy in chronic renal disease. *Arch Neurol* 24:449–461, 1971.
2. Asbury AK, Victor M, Adams RD: Uremic polyneuropathy. *Arch Neurol* 8:413–428, 1963.
3. Asbury AK: Uremic neuropathy, in: Dyck PJ, Thomas PK, Lambert ED, Bunge R (eds): *Peripheral Neuropathy*, 2nd ed. Philadelphia, Saunders, 1984, pp 1811–1825.
4. Avram MM, Feinfeld DA, Huatuco AH: Search for the uremic toxin: Decreased motor nerve conduction velocity and elevated parathyroid hormone in uremia. *N Engl J Med* 298:1000–1003, 1978.
5. Barnes AD, Dukes DC, Robinson BHB, Blainey JD: Neuropathy in renal failure. *Lancet* 2:610, 1971.
6. Bergström J, Bittar EE: The basis of uremic toxicity, in Bittar EE, Bittar N (eds): *The Biological Basis of Medicine*, Volume 6. London, New York, Academic Press, 1969, pp 495–544.
7. Bergström J, Lindblom U, Norée L-O: Preservation of peripheral nerve function in severe uraemia during treatment with low protein high calorie diet and surplus of essential amino acids. *Acta Neurol Scand* 51:99–109, 1975.
8. Bittar EE: Maia muscle fibre as a model for the study of uraemic toxicity. *Nature (London)* 214:310–312, 1967.
9. Bittar EE: The effect of Na^+–K^+-ATPase inhibitors and uraemic plasma on Na^+ efflux from the toad oocyte, in: *Proceedings of the 4th International Congress on Nephrology*, Stockholm 1969, Volume 2. Basel, Munich, New York, Karger, 1970, pp 267.
10. Blumberg A, Esslen E, Bürgi W: Myoinositol—a uremic neurotoxin? *Nephron* 21:186–191, 1978.
11. Bolte HD, Riecker G, Röhl D: Measurements of membrane potential of individual muscle cells in normal man and patients with renal insufficiency, in: *Proceedings of the 2nd International Congress on Nephrology*, Prague 1963, Volume 78. 1963, p 114.
12. Bolton CF: Electrophysiological changes in uremic neuropathy after successful renal transplantation. *Neurology* 26:152–161, 1976.
13. Boudet J, Man NK, Pils P, Sausse A, Funck-Brentano JL: Experimental chronic renal failure in the rat by electrocoagulation of the renal cortex. *Kidney Int* 14:82–86, 1978.
14. Bourgoigne JJ, Klahr S, Bricker NS: Inhibition of transepithelial sodium transport in the frog skin by a low molecular weight fraction of uremic serum. *J Clin Invest* 50:303–311, 1971.
15. Bricker NS, Bourgoigne JJ, Klahr S: A humoral inhibitor of sodium transport in uremic serum. A potential toxin? *Arch Intern Med* 126:860–864, 1970.

16. Caccia MR, Mangili A, Mecca G, Ubiali E, Zanoni P: Effects of hemodialysis treatment on uremic polyneuropathy. *J Neurol* 217:123–131, 1977.
17. Cadilhac J, Mion C, Duday H, Dapres G, Georgesco M: Motor nerve conduction velocities as an index of the efficiency of maintenance dialysis in patients with end-stage renal failure. (A long-term follow-up study), in Canal N, Pozza G (eds): *Peripheral Neuropathies.* Elsevier/North-Holland Biomedical Press, 1978, pp 211–222.
18. Cahalan M: Voltage clamp studies on the node of Ranvier, in Waxman, SG (ed): *Physiology and Pathobiology of Axons.* New York, Raven Press, 1978, pp 155–168.
19. Castaigne P, Cathala H-P, Beaussart-Boulengé L, Petrover M: Effect of ischemia on peripheral nerve function in patients with chronic renal failure undergoing dialysis treatment. *J Neurol Neurosurg Psychiatry* 35:631–637, 1972.
20. Christensen NJ, Orskov H: Vibratory perception during ischaemia in uraemic patients and in subjects with mild carbohydrate intolerance. *J Neurol Neurosurg Psychiatry* 32:519–524, 1969.
21. Clements RS, DeJesus PV, Winegrad AI: Raised plasma myoinisitol levels in uraemia and experimental neuropathy. *Lancet* 1:1137–1141, 1973.
22. Cole CH: Decreased ouabain-sensitive adenosine triphosphatase activity in the erythrocyte membrane of patients with chronic renal disease. *Clin Sci Mol Med* 45:775–784, 1973.
23. Cole CH, Maletz R: Changes in erythrocyte membrane ouabain-sensitive adenosine triphosphatase after renal transplantation. *Clin Sci Mol Med* 48:239–242, 1975.
24. Cole CH, Steinberg R, Guttmann R: Altered erythrocyte sodium efflux following renal transplantation. *Nephron* 20:248–257, 1978.
25. Combined Report on Regular Dialysis and Transplantation in Europe VIII 1977. *Proc Eur Dial Transpl Assoc* 15:4–76, 1978.
26. Cotton JR, Woodard T, Carter NW, Knochel JP: Resting skeletal muscle membrane potential as an index of uremic toxicity. A proposed new method to assess adequacy of hemodialysis. *J Clin Invest* 63:501–506, 1979.
27. Cunningham JN, Carter NW, Rector JC, Seldin DW: Resting transmembrane potential difference of skeletal muscle in normal subjects and severely ill patients. *J Clin Invest* 50:49–59, 1971.
28. Daniel CR, Bower JD, Pearson JE, Holbert RD: Vibrometry and uremic peripheral neuropathy. *South Med J* 70:1311–1316, 1977.
29. Dayan AD, Gardner-Thorpe C, Down PF, Gleadle RI: Peripheral neuropathy in uraemia. Pathological studies on peripheral nerves from 6 patients. *Neurology* 20:649–658, 1970.
30. DeJesus PV, Clements RS, Winegrad AI: Hypermyoinositolemic polyneuropathy in rats. A possible mechanism for uremic polyneuropathy. *J Neurol Sci* 21:237–249, 1974.
31. Delbeke J, Kopec J, McComas AJ: Effects of age, temperature, and disease on refractoriness of human nerve and muscle. *J Neurol Neurosurg Psychiatry* 41:65–71, 1978.
32. Dinn JJ, Crane DL: Schwann cell dysfunction in uraemia. *J Neurol Neurosurg Psychiatry* 33:605–608, 1970.
33. Dyck PJ, Johnson WJ, Lambert ED, O'Brien PC: Segmental demyelination secondary to axonal degeneration in uremic neuropathy. *Mayo Clin Proc* 46:400–431, 1971.
34. Dyck PJ, Johnson WJ, Lambert ED, O'Brien PC, Daube JP, Oviatt KF: Comparison of symptoms, chemistry, and nerve function to assess adequacy of hemodialysis. *Neurology* 29:1361–1368, 1979.
35. Edmondson RPS, Hilton PJ, Jones NF, Patrick J, Thomas RD: Leucocyte sodium transport in uremia. *Clin Sci Mol Med* 49:213–216, 1975.
36. Edwards AE, Kopple JD, Kornfeld CM: Vibrotactile threshold in patients undergoing maintenance hemodialysis. *Arch Intern Med* 132:706–708, 1973.
37. Egan JD, Wells IC: Transketolase inhibition and uremic peripheral sensory neuropathy. *J Neurol Sci* 41:379–395, 1979.
38. Funck–Brentano JL, Vantelon J, Zingraff J: Polynévrite au cours de l'urémie chronique. Evolution aprés transplantation rénale (10 observation personelle). *Nephron* 5:31–42, 1968.
39. Funck-Brentano JL, Boudet J, Sausse A, Cueille G, Man NK: In vitro sural nerve test for the evolution of middle molecule neurotoxicity in uraemia, in Frost H (ed): *Technical Aspects of Renal Dialysis.* Kent, England, Tunbridge, 1978, pp 256–263.

40. Giovanetti S, Barsotti G: Uremic intoxication. *Nephron* 14:123–133, 1975.
41. Goldstein DA, Chui LA, Massry SG: Effect of parathyroid hormone and uremia on peripheral nerve calcium and motor conduction velocity. *J Clin Invest* 62:88–93, 1978.
42. Gregersen G: A study of the peripheral nerves in diabetic subjects during ischaemia. *J Neurol Neurosurg Psychiatry* 31:175–181, 1968.
43. Gregersen G, Pilgaard S: The effect of ischaemia on vibration sense in hypo- and hypercalcaemia and in demyelinated nerves. *Acta Neurol Scand* 47:71–79, 1971.
44. Guiheneuc P, Bathien N: Two patterns of results in polyneuropathies investigated with the H-reflex. Correlation between proximal and distal conduction velocities. *J Neurol Sci* 30:83–94, 1976.
45. Hansen S, Ballentyne JP: A quantitative electrophysiological study of uraemic neuropathy. Diabetic and renal neuropathies compared. *J Neurol Neurosurg Psychiatry* 41:128–134, 1978.
46. Harding AE, Le Fanu J: Carpal tunnel syndrome related to antebrachial Cimino–Brescia fistula. *J Neurol Neurosurg Psychiatry* 40:511–513, 1977.
47. Hille B: Ionic permeability changes in active axon membrane. *Arch Intern Med* 129:293–298, 1972.
48. Ibrahim MM, Barnes AD, Crosland JM, Dawson-Edwards P, Honigsberger L, Newman CE, Robinson BHB: Effect of renal transplantation on uraemic neuropathy. *Lancet* 2:739–742, 1974.
49. Isaacs H: Electromyographic study of muscular weakness in chronic renal failure. *South Am Med J* 43:683–688, 1969.
50. Jefferys JGR, Palmano KP, Sharma AK, Thomas PK: Influence of dietary myoinositol on nerve conduction and phopholipids in normal and diabetic rats. *J Neurol Neurosurg Psychiatry* 41:333–339, 1978.
51. Jennekens FGI, Most Van Spijk D v.d.: Nerve fibre degeneration in uraemic polyneuropathy. *Proc Eur Dial Transpl Assoc* 6:191–197, 1969.
52. Jepsen RH, Tenckhoff HA: Comparison of motor and sensory nerve conduction velocity in early uremic polyneuropathy. *Arch Phys Med* 50:124–126, 1969.
53. Jepsen RH, Tenckhoff HA, Honet JC: Natural history of uremic polyneuropathy and effect of dialysis. *N Engl J Med* 277:327–333, 1967.
54. Kardel T, Nielsen VK: Hepatic neuropathy. A clinical and electrophysiological study. *Acta Neurol Scand* 50:513–526, 1974.
55. Knoll O: Monitoring uremic neuropathy by means of reflex response latency. *Electroenceph Clin Neurophysiol* 43:593, 1977.
56. Kominami N, Tyler HR, Hampers CL, Merrill JP: Variation in motor nerve conduction velocity in normal and uremic patients. *Arch Intern Med* 128:235–239, 1971.
57. Kramer HJ, Bäcker A, Krück F: Inhibition of intestinal (Na^+–K^+)-ATPase in experimental uremia. *Clin Chim Acta* 50:13–18, 1974.
58. Kramer HJ, Gospodinov D, Krück F: Functional and metabolic studies on red blood cell sodium transport in chronic uremia. *Nephron* 16:344–358, 1976.
59. Kussmaul A: Beiträge zur Anatomie und Pathologie des Harnapparats. VI. Zur Lehre von der Paraplegia urinaria. *Würzburger med Zschr* 4:56–63, 1864.
60. Lanceraux E: Troubles nerveux de l'urémie. Thesis. Union Médical, 1887.
61. Lang AH, Forsström J: Transient changes of sensory nerve functions in uraemia. *Acta Med Scand* 202:495–500, 1977.
62. Lang AH, Forsström J, Björkquist S-E, Kuusela V: Statistical variation of nerve conduction velocity. *J Neurol Sci* 33:229–241, 1977.
63. Lonergan ET, Semar M, Lange K: Transketolase activity in uremia. *Arch Intern Med* 126:851–854, 1970.
64. Mallette LE, Patten BM, Engel WK: Neuromuscular disease in secondary hyperparathyroidism. *Ann Intern Med* 82:474–483, 1975.
65. Man NK, Cueille C, Zingraff J, Drueke T, Jungers P, Sausse A, Boudet J, Funck-Brentano JL: Evaluation of plasma neurotoxin concentration in uraemic polyneuropathic patients. *Proc Eur Dial Transpl Assoc* 15:164–170, 1978.

66. Massry SG, Goldstein DA: The search for uremic toxin(s) "X." "X" = PTH. *Clin Nephrol* 11:181–189, 1979.
67. Milutinovic J, Babb AL, Eschbach JW, Follette WC, Graefe U, Strand MJ, Scribner BH: Uremic neuropathy: Evidence of middle molecule toxicity. *Artif Org* 2:45–51, 1978.
68. Minkoff L, Gaertner G, Darab M, Mercier C, Levin ML: Inhibition of brain sodium-potassium ATPase in uremic rats. *J Lab Clin Med* 80:71–78, 1972.
69. Nielsen VK: Sensory nerve conduction studies in uraemic patients. *Proc Eur Dial Transpl Assoc* 4:279–284, 1967.
70. Nielsen VK: The peripheral nerve function in chronic renal failure. V. Sensory and motor conduction velocity. *Acta Med Scand* 194:445–454, 1973.
71. Nielsen VK: The peripheral nerve function in chronic renal failure. VI. The relationship between sensory and motor nerve conduction and kidney function, azotaemia, age, sex, and clinical neuropathy. *Acta Med Scand* 194:455–462, 1973.
72. Nielsen VK: The peripheral nerve function in chronic renal failure. IX. Recovery after renal transplantation. Electrophysiological aspects (sensory and motor nerve conduction). *Acta Med Scand* 195:171–180, 1974.
73. Nielsen VK: The peripheral nerve function in chronic renal failure. X. Decremental nerve conduction in uremia? *Acta Med Scand* 196:83–86, 1974.
74. Nielsen VK: The peripheral nerve function in chronic renal failure. A survey. *Acta Med Scand* (Suppl 573):1–32, 1974.
75. Nielsen VK: Pathophysiological aspects of uraemic neuropathy, in Canal N, Pozza G (eds): *Peripheral Neuropathies*. Elsevier/North-Holland Biomedical Press, 1978, pp 197–210.
76. Nielsen VK: Mechanisms for preserved nerve function with ischemia in peripheral neuropathy, in: Buser PA, Cobb WA, Okuma T (eds): Kyoto Symposia *Electroenceph clin Neurophysiol*, Suppl 36. Amsterdam, New York, Oxford, Elsevier, 1982, pp 70–80.
77. Nielsen VK, Kardel T: Decremental conduction in normal human nerves subjected to ischaemia? *Acta Physiol Scand* 92:249–262, 1974.
78. Nielsen VK, Kardel T: Delayed decrement of the nerve impulse propagation during induced limb ischaemia in chronic hepatic failure. *J Neurol Neurosurg Psychiatry* 38:966–976, 1975.
79. Nielsen VK, Olgaard K, Ladefoged J: Rapid recovery from neuropathy after renal transplantation. *Lancet* 2:1326–1327, 1974.
80. Oh SJ, Clements RS, Lee YW, Diethelm AG: Rapid improvement in nerve conduction following renal transplantation. *Ann Neurol* 4:369–373, 1978.
81. Osler W: *The Principles and Practice of Medicine* (1892), 7th ed. London, Appleton, 1909.
82. Panayiotopoulos CP, Scarpalezos S: F-wave studies on the deep peroneal nerve. Part 2. 1.Chronic renal failure. 2.Limb-girdle muscular dystrophy. *J Neurol Sci* 31:331–341, 1977.
83. Panayiotopoulos CP: F chronodispersion. A new electrophysiologic method. *Muscle Nerve* 2:68–72, 1979.
84. Patten BM, Bilezikian JP, Mallette LE, Prince A, Engel WK, Aurbach GD: Neuromuscular disease in primary hyperparathyroidism. *Ann Intern Med* 80:182–193, 1974.
85. Raskin NH, Fishman RA: Neurological disorders in renal failure. 2nd part. *N Engl J Med* 294:204–210, 1976.
86. Rasminsky M: Physiology of conduction in demyelinated axons, in Waxman SG (ed): *Physiology and Pathobiology of Axons*. New York, Raven Press, pp 361–376.
87. Reznek RH, Salway JG, Thomas PK: Plasma-myoinositol concentrations in uraemic neuropathy. *Lancet* 1:675–676, 1977.
88. Schmidt EKM, Welt LG: The red blood cell as a model for the study of uremic toxins. *Arch Intern Med* 126:827–830, 1970.
89. Seneviratne KN, Peiris OA: Peripheral nerve function in chronic liver disease. *J Neurol Neurosurg Psychiatry* 33:609–614, 1970.
90. Sharma AK, Thomas PK: Peripheral nerve structure and function in experimental diabetes. *J Neurol Sci* 23:1–15, 1974.
91. Sharma AK, Thomas PK, Baker RWR: Peripheral nerve abnormalities related to galactose administration in rats. *J Neurol Neurosurg Psychiatry* 39:794–802, 1976.

92. Spencer PS, Schaumburg HH: Pathobiology of neurotoxic axonal degeneration, in Waxman SG (ed): *Physiology and Pathobiology of Axons.* New York, Raven Press, 1978, pp 265–282.
93. Stanbury SW, Lumb GA: Parathyroid function in chronic renal failure: A statistical survey of the plasma biochemistry in azotaemic renal osteodystrophy. *Q J Med* 35:1–23, 1966.
94. Stanley E, Brown JC, Pryor JS: Altered peripheral nerve function resulting from haemodialysis. *J Neurol Neurosurg Psychiatry* 40:39–43, 1977.
95. Steiness I: Vibratory perception in diabetics during arrested blood flow to the limb. *Acta Med Scand* 163:195–205, 1959.
96. Sterzel RB, Semar M, Lonergan ET, Treser G, Lange K: Relationship of nervous tissue transketolase to the neuropathy in chronic uremia *J Clin Invest* 50:2295–2304, 1971.
97. Sumner A: Physiology of dying-back neuropathies, in Waxman SG: Physiology and Pathobiology of Axons. New York, Raven Press, 1978, pp 349–359.
98. Tackmann W, Ullrich D, Cremer W, Lehmann HJ: Nerve conduction studies during the relative refractory period in sural nerves of patients with uremia. *Eur Neurol* 12:331–339, 1974.
99. Thiele B, Stalberg E: Single fibre EMG findings in polyneuropathies of different aetiology. *J Neurol Neurosurg Psychiatry* 38:881–887, 1975.
100. Thomas PK: Uraemic neuropathy. *Proc Eur Dial Trans Assoc* 13:109–118, 1976.
101. Thomas PK: Screening for peripheral neuropathy in patients treated by chronic hemodialysis. *Muscle Nerve* 1:396–399, 1978.
102. Thomas PK, Hollinrake K, Lascelles RG, O'Sullivan DJ, Baillod RA, Moorhead JF, Mackenzie JC: The polyneuropathy of chronic renal failure. *Brain* 94:761–780, 1971.
103. Tyler HR: Neurological disorders seen in the uremic patient. *Arch Intern Med* 126:781–786, 1970.
104. Welt LG: Erythrocyte transport defect in uremia, in: *Proceedings of the 4th International Congress on Nephrology*, Stockholm 1969, Volume 2. Basel, München, New York, Karger, 1970, pp 263.
105. Welt LG, Sachs JR, McManus TJ: An ion transport defect in erythrocytes from uremic patients. *Trans Assoc Am Physicians* 77:169–181, 1964.

Cardiovascular Complications of Renal Failure

21

Cardiovascular Complications in End-Stage Renal Disease Patients

George A. Porter

As we conclude 20 years of successful treatment of end-stage renal disease (ESRD) with either intermittent hemodialysis or renal transplantation, it seems appropriate to reflect on past accomplishments while identifying future challenges. Although the life expectancy for patients with terminal renal failure has been extended by these therapeutic interventions, premature cardiovascular disease still ranks as the number one threat to the longevity of this patient population. When the rate of cardiovascular mortality for end-stage renal disease patients is compared to that of the United States population, a death rate increase of between 10 and 30 times is evident (Table 1). In this setting this problem will be discussed—from the standpoint of both what is known about the pathophysiology of cardiovascular disease in end-stage renal disease, and what therapeutic manipulations are available that might modify this particular outcome.

The statistical source for the cardiovascular mortality for end-stage renal disease patients was derived from the European Dialysis and Transplant Association.[(1)] Table 2 shows the percent distribution of causes of death for both ESRD and non-ESRD populations. That European data parallel experiences in the United States[(2)] is substantiated from information supplied by Dr. C. Blagg of the Seattle Artificial Kidney Program. (C. Blagg, personal communication). In following more than 1000 chronic dialysis patients they found that 63.4% of all deaths in nondiabetic patients were attributed to cardiovascular disease with 14.2% associated directly with cerebrovascular disease. Likewise, the distribution of transplant deaths shown in Table 2 is very similar to that experienced by our own group in more than 425 live donor and cadaveric transplantations where 44% of deaths were cardiovas-

George A. Porter • Department of Medicine, University of Oregon Health Sciences Center, Portland, Oregon 97201.

Table 1. Comparative Cardiovascular Mortality—ESRD versus Non-ESRD Patients

	Rate/100,000		
		ESRD[b]	
	Non-ESRD[a]	Dialysis (*x*)	Transplant (*x*)
Coronary heart disease	578	8954 (15)	3061 (5)
Cerebrovascular disease	101	3148 (31)	1068 (11)
All cardiovascular disease	802	16045 (20)	6926 (9)
All causes	1621	24833 (15)	19024 (12)

[a] HEW (1975)—age-adjusted death rates, United States, ages 35–74.
[b] EDTA Patient Registry (1970–1977)—60,676 dialysis patients/16,662 transplant patients.

cular related, 11.7% being associated with cerebrovascular disease (J. Barry, personal communication). Of possibly greater interest is the age-related cardiovascular mortality in end-stage renal disease. Shown in Table 3 is a comparison of the distribution of causes of cardiovascular death, by percentage, for three age brackets. For comparison, data[(3)] from the World Health Organization statistics annual reporting of the distribution of deaths in the United States for 1976 are referenced. As one surveys the figures, it is evident that premature cardiovascular death, especially under the age of 55, is the expected outcome for patients treated by either hemodialysis or renal transplantation. However, the incidence of noncardiovascular deaths, principally due to infection, modifies the situation in the case of renal transplant recipients. Although these statistics come as no great surprise to health professionals involved in the care of patients with terminal renal failure, they do present the nephrology community with a major challenge for the 1980s. One approach, which will be discussed in this subpart, relates to the known risk factors for premature cardiovascular disease that have been identified in the population as a whole. From the 7-year experience with non-ESRD patients recently reported from the NIH,[(4)] it is likely that a major emphasis on modifying these risk factors would be rewarded with a significant reduction in cardiovascular mortality for end-stage renal disease patients.

Table 2. Comparative Distribution of Cardiovascular Mortality—ESRD versus Non-ESRD Patients

	Non-ESRD (%)	ESRD (%)	
		Dialysis	Transplant
Coronary heart disease	33.3	36.0	16.1
Cerebrovascular disease	8.1	12.7	5.6
All cardiovascular disease	47.8	63.5	36.4
Other causes	52.2	36.5	63.6

Table 3. Age-Related Cardiovascular Mortality—ESRD versus Non-ESRD[a]

	Age group					
	15–34		35–54		55	
	Non-ESRD	ESRD	Non-ESRD	ESRD	Non-ESRD	ESRD
Coronary heart disease	1.0	34.2/12.0[b]	15.1	35.4/16.8	20.5	38.8/26
Cerebrovascular disease	1.0	10.7/5.6	2.9	12.9/5.6	4.7	13.8/6.8
All cardiovascular disease	3.9	64.9/34.7	21.9	63.4/37.0	29.7	62.2/43.4

[a] Expressed as percent of total.
[b] Hemodialysis/transplant.

Cardiovascular risk factors that have been confirmed from epidemiological studies are summarized in Table 4. The death rate due to cardiovascular disease in the United States has fallen by nearly 30%, and much of this decline has been attributed to a modification of the three major risk factors. Recently, Stamler estimated that reduction in cigarette smoking contributed to 50% of this decline in cardiovascular mortality while the decrease in mean serum cholesterol and the improvement in blood pressure regulation each contributed 25%.[(2)] This subpart will address the pathogenesis and therapeutic manipulation of systemic hypertension and lipid abnormalities as they affect terminal renal failure patients. In addition to hypertension, lipid abnormalities, and cigarette smoking, it is also important to recognize that there are a substantial number of minor cardiovascular risk factors (Table 4). Many of the minor risk factors are present to a substantial degree in patients with ESRD. Those which can be modified by therapeutic introvention include glucose intolerance, obesity, sedentary life-style, hyperuricemia, and dietary sodium intake. Unfortunately, many of the therapeutic and dietary

Table 4. Risk Factors for Premature Cardiovascular Disease

Major
Cigarette smoking
Hypertension
Lipid abnormalities
Minor
Glucose intolerance
Obesity
Sedentary life-style
Hyperuricemia
Dietary sodium
Sex
Family history
Age
Race
Behavior/stress
Alcohol/coffee

manipulations that are applied to patients with intact renal function are constrained in the patient receiving chronic intermittent hemodialysis, while no modifications for sex, family history, age, and race are possible. The evidence, although persuasive, is not conclusive concerning the influence of behavior/stress and alcohol/coffee; thus moderation should be the conventional wisdom. Recently, Haire *et al.*[5] from Seattle have published evidence supporting the adverse effects of smoking, unregulated hypertension, and elevated serum cholesterol on cardiovascular mortality in long-term hemodialysis patients. In this regard, there are four disease states in which a low mean plasma high-density lipoprotein (HDL) cholesterol concentration is associated with a high incidence of coronary heart disease. These include diabetes mellitus, uremia, nephrotic syndrome, and chronic cholestasis. It is noteworthy that three of the four disease categories are frequently encountered in our patients with terminal renal failure, further intensifying cardiovascular risk. A new area of interest and investigation involves the relationship between HDL and atherosclerosis. Support is growing to substantiate the inverse relationship between HDL cholesterol concentrations and the rate of progression of atherosclerosis in man.[6]

Within the group of patients with end-stage renal disease, there are subsets that are a special risk to vascular disease based on their underlying systemic illness. We have already referred to the increased risk of the diabetic, and this can be confirmed when one looks at the mortality rate for diabetic patients compared to nondiabetic patients treated either by chronic intermittent hemodialysis (C. Blagg, personal communication) or by renal transplantation.[7] Recently, Nanra *et al.*[8] from Australia have reported an increased incidence of cardiovascular mortality in patients with analgesic nephropathy undergoing long-term hemodialysis management. Obviously, this latter group raises the question about the contribution of chronic prostaglandin inhibition as a contributor to progressive atherosclerosis in terminal renal failure.

What will be the challenge for the 1980s? At least two points come to mind with regard to the influence and the impact of cardiovascular disease in patients with end-stage renal failure. The first relates to the psychology of living with a predictable fatal illness. How does one motivate behavioral changes which have a hypothetical, but as yet unproven, long-term benefit to the patient in question? Second, the multifactorial character of cardiovascular disease challenges the development and testing of effective programs of prevention.

References

1. *Proc Eur Dial Transpl Assoc* 15:40–53, 1978.
2. *Proceedings of National Heart, Lung, and Blood Institute Conference on Coronary Heart Disease Mortality*, October 24–25, 1978.
3. *World Health Organization Statistics Annual*, 1979, pp 135–141.

4. Cooper R, Stamler J, Dyer A, Garside D: The decline in mortality from coronary heart disease, USA, 1968–1975. *J Chron Dis* 31:709–720, 1978.
5. Haire HM, Sherrard DJ, Scardapane D, Curtis FK, Brunzell JD: Smoking, hypertension, and mortality in a maintenance dialysis population. *Cardiovasc Med* 3:1163–1168, 1978.
6. Kannel WB, Castelli WP, Gorden T: Cholesterol in the prediction of atherosclerotic disease. *Ann Intern Med* 90:85, 1979.
7. Bennet WM, Kloster F, Rosch J, Barry J, Porter GA: Natural history of asymptomatic coronary arteriorgraphic lesions in diabetic patients with end-stage renal disease. *Am J Med* 65:779–784, 1978.
8. Nanra RS, Stuart–Taylor J, deLeon AH, White KH: Analgesic nephropathy: Etiology clinical syndrome and cliniopathologic correlations in Australia. *Kidney Int* 13:79–92, 1978.

22

Renal Function, Sodium, Volume, and Arterial Pressure Relationships

Allen W. Cowley, Jr.

Nephrologists have a greater awareness of the important relationships between the kidneys and the cardiovascular system than any other group of clinicians. This association between renal function and the cardiovascular system was recognized by Richard Bright nearly a century ago. It was logical for investigators in the early twentieth century to assume that if the kidneys were unable to excrete sodium and water at a rate equivalent to daily intake, blood volume would expand with a resultant rise of cardiac output and arterial pressure. Curiously, however, as technology progressed through the 1930s to the present time, this basic notion became increasingly difficult to accept. It was found that even with decreased excretory ability of the kidneys and associated hypertension, blood volume and cardiac output could be either normal, low, or elevated.[1,2] The extracellular fluid volume was found to be inversely related to the level of arterial pressure in patients with essential hypertension. Elevation of peripheral vascular resistance appeared to be the only hemodynamic variable that hypertensive patients had in common, even those with clear evidence of decreased renal excretory capacity.

Interest in the factors that influence systemic vascular resistance was further stimulated by the experiments of Goldblatt in the 1930s, leading to the elucidation of the renin–angiotensin system. The prodigious research on the renin–angiotensin system was matched only by the research on the automatic nervous system and associated efforts to develop clinically effective sympathetic blocking agents. Successful treatment of hypertension with chronic blockade of the sympathetic nervous system naturally provided even greater impetus for the notion that hypertension was basically a disease of

Allen W. Cowley, Jr. • Department of Physiology and Biophysics, University of Mississippi Medical Center, Jackson, Mississippi 39216.

increased vascular resistance having little to do with abnormalities of the fluid volume control systems.

How, then, do renal excretory ability and the control of body fluid volumes relate to arterial pressure and the cardiovascular system? What was wrong with the early notion that cardiac output and arterial pressure were directly related to fluid volume, and more specifically to blood volume? After considerable experimental and theoretical examination of this question, we have concluded that there was *nothing* inherently *wrong* with this concept.

1. Relationships between Renal Function, Fluid Volumes, and Arterial Pressure

A sound theoretical framework has been developed which appears to unify much of the seemingly paradoxical observations just cited. I have chosen a simple schematic representation of the cardiovascular and renal fluid volume system to focus attention on some of the basic mechanisms with which one must deal when considering the relationships between renal function, fluid volumes, and arterial pressure (Fig. 1). It includes the continuous "intake" and "loss" of sodium and water, in and out of compliant and resistive arterial and venous vascular segments; a pump; and a central nervous system. An integrating type of system is represented whereby in time, if the amount of salt and water entering exceeds the amount leaving, fluid will accumulate and the filling pressure of the system will rise within all segments of the container and raise the cardiac output. Pressure within the system is generated by a cardiac pump normally capable of recirculating all of the volume that is returned to it. The magnitude of this pressure elevation will depend on the ability of the vessel walls to distend and accommodate fluid in excess of that required to fill the system.

A key element in this system is the renal excretory system. Since environment and dietary habits normally determine the amount of sodium and water intake to the system, it remains a function of the kidneys to control the rate of excretion and thereby the amount of volume expansion that will occur. A paramount physical feature of this system is that glomerular filtration and the loss of sodium and water are dependent fundamentally on the hydraulic forces within the vascular system. Acting on the enormous daily volume of filtered fluid and solutes are many finely tuned biochemical–neurohumoral mechanisms which exert a major influence to regulate the rate of tubular reabsorption necessary to conserve appropriate amounts of water, electrolytes, and other substances.

The basic hydraulic relationship between renal perfusion pressure and overall urinary excretion has been determined using isolated blood-perfused kidneys that exhibited normal autoregulatory ability (Fig. 2). As renal arterial perfusion pressure is increased from 100 to 200 mm Hg, urine output rises nearly six- to sevenfold.[3,4] Unfortunately, these direct hydraulic effects on urinary excretion are difficult to demonstrate in normal, conscious animals

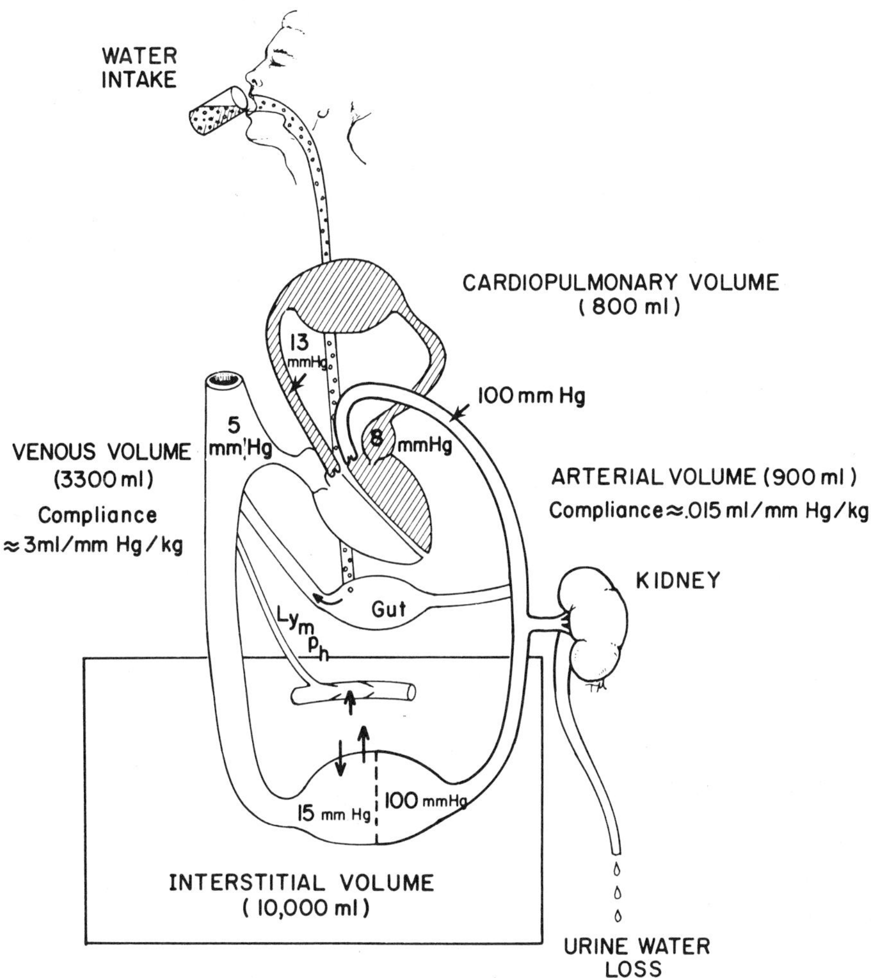

Figure 1. Schematic diagram of the renal–fluid volume–cardiovascular relationships. (Reprinted from ref. 19.)

or man. It has not been technically feasible to independently raise renal perfusion pressure for prolonged periods while measuring the rate of urine excretion. It has been possible, however, to determine the level of renal arterial perfusion pressure required to eliminate variously administered daily loads of sodium and water. Studies of this type have shown that *in situ* kidneys normally can increase excretion of sodium and water nearly six- to sevenfold while mean arterial pressure increases only 8–10 mm Hg.[5,6] The vertical axis in Fig. 2 represents urinary sodium output. But since it is axiomatic that in steady-state conditions (3–4 days) total sodium and water lost through all sources must equal their intake, under these steady-state conditions values on the ordinate represent both sodium intake and loss,

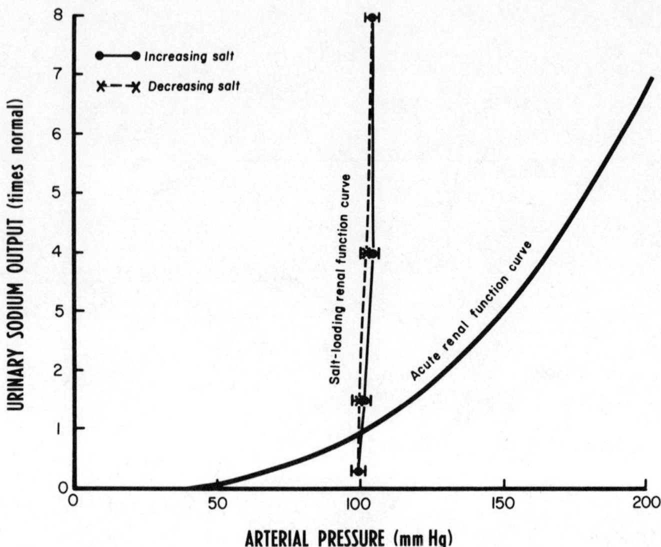

Figure 2. Effect of arterial pressure on urinary output of sodium when arterial pressure is changed acutely or chronically. (Reprinted from ref. 20.)

correcting for extrarenal sources of loss. It is clear that the slope of the chronic relationship is considerably steeper than the acute changes observed in the isolated kidney. This has led some people to conclude that arterial pressure is unimportant in controlling renal excretion, but nothing could be further from reality. There has now been a great amount of experimental and theoretical support presented for the importance of arterial pressure in renal excretion.[7,8] First is the clear relationship between renal perfusion pressure and renal excretion observed in the isolated kidney. Second is the inescapable consequence of the fact that the fluid volume systems of all organisms are integrating-type systems. This concept is illustrated in Fig. 3 in which is it clear that if the net rate of urine output does not equal the net rate of daily intake (plus extrarenal water loss), there will be a continuous change of the extracellular fluid volume. If intake exceeds output, volumes will expand raising filling pressures and finally raising arterial pressure. It is an integrating system because as long as intake exceeds output, the volume will continue to increase either until pressure rises to sufficient levels to make urinary output equal to input or until the heart fails. Finally, the overriding role of arterial pressure in renal excretion is necessary because of the nature of other known mechanisms involved in the control of renal excretion, that is, the neurohumoral systems. None of these systems are capable of making a 100% correction following a step change in fluid volume intake. The consequence of a slight remaining deviation from normal is readily apparent if we consider what would happen if only 99.9% of our daily water intake was removed by the rapid neurohumoral systems. In 1

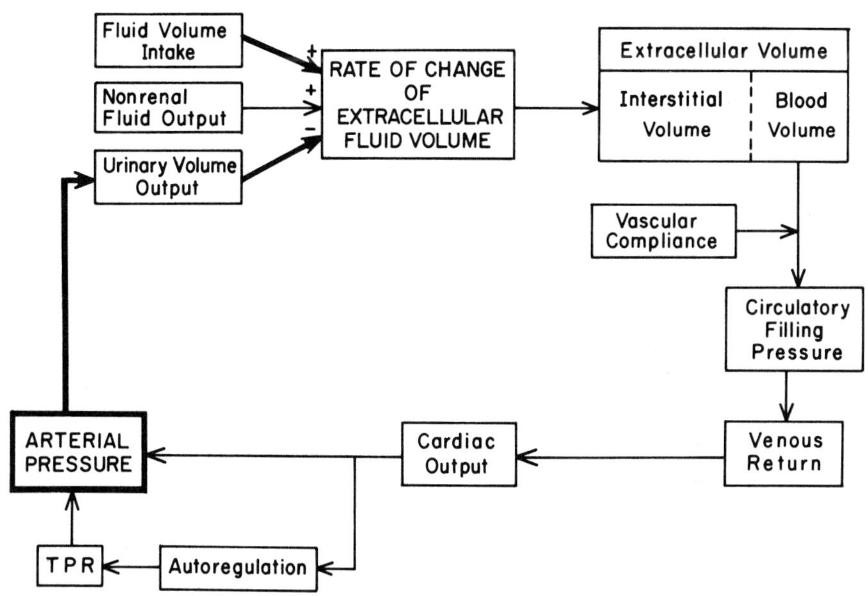

Figure 3. Diagram of the circular relationship between arterial pressure, urinary volume output, and body fluids. (Reprinted from ref. 21.)

year, we would accumulate 430 ml and over a lifetime, provided we had the capacity to store it, about 30 liters of fluid. It is therefore the unique integral function of the kidneys that makes this organ the prevailing factor in the long-term control of arterial pressure. The kidneys become the final common pathway for the control of arterial pressure in both normal and pathological states.

Despite the importance of the circular fluid–volume–arterial pressure–urinary output relationship, it is difficult to demonstrate in normal intact subjects. One reason for this is because of the consequences of local tissue autoregulation, which I will discuss shortly. The other reason is because of the many complex and well-known extrinsic factors that influence renal function. The most important of these is the renin–angiotensin–aldosterone system and the low-pressure stretch receptor reflex mechanisms in the atria of the heart and the arterial baroreceptor reflexes. It is, of course, these neurohumoral systems that are most easily studied and with which we are all generally familiar that enable the organism to respond *rapidly* to changes in fluid and electrolyte status while arterial pressure is controlled relatively constant.

To demonstrate the basic importance of arterial pressure in long-term regulation of salt and water excretion, one need only look at what happens to the relationship between arterial pressure and urinary excretion when one of the major endocrine systems controlling sodium and water excretion is inoperative. Look, for example, at the consequences of sustained increases

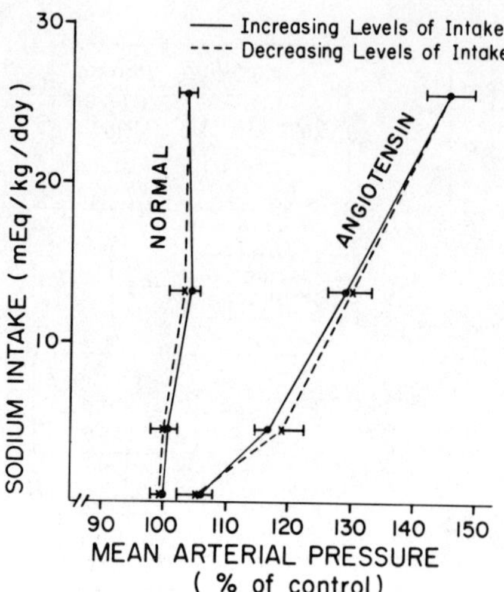

Figure 4. Renal function curves: steady-state relationship between mean arterial pressure and sodium intake (equal to excretion in steady state). Mean arterial pressure was recorded in six dogs infused with normal saline beginning at a very low sodium intake per day and increasing in steps to a very high intake, then returning to the very low levels. Each step required 3 or more days of infusion. After the series in normal dogs was completed, the protocol was repeated several weeks later in the same animals while angiotensin II, 5 ng/kg per minute, was infused continuously during the entire saline infusion period.

of sodium and water intake when the renin–angiotensin system is maintained at a constant level and cannot respond as usual. The normal suppression with excess sodium can be prevented by infusing angiotensin at a constant level throughout the period of increasing sodium and water intake. It can be seen in Fig. 4 that without suppression of the renin–angiotensin system, arterial pressure must rise to very high levels before a steady-state sodium and water balance can be achieved.[5,9] On the other hand, under normal conditions, demonstrated by the curve on the left, suppression of renin secretion occurs with increasing levels of sodium and water intake. This permits the highly efficient renal excretion of sodium and water while body fluid volumes and arterial pressure are maintained at a relatively constant level. Similarly, it has also been shown that when the renin-angiotensin system is prevented from operating by continuous infusion of the angiotensin I-converting enzyme inhibitor SQ 14,225, arterial pressure must again rise to enable excretion of increased amounts of administered sodium and water.[10]

The participation of other factors that can importantly influence the arterial pressure–urinary output relationship has been similarly studied. There are three major renal sites of action where various physiological and pathological factors can act to alter glomerular tubular balance in such a way as to change the normal relationship between arterial pressure and renal excretion. These include, first, preglomerular sites, which can be influenced by direct stenosis of the renal artery or by diffuse vasoconstriction of afferent arterioles; second, glomerular filtration *per se*, which can be altered in various disease states; and third, the rate of tubular reabsorption of sodium and water as influenced by angiotensin, aldosterone, and vasopressin. Alteration of renal function at each of these particular sites has been shown to result in characteristic alterations of the steady-state arterial pressure–urinary output curves.[6]

Those factors that act predominantly on preglomerular sites shift the renal function curve upward from normal in a nearly parallel fashion. This has been shown in one-kidney, one-clamp, Goldblatt hypertension where glomerular and tubular function become essentially normal after aortic pressure has risen to sufficient levels to overcome the imposed vascular resistance.[11] It has been observed that chronic intrarenal infusion of norepinephrine will also shift the relationship in a somewhat parallel manner, suggestive of predominantly afferent arteriolar resistance changes, although this situation is complicated with mildly elevated levels of renin.[12] It is particularly interesting that spontaneously hypertensive rats also exhibit a nearly parallel shift in their renal function curve, suggesting a predominant role for the afferent preglomerular resistance vessels in this genetic strain of hypertensive rats.[11]

Factors that act predominantly on renal tubules, such as aldosterone, depress the slope of the renal function curve so that a higher level of pressure is required at each increased amount of sodium and water load to achieve balance.

Reduction in the total number of functional nephrons which has been experimentally induced by surgical reduction of renal mass to one third normal serves to clearly demonstrate an inability of these kidneys to excrete increasing loads of sodium and water without a rise in arterial perfusion pressure.[6] Many other examples demonstrating the basic relationship between renal excretory ability and arterial pressure could be sited, and efforts are presently being made to characterize the renal function curves that are associated with identifiable renal alterations. I offer these examples only to demonstrate that *clearly an important relationship does exist between renal excretory ability and arterial pressure.*

2. *Relationship of Body Fluid Volume to Arterial Pressure*

To complete the link between renal excretory function and arterial pressure, however, it is necessary to now explain how body fluid volumes and blood volume in particular are related to arterial pressure. Curiously, this has been a very difficult thing to explain. Even when renal excretory function is seriously compromised by the surgical reduction of renal mass to one third normal and the continuous administration of six times the normal level of sodium and water intake, it is difficult after 7–10 days to demonstrate an elevation of either blood volume or cardiac output; only arterial pressure and vascular resistance are elevated.[13] Likewise, in established one-kidney Goldblatt hypertension where renal perfusion pressure is experimentally lowered and urinary excretion is slowed for several days with increased drinking, it has not been possible to demonstrate that the chronic state of hypertension is associated with expanded fluid volumes.[14]

Sequential studies of the alterations of fluid volumes, renal excretion, and hemodynamic variables during the developmental stages of these two

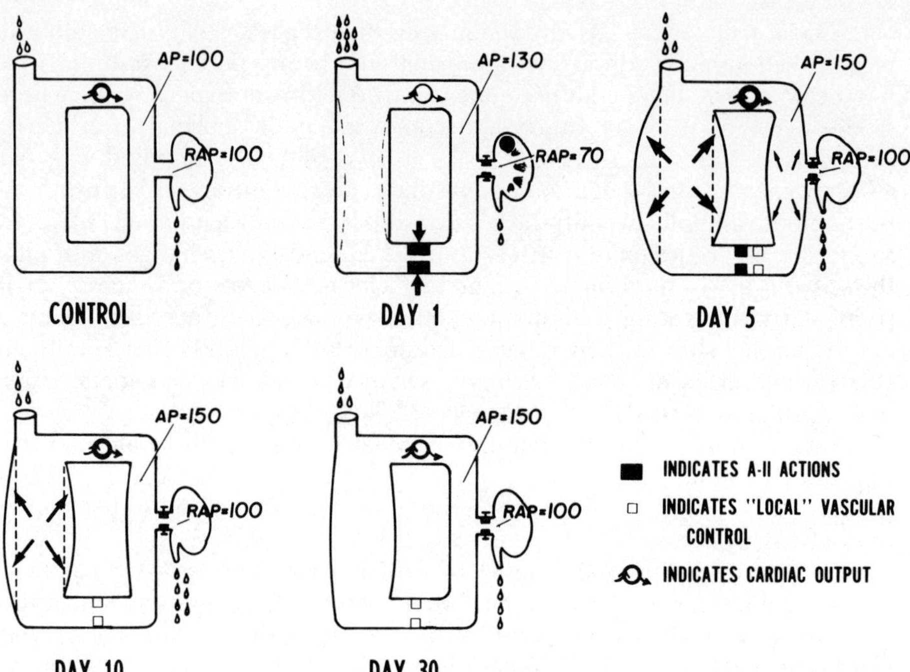

Figure 5. Sequential changes in body fluid volumes and arterial pressure observed during the development of one-kidney, one-clip Goldblatt hypertension (normal sodium intake). (Reprinted from ref. 22.)

experimental models of hypertension have greatly contributed to our understanding of these disturbing observations.

Figure 5 illustrates the major sequence of events observed during the development of one-kidney, one-clip Goldblatt hypertension. Constriction of the renal artery immediately releases renin, and renal excretion of sodium and water is decreased because of a fall in renal perfusion pressure. Arterial pressure promptly rises with angiotensin-induced vasoconstriction. Soon, a large increase in water intake occurs owing to an angiotensin-induced thirst stimulus. The consequent expansion of blood volume by the fifth day results in an increase of cardiac output which raises arterial pressure yet higher. By the fifth day following occlusion, renal perfusion pressure beyond the clamp rises to a level adequate to maintain renal function where balance can be achieved between fluid intake and excretion. As a result of this, the stimulus for renin release diminishes, and plasma levels of angiotensin and aldosterone return to nearly normal levels. Hypertension at this point is supported by an obviously expanded blood volume, as indicated by the diagram. Over the next week or two, the blood volume, extracellular fluid volume, and cardiac output return toward normal. This occurs in association with an increase in total peripheral resistance. It is this gradual increase of vascular resistance on which we need to focus our attention.

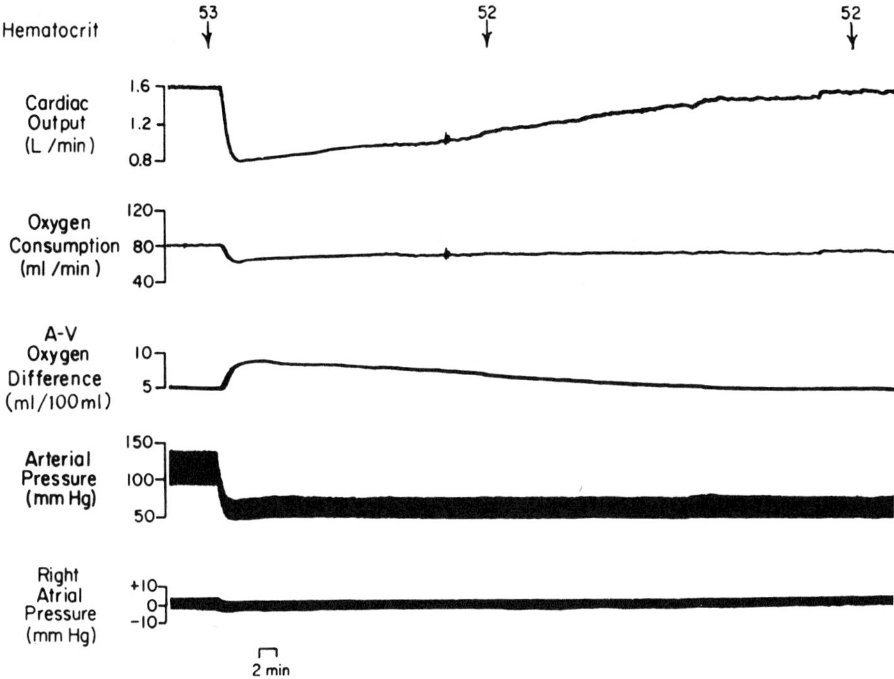

Figure 6. Whole-body autoregulation demonstrated in a dog after total removal of the central nervous system. Cardiac output was decreased by removal of blood, and arterial pressure was maintained at 55 mm Hg. Note the initial fall in arterial pressure as cardiac output fell. This was followed by a gradual rise in cardiac output as total peripheral resistance (not shown) decreased by autoregulation.(17)

The underlying mechanisms for these changes in resistance are poorly understood, but the most plausible hypothesis is based on the concept of whole-body autoregulation. This concept, suggested in 1963 by Borst and Borst-de-Geus(15) and Ledingham and Cohen,(16) proposes that expansion of body fluid volumes with consequent elevation of cardiac output results in overperfusion of the peripheral tissues, which in turn vasoconstrict to normalize tissue blood flow. As a result, cardiac output would return toward normal owing to an increased resistance to venous return and because of the contraction of blood volume secondary to renal pressure diuresis.

Evidence of the participation of whole-body autoregulation as a determinant of vascular resistance has been presented by a number of different laboratories. A dramatic example of regulation of total flow or cardiac output at the local tissue level is that seen in dogs in which the entire nervous system was surgically eliminated (Fig. 6).(17) In these animals, the total blood flow through the circulation was decreased by removal of whole blood while the arterial pressure was recorded and total peripheral resistance was calculated. It was observed that arterial pressure fell initially because cardiac output immediately fell, but over a period of 30 min total peripheral resistance gradually decreased because of tissue underperfusion until the decrease in resistance exceeded the decrease in cardiac output by 4.5× while arterial pressure was maintained at 55 mm Hg.

A number of theories have been proposed to explain the mechanisms of local autoregulation, but these are beyond the scope of this chapter. It is relevant, however, that experiments have thus far examined this mechanism only over brief time periods of minutes to hours. But the volume–pressure relationships we have been discussing, and which are clinically related to hypertension, develop slowly over days and months. A striking example of long-term tissue autoregulation in man is the adjustment of blood flow observed in patients with coarctation of the aorta. Measurements have shown that despite elevated arterial pressure in the upper extremities, with normal or below normal pressure in the lower extremities, the blood flow per unit mass of tissue is nearly equal in both locations.[18] Such opposite adjustments in vascular resistance between upper and lower extremities in the presence of the same hormonal milieu cannot be explained on the basis of any circulating substance nor by any known neural mechanisms. The mechanisms are unclear, but the most striking adjustment of the vasculature is the gradual alteration of vascular architecture by changes in wall thickness and length, and the growth or retardation of new or existing vessels. Such changes are well known to accompany normal growth and maturation, and it should not be surprising that similar changes also accompany various types of chronic stress such as volume overloading to the system. It is these slowly developing structural changes that appear to contribute in large measure to the adjustments in total peripheral resistance that have been observed during the development of volume-induced types of hypertension.

It is important to know the overall strength or ability of the autoregulatory mechanisms to return tissue blood flow toward normal, for this determines the extent to which the blood volume and cardiac output will be altered during volume overloading in hypertension. The degree of arterial pressure elevations that can be achieved with a 10% rise of cardiac output has been estimated at three different strengths of autoregulation. The changes seen in Fig. 7 were estimated using a mathematical model of the circulation in which the strength of autoregulation was adjusted to simulate the three steady-state values observed in volume-expanded, partially nephrectomized animals, assuming the long-term resistance changes were autoregulatory. In the *absence* of autoregulation, a 10% elevation of cardiac output would sustain approximately a 10% elevation of arterial pressure. This is the type of response observed with rapid blood volume expansion (10 min) in the absence of baroreceptor reflex mechanisms. However, in the presence of an autoregulatory response equivalent to that which has been shown to occur over a time period of 1–2 hr, a comparable steady-state rise of cardiac output (10%) is associated with a 43% elevation of arterial pressure after several hours.

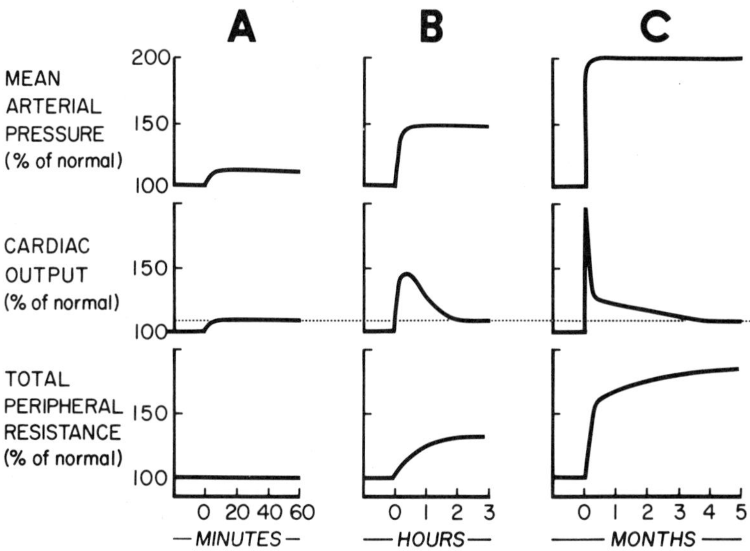

Figure 7. The response to expansion of blood volume with an associated rise in cardiac output under three conditions. (A) With no autoregulation the rise of arterial pressure is directly proportional to the rise in cardiac output. (B) With strength of autoregulation exhibited over a short period, arterial pressure is directly related only initially to the rise in cardiac output. After several hours, a cardiac output elevation of only 10% sustains arterial pressure at 100% of normal. (C) Long-term autoregulation after several months enables the same elevation of cardiac output (10%) that resulted in only a slight pressure elevation in the short-term state seen in A, to now sustain pressure at 200% of normal. (Reprinted from ref. 23.)

The long-term strength of the autoregulatory mechanism which develops over days and weeks far exceeds that observed acutely. On the basis of evidence from patients with coarctation of the aorta and a variety of animal studies, it appears that the system is capable in time of sustaining a 100% increase in arterial pressure with only a 10% increase in cardiac output.

Recall that even with a large sustained volume overload, such as occurs when fluid intake is increased to 7 times normal in subjects with reduced renal mass, or after a step decrease in renal perfusion pressure with a Goldblatt clamp, the initially large rise of cardiac output is nearly normal at the end of several weeks. Experimentally, it has been necessary to induce *rapid and large volume overloads* to demonstrate the transient elevations of fluid volumes and cardiac output. The autoregulatory events cannot be unmasked using a very slow expansion of body fluids since the long-term autoregulatory adjustments occur at nearly the same rate as body fluid accumulation, and consequently large changes in fluid volumes or cardiac output do not occur. Since even massive sustained volume loading is associated with less than a 10% elevation of cardiac output and fluid volume at the end of 1–2 weeks, one would not expect to be able to detect clinically, using any available means, alterations of cardiac output or volumes during hypertensive states associated with slow accumulation of salt and water. The preceding analysis indicates that an overexpansion of blood flow of only 5%, clinically undetectable, could sustain an elevation of arterial pressure in excess of 50% of normal. Thus, the amount of excess volume and flow needed to initiate the long-term autoregulatory changes in resistance is probably extremely small.

It should be apparent that there are invariably many types of hypertension in which these mechanisms could play a significant role in the long-term adjustment of total peripheral resistance. These include in particular those situations in which renal function is some way chronically impaired resulting in fluid retention. These include renal artery constriction, reduction of functional renal mass, glomerulonephritis, and pressure-induced nephrosclerosis. In all these situations, expansion of blood volume and elevation of cardiac output may occur at some stage of development of hypertension, albeit slowly and undetectably.

Unfortunately, the concept of autoregulation has often been inappropriately applied. Some investigators have attempted to use the concept to account for increased total peripheral resistance in all forms of hypertension. Others have tried to apply it to all situations of acute and chronic volume overload. When the observed hemodynamic changes have not been in agreement with what might be predicted by autoregulation, the validity of the theory has been questioned. For this reason, it is important to understand some of the conditions that must be met in order to observe autoregulation.

First, an autoregulatory increase in vascular resistance can occur only when the expansion of blood volume results in overperfuson of body tissues. This volume expansion may be *real* or may be reflected as only a change in the "effective volume" whereby the same absolute volume is confined to a vascular compartment of reduced size or compliance. Since such a real or "effective" volume change can equally affect cardiac output, measurements of the total blood volume *per se* are of limited value in studying the hemodynamic mechanisms of hypertension. Unfortunately, the "effective volume" or the degree of filling of the vasculature cannot be clinically determined so that interpretation of clinical volume data is at the present time very difficult.

The second condition to be met if autoregulation is to be observed is that the heart must be capable of converting an expanded volume into an elevated cardiac output. In cardiac failure, even a large overexpansion of total blood volume need not result in increased cardiac output or tissue overperfusion.

Third, all the systems responsible for delivery of tissue oxygen and other tissue nutrients must be normal. If the oxygen-carrying capabilities of the blood are depressed as in anemia, an elevated tissue blood flow would not be perceived as excessive and increased vascular resistance by autoregulation would not result.

Fourth, the metabolic needs of the tissue must remain unchanged since metabolic rate changes alter tissue flow requirements which can alter tissue blood flow independently of the blood volume status. Many substances can exert this influence including the thyroid hormones, corticosteroids, catecholamines, insulin, certain vitamins, and many other hormones and drugs.

Fifth, the fluids that have initiated the expansion of blood volume must be held within the vasculature. Situations that lead to increased capillary filtration or renal diuresis can rapidly obscure changes in vascular resistance expected on the basis of autoregulation. Dilution of plasma proteins must always be considered in this regard.

Thus, there are many events that can obscure what at first might be expected to result in a predictable autoregulatory response. Finally, it should be recognized that volume expansion with consequent autoregulation is certainly not the only mechanism that could increase vascular resistance during the development of hypertension. Some forms of hypertension appear to be initiated solely by constriction of both renal and peripheral arterioles with changes in body fluid volumes and cardiac output being only *secondary* consequences of a high total peripheral resistance. Examples of such situations are renal tumors or trauma with release of renin and formation of angiotensin or pheochromocytoma with abrupt release of norepinephrine.

In summary, the core of the information I have tried to convey in this chapter is basically simple. That is, that the long-term level at which arterial pressure is regulated is ultimately determined by the ability of the kidney to produce urine at a given perfusion pressure and by the total volume load presented to the kidney. Alterations of normal renal function necessitate alterations of renal perfusion pressures in order to permit the kidney to respond to the varying amounts of daily sodium and water intake. If the arterial pressure level is not sufficient, fluid will accumulate until such a renal perfusion pressure is achieved. Since we have seen that autoregulatory mechanisms appear to possess considerable compensatory strength, only a small amount of fluid retention and cardiac output elevation is required to ultimately increase systemic vascular resistance, so small in fact that in the steady-state condition changes in cardiac output and blood volume are nearly undetectable.

The renal–fluid volume mechanism for determining arterial pressure occurs slowly and is often masked by more rapidly acting reflex and hormonal mechanisms. However, in time the pressure–diuresis system prevails over all systems and determines the long-term level of arterial pressure. Clearly, Richard Bright was correct when he emphasized an intimate relationship between renal function and the cardiovascular system.

References

1. Birkenhager WH, Schalekamp ADH, Krauss XH, Kolsters G, Schalekamp–Kuyken MPA, Kroon BJM, Teulings FAG: Systemic and renal hemodynamics, body fluids and renin in benign essential hypertension with special reference to natural history. *Eur J Clin Invest* 2:115, 1972.
2. Safar ME, Chau NP, Weiss YA, London GM, Simon ACH, Milliez PP: The pressure–volume relationship in normotensive and permanent essential hypertensive patients. *Clin Sci Mol Med* 50:207, 1976.

3. Selkurt EE: Effects of pulse pressure and mean arterial pressure modification on renal hemodynamics and electrolyte and water excretion. *Circulation* 4:541, 1951.
4. Thuraw K, Deetzen P: Diuresis in arterial pressure increases. *Pflugers Arch ges Physiol* 274:567, 1962.
5. DeClue JW, Guyton AC, Cowley AW Jr., Coleman TG, Norman RA, McCaa RE: Subpressor angiotensin infusion, renal sodium handling, and salt-induced hypertension in the dog. *Circ Res* 43:503, 1978.
6. Guyton AC, Cowley AW Jr., Coleman TG, Liard JF, McCaa RE, Manning RD, Norman RA, Young DB: Pretubulus versus tubulus mechanisms of renal hypertension, in Sambhi MP (ed): *Mechanisms of Hypertension*, Proceeding of International Workshop. Amsterdam, Excerpta Medica, 1973.
7. Guyton, AC, Coleman TG, Cowley AW Jr., Scheel KW, Manning RD, Norman RA: Arterial pressure regulation. *Am J Med* 52:584, 1972.
8. Guyton AC, Coleman TG, Granger HJ: Circulation: Overall regulation. *Ann Rev Physiol* 34:13, 1972.
9. Cowley AW Jr., McCaa RE: Acute and chronic dose-response relationships for angiotensin, aldosterone, and arterial pressure at varying levels of sodium intake. *Circ Res* 39:788–797, 1976.
10. Hall JE, Guyton AC, Coleman TG, McCaa RE: Long-term relationships between arterial pressure, urinary output and renal hemodynamics after converting enzyme inhibition. *Kidney Int* 14:696, 1978.
11. Norman RA, Enobakhare JA, DeClue JN, Douglas BH, Guyton AC: Arterial pressure–urinary output relationship in hypertensive rats. *Am J Physiol* 234:R98, 1978.
12. Cowley AW Jr., Lohmeier TE: Changes in renal vascular sensitivity and arterial pressure associated with sodium intake during long-term intrarenal norepinephrine infusion in dogs. *Hypertension* 1:549, 1979.
13. Cowley AW Jr., Guyton AC: Baroreceptor reflex effects on transient and steady-state hemodynamics of salt-loading hypertension in dogs. *Circ Res* 36:536–546, 1975.
14. Bianchi G, Baldoli E, Lucca R., Barbin P: Pathogenesis of arterial hypertension, after the constriction of the renal artery, leaving the opposite kidney intact, both in the anesthetized and in the conscious dog. *Clin Sci* 40:651, 1972.
15. Borst JGG, Brost-de-Geus A: Hypertension explained by Starling's theory of circulatory homeostasis. *Lancet* 1:677, 1963.
16. Ledingham JM, Cohen RD: Autoregulation of the total systemic circulation and its relation to control of cardiac output and arterial pressure. *Lancet* 1:887, 1963.
17. Granger HJ, Guyton AC: Autoregulation of the total systemic circulation following destruction of the central nervous system in the dog. *Circ Res* 25:379, 1969.
18. Wakin KG, Slaughter O, Clagett DT: Studies on the blood flow in the extremities in cases of coarctation of the aorta; determination before and after excision of the coarcted region. *Proc Mayo Clin* 23:347, 1948.
19. Cowley AW Jr: Perspectives on the physiology of hypertension, in Onesti G, Brest AN (eds): *Cardiovascular Clinics—Hypertension: Mechanisms, Diagnosing, and Treatment.* Philadelphia, F. A. Davis, 1978.
20. Guyton AC: *Circulation Physiology; Arterial Pressure and Hypertension.* Philadelphia, Saunders, 1980.
21. Onesti G, Brest AN (eds): *Cardiovascular Clinics—Hypertension: Mechanisms, Diagnosis, and Treatment.* Philadelphia, F. A. Davis, 1978.
22. Cowley AW Jr, Coleman TG, Lohmeier TE: Renal hypertension; A unifying theory, in Villarceal H (ed): *Hypertension.* New York, John Wiley & Sons, 1981, pp 99–108.
23. Cowley AW Jr: The concept of autoregulation of total blood flow and its role in hypertension. *Am J Med* 68:906–916, 1980.

23

Abnormal Carbohydrate and Lipoprotein Metabolism in Uremia

Possible Relationship to Atherogenesis

Gerald M. Reaven

1. Introduction

There is a good deal of evidence which indicates that abnormalities of carbohydrate and lipid metabolism occur frequently in patients with chronic renal failure (CRF). Given the increased incidence of atherosclerotic heart disease (ASHD) in patients with diabetes and/or hyperlipoproteinemia, it seems reasonable to wonder if the accelerated atherogenesis described in patients with CRF is related to the coexistence of abnormal carbohydrate and lipid metabolism in these patients. In this chapter I will attempt to approach this question by defining the effects of the uremic syndrome on carbohydrate and lipid metabolism and then suggesting possible mechanisms by which these changes could lead to atherosclerosis.

2. Effect of Uremia on Carbohydrate Metabolism

2.1. Insulin Catabolism

A delay in the removal of insulin from plasma is probably the most profound change in carbohydrate metabolism seen in patients maintained on chronic hemodialysis. This phenomenon is clearly seen in Fig. 1, which compares the rate at which normal individuals and anephric patients remove

Gerald M. Reaven • Department of Medicine, Stanford University School of Medicine, and Geriatric Research, Education and Clinical Center, Veterans Administration Medical Center, Palo Alto, California 94304. Work supported by the Research Services of the Veterans Administration.

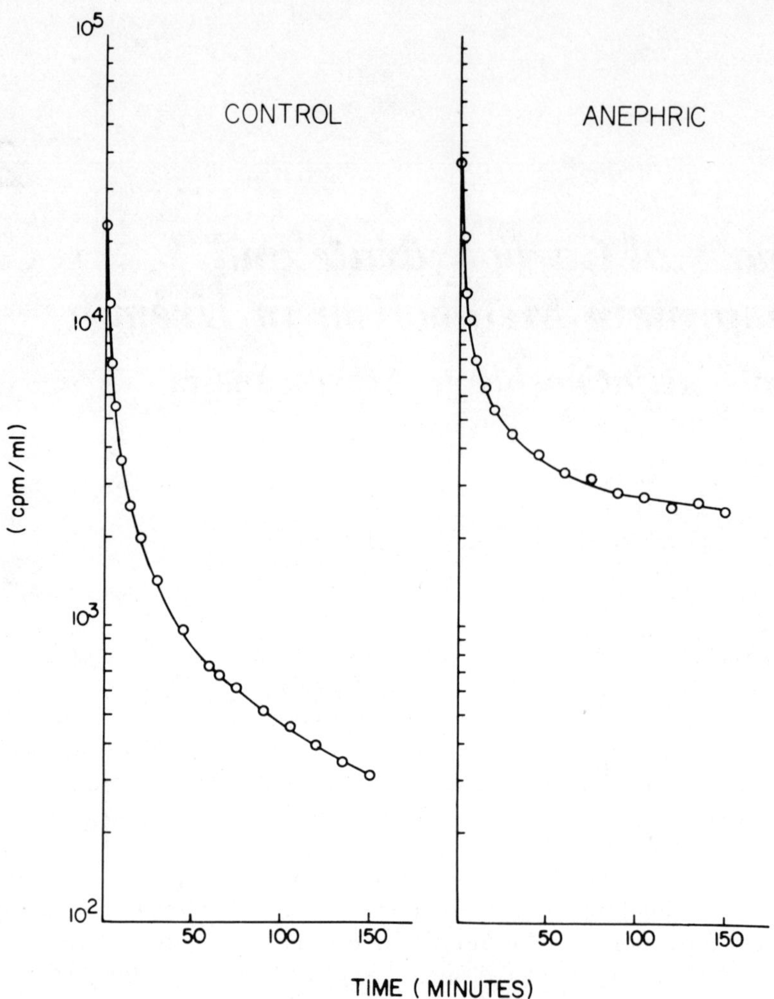

Figure 1. Disappearance curves from plasma of immunoprecipitate ^{131}insulin in a normal subject and in an anephric patient. (Reprinted from ref. 1, with permission of the authors.)

a tracer dose of iodinated insulin from plasma. These results emphasize the important role that the kidney plays in removal of insulin from the systemic circulation, and this point has been appreciated for some time.[(1)]

On the other hand, recent results suggest that the delay in removal of insulin from plasma seen in patients with CRF may not be due entirely to loss of normal renal parenchyma.[(2)] Evidence for this is seen in Fig. 2, which illustrates the rate at which insulin is cleared by perfused hindlimbs of control and acutely uremic rats. It is obvious from these data that acute uremia results in an inhibition of insulin removal by muscle. A similar defect

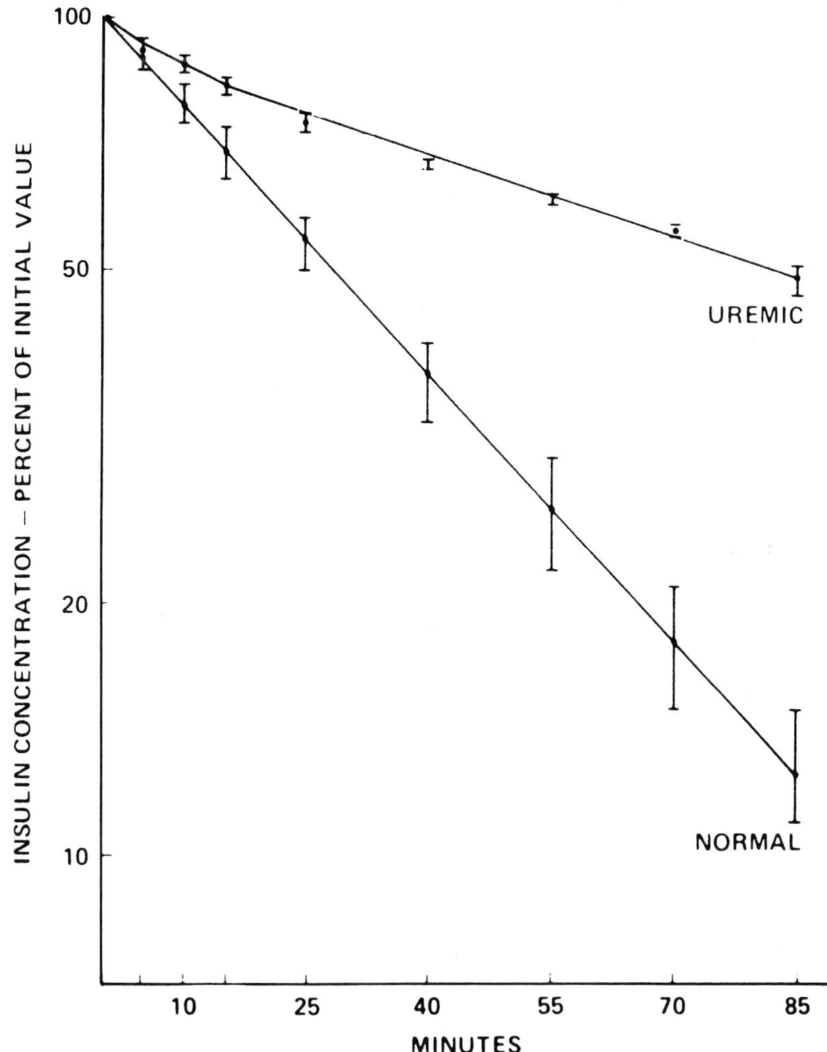

Figure 2. Percentage of initial insulin concentration remaining during 90 min recirculation of normal and uremic hindlimb. Insulin concentration at 5 min was taken as 100%, and each point represents the mean ± SEM of nine experiments. (Reprinted from ref. 2, with permission of the authors.)

in insulin catabolism by muscle of chronically uremic rats has recently been reported by Rabkin *et al.*[3]

In contrast, hepatic catabolism of insulin appears to be unaffected by uremia.[2] Evidence for this conclusion is seen in Fig. 3, which indicates that hepatic extraction of insulin by perfused livers of acutely uremic and control rats is identical over a wide range of perfusate insulin concentrations. This question has also been addressed by Rabkin *et al.*,[3] and their data add

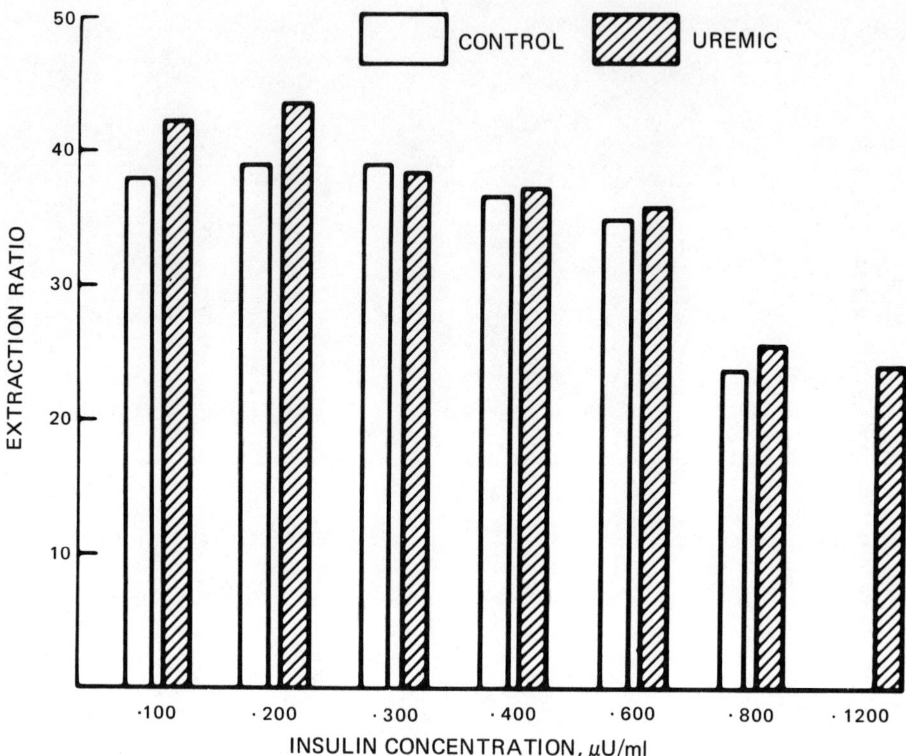

Figure 3. Extraction ratios of insulin at different perfusate insulin concentrations by perfused livers from control and acutely uremic rats.

further support to the conclusion that hepatic catabolism of insulin is normal in uremia.

Thus, there is general agreement that uremia is associated with a prolongation of insulin removal from plasma. A major cause of this defect is certainly the loss of normal renal parenchyma. However, it also seems clear that uremia leads to a defect of insulin catabolism by muscle. Given the quantity of body tissue that is muscle, it is likely that altered muscle insulin catabolism plays a role in prolonging the clearance of insulin from plasma in uremic subjects.

2.2. *Plasma Glucose and Insulin Responses*

Glucose intolerance is another well-recognized effect of uremia,[1] and this phenomenon is illustrated in Fig. 4. These results are characteristic of the plasma glucose and insulin responses of patients maintained on hemodialysis. When patients with CRF are compared to normal subjects, it is clear that their plasma glucose levels are moderately, but significantly greater at every time interval during the glucose tolerance test. Furthermore, it is clear from

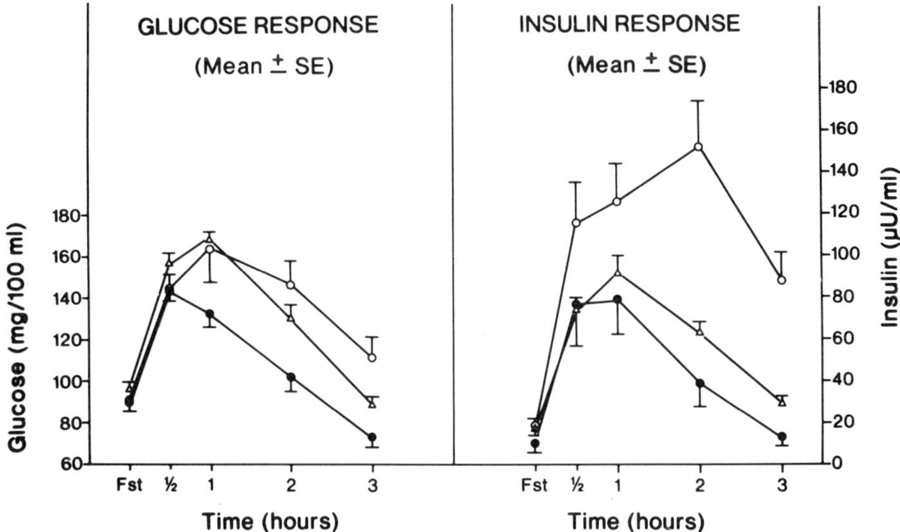

Figure 4. Mean (±SEM) plasma glucose and insulin responses during an oral glucose tolerance test (40 g/m^2) of normal subjects (•), patients with CRF (○), and individuals with slightly impaired glucose tolerance (△).

these data that the plasma insulin response of patients with CRF is much greater than that of normal subjects.

The plasma insulin response to an oral glucose load is a complex function of the rate at which insulin is entering and leaving the circulation. Given the profound effect that uremia has on insulin catabolism, it is possible that the observed hyperinsulinemia is secondary to delayed insulin removal from plasma. On the other hand, since uremic subjects were glucose intolerant, the hyperinsulinemia may also be a reflection of their higher plasma glucose levels. In order to gain some insight into the relative importance of glucose intolerance and impaired insulin removal in the hyperinsulinemia of patients with CRF, the insulin response of a group of subjects with normal renal function, but impaired glucose tolerance, is also included in Fig. 4. It is obvious that the plasma insulin response of these subjects is lower than that of patients with CRF, in spite of the fact that the two groups had essentially similar glucose responses. These results demonstrate that the glucose intolerance of patients with CRF is associated with hyperinsulinemia, part of which may reflect the development of glucose intolerance, but part of which also appears to be a consequence of defective insulin catabolism.

2.3. *Insulin Sensitivity*

Uremic patients respond to an oral glucose load with hyperglycemia and hyperinsulinemia (see Fig. 4). The fact that glucose intolerance occurs in the face of plasma insulin levels that are greater than those of normal subjects

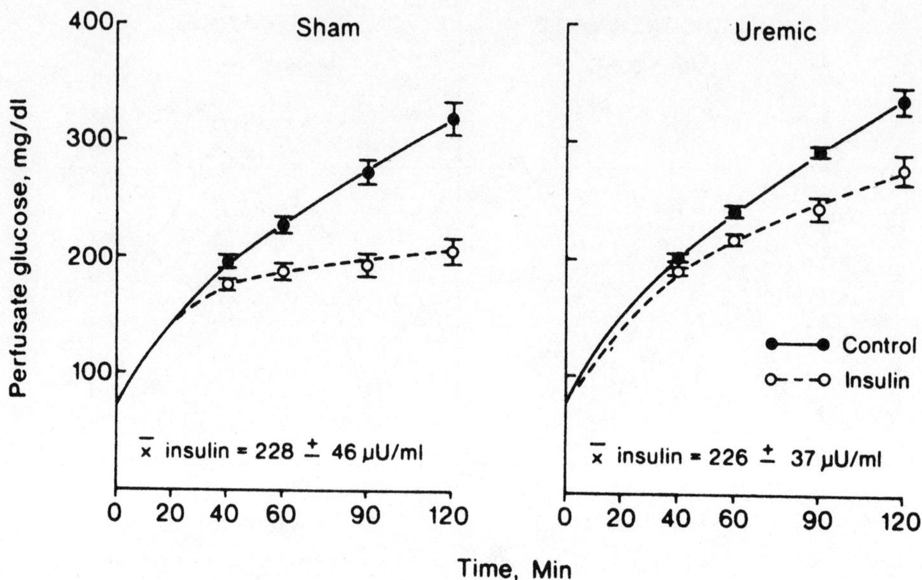

Figure 5. Effect of insulin on disappearance of glucose from perfusing medium during perfusion of hindlimbs from sham-operated and uremic rats. Mean ($\bar{x}$) insulin was calculated from average perfusate concentration between 20 and 120 min. The effect of insulin on lowering perfusate glucose concentration was significant to $p < 0.005$ at 60, 90, and 120 min in both sham-operated and uremic perfusions. (Reprinted from ref. 5, with permission of the authors.)

is indirect evidence that the biological effect of insulin is blunted in uremic subjects. Direct evidence that uremia leads to loss of normal insulin sensitivity has been furnished by recent studies in acutely uremic dogs[4] and rats[5] and in chronically uremic man.[6] Although the mechanism of this insulin resistance remains to be fully defined, recent studies have greatly helped in locating the tissue site of the abnormality.[5,6]

The data in Fig. 5 compare the ability of insulin to stimulate glucose uptake in perfused hindlimb muscle of acutely uremic and control rats. It is apparent that the effect of insulin to augment glucose uptake was attenuated in the acutely uremic rats. A quantitative estimate of this difference is seen in Table 1, and it is clear from these data that perfused muscle of acutely uremic rats did not respond to insulin with a significant increase in glucose uptake.

On the other hand, the ability of insulin to inhibit glucose production by perfused liver was not impaired in acutely uremic rats. These data are shown in Fig. 6 and demonstrate that the effect of adding either minimally or maximally effective doses of insulin to the perfusate led to comparable suppression of glucose outflow from livers of control or uremic rats.

These results suggest that the glucose intolerance of uremia is due to insulin resistance in the muscle, with the liver maintaining normal insulin sensitivity. However, studies in both chronically uremic man[7] and rat[8] have suggested that uremia may lead to an enhancement of the glycogenolytic

Table 1. Effect of Insulin on Glucose Uptake in Perfused Hindlimbs of Sham-Operated and Uremic Rats[a]

	Glucose uptake (nmoles/muscle per min)	
	Sham (7)	Uremic (8)
Control	160 ± 9	156 ± 13
Insulin	222 ± 12	189 ± 7
Δ I-C	62 ± 15	23 ± 15
p	<0.005	N.S.

[a] Numbers of control and insulin-treated experiments are listed in parentheses. Values are expressed as means ± SEM. (Reprinted from ref. 5, with permission of the authors.)

effect of glucagon, which raises the possibility that the liver may play a role in the glucose intolerance of uremia. On the other hand, DeFronzo[(6)] has indicated that hepatic glucose production is normally suppressed by insulin, and we have not found perfused livers from acutely or chronically (unpublished) uremic rats to be uniquely sensitive to glucagon. Obviously, this question remains to be settled definitively.

3. Effect of Uremia on Lipoprotein Metabolism

3.1. Triglyceride Concentration

It is well recognized that patients with chronic uremia have elevated plasma triglyceride (TG) concentrations.[(10,11)] A quantitative estimate of this

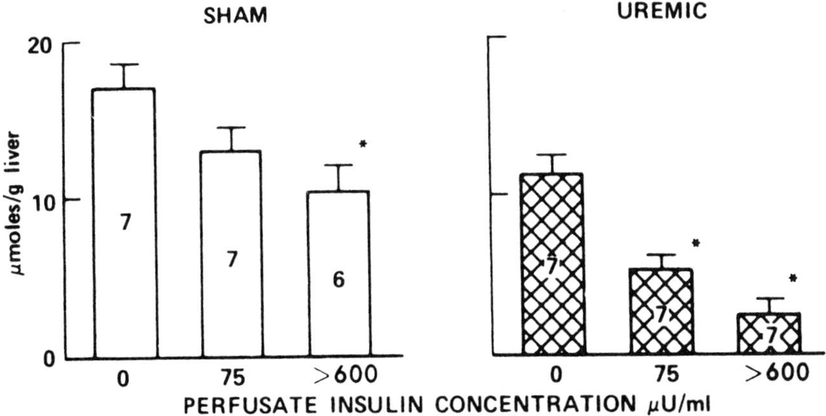

Figure 6. Effect of physiologic (<75 μU/ml) and maximal (>600 μU/ml) perfusate insulin concentration on suppression of glucose outflow by sham-operated and uremic rats after 120 min perfusion. Number of experiments in each group are listed in the bars, and significance of differences from control perfusions are indicated by $*p < 0.02$ sham and $*p < 0.005$ uremic. (Reprinted from ref. 5, with permission of the authors.)

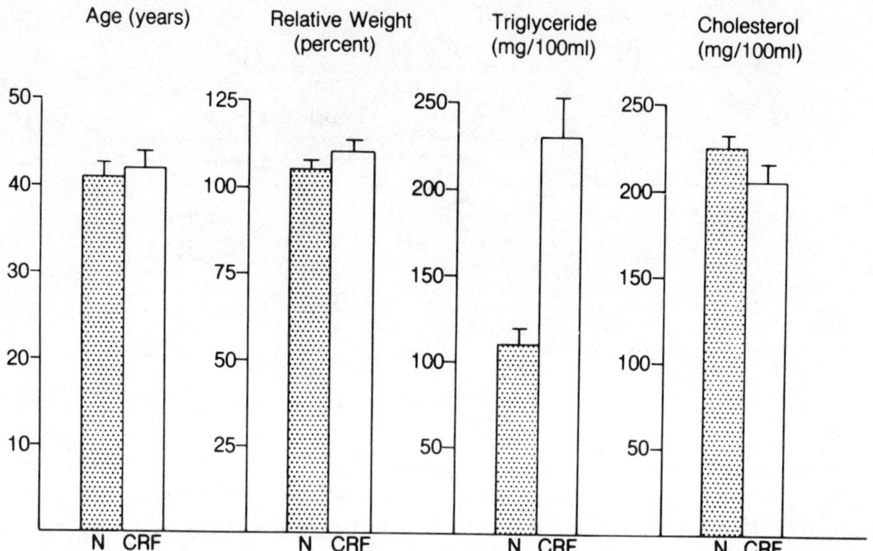

Figure 7. Mean (±SEM) age, relative weight, triglyceride, and cholesterol concentration in 27 patients with CRF. The values in these patients are compared to those obtained in 125 normal (N) subjects. (Reprinted from ref. 9, with permission of the authors.)

phenomenon is shown in Fig. 7, which illustrates the plasma TG concentration of a group of patients with CRF. It is obvious from these data that patients with CRF are hypertriglyceridemic. Parenthetically, it should be noted that uremia does not lead to hypercholesterolemia.

Hypertriglyceridemia can result from increases in very low-density lipoprotein (VLDL)–TG secretion rate and/or decreases in VLDL–TG removal from plasma. In order to approach this question, we determined the relationship between VLDL–TG secretion rate and plasma TG concentration in patients with CRF and compared it to the relationship seen in normal individuals.[12] These data appear in Fig. 8, in which the results from normal individuals are depicted by the stippled area. It is apparent that most of the patients with CRF, the filled circles, lie below the stippled area. Thus, for a given VLDL–TG secretion rate, they had a higher plasma TG concentration. In other words, they removed VLDL–TG from plasma less efficiently than did normal subjects. However, it should also be noted that the higher the secretion rate, the higher the plasma TG concentration in both groups, and that some patients with renal failure have very high VLDL–TG secretion rates.

The VLDL–TG removal defect seen in patients with CRF has been generally attributed to a decrease in the activity of the enzyme lipoprotein lipase (LPL).[13–15] However, this conclusion, which was based on measurement of plasma postheparin lipolytic activity (PHLA), is currently being reexamined. It is now recognized that total PHLA activity is a combination

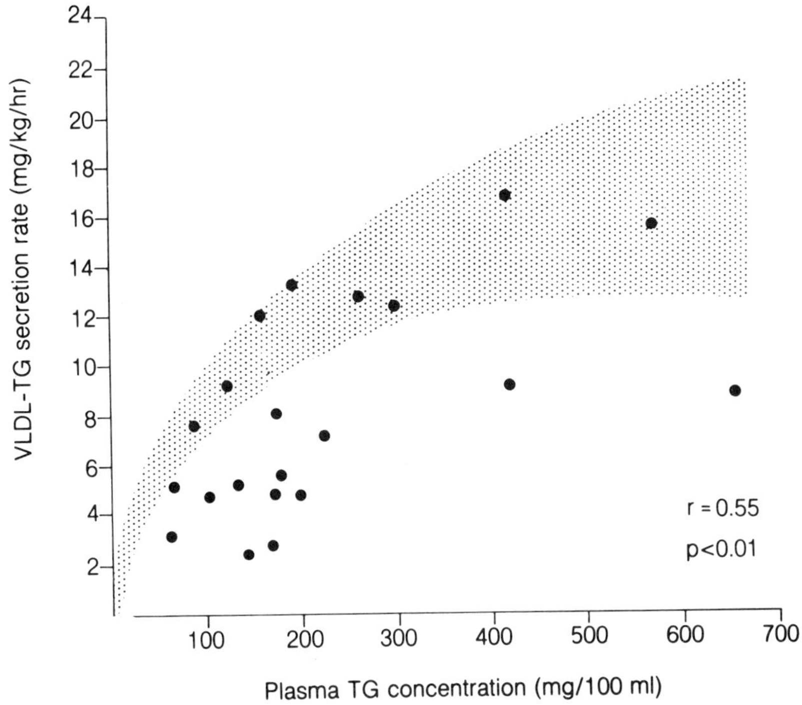

Figure 8. Relationship between VLDL–TG secretion rate and TG concentration in 21 patients with chronic renal failure. The stippled area defines the relationship between these two variables (mean and 95% confidence interval) seen in a group of 95 subjects with normal renal function and fasting plasma glucose concentration. (Reprinted from ref. 9 with permission of the authors.)

of at least two enzymes, hepatic triglyceride lipase (HTG) and LPL,[16,17] and specific measurements of LPL raise questions as to the role of this enzyme in uremic hypertriglyceridemia. Thus, the results of recent studies have indicated that LPL activity either is normal[18,19] or, if reduced,[20] is unrelated to hypertriglyceridemia in patients with CRF.

We have tried to approach this question by directly measuring tissue LPL activity in chronically uremic rats. These results are shown in Fig. 9, in which we have related plasma TG concentrations to adipose tissue LPL activity. Uremic rats, which had a sixfold elevation of BUN level, were divided into two groups on the basis of their plasma TG concentrations. Both groups had decreased tissue LPL activity, but the changes in enzyme activity were obviously unrelated to the changes in plasma TG concentration. Thus, although there is general agreement that hypertriglyceridemia in patients with CRF is due to a defect in VLDL removal, the cause of this abnormality remains to be defined.

3.2. High-Density Lipoprotein (HDL) Concentration

Several recent reports have indicated that patients with CRF, both dialyzed and undialyzed, have HDL–cholesterol levels that are lower than

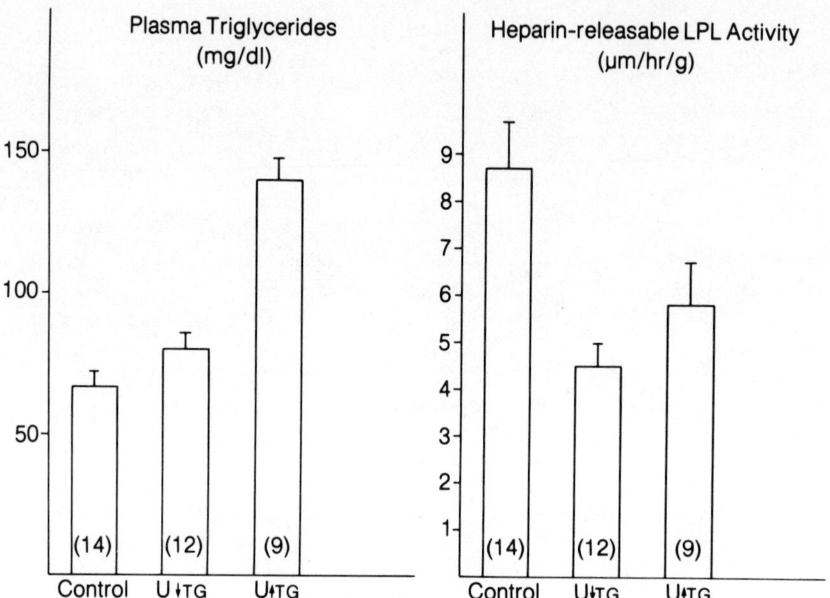

Figure 9. Mean (±SEM) plasma TG (mg/dl) and heparin-releasable LPL activity (μm FFA/hr per g wet weight) in control and chronically uremic (U) rats. U rats were subdivided into two groups on the basis of their plasma TG concentrations—those with TG concentrations below ($U\downarrow_{TG}$) and above ($U\uparrow_{TG}$) 100 mg/dl. Mean (±SEM) BUN concentrations of the three groups were as follows: control = 12 ± 1 mg/dl; $U\downarrow_{TG}$ = 63 ± 10 mg/dl; $U\uparrow_{TG}$ = 64 ± 8 mg/dl. Numbers in parentheses refer to the number of animals per group.

normal.[21–23] Reduced HDL–cholesterol levels have also been described[21] after successful renal transplantation, suggesting that renal failure *per se* may not be totally responsible for the lowered HDL–cholesterol levels. In this regard, it is interesting to note that a significant correlation exists between increased TG levels and decreased HDL–cholesterol levels in chronically dialyzed patients.[22] This observation is consistent with the possibility that changes in HDL metabolism are secondary to changes in VLDL metabolism, and this relationship has been noted in a variety of hypertriglyceridemic situations.[24] On the other hand, HDL–cholesterol levels in patients with CRF appear to be lower than can be accounted for by the degree of hypertriglyceridemia,[22] and the cause for the reduced HDL–cholesterol levels remains to be worked out.

4. *Relationship between Abnormal Carbohydrate and Lipid Metabolism and Development of ASHD in Patients with CRF*

The development of ASHD is certainly multifactorial, and risk factors such as hypertension and smoking, which have a harmful effect on normal individuals, will obviously also have an impact on patients with CRF. No

Table 2. Possible Metabolic Causes of ASHD in CRF

1. Impaired glucose tolerance
2. Elevated postprandial insulin concentrations
3. Hypertriglyceridemia
4. Reduced HDL–cholesterol concentrations

attempt will be made in this section to discuss all the possible factors that might contribute to accelerated atherogenesis in patients with CRF. Instead, an attempt will be made to select those abnormalities of carbohydrate and lipid metabolism which are both known to occur in patients with CRF and which might play a role in the development of cardiovascular disease. Four such factors are listed in Table 2: glucose intolerance, postprandial hyperinsulinemia, hypertriglyceridemia, and reduced levels of HDL–cholesterol. There is evidence that all these metabolic abnormalities are associated with accelerated atherogenesis, and in the remainder of the chapter an attempt will be made to briefly summarize this information.

4.1. *Impaired Glucose Tolerance*

There is no doubt that the incidence of ASHD is increased in patients with frank diabetes mellitus. However, the deleterious effect of minor abnormalities of glucose intolerance, similar to that seen in patients with CRF, is less clear. Indeed, one of the major difficulties is that studies that have attempted to deal with this issue have too often grouped together patients with widely varying degrees of glucose intolerance under the general heading of diabetes. On the other hand, there is substantial support for the notion that minor impairments of glucose tolerance can lead to accelerated atherogenesis. Thus, there is a good deal of evidence that impaired glucose tolerance is a common finding in patients with clinical evidence of ASHD.[(25–29)] Second, prevalence studies have reported a significant association between glucose intolerance and vascular disease in unselected population groups.[(30–32)] Finally, there is evidence from prospective studies that patients with glucose intolerance develop significantly more atherosclerosis.[(33–35)]

4.2. *Postprandial Hyperinsulinemia*

The evidence that hyperinsulinemia may play a role in the development of atherosclerosis has recently been reviewed,[(36)] and the argument can be summarized as follows. Nondiabetic patients with atherosclerosis respond to an oral glucose challenge with an elevated insulin response.[(37–42)] Furthermore, patients with diabetes and atherosclerosis frequently have plasma insulin levels that are higher than in normal subjects. Thus, the argument that hyperinsulinemia can lead to accelerated atherogenesis is based primarily on the observation that hyperinsulinemia is a common finding in subjects with vascular disease. However, there is a recent report of a prospective study from Paris[43] which identifies hyperinsulinemia as a primary risk factor in the development of ASHD. This finding provides additional support for the idea that elevated insulin levels may be important in atherogenesis and makes it mandatory that this possibility receive further study.

4.3. *Hypertriglyceridemia*

The incidence of hypertriglyceridemia is significantly greater in both diabetic and nondiabetic patients with ASHD.[25–27,34,35,44–46] Furthermore, several prospective studies have demonstrated that there is a significant relationship between hypertriglyceridemia and ASHD in unselected populations.[47–50] Indeed, there seems to be general agreement concerning this point, and the only issue in question is whether or not hypertriglyceridemia is a primary risk factor. In other words, when one takes into account associated changes in HDL and LDL metabolism, is hypertriglyceridemia a risk factor for atherosclerosis? This question cannot be dealt with fully in the context of this chapter; however, it is essential to realize that there is a very intimate relationship between the metabolism of all three classes of lipoproteins. Thus, the argument over what is a primary risk factor may be irrelevant in therapeutic efforts to treat the lipoprotein abnormality of patients with CRF. This conclusion may be particularly relevant in view of the recent report of a prospective study that found hypertriglyceridemia to be significantly associated with ASHD in patients with CRF.[51]

4.4. *Reduced HDL–Cholesterol*

Several recent studies[49,52,53] have confirmed the earlier observation[54] that ASHD and HDL–cholesterol concentrations are inversely related; i.e., the lower the HDL–cholesterol concentration, the greater the incidence of ASHD. Consequently, considerable attention is currently being directed toward study of HDL metabolism. As a result of this we have learned a great deal about the relationship between VLDL and HDL metabolism, as well as information concerning factors that can modify HDL–cholesterol concentration. Thus, we are in a position to modulate HDL–cholesterol levels in an effort to see if this would benefit patients at risk for developing ASHD.

5. *Conclusion*

In conclusion, profound abnormalities of carbohydrate and lipid metabolism are seen in patients with CRF. There is general agreement about the nature of the changes that do occur, and a good deal of understanding exists as to their pathogenesis. There is reason to believe that at least four distinct metabolic abnormalities are associated with the uremic syndrome, the presence of which may help explain the accelerated atherogenesis that occurs in this situation. Understanding of the mechanism by which these abnormalities develop has reached a point where thoughtful therapeutic intervention is possible. The time may now be ripe to begin a multiple-risk intervention trial to see if it would be possible to inhibit the development of ASHD in patients with CRF.

References

1. Reaven GM, Weisinger JR, Swenson RS: Insulin and glucose metabolism in renal insufficiency. *Kidney Int* 6:563–569, 1974.
2. Mondon CE, Dolkas CB, Reaven GM: Effect of acute uremia on insulin removal by the isolated perfused rat liver and muscle. *Metabolism* 27:133–142, 1978.
3. Rabkin R, Unterhalter SA, Duckworth WC: Effect of prolonged uremia on insulin metabolism by isolated liver and muscle. *Kidney Int* 16:433–439, 1979.
4. Swenson RS, Peterson DT, Eshleman M, Reaven GM: Effect of acute uremia on various aspects of carbohydrate metabolism in dogs. *Kidney Int* 4:267–272, 1973.
5. Mondon CE, Dolkas CB, Reaven GM: The site of insulin resistance in acute uremia. *Diabetes* 25:571–576, 1978.
6. DeFronzo RA: Pathogenesis of glucose intolerance in uremia. *Metabolism* 27:1866–1880, 1978.
7. Sherwin RS, Bastle C, Finkelstein FO, Fisher M, Black H, Hendler R, Felig P: Influence of uremia and hemodialysis on the turnover and metabolic effects of glucagon. *J Clin Invest* 57:722–731, 1976.
8. Soman J, Felig P: Glucagon and insulin binding to liver membranes in a partially nephrectomized uremic rat model. *J Clin Invest* 60:224–232, 1977.
9. Mondon CE, Reaven GM: Evaluation of enhanced glucagon sensitivity as the cause of glucose intolerance in acutely uremic rats. *Am J Clin Nutr* 33:1456–1460, 1980.
10. Sanfelippo ML, Swenson RS, Reaven GM: Reduction of plasma triglycerides by diet in subjects with chronic renal failure. *Kidney Int* 11:54–61, 1977.
11. Sanfelippo ML, Swenson RS, Reaven GM: Response of plasma triglycerides to dietary changes in patients on hemodialysis. *Kidney Int* 14:180–186, 1978.
12. Reaven GM, Swenson RS, Sanfelippo ML: An inquiry into the mechanism of hypertriglyceridemia in patients with chronic renal failure. *Am J Clin Nutr* 33:1476–1484, 1980.
13. Bagdade JE, Porte D Jr, Bierman EL: Hypertriglyceridemia. A metabolic consequence of chronic renal failure. *N Engl J Med* 279:181–185, 1968.
14. Bagdade JD: Uremic lipemia. *Arch Intern Med* 126:875–881, 1970.
15. Boyer JL, Scheig RL: Inhibition of postheparin lipolytic activity in uremia and its relationship to hypertriglyceridemia. *Proc Soc Exp Biol Med* 134:603–605, 1970.
16. Fielding CJ: Further characterisation of lipoprotein lipase and hepatic post-heparin lipase from rat plasma. *Biochim Biophys Acta* 280:569–578, 1972.
17. Krauss RM, Levy RI, Fredrickson DS: Selective measurement of two lipase activities in postheparin plasma from normal subjects and patients with hyperlipoproteinemia. *J Clin Invest* 54:1107–1124, 1974.
18. Mordasini R, Frey F, Flury W, Klose G, Greten H: Selective deficiency of hepatic triglyceride lipase in uremic patients. *N Engl J Med* 297:1362–1366, 1977.
19. Bolzano K, Krempler F, Sandhofer F: Hepatic and extrahepatic triglyceride lipase activity in uraemic patients on chronic haemodialysis. *Eur J Clin Invest* 8:289–293, 1978.
20. Crawford GA, Savdie E, Stewart JH: Heparin-released plasma lipases in chronic renal failure and after renal transplantation. *Clin Sci* 57:155–165, 1979.
21. Bagdade, JD, Albers JJ: Plasma high-density lipoprotein concentrations in chronic-hemodialysis and renal-transplant patients. *N Engl J Med* 296:1436–1439, 1977.
22. Brunzell DD, Albers JJ, Haas LB, Goldberg AP, Agadoa L, Sherrard DJ: Prevalence of serum lipid abnormalities in chronic hemodialysis. *Metabolism* 26:903–910, 1977.

23. Rapoport J, Aviram M, Chaimovitz C, Brook JG: Defective high-density lipoprotein composition in patients on chronic hemodialysis. *N Engl J Med* 299:1326–1329, 1978.
24. Nikkilä EA: Metabolic regulation of plasma high density lipoprotein concentrations. *Eur J Clin Invest* 8:111–113, 1978.
25. Reaven GM, Calciano A, Cody R, Lucas C, Miller R: Carbohydrate intolerance and hyperlipemia in patients with myocardial infarction without known diabetes mellitus. *J Clin Endocrinol Metab* 23:1013–1023, 1963.
26. Heinle RA, Levy RI, Frederickson DS, Gorlin R: Lipid and carbohydrate abnormalities in patients with angiographically documented coronary artery disease. *Am J Cardiol* 24:178–186, 1969.
27. Falsetti HL, Schnatz JD, Greene DG, Bunnell IL: Serum lipids and glucose tolerance in angiographically proved coronary artery disease. *Chest* 58:111–115, 1970.
28. Kingsbury KJ: The relation between glucose tolerance and atherosclerotic vascular disease. *Lancet* 2:1374–1379, 1966.
29. Sloan JM, Mackay JS, Sheridan B: Glucose tolerance and insulin response in atherosclerosis. *Br Med J* 4:586–588, 1970.
30. Keen H, Jarrett RJ: Macroangiopathy—its prevalence in asymptomatic diabetes. *Adv Metab Disord* 2:(suppl)3–9, 1973.
31. Ostrander LD, Francis T, Hayner NS, Kjelsberg MO, Epstein FH: The relationship of cardiovascular disease to hyperglycemia. *Ann Intern Med* 62:1188–1198, 1965.
32. Epstein FH, Ostrander LD, Johnson BJ, Payne MW, Hayner NS, Keller JB, Francis T: Epidemiological studies of cardiovascular disease in a total community—Tecumseh, Michigan. *Ann Intern Med* 62:1170–1187, 1965.
33. Gordon T, Kannel, WB: Predisposition to atherosclerosis in the head, heart, and legs. *JAMA* 221:661–666, 1972.
34. Garcia MJ, McNamara PM, Gordon T, Kannel WB: Morbidity and mortality in diabetics in the Framingham population. Sixteen year follow-up study. *Diabetes* 23:105–111, 1974.
35. Gordon T, Castelli WP, Hjortland MC, Kannel WB, Dawber TR: Diabetes, blood lipids, and the role of obesity in coronary heart disease risk for women. The Framingham Study. *Ann Intern Med* 87:393–397, 1977.
36. Stout RW: Diabetes and atherosclerosis—the role of insulin. *Diabetologia* 16:141–150, 1979.
37. Peters N, Hales CN: Plasma insulin concentrations after myocardial infarction. *Lancet* 1:1144–1145, 1965.
38. Nikkilä EA, Miettinen TA, Vesenne MR, Pelkonen R: Plasma insulin in coronary heart disease. *Lancet* 2:508–511, 1965.
39. Tzagournis M, Chiles R, Ryan JM, Skillman TG: Interrelationships of hyperinsulinism and hypertriglyceridemia in young patients in coronary heart disease. *Circulation* 38:1156–1163, 1968.
40. Malherbe C, deGasparo M, Berthet P, deHertogh R, Hoet JJ: The pattern of plasma insulin response to glucose in patients with a previous myocardial infarction—the respective effects of age and disease. *Eur J Clin Invest* 1:265–270, 1970.
41. Gertler MM, Leetma HE, Saluste E, Rosenberger JL, Guthrie RG: Ischemic heart disease. Insulin, carbohydrate and lipid interrelationships. *Circulation* 46:103–111, 1972.
42. Sorge F, Schwartkopff W, Neuhaus GU: Insulin response to oral glucose in patients with a previous myocardial infarction and in patients with peripheral vascular disease. *Diabetes* 25:586–594, 1976.
43. Eschwege E, Ducimetiere P, Rosselin GE, Claude JR, Richard JL: 0–2 hr OGTT plasma glucose and insulin levels as coronary heart disease risk factors in middle-aged active men. Abstracts, 10th Congress of the IDF, 1979, p 59.
44. Albrink MJ, Man EB: Serum triglycerides in coronary heart disease. *Arch Intern Med* 103:4–8, 1959.
45. Ostrander LD, Neff BJ, Block WD, Francis T, Epstein FH: Hyperglycemia and hypertriglyceridemia among persons with coronary heart disease. *Ann Intern Med* 67:34–41, 1967.
46. Santen RJ, Willis PW, Fajans SS: Atherosclerosis in diabetes mellitus. *Arch Intern Med* 130:833–843, 1972.

47. Kannel WB, Castelli WP, Gordon T, McNamara PM: Serum cholesterol, lipoproteins, and the risk of coronary heart disease. The Framingham study. *Ann Intern Med* 74:1–12, 1971.
48. Carlson LA, Böttiger LE, Ischaemic heart-disease in relation to fasting values of plasma triglycerides and cholesterol. Stockholm prospective study. *Lancet* 1:865–868, 1972.
49. Castelli WP, Doyle JT, Gordon T, Hames CG, Hjortland MC, Hulley SB, Kagan A, Zukel WJ: HDL-cholesterol and other lipids in coronary heart disease. The cooperative lipoprotein phenotyping study. *Circulation* 55:767–772, 1977.
50. Logan RL, Thomson M, Riemersma RA, Oliver MF, Olsson AG, Rossner S, Callmer E, Walldius G, Kaijser L, Carlson LA, Lockerbie L, Lutz W: Risk factors for ischaemic heart-disease in normal men aged 40. Edinburgh-Stockholm study. *Lancet* 1:951–954, 1978.
51. Brunzell JD, Sherrard DJ: Atherosclerotic risk factors in a chronic dialysis population. Abstract, American Society of Nephrology, 12th Annual Meeting, 1979, p 118A.
52. Miller GJ, Miller NE: Plasma high density lipoprotein concentration and development of ischaemic heart-disease. *Lancet* 1:16–19, 1975.
53. Rhoads GG, Gulbrandsen CL, Kagan A: Serum lipoproteins and coronary heart disease in a population study of Hawaiian Japanese men. *N Engl J Med* 294:293–298, 1976.
54. Barr DP, Russ EM, Eder HA: Protein–lipid relationships in human plasma. II. In atherosclerosis and related conditions. *Am J Med* 11:480–493, 1951.

24

The Role of Blood Pressure Regulation in Uremia

Donald J. Sherrard

The risks of high blood pressure and the benefits of its control are well established in the nonuremic population.[1,2] Less well-controlled, older studies strongly support the benefits of blood pressure reduction in patients with moderate renal insufficiency.[3] There is little reason to doubt that treatment of hypertension is an important facet of the care of patients with end-stage renal disease. Indeed, attempts to prove this contention with studies that included a control group of untreated hypertensives would not be ethically defensible.

The pathophysiology of elevated blood pressure centers around an expanded extracellular volume in the great majority of uremic patients. A minority of 10–15% are primarily renin dependent.[4] In both groups there is an abnormality in volume-mediated renin feedback inhibition.[5]

Control of hypertension in this group of subjects therefore must be based on extracellular volume reduction (i.e., by limited salt intake and enhanced elimination). Renin suppression usually plays a secondary role.[6] For the occasional extremely refractory patient minoxidil, a potent vasodilator, may be necessary.[7] Recently, the value of exercise in reducing blood pressure and serum triglycerides as well as elevating hematocrit has been documented in patients on dialysis.[8]

In the general population it is established that hypertension is the most important and the most reversible risk factor for cardiovascular disease.[9] Accelerated atherosclerosis is generally accepted to be the major cause of death in the dialysis population,[10,11] two recent studies notwithstanding.[12,13]

Donald J. Sherrard • Dialysis Unit, Veterans Administration Medical Center, Seattle, Washington 98108. Supported by the Medical Research Service of the Veterans Administration.

In reviewing subsequent patient data from a group reported earlier[10] we found that hypertension was a major factor in early mortality. Of the 14 patients who survived more than 10 years of dialysis only one was hypertensive (diastolic blood pressure over 95). In sharp contrast are the 23 patients who survived less than 10 years; ten were hypertensive. Finally 7 of 14 patients dying from cardiovascular events were hypertensive.

With this retrospective evaluation suggesting the importance of hypertension we then assessed a Veterans Administration (VA) dialysis population in whom risk factor data had been prospectively collected over 11 years.[14] Again the deleterious effect of hypertension was striking with a 2-year survival of only 45% in the hypertensive group ($n = 35$) vs. 81% ($p < 0.01$) in the 88 normotensive subjects.

Ongoing assessment of dialysis mortality continues to implicate hypertension. In a recent report we again noted the hazards of hypertension.[15] When combined with either smoking or elevated triglycerides it may be particularly deleterious.[14,15]

As pointed out by Burke *et al.*,[11] the status of a patient's vascular tree prior to starting dialysis may have an important influence on outcome. Both Vincenti *et al.*[16] and Goodman *et al.*[17] have been able to relate blood pressure control prior to dialysis treatment to overt vascular disease after the onset of dialysis. Thus, the control of blood pressure must be aggressively pursued throughout the course of renal disease. It is not enough to treat hypertension after the patient is on dialysis.

The preceding discussion has emphasized the importance of hypertension in end-stage uremic and dialysis patients. Transplant recipients are also at great risk. Hypertension may impair a patient's health to such an extent that he is not a transplant candidate. One report[16] noted such severe vascular disease in two hypertensive transplant candidates that the vascular anastamoses could not be made.

In addition to reducing the possibility of a patient's obtaining a transplant, hypertension may seriously affect life after transplantation. Hypertension may be a result of transplantation[18] or may damage the transplanted organ or other organs at risk. Atherosclerotic complications are, in fact, the second most common cause of death in renal transplant recipients.[19]

In summary, blood pressure control should be an integral part of the management plan of all patients with renal disease. No matter how mild the patient's renal disease or what type of therapy is being used, hypertension frequently accompanies the renal disorder. Control of blood pressure may slow the progression of renal disease. It will certainly protect other organs at risk.

References

1. Veterans Administration Cooperative Study on Antihypertensive agents: Effects of treatment on morbidity in hypertension: Results in patients with diastolic blood pressures averaging 115 through 129 mm Hg. *JAMA* 202:116–122, 1967.

2. Veterans Administration Cooperative Study on Antihypertensive Agents: Effects of treatment on morbidity in hypertension: II—Results in patients with diastolic blood pressure averaging 90 through 114 mm Hg. *JAMA* 213:1143–1152, 1970.
3. Harrington M, Kincaid-Smith P, McMichael J: Results of treatment in malignant hypertension. *Br Med J* 2:969–980, 1959.
4. Vertes V, Cangiano JL, Berman LB, Gould A: Hypertension in end-stage renal disease. *N Engl J Med* 280:978–981, 1969.
5. Brunner HP, Wauters J-P, McKintry D, Waeber B, Gustave-Turini A, Gavras H: Inappropriate renin secretion unmasked by captopril in hypertension of chronic renal failure. *Lancet* 2:704–707, 1978.
6. Lindner A, Douglas SW, Adamson JW: Effects of propranolol in long term hemodialysis patients with renin-dependent hypertension. *Ann Intern Med* 88:457–462, 1978.
7. Limas CJ, Fries ED: Minoxidil in severe hypertension with renal failure: Effect of its addition to conventional antihypertensive drugs. *Am J Cardiol* 31:355–361, 1973.
8. Goldberg AP, Hagberg JM, Delmeg JA, Haynes ME, Harter HR: Metabolic effects of exercise training in hemodialysis patients. *Kidney Int* 18:754–761, 1980.
9. Page IH: Two cheers for hypertension. *JAMA* 242:2559–2560, 1979.
10. Lindner A, Charra B, Sherrard DJ, Scribner BH: Accelerated atherosclerosis in prolonged maintenance hemodialysis. *N Engl J Med* 290:697–701, 1974.
11. Gurland HJ, Brunner FP, von Dehn H, Härlen H, Parsona FM, Scharer K: Combined report on regular dialysis and transplantation in Europe. *Proc Eur Dial Transpl Assoc* 10:17–57, 1973.
12. Burke JF, Francos GC, Moore LL, Cho SY, Lasker N: Accelerated atherosclerosis in chronic dialysis patients—another look. *Nephron* 21:181–187, 1978.
13. Rostand SG, Gretes JC, Kirk KA, Rutsky EA, Andreoli TE: Ischemic heart disease in patients with uremia undergoing maintenance hemodialysis. *Kidney Int* 16:600–611, 1979.
14. Haire HM, Sherrard DJ, Scardapane D, Curtis FK, Brunzell JD: Smoking, hypertension and mortality in a maintenance dialysis population. *Cardiovasc Med* 3:1163–1168, 1978.
15. Haas LB, Brunzell JD, Sherrard DJ: Atherosclerotic risk factors in a chronic dialysis population. *Kidney Int* 16:888A, 1979.
16. Vincenti F, Amend WJ, Abele J, Feduska NJ, Salvatierra O: The role of hypotension in hemodialysis-associated atherosclerosis. *Am J Med* 68:363–369, 1980.
17. Goodman WG, Haas LB, Sherrard DJ: Left ventricular hypertrophy and dialysis survival. *Clin Res* 27:61A, 1979.
18. Guttman RD: Renal transplantation. *N Engl J Med* 301:1038–1048, 1979.
19. The Advisory Committee to the Renal Transplant Registry: The 12th report of the human renal transplant registry. *JAMA* 233:787–796, 1975.

25

The Role of Manipulating Lipids in Uremia

Thomas A. Golper

Since the manipulation of lipids is such a broad subject, this chapter will specifically address the issue of hyperlipidemia (HL) associated with maintenance dialysis therapy.

1. *Introduction*

The incidence of HL in dialysis populations varies from 30 to 70%.[1–5] The predominant pattern is that of type IV, consisting of increased total triglycerides (TG), an increased very low-density lipoprotein (VLDL) fraction, and near-normal total cholesterol (Chol). Prospective studies in patients without renal disease indicate that the type IV pattern is associated with an increased incidence of ischemic heart disease.[6–8] Both direct and indirect evidence confirms this association in patients with end-stage renal disease (ESRD). In a prospective longitudinal study the Seattle group has shown that males less than 60 years of age with high triglyceride levels on dialysis are at a greater risk for premature cardiovascular disease than are normotriglyceridemic patients of the same age.[9] Once a patient is on dialysis, his lipids tend to remain stable.[10,11] However, when group means are examined after years on dialysis, TG levels have fallen.[2,11] This may be due to weight loss, decreased food intake, or a selection process in which those patients with high TG die, and those patients with lower TG survive and form the group studied at a later time. The appearance of HL coincides with the creatinine clearance declining to 50 ml/min. When dialysis is finally initiated, years of HL may have transpired.

In ESRD, a decrease in the high-density lipoprotein (HDL) fraction of cholesterol accompanies the type IV pattern.[1] This, by itself, is associated

Thomas A. Golper • University of Oregon Health Sciences Center, Portland, Oregon 97201.

with an increased incidence of ischemic heart disease in both renal and nonrenal patients.[10,12]

Since both type IV HL and a decreased HDL-Chol are atherosclerotic risk factors, can correcting them improve the prognosis? In the Coronary Drug Project, nicotinic acid did decrease the incidence of further events.[13] However, the drug was associated with side effects and was not recommended for use in patients with known heart disease. In the World Health Organization study, the patients were selected because of increased Chol, but therapy with clofibrate did decrease the incidence of nonfatal ischemic cardiac events.[14] Of the three most often quoted diet studies,[15–17] only Dayton and colleagues report a reduction in both Chol and total lipids, as well as a reduction in cardiovascular morbidity and mortality. Regression of atherosclerosis has been observed in patients specifically treated for their HL.[18,19]

I have found no evidence that specific correction of the type IV pattern reduces the incidence of ischemic cardiac events in the presence or absence of renal disease. Since uremia accelerates the atherosclerotic process,[20,21] uremic patients appear ideally suited to be the subjects of studies to investigate the hypothesis that correcting the type IV abnormality decreases ischemic cardiac events. The task would be to try to reverse the lipid abnormality in these patients. The remainder of this chapter deals with how this might be accomplished and emphasizes certain areas of controversy where further research is indicated.

2. Manipulations Primarily by the Patient

2.1. Ideal Weight

Under the physician's guidance there are several manipulations that are still primarily the responsibility of the patient. First among these is achievement of the ideal body weight. This is the first step in the management of elevated VLDL.[22] Correlations between weight and elevated TG in dialysis patients have been reported.[4,23] We should strongly encourage our patients with HL to achieve their ideal body weight.

2.2. Exercise

A graded exercise program should accompany the weight reduction. Goldberg *et al.* demonstrated improvement in HDL-Chol, elevated TG, glucose disappearance, oxygen uptake, anemia, and hypertension in hemodialysis (HD) patients who participated in aerobic exercise training.[24,25]

2.3. Diet

There are several beneficial changes that patients can make in their dietary habits that may contribute to their overall lipid-lowering efforts.

2.4. *Phosphate*

Phosphate control and avoidance of hyperparathyroidism may prove beneficial in ESRD atherosclerosis. Hypercalcemia accompanying hyperparathyroidism is associated with reduced tissue sensitivity to insulin,[26] and this is potentially lipogenic. Animal, human and *in vitro* studies have demonstrated parathyroid hormone (PTH) effects on the lipolytic system,[27–29] and this may have clinically significant effects on lipid mobilization in ESRD. In contrast are the findings of Lazarus and colleagues.[21] Seven HD patients were evaluated pre- and postparathyroidectomy with a significant decrement in PTH levels after surgery but no significant change in carbohydrate metabolism, fasting insulin, TG, or Chol. In addition, Ponticelli and colleagues found no correlation between PTH and lipid levels.[5] However, this still leaves unexplained Cantin's observations on the interactions of PTH, lipids, and uremia.[30] He demonstrated that anephric or bilateral ureteral-ligated rats had more severe hyperlipidemia in the presence of PTH, either from functioning parathyroid tissue or, in the postparathyroidectomized rats, from parathyroid extract. Independent of lipids, PTH may have an effect on the acceleration of atherosclerosis through its effects on cellular calcium movement, particularly in vascular smooth muscle.[31,32] The relationship between uremic hyperparathyroidism and HL is still unclear and needs to be resolved.

2.5. *Carbohydrates and Fats*

Although uremic HL may not be directly correlated with carbohydrate intake,[33,34] there is a tendency for TG to rise with protein restriction and increased carbohydrate compensation.[35] Gutman and colleagues have commented that proper nourishment is probably a prerequisite for hypertriglyceridemia to manifest itself.[3]

Heuck *et al.* demonstrated in uremic rats that TG rose when the animals were fed diets rich in protein, fat, or carbohydrate.[36] With the protein-rich diet the animals died. With the carbohydrate-rich diet the TG were higher than with the fat-rich diet. This exacerbation of HL with short-term carbohydrate-rich diets was confirmed in ESRD patients by Sorge *et al.*[37]

Two types of dietary intervention have been described for the HL of ESRD in humans. The Stanford group has shown that a low-carbohydrate, relatively high-fat diet, regardless of the saturated fat or Chol content, significantly lowers TG in HD patients.[38] These patients did not suffer from HL and the diet period ran for only 10 days. Gokal *et al.* evaluated a high-carbohydrate, low-fat, low-Chol, low-saturated-fat diet in 20 patients with two forms of uremic HL.[39] TG fell in all patients; Chol fell in those with the IIB abnormality. Posttreatment values returned toward baseline.

At the University of Oregon we are utilizing a diet similar to that of Gokal, where complex carbohydrates are used to maintain a eucaloric state and the total cholesterol intake is further reduced to 100 mg/day.[40]

Long-term studies using these various diets need to be completed. In the meantime, our HL patients should achieve their ideal weight, and regardless of the diet regimen, unnecessary simple carbohydrates and alcohol should be avoided.

3. Manipulations Primarily by the Physician

The next major category of manipulations to lower lipids in uremic patients is that of physician-controlled adjustments. These can be subcategorized into dialytic and medicinal.

3.1. Dialytic Manipulations

3.1.1. Acetate

Uremic patients have HL before they come to dialysis therapy.[3,4] Therefore, dialysis or dialysate composition does not cause HL, but it may contribute to or exacerbate the preexisting condition. Part of the problem may be the use of acetate as the dialysate buffer. Acetate is a source of calories as well as a precursor of fatty acids and cholesterol. Savdie *et al.* employed two 3- to 5-week crossover periods using acetate, then bicarbonate.[41] One of eight patients showed a clear fall in TG during the bicarbonate, as compared to the acetate, period. Kluge *et al.* report a significant fall in TG (367 mg% to 244 mg%) when using bicarbonate in their crossover study consisting of 2-month treatment periods.[42] After 8 months of bicarbonate dialysis, 9 of 12 patients with type IV HL had a TG fall from 273 to 122 mg% with a rebound to 305 mg% after restarting acetate.[43]

Very short studies of acetate administration yield mixed results. Whereas Port *et al.* found no evidence to suggest a role for acetate in HL,[44] Davidson *et al.* have shown that labeled acetate can be recovered in tissue and plasma lipids.[45] Perez-Garcia *et al.* have found free-fatty-acid levels to be higher during acetate dialysis than during either a heparin or glucose infusion.[46]

Furthermore, the Heidelberg group has shown that despite the fall in TG after 2 months of bicarbonate,[42] the HDL–Chol also fell.[47] This could negate any beneficial effect of lowering TG in regard to ischemic heart disease.

As Davidson *et al.* point out, over time even a small contribution to lipid production and deposition by acetate may contribute to HL and atherosclerosis.[45] In light of the evidence outlined as well as the awareness that dialysis well-being is improved with bicarbonate,[48] I recommend changing HL patients to bicarbonate-buffered dialysate.

3.1.2. Glucose

The role of glucose dialysate (GD) in uremic HL is also unsettled, a situation attributable, in large part, to poorly designed studies. Because patients dialyzed at centers where GD was used had lower TG than patients at centers where glucose-free dialysate (GFD) was used, Hubner *et al.* concluded that GD did not contribute to HL.[49] Dombeck *et al.*, in the course of studies on the effects of androgens, noted no changes in lipids when GFD was used instead of GD.[50] Novarini *et al.* sequentially evaluated GFD and then 200 mg% GD for 2 months.[51] No individual patient's data are reported.

Some prospective studies have yielded different results. In a 15-day study, Daubresse *et al.* demonstrated a mean TG rise of 30 mg% when a 200-mg% GD was used in lieu of a GFD.[34] Swamy *et al.* compared a 500-mg% GD to a GFD, each administered for 6 months.[52] For the group TG did not change, but 4 of the 16 patients clearly had a fall in TG in the GFD period.

The presence of glucose in the dialysate has significant metabolic effects.[53] The absence of glucose leads to intradialytic gluconeogenesis, and this could be beneficial or not, depending on the patient's overall status. In marginally nourished patients, modest GD (100–200 mg%) may be beneficial. In obese HL patients, a 4- to 6-month trial of GFD is a simple, cheap, and easy maneuver to attempt to lower lipids.

3.1.3. Heparin

Heparin stimulates the release of several lipolytic enzymes that help clear the plasma of chylomicrons and VLDL. Since decreased postheparin lipolytic activity (PHLA) is a common defect in uremic patients, the question arises as to whether or not the heparin used during dialysis may play a role in uremic HL. As mentioned earlier, the majority of uremic patients have HL before they need dialysis and are exposed to heparin. Furthermore, patients on chronic peritoneal dialysis (CPD) do not receive heparin but also suffer from HL.[54] Felts and colleagues have shown that after repeated exposure to heparin on dialysis, a resistance to activation of lipoprotein lipase develops, possibly on an immunologic basis.[55] Daily dialysis does lower PHLA but TG levels do not rise.[56] In a given dialysis, TG levels fall because of heparin-induced activation of lipoprotein lipase, although this change can be negated by protamine.[3] In conclusion, heparin does not appear to play a significant role in the HL of dialysis patients.

3.1.4. m^2-Hours, Dialysis Efficiency

Bagdade first observed that by increasing dialysis time from 18 to 40 hr per week, TG fell and PHLA increased.[57] In a prospective study involving only three patients, Samar *et al.* observed a worsening of the HL with increased m^2-hr[58] although, in this study, the dialysate contained acetate. In contrast, Cattran *et al.* studied three patients after increasing m^2-hr and lowering predialysis creatinine from 14 to 8.5 mg%.[54] TG turnover was increased by this manuever. Novarini *et al.* compared the lipid levels of patients on short and long dialysis and found the group means to be the same.[51] Delavelle *et al.* found a positive correlation between HDL–Chol and nerve conduction velocity, implying that better adequacy of dialysis may improve that risk factor.[33]

Since more efficient dialyzers are becoming available, we must learn about the metabolic consequences of increased m^2-hr, particularly involving HL.

3.1.5. *Peritoneal Dialysis*

Peritoneal dialysis more efficiently removes middle and large molecules but is less efficient in small solute removal when compared to HD. Acetate or lactate is the major buffer and carbohydrate loads are greater than in HD. The HL associated with CPD may be more prevalent and more severe than in HD.[54] Both TG and Chol are reported to progressively rise over the course of continuous ambulatory peritoneal dialysis.[59] An exacerbation of uremic HL appears to be a real, yet unexplained, finding in CPD. Whether this is due to the transperitoneal loss of lipid-regulating proteins is an intriguing speculation.

3.1.6. *Hemofiltration*

A potential therapeutic intervention regarding HL may be hemofiltration (HF). Sanfelippo and colleagues have observed that five of six patients on HF for 3 months lowered their TG and all six lowered their Chol.[60] TG transport and fractional clearance rates were improved by HF.[61] These data are exciting and currently unexplained.

3.2. Medicinal Manipulations

The final group of manipulations primarily by the physician involve the use or avoidance of drugs.

3.2.1. *Drugs to Avoid*

Both propranolol and androgens are associated with higher TG in dialysis patients than in HD patients not taking these drugs.[11,50] Estrogens, glucocorticoids, diuretics, and ethyl alcohol all have a tendency to exacerbate a predisposition to HL,[4,22,62] and their avoidance is recommended in patients with HL, if possible.

3.2.2. *Specific Drug Therapy for Hyperlipidemia*

Friedman *et al.* have reported their initial success with activated charcoal, ingested as a slurry four times a day.[63] Lipids were the only biochemical parameters to change with significant reductions in both Chol and TG. Acceptance of this agent may limit its use (T. Manis, personal communication).

Nicotinic acid is effective in uremic HL but its side effects may also limit its usefulness.[64]

Since Goldberg and colleagues established a safe regimen for the use of clofibrate in ESRD,[65] they and several others have reported wide success in lowering lipids in patients with ESRD.[5,66,67] Of additional benefit is the rise in HDL–Chol seen in these patients taking clofibrate.[66] Others have not enjoyed as much success with clofibrate[68] and a large prospective study with this agent is warranted. The World Health Organization study noted an increased mortality from gastrointestinal malignancies in patients on clofibrate.[14] For this reason, the agent is not recommended for communitywide prevention of ischemic heart disease. In ESRD patients with accelerated atherosclerosis, VLDL elevations, low HDL–Chol, and decreased lipoprotein lipase activity, all of which clofibrate may improve, I cannot recommend withholding a drug as useful as clofibrate.

4. Conclusion/Recommendations

I am persuaded that our patients with ESRD suffer from accelerated atherosclerosis. The course of their atherosclerosis is collapsed into a time frame of usually less than a decade. Therefore, these patients are the ideal subjects in which to evaluate the effects of lipid lowering by any of the methods I have discussed. I have attempted to outline areas where explanations are still forthcoming. These deserve our highest research priorities.

References

1. Bagdade JD, Albers JJ: Plasma high-density lipoprotein concentrations in chronic-hemodialysis and renal-transplant patients. *N Engl J Med* 296:1436, 1977.
2. Frank WM, Rao TKS, Manis T, Delano BG, Avrom MM, Saxene AK, Carter AC, Friedman EA: Relationship of plasma lipids to renal function and length of time on maintenance hemodialysis. *Am J Clin Nutr* 31:1886, 1978.
3. Gutman RA, Uy A, Shalhoub RJ, Wade AD, O'Connell JMB, Recont L: Hypertriglyceridemia in chronic nonnephrotic renal failure. *Am J Clin Nutr* 26:165, 1973.
4. Ibels LS, Simons LA, King JO, Williams PF, Neale FC, Stewart JM: Studies on the nature and causes of hyperlipidemia in uraemia, maintenance dialysis, and renal transplantation. *Q J Med* 44:601, 1975.
5. Ponticelli C, Barbi G, Cantaluppi A, Donati C, Annoni G, Brancaccio D: Lipid abnormalities in maintenance dialysis patients and renal transplant recipients. *Kidney Int* 13 (suppl 8):S-72, 1978.
6. Brown DF, Kinch SH, Doyle JT: Serum triglyceride in health and in ischemic heart disease. *N Engl J Med* 273:947, 1965.
7. Carlson LA, Bottiger LE: Ischaemic heart diseases in relation to fasting values of plasma triglycerides and cholesterol. *Lancet* 1:865, 1972.
8. Rosenmann RH, Brand RJ, Jenkins CD, Friedman M, Straus R, Wurm M: Coronary heart disease in the Western Collaborative Group Study. *JAMA* 233:872, 1975.
9. Haas LB, Sherrard DJ, Brunzell JD: Hypertriglyceridemia and premature cardiovascular disease in patients on maintenance hemodialysis. *Clin Res* 27:416A, 1979.

10. Henriquez M, Raja R, Kramer M, Rosenbaum JL: Role of high density lipoproteins in cardiovascular disease in hemodialyzed patients. *Am Soc Artif Int* Organs, 44, 1979 (abstr).
11. Brunzell JD, Albers JJ, Haas LB, Agadoa L, Goldberg AP, Sherrard DJ: Prevalence of serum lipid abnormalities in chronic hemodialysis. *Metabolism* 26:903, 1977.
12. Kannel WB, Castelli WP, Gordon T: Cholesterol in the prediction of atherosclerotic disease: New perspectives based on the Framingham study. *Ann Intern Med* 90:85, 1979.
13. Stamler J: The coronary drug project (clofibrate and niacin in coronary heart disease). *JAMA* 231:360, 1975.
14. Committee of Principal Investigators: A cooperative trial in the primary prevention of ischaemic heart disease using clofibrate. *Br Heart J* 40:1069, 1978.
15. Dayton S, Pearce WL, Hashimoto S, Dixon WJ, Tomiyasu U: A controlled clinical trial of a diet high in unsaturated fat in preventing complications of atherosclerosis. *Circulation* 39, 40 (suppl 2):II-1, 1969.
16. Miettinen M, Turpeinen O, Karvonen MJ, Elosno R, Paavilainen E: Effect of cholesterol-lowering diet on mortality from coronary heart disease and other causes (12 year clinical trial in men and women). *Lancet* 2:835, 1972.
17. Leren P: The effect of plasma cholesterol lowering diet in male survivors of myocardial infarction. *Acta Med Scand* (suppl) 466:5, 1966.
18. Barndt R, Blankenhorn DH, Crawford DW, Brooks SH: Regression and progression of early femoral atherosclerosis in treated hyperlipoproteinemic patients. *Ann Intern Med* 86:139, 1977.
19. Basta LL, Williams C, Kioschos JM, Spector AA: Regression of atherosclerotic stenosing lesions of the renal arteries and spontaneous cure of systemic hypertension though control of hyperlipidemia. *Am J Med* 61:420, 1976.
20. Lindner A, Charra B, Sherrard DJ, Scribner BH: Accelerated atherosclerosis in prolonged maintenance hemodialysis. *N Engl J Med* 290:697, 1974.
21. Lazarus JM, Lowrie EG, Hampers CL, Merrill JP: Cardiovascular disease in uremic patients on hemodialysis. *Kidney Int* 7 (suppl 2):S-167, 1975.
22. Levy RI, Morganroth J, Rikfind BM: Treatment of hyperlipidemia. *N Engl J Med* 290:1295, 1974.
23. Swamy AP, Cestero RVM, Campbell RG: Lipid changes in maintenance hemodialysis. *Am Soc Nephrol.* 54A, 1978 (abstr).
24. Goldberg AP, Hagberg JM, Delmez JA, Heath GW, Hartes HR: Exercise training corrects abnormal lipid and carbohydrate metabolism in hemodialysis patients. *Trans Am Soc Artif Int Organs* 25:431, 1979.
25. Goldberg AP, Hagberg JM, Delmez JA, Carney RM, McKenitt PM, Ehsani AA, Harter HR: The metabolic and psychological effects of exercise in hemodialysis patients. *Am J Clin Nutr* 33:1620, 1980.
26. Amend WJC, Steinberg SM, Lowrie EG, Lazarus JM, Soeldner JC, Hampers CL, Merrill JP: The influence of serum calcium and parathyroid hormone upon glucose metabolism in uremia. *J Lab Clin Med* 86:435, 1975.
27. Hallberg D, Werner S: Circulatory and lipolytic effects of parathyroid hormone. *Hormone Metab Res* 9:424, 1977.
28. Sinha TK, Thajchayapong P, Queener SF, Allen DO, Bell NH: On the lipolytic action of parathyroid hormone in man. *Metabolism* 25:251, 1976.
29. Kather H, Heuck CC, Tschope W, Ritz E, Simon B: Unchanged hormone sensitivity of rat fat cell adenylate cyclase in uremia. *Clin Nephrol* 8:324, 1977.
30. Cantin M: Kidney, parathyroid and lipemia. *Lab Invest* 14:1691, 1965.
31. Tuma SN, Seidel CL, Entman ML: Relaxing effect of parathyroid extract on the smooth muscle of rabbit aorta. *Am Soc Nephrol,* p. 90A, 1979.
32. Ibels LS, Alfrey AC, Huffer WE, Craswell PW, Anderson JT, Weil R: Arterial calcification and pathology in uremic patients undergoing dialysis. *Am J Med* 66:790, 1979.
33. Delavelle F, Trombert JC, Canarelli G: HDL cholesterol as cardiovascular risk factor in uremia. *Kidney Int* 16:94, 1979.

34. Daubresse JC, Lerson G, Plamteux G, Rorive G, Luyckx AS, Lefebure PJ: Lipids and lipoproteins in chronic uremia. A study of the influence of regular haemodialysis. *Eur J Clin Invest* 6:159, 1976.
35. Wochos DN, Anderson CF, Mitchell JC: Serum lipids in chronic renal failure. *Mayo Clin Proc* 51:660, 1976.
36. Heuck CC, Ritz E, Liersch M, Mehls O: Serum lipids in renal insufficiency. *Am J Clin Nutr* 31:1547, 1978.
37. Sorge F, Castro LA, Nagel A, Kessel M: Serum glucose, insulin, growth hormone, free fatty acids and lipids responses to high carbohydrate and to high fat isocaloric diets in patients with chronic, non-nephrotic renal disease. *Hormone Metab Res* 7:118, 1975.
38. Sanfelippo ML, Swenson RS, Reaven GM: Response of plasma triglycerides to dietary changes in patients on hemodialysis. *Kidney Int* 14:180, 1978.
39. Gokal R, Mann JI, Oliver O, Ledingham JGG: Dietary treatment of hyperlipidemia in chronic hemodialysis patients. *Am J Clin Nutr* 31:1915, 1978.
40. Connor WE, Connor SL: Dietary treatment of hyperlipidemia, in Rifkind BM, Levy RI (eds): *Hyperlipidemia: Diagnosis and Therapy*. New York, Grune & Stratton, 1977.
41. Savdie E, Mahony JF, Steward JH: Effect of acetate on serum lipids in maintenance hemodialysis. *Trans Am Soc Artif Int Organs* 23:385, 1977.
42. Kluge R, Heuck C. Wildberger D, Wirth A, Ritz E: Dialysate bicarbonate and hyperlipidemia. *Am Soc Artif Int Organs* p. 73, 1979 (abstr).
43. Giorcelli G, Dalmasso F, Bruno M, Pellegrino S, Sirkka M, Vacha G: RDT with acetate-free bicarbonate buffered dialysis fluid: Long-term effects on lipid pattern, acid-base balance and oxygen delivery. *Kidney Int* 16:223, 1979.
44. Port FK, Easterling RE, Barnes RV: Effect of acetate administration on blood lipids. *Am J Clin Nutr* 31:1893, 1978.
45. Davidson WD, Rorke SJ, Guo LSS, Morin RJ: Comparison of acetate-1-^{14}C metabolism in uremic and nonuremic dogs. *Am J Clin Nutr* 31:1897, 1978.
46. Perez-Garcia A, Breto M, Alvarino J, Alegre B, Cruz JM: The influence of several factors that intervene in hemodialysis on serum levels of triglycerides and free fatty acids. *Clin Nephrol* 12:14, 1979.
47. Heuck CC, Ritz E, Kluge R, Wildeberger D, Wirth A: High density lipoprotein composition in chronic hemodialysis. *N Engl J Med* 300:1055, 1979.
48. Graefe U, Milutinovich J, Follette WC, Vizzo JE, Babb AL, Scribner BH: Less dialysis-induced morbidity and vascular instability with bicarbonate in dialysate. *Ann Intern Med* 88:332, 1978.
49. Hubner W, Sieberth HG, Diemer A, Finke K, Prange E: Effects of regular haemodialysis with glucose and glucose free dialysate on hyperlipidemia. *Proc Eur Dial Transpl Assoc* 8:174, 1971.
50. Dombeck DH, Lundholm DD, Vieira JA: Lipid metabolism in uremia and the effects of dialysate glucose and oral androgen therapy. *Trans Am Soc Artif Int Organs* 19:150, 1973.
51. Novarini A, Zuliani U, Bandini L, Laronna S, Montanari A, Perinotto P: Observations on lipid metabolism in chronic renal failure, during conservative and haemodialysis therapy. *Eur J Clin Invest* 6:473, 1976.
52. Swamy AP, Cestero RUM, Campbell RG, Freeman RB: Long-term effect of dialysate glucose on the lipid levels of maintenance hemodialysis patients. *Trans Am Soc Artif Int Organs* 22:54, 1976.
53. Wathen R, Keshaviah P, Hommeyer P, Cadwell K, Comty G: Role of dialysate glucose in preventing gluconeogenesis during hemodialysis. *Trans Am Soc Artif Int Organs* 23:393, 1977.
54. Cattran DC, Fenton SSA, Wilson DR, Steiner G: Defective triglyceride removal in lipemia associated with peritoneal dialysis and haemodialysis. *Ann Intern Med* 85:29, 1976.
55. Felts JM, Zacherle B, Staprans I, Itakura H: Mechanisms of hyperlipidemia in chronic renal failure. Contract NO-1-AM-4-2220, 10th Annual Contractor's Conference, NIAMDD:10, 1977.
56. Ibels LS, Reardon MF, Nestel PJ: Plasma post-heparin lipolytic activity and triglyceride clearance in uremic and hemodialysis patients and renal allograft recipients. *J Lab Clin Med* 87:648, 1976.

57. Bagdade JD. Uremic lipemia: An unrecognized abnormality in triglyceride production and removal. *Arch Intern Med* 126:875, 1970.
58. Samar RE, Moncrief JW, Decherd JF, Popovich RP: Lipoprotein binding and hypertriglyceridemia in chronic uremia. *Trans Am Soc Artif Int Organs* 21:455, 1975.
59. Roncari DAK, Breckenridge WC, Ogilvie R, Katirtzoglan A, Oreopoulos DG: Lipoprotein metabolism in patients treated with continuous ambulatory peritoneal dialysis. *Am Soc Nephhol,* 184A, 1979 (abstr).
60. Sanfelippo M, Barg A, Henderson L: Altered lipid and insulin response in hemodialysis patients after hemofiltration. *Am Soc Nephrol,* 128A, 1979 (abstr).
61. Sanfelippo M, Grundy S, Henderson L: Transport of very low density lipoprotein triglyceride: Comparison of hemodialysis and hemofiltration. *Am Soc Nephrol,* p 96A, 1979 (abstr).
62. Rosenthal T, Holtzman E, Segal P: The effect of chlorthalidone on serum lipids and lipoproteins. *Atherosclerosis* 36:111, 1980.
63. Friedman EI, Feinstein EI, Beyer MM, Galonsky RS, Hirsch SR: Charcoal-induced lipid reduction in uremia. *Kidney Int* 13 (suppl 8):S-170, 1978.
64. Gokal R, Mann JI, Oliver DO, Ledingham JGG: Treatment of hyperlipidemia in patients on chronic haemodialysis. *Br Med J* 1:82, 1978.
65. Goldberg AP, Sherrard DJ, Haas LB, Brunzell JD: Control of clofibrate toxicity in uremic hypertriglyceridemia. *Clin Pharmacol Ther* 21:317, 1977.
66. Goldberg AP, Applebaum-Bowden DM, Bierman EL, Hazzard WR, Haas LB, Sherrard DJ, Brunzell JD, Huttunen JK, Einholm CJ, Nikkila EA: Increase in lipoprotein lipase during clofibrate treatment of hypertriglyceridemia in patients on hemodialysis. *N Engl J Med* 301:1073, 1979.
67. di Giulio S, Boulu R, Drueke T, Nicolai A, Zingraff J, Crosnier J: Clifobrate treatment of hyperlipidemia in chronic renal failure. *Clin Nephrol* 8:504, 1977.
68. Comty CM, Hemphill G, Wathen RL: Use of clofibrate in treatment of hyperlipidemia of chronic hemodialysis patients. *Am Soc Artif Int Organs,* p 15, 1977 (abstr).

26

Coronary Artery Disease in Diabetic Patients with End-Stage Renal Disease

William M. Bennett

1. Introduction

Diabetes mellitus is no longer considered a contraindication for end-stage renal disease care. In fact, in some centers approximately 20% of all new patients with uremia accepted into treatment programs have diabetic nephropathy as a primary diagnosis. Although some investigators have reported excellent patient survival in diabetic patients undergoing renal transplantation,[1] other recent data have been less favorable, pointing out some selection bias in the previous results. It is uniformly accepted that both maintenance hemodialysis and renal transplantation in diabetic patients are associated with excessive mortality over that expected in nondiabetic subjects.[1–4] Much of the mortality observed in this high-risk group of patients is attributable to cardiovascular disease despite the relatively young age of many of these patients.

In order to ascertain the role of cardiovascular disease in treatment outcome, a group of patients carefully selected because of absence of clinical coronary or cerebrovascular disease was studied and followed prospectively. This group of patients should represent individuals who would be predicted to have the best chance of longevity with currently available technology.

2. Patients and Methods

All 22 patients with insulin-dependent juvenile diabetes mellitus (onset less than age 20) who presented to the University of Oregon Health Sciences

William M. Bennett • Division of Nephrology, Department of Medicine, Oregon Health Sciences University, Portland, Oregon 97201.

Center for renal transplant recipient evaluations from January 1973 through December 1976 were considered for the study. The University is the sole transplant facility in a state of 2.3 million people. Seven patients were excluded because of either a history of angina pectoris, a previous myocardial infarction, or pathological Q waves on electrocardiogram. Eleven of the fifteen patients with none of the cited evidence of arteriosclerotic heart disease gave their informed consent for coronary arteriograms and left ventricular angiograms. Selected patients had echocardiograms and stress electrocardiography. The four patients who refused arteriography were followed clinically. All patients had been accepted as candidates for end-stage renal disease management prior to entering the study by virtue of having a need for imminent dialysis or transplantation. Renal function as measured by endogenous creatinine clearance was less than 10 ml/min in all patients. There were seven females and four males who underwent arteriography with a mean age of 32 (21–50). All had medically treated hypertension and each had known insulin-dependent diabetes for at least 15 years. The clinical characteristics of the study population are depicted in Table 1.

Left ventricular function was determined by measuring left ventricular end diastolic pressure and calculating the ejection fraction from the left ventricular angiograms.

Seven patients underwent renal transplantation shortly after this study with 11 grafts done over the study period. Three were from living related donors and eight from cadaver donors. Eight patients entered chronic dialysis programs. Patients were followed at monthly intervals with clinical examinations and electrocardiograms.

3. *Results*

Findings of the coronary angiography and other special studies are shown in Table 2. All 11 patients studied by angiography had evidence of multifocal coronary atherosclerosis. The studies themselves produced no detectable deterioration in cardiac or renal function. A life table showing cumulative survival of these patients with respect to cardiovascular disease is shown in Fig. 1. Over the period of follow-up through December 1979 only three patients remain alive. Only one patient remains free of symptomatic cardiac or cerebrovascular disease. The other two surviving patients have functional class 3 angina and a disabling stroke, respectively. Only 2 of those 15 patients died from causes related to treatment given for renal failure. One patient died of sepsis after a successful living-related-donor transplant, and another discontinued dialysis because of depression over his quality of life.

4. *Discussion*

During the past decade indications for treatment of end-stage renal disease by long-term dialysis and renal transplantation have expanded to

Table 1. Clinical Characteristics of the Patient Population[a]

Patient	Age	Sex	Known duration of hypertension (years)	Blood pressure at time of study	Smoking history (years)	Duration of diabetes mellitus	Endogenous creatinine clearance (ml/min)	Chest x-ray
1	24	M	7	152/100	8	17	6	Normal
2	36	M	3	162/82	None	22	8	Mild cardiomegaly
3	22	F	3	155/96	6	17	4	Normal
4	32	F	5	136/84	10	20	6	Normal
5	42	F	10	180/100	26	30	3	Normal
6	50	F	4	155/100	30	31	6	Normal
7	25	F	3	140/82	7	18	8	Normal
8	38	F	3	160/100	None	22	4	Cardiomegaly
9	21	M	1	130/72	4	15	2	Normal
10	28	F	2	152/96	None	16	3	Normal
11	34	M	6	162/100	25	19	8	Normal
12[b]	30	F	7	180/110	36	20	4	Normal
13[b]	22	M	2	140/60	None	15	6	Normal
14[b]	35	M	6	162/100	15	17	5	Normal
15[b]	28	F	2	166/90	None	16	7	Normal

[a] Adapted from ref. 11.
[b] Not studied with arteriography.

Table 2. Findings of Coronary Angiography and Other Special Studies[a]

			Coronary angiography				
Pt.	Left ventricular end diastolic pressure	Ejection fraction	Left anterior descending	Right coronary	Circumflex	Stress electrocardiography	Echocardiogram
1	12	0.66	Minimal, diffuse	Minimal, diffuse	Minimal, diffuse	Inadequate rate due to fatigue	Left ventricular hypertrophy
2	20	0.72	Minimal, diffuse; 30% stenosis	Normal	Normal	Inadequate rate due to fatigue	Minimal pericardial effusion
3	9	0.72	Minimal, diffuse	Normal	Minimal, diffuse	—	Left ventricular hypertrophy
4	10	0.55	Minimal, diffuse	Minimal, diffuse	Minimal, diffuse	—	—
5	5	0.69	75% stenosis	75% stenosis	30% stenosis	Positive	Left ventricular hypertrophy
6	6	0.81	50% stenosis	Normal	50% stenosis	—	Reduced left ventricular compliance
7	24	0.51	50% stenosis	70% stenosis	50% stenosis	Inadequate rate due to fatigue	Moderate pericardial effusion, left ventricular hypertrophy
8	15	0.76	60% stenosis	60% stenosis	50% stenosis	Positive	Reduced left ventricular compliance
9	15	0.59	80% stenosis	Occluded	Moderate diffuse involvement	Positive	Left atrial enlargement
10	14	0.65	25% stenosis	Minimal, diffuse	20% stenosis	—	—
11	15	0.64	70% stenosis	60% stenosis	Minimal diffuse involvement	Positive	Left ventricular hypertrophy

[a] Adapted from ref. 11.

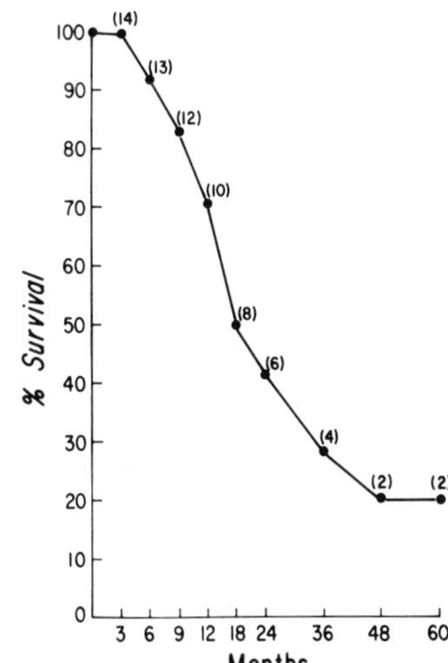

Figure 1. Life table showing cumulative survival of patients with asymptomatic coronary disease. Numbers in parentheses indicate patients entering observation interval. Deaths from noncardiovascular causes are excluded.

include patients with end-stage diabetic nephropathy. Since approximately half of the deaths in nondiabetic dialysis and transplant patients are due to cardiovascular disease, it is of interest to know the significance of coronary artery disease in diabetics, a group of patients known to be at high risk.[(5)] The data from our long-term observation of 15 patients asymptomatic for clinical coronary artery disease confirms the high risk of arteriosclerotic heart disease in the diabetic patient with end-stage renal disease. A cumulative morality rate due to cardiovascular causes of 80% at 5 years is of concern since patients were young and were selected because of lack of prior disease. Weinrauch *et al.* reported a high incidence of asymptomatic coronary artery lesions in 21 similar patients.[(6)] Their series differed from ours in that 57% of patients were designated as having no coronary artery disease if they had less than a 50% obstructive lesion in any coronary vessel. Thus, small multiple vessel lesions might be considered as no disease, whereas in our patients, any lesions were considered as evidence for the presence of atheroma. Their 2-year survival of 22% in those with major coronary lesions is worse than our data. This contrasts with the situation in symptomatic nondiabetic subjects reported by Bruschke *et al.* who reported a 5-year survival of 66% in 590 patients with coronary arteriographic lesions.[(7)] It is not known whether a similar degree of arteriographic abnormalities might be discovered in age and sex-matched, nondiabetic patients with end-stage renal disease.

Diabetic subjects in a 16-year follow-up of the Framingham study showed an increased morbidity and mortality from all cardiovascular causes.[(5)] Coronary deaths were most increased in insulin-treated diabetic women. Known risk factors could not explain the increased mortality; however, renal function was not specifically assessed.[(5)] Recent data have cast some doubt, however, on renal dysfunction *per se* in promoting accelerated atherosclerosis in nondiabetic patients on dialysis. It is not clear if this is also true of diabetics.[8]

The lack of cardiac symptoms in these diabetic patients is not easily explained. Autonomic neuropathy may preclude perception of pain due to coronary ischemia. An increased incidence of silent myocardial infarcts has been reported in diabetics.[9] Alternatively, small-vessel disease might predispose to arrhythmia and death without large-vessel ischemic symptoms. Application of new noninvasive techniques to diagnose and follow these patients would appear warranted. The role of aortocoronary bypass surgery in asymptomatic patients with angiographic lesions or perfusion defects by myocardial radionuclide imaging is unclear at present. Careful randomized studies in high-risk patients such as those in this study might help ascertain whether a surgical approach might improve long-term survival in diabetic and nondiabetic patients.

5. *Critique of Previous Data Concerning Mortality in Diabetics Treated for End-Stage Renal Failure*

Many reports do not precisely define the patient population in terms of the nature of the diabetic state. Although most patients in these reports require insulin, this has not uniformly been the case.[4] In addition, most series combine patients whose disease begins in childhood (age less than 20 years) with those who develop hyperglycemia in adult life. This tendency to lump patients with juvenile and maturity-onset diabetes together makes data concerning causes of death difficult to compare from study to study.[3,10] To be meaningful, survival statistics from various treatment centers must explicitly define the patient population.

Selection criteria for the renal treatment modality are not always stated. These criteria, as well as the extent of vascular disease present in organ systems which might impair patient survival exclusive of treatment of renal failure, are needed. For example, one recent favorable report includes patients who were treated with renal transplantation prior to the medical need for dialysis therapy and excludes from analysis of posttransplant patient survival some patients who died prior to transplantation from pretransplant surgery.[1] Ideally, time of diabetic patient entry into end-stage renal disease, type of diabetes, and extent of vascular disease will be controlled in future investigations concerning proper management of end-stage diabetic nephropathy.

The experience with treatment of end-stage diabetic nephropathy in our center, as well as in others during the past 2 years, shows a mortality greater than that expected for nondiabetics.[3,11] This occurs primarily in patients treated by hemodialysis. This may simply reflect selection of better risk patients for renal transplantation, other bias such as transplantation prior to reaching end-stage uremia, or use of large numbers of living related donors. The high incidence of both symptomatic and asymptomatic coronary disease in this population and its eventual role in patient mortality demands attention by all those involved in the care of these patients. It is clear that, under some circumstances, treatment by transplantation can achieve rehabilitation from renal failure equal to that achieved by nondiabetics.[1] Progress in understanding the basic pathophysiology and management of diabetes is necessary if excessive patient mortality is to be avoided and expensive resources are to be saved. It is possible that the true ravages of coronary artery disease in diabetics might even be underestimated by our survey if patients die of heart disease prior to reaching end-stage renal disease referral centers.

References

1. Najarian JS, Sutherland DER, Simmons RL, Howard RJ, Kjellstrand CM, Mauer SM, Kennedy W, Ramsey R, Barbosa J, Goetz FC: Kidney transplantation for the uremic diabetic patient. *Surg Gynecol Obstet* 144:682–690, 1977.
2. End stage diabetic nephropathy. *Br Med J* 2:1175–1176, 1978.
3. Avram MM, Slater PA, Fein PA, Altman E: Comparative survival of 673 patients with chronic uremia treated with renal transplantation and maintenance hemodialysis. *Trans Am Soc Artif Intern Organs* 25:391–393, 1979.
4. Goldstein DA, Massry SG: Diabetic nephropathy. *Nephron* 20:286–296, 1978.
5. Garcia MJ, McNamara PM, Gordon T, Kannell WBJ: Morbidity and mortality in diabetics in the Framingham population. *Diabetes* 23:105–111, 1974.
6. Weinrauch LA, D'Elia JA, Healy RW, Gleason RE, Takacs FJ, Libertino JA, Leland OS: Asymptomatic coronary artery disease: Angiography in diabetic patients before renal transplantation. *Ann Intern Med* 88:346–348, 1978.
7. Bruschke AVG, Proudfit WL, Sones FM: Progress study of 590 consecutive non-surgical cases of coronary disease followed 5–9 years. *Circulation* 47:1147–1154, 1973.
8. Rostand SG, Gretes JC, Kirk K, Rutsky EA, Andreoli TE: Ischemic heart disease in patients with uremia undergoing maintenance hemodialysis. *Kidney Int* 16:600–611, 1979.
9. Bradley RF, Schonfield A: Diminished pain in diabetic patients with acute myocardial infarction. *Geriatrics* 17:322–326, 1962.
10. Jacobs C, Rottembourg J, Frantz P, Slama G, Legrain M: Treatment of end stage renal failure in the insulin-dependent diabetic patient. *Adv Nephrology* 8:101–126, 1979.
11. Bennett WM, Kloster F, Rosch J, Barry J, Porter GA: Natural history of asymptomatic coronary arteriographic lesions in diabetic patients with end stage renal disease. *Am J Med* 65:779–783, 1978.

27

Indicators for Cardiovascular Catastrophe in Diabetic Patients with Renal Failure

C. M. Kjellstrand

Cardiovascular catastrophes are the most common cause of death in dialyzed patients and account for 50% of all patient deaths. Although there has been no change in *relative* death rate from cardiovascular diseases in hemodialyzed patients, there has been an astounding absolute decrease, particularly early in the first-year mortality, from 50% to 14% over the last decade.[1,2] This has occurred in spite of the marked rise in the age of patients when accepted into dialysis in spite of the fact that more patients with serious systemic diseases are now treated.[2] Actually, recent papers question whether there is still an increased incidence of cardiovascular deaths.[3,4]

In diabetic patients, the absolute death rate is at least two or three times that of nondiabetic patients on dialysis, and the relative cardiovascular death rate is even higher, being close to 70% of all deaths.[5] Also, cardiovascular deaths are many times more common in transplanted diabetic patients than in transplanted nondiabetic patients.[6,7] Beyond the first posttransplant year, cardiovascular deaths are more common than septic deaths in diabetic transplanted patients.[8] It is obviously of great importance to identify any clinical markers predicting cardiovascular catastrophes in such patients. It is a waste of resources to start dialysis or transplant a patient who dies soon thereafter. It also prolongs the patient's agony and dashes the hopes of the patient's family. The following methods have been evaluated in predicting cardiovascular deaths in patients on dialysis and following transplantation: (1) history of angina, congestive heart failure, or myocardial infarct, (2) electrocardiogram (EKG), (3) stress EKG, (4) blood lipid levels, (5) angiography, and (6) stress EKG, plus before and after ^{201}Tl imaging.

C. M. Kjellstrand • Division of Nephrology, Department of Medicine, Hennepin County Medical Center, Minneapolis, Minnesota 55415.

Table 1. *Heart Disease and First-Year Mortality*[a]

	All	ASHD	Angina or MI
Pre-1972	43%	56%	80%
Post-1972	27%	40%	29%

[a] Reprinted from ref. 9.

1. *History of Heart Disease*

The most thorough evaluation of the predictive value of a history of heart disease in diabetic patients has been performed by Comty and co-workers.[9] Table 1 summarizes their findings. Evaluating more than 100 diabetic patients starting chronic dialysis, they had an overall first-year mortality rate of 43% in patients started before 1972 versus 17% of those started thereafter. Before 1972, a patient with a history of angina or myocardial infarct had twice the death rate, but after 1972 there was no difference in mortality. Their findings suggest that technologic advances modify predictive factors. Indirect evidence that preexisting cardiac arterio-sclerosis is of predictive value of the survival of nondiabetic patients has been presented by Blagg.[10] The 1-year death rate in patients with a diagnosis other than nephrosclerosis was less than 10%, whereas in patients with nephrosclerosis it approached 50%. Three-year survival rates were 80% and 40%, respectively. On the other hand, a history of heart disease was not a bad prognostic marker in patients started on dialysis according to a report summarizing the overall United States experience since 1975. The 3-year survival in patients with heart disease was 70%, the same as in *all* dialysis patients.[11] The impact of a history of heart disease on the prognosis of dialyzed patients is thus contradictory but appears to be of little importance. No analysis of the prognosis of transplant survival relative to a history of heart disease has been reported.

2. *EKG or EKG Combined with History*

When Comty and co-workers combined a history of angina or myocardial infarct with grossly abnormal EKG, they found an increase in death rate of diabetic patients started on dialysis (Table 1). Thus, the death rates in patients with such findings were 56% and 40% versus 43% and 27%, respectively, before and after 1972.[9] In 132 transplanted diabetic patients, we evaluated the prognostic importance of grossly abnormal EKG and/or a history of angina. Sixty-eight patients had evidence of heart disease by these criteria. Two had had fatal myocardial infarcts and three nonfatal myocardial infarcts for an overall incidence of five (7.4%). In patients without such markers (64 patients), four had fatal myocardial infarcts and five had nonfatal myocardial infarcts for an overall incidence of nine (14%). Obviously, there is no difference.[7] Also, when a more sophisticated evaluation was done of EKG alone, this failed to differentiate patients who survived versus those who experienced myocardial infarct.[6] Three out of twenty-three patients with a normal EKG had myocardial infarct versus 2 of 17 with ST abnormalities only and 3 of 20 with left ventricular hypertrophy on EKG. None of three patients with clear-cut evidence of previous myocardial infarct had a recurrence after transplantation. Thus, we could not substantiate that a history of angina combined with EKG predicted myocardial infarctions after transplantation. However, an article from Scandinavian transplant centers reported that blind patients with a history of heart disease had a much worse survival after cadaver transplantation than those patients without heart disease and with good eyesight. The reported 1-year survival was only 20% versus 65%, and the four-year survival 10% vs. 50%.[12] This is contrary to our finding but may represent differences in total patients included and method of analysis. Thus, although an abnormal EKG and a history of heart disease carry a bad prognosis for dialysis, this probably is not as significant for transplantation.

3. *Blood Lipid Levels*

Haas and co-workers[13] report that the triglyceride level was significantly higher for dialysis patients who died of cardiovascular events than for those who survived or died of other causes. No similar study has been reported in diabetic patients although Goetz at our institution is presently conducting such an evaluation. A most interesting study was done by Goldberg and co-workers.[14] They speculated that the reason for many abnormalities, including elevated triglyceride and reduced HDL levels in dialyzed patients, might be that physicians and dialysis personnel reinforced that dialysis patients are "sick" and should be discouraged from exercise. When a number of their patients underwent a vigorous exercise program, there was an improvement in hematocrit, triglyceride levels, HDL levels, immune reactive insulin, and the glucose disappearance curve. In view of these findings, prognostic implications of blood lipid levels in dialyzed diabetic patients need to be reassessed.

4. *Angiography*

Two groups have used coronary angiograms and left ventriculography in diabetic patients with end-stage renal failure to study whether abnormalities of this test had prognostic importance. Weinrauch and co-workers[15] performed coronary angiogram and left ventriculography in 21 patients with diabetes. Twelve had less than 50% narrowing of their coronary arteries; 12 underwent transplantation, three receiving kidneys from cadavers, and nine receiving kidneys from living related donors; four patients died, and none

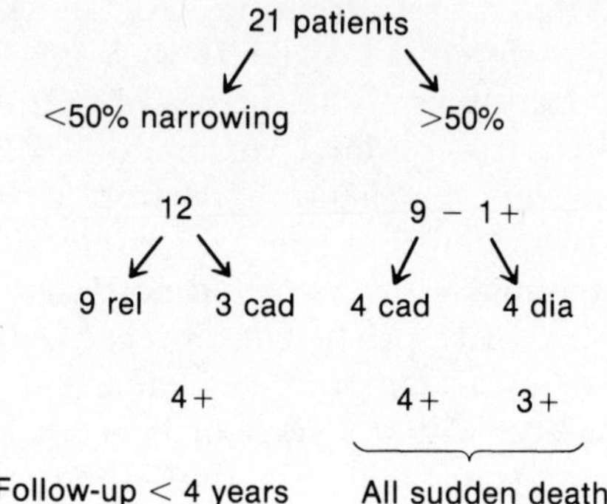

Figure 1. Flow diagram of 21 patients studied with coronary angiograms by Weinrauch *et al.*[15] For explanation, see the text.

of those were sudden deaths; nine patients had more than 50% stenosis, and one of these died before dialysis; four patients went on long-term dialysis, and four received cadaver transplantation. All four cadaver recipients died sudden deaths as did three of the patients started on dialysis[15] (Fig. 1).

Bennett and co-workers[16] studied 22 juvenile-onset diabetic patients. Seven of these patients had a positive history of EKG or heart disease and were excluded from the study. The 15 remaining patients had only minimal EKG changes and a negative history. Four of those patients refused to have coronary angiograms and the other 11 underwent elective angiography. All patients who underwent angiography had gross abnormalities. Of three patients who received transplants from related donors, one is alive. Of two who underwent cadaver transplantation, one is alive on dialysis after rejection of two cadaver transplants. Of six patients who went on to long-term hemodialysis, one is alive. Of the eight patients who died, six died coronary deaths, one had a cerebral vascular accident, and one died of sepsis. Of the patients who refused angiograms, two are alive, one with cerebral thrombosis. Two died of suicide and arrhythmia[16] (Fig. 2). It is obvious that these studies are very difficult to interpret. Both studies are uncontrolled, the series are obviously very small, follow-up time is short, and the death rates are much higher than those reported by almost anyone else treating diabetic patients either with transplantation or by dialysis. For example, the survival of Weinrauch's nine patients who underwent transplantation and who had relative normal angiography is no better than that of all of our patients, over half of whom had indicators of severe heart disease by history and EKG. Coronary angiogram has a considerable mortality and morbidity rate and is invasive and particularly dangerous to a patient who cannot defend himself against a volume overload caused by the markedly hyperosmolar dye used. It is also well known that patients with diabetes and renal failure have a very high incidence of exacerbation of their renal failure after contrast studies. This seems to occur in at least 75% of such patients after IVP.[17,18] In

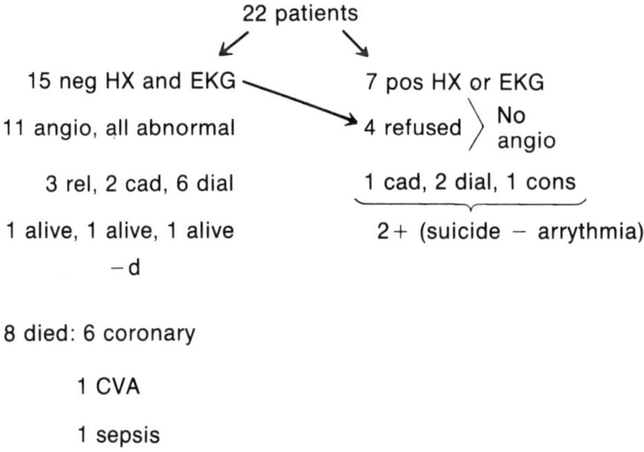

Figure 2. Flow diagram of 22 patients investigated by Bennett *et al.*[16] For explanation, see the text.

Weinrauch's series of 13 patients, 12 patients had a serious problem from their kidneys, two developed hyperkalemia, and six needed emergency dialysis.[19] It can be argued that one can wait until the patient's renal function has deteriorated and dialysis is required before doing the angiogram. Still, the risk of the procedure is substantial. We believe that transplantation should be performed before dialysis is necessary, a policy that obviously rules out coronary angiograms as a prognostic tool.

5. ^{201}Tl Imaging

^{201}Tl imaging can be used to improve the diagnosis of myocardial ischemia.[20–23] We are presently combining ^{201}Tl imaging with stress EKG as a prognostic test in all our diabetic patients. Technical problems of exercising blind diabetic patients have been overcome. During the 2 years of our study, 57 patients have undergone testing. The mean age of these 57 patients was 34 years, and the peak pulse rate of 131/min was obtained during exercise. Thirteen (23%) of these patients had a positive EKG and/or positive ^{201}T1 test, and eight (14%) had a positive ^{201}T1 test alone. So far, we have not performed follow-up studies on these patients, but continue to observe these patients closely for future reference.

6. Conclusions

Cardiovascular accidents are the most common cause of death in diabetic patients on dialysis and after transplantation. It is important to search for prognostic indices for these accidents.

A history of heart disease combined with EKG seems to be of moderate prognostic significance in dialysis patients but less so in transplanted patients. Blood lipid levels are of some importance in nondiabetic patients, but their prognostic importance has not been studied in diabetic patients on dialysis or after transplantation. Two studies of coronary angiograms in diabetic patients with end-stage renal failure are inconclusive and have an unacceptably high complication rate. We are presently studying pretransplant screening with ^{201}Tl imaging in combination with stress EKG. At present, there do not seem to be any reliable, simple clinical markers for predicting success or failure of dialysis and transplantation in diabetic patients.

References

1. Alberts, C, Drukker W: Report on regular dialysis treatment in Europe. *Proc Eur Dial Transpl Assoc* 2:82–87, 1965.
2. Wing AJ, Brunner FP, Brynger H, Chantler C, Donckerwolcke RA, Gurland HJ, Hathway RA, Jacobs C: Combined report on regular dialysis and transplantation in Europe, VIII, 1977. *Proc Eur Dial Transpl Assoc* 15:3–76, 1978.
3. Burke JF, Francos GC, Moore LL, Cho SY, Lasker N: Accelerated atherosclerosis in chronic-dialysis patients—another look. *Nephron* 21:181–185, 1978.
4. Rostand SG, Gretes JC, Kirk KA, Rutsky EA, Andreoli TE: Ischemic heart disease in patients with uremia undergoing maintenance hemodialysis. *Kidney Int* 16:600–611, 1979.
5. Kjellstrand CM: Dialysis in diabetics, in Friedman E (ed): *Strategy in Renal Failure*. New York, Wiley, 1977, pp 345–391.
6. Kjellstrand CM, Shideman JR, Simmons RL, Buselmeier TJ, von Hartitzsch B, Goetz FC, Najarian JS: Renal Transplantation in insulin-dependent diabetic patients. *Kidney Int* 6:S15–S20, 1974.
7. Najarian JS, Sutherland DER, Simmons RL, Howard RJ, Kjellstrand CM, Mauer SM, Kennedy W, Ramsay R, Barbosa J, Goetz FC: Kidney transplantation for the uremic diabetic patient. *Surg Gynecol Obstet* 144:682–690, 1977.
8. Najarian JS, Sutherland DER, Simmons RL, Howard RJ, Kjellstrand CM, Ramsay RC, Goetz FC, Fryd DS, Sommer BG: Ten year experience with renal transplantation in juvenile onset diabetics. *Ann Surg* 190:487–500, 1979.
9. Comty CM, Kjellsen D, Shapiro FL: A reassessment of the prognosis of diabetic patients treated by chronic hemodialysis. *Trans Am Soc Artif Intern Organs* 22:404–411, 1976.
10. Blagg CR: Visual and vascular problems in dialyzed diabetic patients. *Kidney Int* 6:S27–S31, 1974.
11. Bryan FA: *Seventh Annual Progress Report* (Report No. AK-7-7-1387), October 1, 1974–October 1, 1975. Artificial Kidney Chronic Uremia Program, Research Triangle Institute, Research Triangle Park, North Carolina, October 1975.
12. Scandinavian Report: Renal transplantation in insulin-dependent diabetics. *Lancet* 2:915–917, 1978.
13. Haas LB, Brunzell JD, Sherrard DJ: Atherosclerotic risk factors in a chronic dialysis population. *Abstr Am Soc Nephrol* 12:118A, 1979.
14. Goldberg AP, Hagberg JM, Delmez JA, Heath GW, Harter HR: Exercise training improves abnormal lipid and carbohydrate metabolism in hemodialysis patients. *Trans Am Soc Artif Intern Organs* 25:431–437, 1979.
15. Weinrauch LA, D'Elia JA, Healy RW, Gleason RE, Takacs FJ, Liberitino JA, Leland OS: Asymptomatic coronary artery disease: Angiography in diabetic patients before renal transplantation. *Ann Intern Med* 88:346–348, 1978.

16. Bennett WM, Kloster F, Rosch J, Barry J, Porter GA: Natural history of asymptomatic coronary arteriographic lesions in diabetic patients with end-stage renal disease. *Am J Med* 65:779–784, 1978.
17. Harkonen S, Kjellstrand CM: Exacerbation of diabetic renal failure following intravenous pyelography. *Am J Med* 63:939–946, 1977.
18. Harkonen S, Kjellstrand CM: Intravenous pyelography in nonuremic diabetic patients. *Nephron* 24:268–270, 1979.
19. Weinrauch LA, Healy RW, Leland OS, Goldstein HH, Kassissieh SD, Libertino JA, Takacs FJ, D'Elia JA: Coronary angiography and acute renal failure in diabetic azotemic nephropathy. *Ann Intern Med* 86:56–59, 1977.
20. Wackers FJ, Solcole IB, Samson G, *et al*: Value and limitations of thallium-201 scintigraphy in the acute phase of myocardial infarction. *N Engl J Med* 295:1, 1976.
21. Bailey IJ, Griffith LSC, Rouleau J, *et al*: Thallium-201 myocardial perfusion: Imaging at rest and during exercise. *Circulation* 55:79, 1977.
22. Ritchie JL, Trobaugh CG, Hamilton GW, *et al*: Myocardial imaging with thallium-201 at rest and during exercise. *Circulation* 56:66, 1977.
23. Botvinick EH, Taradash MR, Shames DM, Parmley WW: Thallium-201 myocardial perfusion scintigraphy for the clinical clarification of normal, abnormal and equivocal electrocardiographic stress tests. *Am J Cardiol* 41:43, 1978.

III

UNIQUE PROBLEMS OF THE CHILD WITH RENAL FAILURE

28

The Child with Renal Failure

An Overview

Robert L. Vernier

Chronic renal failure is an uncommon problem in children. The data available on incidence show considerable variation because of differing definitions and sources of information. The total incidence in Great Britain has been estimated at 3.5 cases per million total population per year (Meadow *et al.*, 1970); in Germany at 3.0 (Schärer, 1971); and in the United States at 4.8 (Zilleruelo *et al.*, 1980). Studies from dialysis and transplantation centers indicate that 1–1.6 children per million population present for treatment annually (Cameron, 1973; Potter *et al.*, 1980). Thus about one of three children with chronic renal failure survive to be considered for treatment by the current selection criteria. The feasibility of dialysis and transplantation as techniques for prolongation of life in children with renal failure has been well demonstrated. The results of several large published series suggest that children fare as well as or better than adults. The availability of partial funding for the enormous costs of end-stage renal disease (ESRD) treatment through federal programs and the wider application of this new technology require increased attention to a growing list of new problems, some of which are considered in this section.

The data cited indicated that many young children with chronic renal failure are not considered suitable candidates for dialysis or transplantation. Some are severely mentally retarded or have other congenital malformations which are believed to preclude their selection for these modalities of treatment. Others are very young and are not judged to be salvageable by present criteria. Presumably their parents are told that nothing can or should

Robert L. Vernier • Department of Pediatrics, University of Minnesota Health Sciences Center, Minneapolis, Minnesota 55455.

be done—a self-fulfilling prophecy. Such decisions are not made lightly by either the physicians or the parents, for very difficult moral, ethical, social, and financial considerations are involved—and there are few guidelines. The parents are usually young, often have other children for whom they are responsible, and nearly always have serious financial problems prior to the time that the question of management of renal failure arises. The issue of a living related (parental) donor may have been raised to further complicate their lives. What are the obligations and appropriate priorities of the parents to the affected child, to their other children, and to each other?

The remaining technical problems of transplantation largely limit the application of this method to children of greater than 7–10 kg body weight. Hemo- or peritoneal dialysis is feasible in very small children, but survival and growth to an age and size that will permit successful transplantation have rarely been described. More often the practical problem is how to handle the young child with moderate renal failure and an irreversible kidney lesion. The physician must make a "best guess" of the probability that the child, with extraordinary medical care, might survive and grow to a size sufficient to receive an adult donor kidney. The physician team may present to the parents a plan for care necessary to achieve that goal. On the other hand, they may, for perfectly rational reasons (as we now understand the issues), decide to discourage extraordinary measures, in which case the natural history of the disease process will continue. The parents of the child have several choices in either case. In my experience and that of others (Matthews *et al.*, 1981), parents offered the opportunity to participate in a plan for survival of the child almost always agree to proceed. Parents may either accept the natural history concept and agree that nothing extraordinary should be done, or they may seek another opinion. I believe that the latter attitude is growing among well-educated parents who are increasingly aware of the potential of high-technology medicine, and who will increasingly demand consideration for their very young children. We must develop improved understanding of the moral and ethical issues involved and guidelines which are acceptable to society.

The causes of chronic renal failure in children differ greatly from those commonly reported by centers treating adults. Renal dysplasia, obstructive uropathy, vesicoureteral reflux, and chronic atrophic pyelonephritis account for 20–40% of several series and surveys (Schärer, 1971; Cameron, 1973; Potter *et al.*, 1980; Zilleruelo *et al.*, 1980). This unique distribution of diagnoses and the contrast with reports in adults are especially striking among younger children. In our renal transplantation experience at the University of Minnesota involving 89 children less than 10 years of age, 24% had obstructive uropathy dysplasia and 22% had congenital nephrosis (Lum *et al.*, 1981). These unique medical problems of childhood offer special research opportunities to the scientist–physician caring for these children and ultimately may be shown to be partially preventable diseases. In this subparts, Dr. Winberg reviews the problem of chronic atrophic pyelonephritis and the remarkable progress that has been made in reducing the incidence of this disease as a cause of renal failure in children in Sweden.

Since a minimal body size and weight limitation exists for optimal-risk renal transplantation, the problem of growth retardation continues to be a major concern of physicians caring for children with chronic renal failure. Optimal nutrition in a child with reduced renal function, and special attention to protein nutrition, total calories, acidosis, calcium and phosphorus, vitamin D, and other essential nutrients, constitute a unique field of research of great importance. Drs. Holliday and Grupe discuss the current status and new developments in this area.

Renal osteodystrophy is almost invariably a consequence of chronic renal failure in the growing child. It is also likely that the severity of the failure of growth in most children with renal failure is determined to a large extent by the severity of the disturbances in metabolism at the growing ends of bones. In spite of a virtual explosion in new knowledge regarding bone disease, calcium absorption and metabolism, and vitamin D chemistry, optimal treatment of osteodystrophy in children with renal failure remains elusive. Dr. Chesney reviews the new developments in this important area.

Finally, a group of European and American experts in the field of dialysis and transplantation of children review their personal experiences and project their views of the future. Our hope is that this review of the concepts, attitudes, and concerns regarding dialysis and transplantation in children will help the reader with specific interests in pediatric nephrology to formulate some guidelines for optimal management of end-stage renal failure in children. Given the current estimate of 1.6 children per million population with treatable renal failure, only 300 children will present for management each year. According to Potter's estimate (1980), only about 160 children less than 11 years of age will be included per year. It seems clear that some attempt to regionalize the care of these smaller children must be made in order to provide for them the best care available. The medical community and the federal government, which pays much of the cost, must also deal effectively with this important problem.

References

Cameron, J. S., 1973, The treatment of chronic renal failure in children by regular dialysis and by transplantation, *Nephron* **11:**221–251.

Lum, C. T., Fryd, D. S., Polta, T. A., and Najarin, J. S., 1982, Renal transplantation in children 0–10 years of age, *Current Surgery* **39:**27.

Matthews, D. E., Van Leeuwen, J. J., and Christensen, L., 1981, Psychological problems of young children and their families in dialysis–transplant program, *Dialysis Transplantation,* **10:**73–80.

Meadow, S. R., Cameron, J. S., and Ogg, C. S., 1970, Regional service for acute and chronic dialysis of children, *Lancet* **2:**707–710.

Potter, D. E., Holliday, M. A., Piel, C. F., Feduska, N. J., Belzar, F. O., and Salvatierra, O., Jr., 1980, Treatment of end-stage renal disease in children: A 15-year experience, *Kidney Int.* **18:**103–109.

Schärer, K., 1971, Incidence and causes of chronic renal failure in childhood, *Proc. Eur. Dial. Transpl. Assoc.* **8**:211–214.

Zilleruelo, G., Andia, J., Gorman, H.—M., and Strauss, J., 1980, Chronic renal failure in children: Analysis of main causes and deterioration rate in 81 children, *Int. J. Pediatr. Nephrol.* **1**:30–33.

29

Prevention of Renal Damage by Early Recognition of Urinary Tract Infections in Childhood

Jan Winberg

1. Introduction

The ultimate goal of the care of children with urinary tract infections (UTI) is to prevent progressive renal damage with its consequences such as hypertension, complications of pregnancy, and end-stage renal disease. This will be a selected review of this subject, based mainly on an epidemiological study of the occurrence of acute, clinical pyelonephritis among children in a defined population and the long-term prognosis of these cases (Winberg *et al.*, 1974, 1975).

Recent studies of bacterial attachment have brought research on UTI down to a molecular level. Since such studies probably will contribute to a better understanding of the pathogenesis of UTI and renal damage, I will try to put these studies into their clinical context.

2. The Göteborg Epidemiological Study, 1960–1966 (Winberg et al., 1974, 1975)

Göteborg was a city very suitable for true epidemiological research. It had about half a million inhabitants, one single pediatric hospital, and very few private practitioners. The medical care was so organized that when a child fell acutely ill with fever or other symptoms, he was brought to the hospital for examination. This provided us with a large group of acutely ill

---

Jan Winberg • Department of Pediatrics, Karolinska Hospital, S-104 01 Stockholm, Sweden.
Supported by Swedish Medical Research Council (project no. 19X-765).

Table 1. Renal Scarring in Males at "First" Infection and at Follow-up

		Percent with scars	
Age at "first" UTI	No.	At "first" infection	At follow-up[a]
1–30 days	54	0	4
2–12 months	62	1	6
1–16 years	44	25	0

[a] In earlier undamaged kidneys.

patients aged 0–16 years from which we could draw those who had acute clinical pyelonephritis or other types of UTI. We also controlled the health care of all newborns, while they were in the maternity clinic—usually the first week of life. This provided a large source of patients with neonatal UTI (Bergström *et al.*, 1972). The collection period started in 1960 and was completed by the end of 1966. All patients who had a history of one or several earlier infections were excluded from the epidemiological study, as were all patients with malformations or neurogenic bladder. Patients with vesicoureteral reflux (VUR) were included. In this way 596 children: 440 girls and 156 boys, with a presumed "first" infection were collected consecutively. During follow-up, 38 children developed renal scars after the infection or had such scars already at the first infection.

3. Main Determinants of Renal Damage

3.1. Obstruction

The role of obstruction, especially when associated with infection, in occurrence of severe renal damage is well established in the literature and will not be discussed here. Generous use of intravenous pyelography in infants and small children with febrile infections as well as in patients with recurrent infections is recommended.

3.2. Age

Table 1 shows that among boys under 1 year of age only 1/116 had a scar at the time of the first infection, whereas approximately 5% developed a scar during follow-up. Among those who were more than 1 year old at the time of the so-called "first infection," a focal scar was present in one fourth at the time the first infection was diagnosed. This table indicates three things. First, it suggests that when infections are diagnosed during the first year of life, immediately treated, and followed up carefully, the infection carries a good prognosis with few patients developing scars. Second, when UTI is

Table 2. Sex Distribution of "First" UTI and of Focal Scarring at Follow-up in Göteborg 1960–1966

	UTI	Scars
0–16 years		
Males	156	18
Females	440	20
0–12 months		
Males	113	
Females	145	
0–6 months		
Males	102	
Females	91	

diagnosed after the first year of life, patients have often had at least one earlier unrecognized and untreated infection causing scarring and renal growth retardation in a high percentage of the cases. The table also indicates that infections occurring after the first year of life seem to carry a small risk for scar development. Girls seemed, as a group, to have a later onset of initial infections than do boys. Girls developed scars usually up to about 3–4 years of age, or later.

McLachlan *et al.* (1975), studying asymptomatic bacteriuria in British schoolgirls, found that after the age of 5, the prevalence of radiological evidence of pyelonephritis is independent of age. Thus, the frequency of scarring was similar at 5 years and at 12 years. These findings emphasize the fact that efforts to prevent renal damage should be directed toward very young children.

Postmortem examinations of adults show that focal renal scars are as common in males as in females. Since UTI are about 10 times more common in females than in males, it has been questioned whether infections are causally related to such scars (Freedman, 1967; Kleeman and Freedman, 1968).

Table 2 shows that in the 1960–1966 study group the male/female ratio for scars among 0- to 16-year-olds was close to one. The infection ratio was 1 : 3 in the whole material but, among 0- to 12-month-olds, it was 0.8, and among 0- to 6-month-olds, it was 1.1. If the age before 1 year is the most vulnerable period the sex ratio of 1 : 1 for pyelonephritic scarring makes sense.

Increased attention to the possibility of pyelonephritis in infants and children with fever, for which there is no other obvious cause, is necessary. For example, in the Göteborg study the number of infections recognized during the first 4 years were only half as frequent as during the last 3 years.

Thus, age is an important factor in the development of a renal scar. Early infections often cause renal damage if they are unrecognized and untreated. Late infections carry a better prognosis. The most important populations to screen for bacteriuria are infants and toddlers with fever.

Table 3. *Effect of Therapeutic Delay on Scar Development*

	UTI (No.)	Scarring (No.)	Scarring %
Adequate care[a] at first infection	440	20	4.5
Adequate care[b] only at second infection	41	7	17

[a] Early diagnosis and treatment; follow-up after treatment.
[b] First infection: therapeutic delay for various reasons.

This might be the way to recognize infantile pyelonephritis and thus to prevent subsequent severe renal damage.

3.3. *Therapeutic Delay*

One important determinant of renal damage is the duration of infection before treatment begins. A few days of persistent infection may be enough to cause persistent renal and ureteral damage. During the Göteborg study we were able to collect 41 girls in whom the first known infection was treated inadequately. The incidence of renal damage was four times as high in this group with therapeutic delay as in the group of 440 girls who were diagnosed and treated promptly and adequately (Table 3).

In an analysis of causes of ureteral and renal damage, attention should be given to the duration of the first febrile infection before treatment begins. This has rarely—if ever—been done systematically in the many studies of determinants of renal damage, especially those of reflux and its operative correction. The impact of the therapeutic delay is demonstrated beautifully in a recent study by Miller and Phillips (1981). They induced pyelonephritis in rats by a very precise method and delayed therapy for varying periods. With each prolongation of the treatment-free interval, from 8 hr to 7 days, the renal damage became more and more severe. These findings have their obvious human counterpart.

3.4. *Bacterial Virulence*

Host and aggressor characteristics and their interaction deserve attention with regard to pathogenesis of renal scarring. Some infecting *E. coli* are extremely sensitive to the bactericidal action of normal serum. Such bacteria are stripped of nearly all virulence factors. When they appear in the urinary tract, usually in patients with asymptomatic bacteriuria, they seem to do no harm (Lindberg *et al.*, 1975). In fact, their elimination by treatment may do more harm than good.

The first step in initiation and propagation of any infection seems to be an adherence between the bacteria and epithelial cells (Jones, 1977). This adhesion is mediated by pili or fimbriae extending from the bacterial wall.

Table 4. Demonstration of VUR at the time of the First Infection in 23 Kidneys Developing Focal Scarring

Reflux	
Grade	%
0–1	39
2	26
3	35
4	0

They are of protein nature and appear in a frequency of 100–200 per bacteria.

Bacteria causing pyelonephritis seem to adhere better to uroepithelial cells than bacteria causing cystitis or asymptomatic bacteriuria (Svanborg-Edén *et al.*, 1976). On the host side, uroepithelial cells from patients prone to infections seem to bind pyelonephritogenic bacteria better than cells from controls (Fowler and Stamey, 1977; Källenius and Winberg, 1978; Svanborg-Edén and Jodal, 1979).

Källenius, Möllby, and others in our group have recently been able to identify the structure of the minimal receptor on the cell surface which binds the fimbriae of pyelonephritogenic bacteria (Källenius and Möllby, 1979; Källenius *et al.*, 1980a–c; Källenius *et al.*, 1981a,b). This receptor has been identified as a galactose–galactose (gal–gal) moiety, which is related to the antigens of the P blood group system. Bacteria with fimbriae recognizing this structure thus have a virulence factor.

Such P-fimbriated bacteria seem to cause about 90% of acute pyelonephritis in childhood but are much less common in other types of UTI. This observation fits well with Svanborg–Edén's demonstration that adhesive properties of bacteria were related to the symptomatology of the infection.

3.5. Ureteral Dysfunction and VUR

The association of gross VUR and renal damage is well established in retrospective studies emanating from referral clinics. Bacterial invasion of the kidney by pyelorenal backflow seems to play a decisive role in the induction of renal damage. Gross VUR with intrarenal reflux (IRR) has been claimed to be operative in such instances (Hodson and Edwards, 1960; Filly *et al.*, 1974; Rolleston *et al.*, 1974; Smellie and Normand, 1975; Ransley and Risdon, 1975a,b). In the prospective Göteborg study, it was clearly shown that reflux with dilatation at the time of infection was found in only one third of those children who developed a focal renal scar (Table 4).

The discrepancies between this study and others may be explained by a series of elegant experiments in monkeys performed by Roberts and coworkers (Roberts, 1974, 1975; Roberts and Riopelle, 1977, 1978; Fussell and

Table 5. Effects of Ureteric Instillation of Gal–Gal-Recognizing E. coli 04 and Non-Gal–Gal-Recognizing E. coli 06 and 0111[a]

Ureteral function	Strain	
	04	06, 0111
Ureteritis	+ + +	±
Peristalsis abnormal	+ + +	±
Slow passage of dye	+ + +	±
Increased ureteral pressure	+ + +	±

[a] From Roberts (1975) and Roberts *et al.* (1984).

Roberts, 1979; Angel *et al.*, 1979). They found that some *E. coli* induced ureteritis leading to a functional obstruction of the urinary flow with increased intraureteral pressure. This could amount to approximately 35 mm Hg, roughly corresponding to the voiding pressure that is transmitted to the kidney in gross VUR (cf. Table 5).

The *E. coli* strains used in these experiments were sent to us by Roberts. An *E. coli* 04, which regularly caused ureteritis and pyelonephritis, was shown to recognize the gal–gal receptor (Table 5). Less virulent strains did not show this binding specificity (Roberts *et al.*, 1984).

The functional obstruction of urinary excretion associated with infection with gal–gal-recognizing *E. coli* may be as effective as gross VUR with IRR to cause infection of the renal tissue. In fact, such changes of ureteral function seem to be the "missing link," which, looking on the problem from an epidemiological point of view, can explain the fact that more scars are found to develop in the absence than in the presence of gross reflux.

4. *Hypothesis for Renal Damage*

The following hypothesis for ureteral and renal damage is advanced: (1) Ascending infection with gal–gal-recognizing *E. coli* causes ureteral infection (by means of minute reflux?). (2) Ureteritis results in ureteral "holdup" in excretion and consequent increased perfusion pressure. This might be due to structural damage of the ureter (Fussell and Roberts, 1979) or to endotoxin inhibition of norepinephrine-mediated transmission in ureteral synapses (cf. Nergardh, 1974; Long and Nergardh, 1978; Nergårdh *et al.*, 1977). (3) Pyelorenal backflow and renal tissue inflammation follow. Confounding factors involve quality of care, gross VUR and compound papillae. When diagnosis and treatment are immediate, damage may be avoided even when there is gross intrarenal reflux.

Figure 1 is an attempt to demonstrate graphically two different views about factors of importance for renal damage. The reflux nephropathy hypothesis (upper part) puts gross VUR in the center. In association with

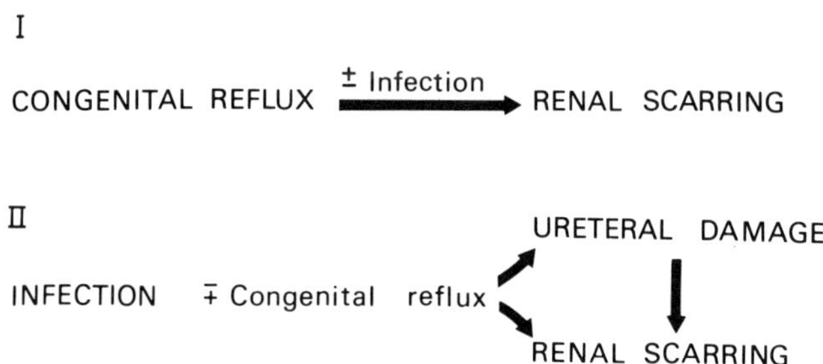

Figure 1. Two views on the relationship among infection, vesicoureteral reflux, and ureteral damage and scarring (see text).

infection (sometimes without infection) and IRR, VUR causes renal damage. This hypothesis cannot explain the fact that many children developing scarring have never had demonstrable gross reflux or any reflux at all.

Our current view is that infection with virulent bacteria causes ureteral damage which facilitates renal damage by means of functional obstruction and pyelorenal backflow of infected urine (lower part of Fig. 1). If gross VUR is present, renal scarring can occur whether ureteral damage is present or not.

5. Summary

Disregarding anatomical obstruction of the urinary flow, at ages of less than 1 year, therapeutic delay, and bacterial virulence seem to be the most important determinants of renal damage following UTI. The importance of the interval between onset of infection and onset of therapy has often been neglected.

References

Angel, J. R., Smith, T. W. Jr., and Roberts, J. A., 1979, The hydrodynamics of pyelorenal reflux, *J. Urol.* **122:**20.

Bergström, T., Larson, H., Lincoln, K., and Winberg, J., 1972, Studies of urinary tract infections in infancy and childhood. XII. Eighty consecutive patients with neonatal infection, *J. Pediatr.* **80:**858.

Filly, R., Friedland, G. W., Govan, E. D., and Fair, W. R., 1974, Development and progression of clubbing and scarring in children with recurrent urinary tract infections, *Radiology* **113:**145.

Fowler, J. E., and Stamey, T. S., 1977, Studies of introital colonization in women with recurrent urinary infections. VII. The role of bacterial adherence, *J. Urol.* **117:**472.

Freedman, L. R., 1967, Chronic pyelonephritis at autopsy, *Ann. Intern. Med.* **66:**697.

Fussell, E. N., and Roberts, J. A., 1979, Chronic pyelonephritis. Electron microscopic study. III. The ureter, *Invest. Urol.* **17:**108.

Hodson, C. J., and Edwards, D., 1960, Chronic pyelonephritis and vesicoureteric reflux, *Clin. Radiol.* **11:**219.

Jones, G. W., 1977, The attachment of bacteria to the surfaces of animal cells, in: *Receptors and Recognition,* series B, Volume 3, *Microbial Interactions* (J. L. Reissing, ed.), Chapman & Hall, London, pp. 139–176.

Källenius, G., and Möllby, R., 1979, Adhesion of *Escherichia coli* to human periurethral cells correlated to mannose-resistant agglutination of human erythrocytes, *FEMS Microbiol. Lett.* **5:**295.

Källenius, G., and Winberg, J., 1978, Bacterial adherence to periurethral epithelial cells in girls prone to urinary tract infections, *Lancet* **2:**540.

Källenius, G., Möllby, R., Svenson, S. B., Winberg, J., Lundblad, A., Svensson, S., and Cedergren, B., 1980a, The pk antigen as receptor for the haemagglutinin of peylonephritic *Escherichia coli, FEMS Microbiol. Lett.* **7:**297.

Källenius, G., Möllby, R., and Winberg, J., 1980b, *In vitro* adhesion of uropathogenic *Escherichia coli* to human periurethral cells, *Infect. Immunol.* **28:**972.

Källenius, G., Möllby, R., Svenson, S. B., Hultberg, H., and Winberg, J., 1980c, Identification of a carbohydrate receptor recognized by uropathogenic *Escherichia coli, Infection* **8**(suppl 3):288.

Källenius, G., Svenson, S. B., Möllby, R., Cedergren, B., Hultberg, H., and Winberg, J., 1981a, Structure of carbohydrate part of receptor on human uroepithelial cells for pyelonephritogenic *E. coli, Lancet* **2:**604.

Källenius, G., Möllby, R., Svenson, S. B., Helin, I., Hultberg, H., Cedergren, B., and Winberg, J., 1981b, Occurrence of P-fimbriated *Escherichia coli* in urinary tract infections, *Lancet* **2:**1369.

Kleeman, S. E. T., and Freedman, L. R., 1968, The finding of chronic pyelonephritis in males and females at autopsy, *N. Engl. J. Med.* **263:**988.

Lindberg, U., Hanson, L. Å., Jodal, U., Lidin–Janson, G., Lincoln, K., and Olling, S., 1975, Asymptomatic bacteriuria in schoolgirls. II. Differences in *Escherichia coli* causing asymptomatic and symptomatic bacteriuria, *Acta Paediatr. Scand.* **64:**432.

Long, S., and Nergardh, A., 1978, Autonomic receptor functions of the human ureter: An *in vitro* study, *Scand. J. Urol. Nephrol.* **12:**23.

McLachlan, M. S. F., Meller, S. T., Verrier Jones, E. R., Asscher, A. W., Fletcher, E. W. L., Mayon–White, R. T., Ledingham, J. G. G., Smith, J. C., and Johnston, H. H., 1975, The urinary tract in schoolgirls with covert bacteriuria, *Arch. Dis. Child.* **50:**253.

Miller, T., and Phillips, S., 1981, Pyelonephritis: The relationship between infection, renal scarring and antimicrobial therapy, *Kidney Int.* **19:**654.

Nergardh, A., 1974, The functional role of adrenergic receptors in the outlet region of the urinary bladder, *Scand. J. Urol. Nephrol.* **8:**100.

Nergårdh, A., Boréus, L. O., and Holme, T., 1977, The inhibitory effect of coli-endotoxin on alpha-adrenergic receptor functions in the lower urinary tract. An *in vitro* study in cats, *Scand. J. Urol. Nephrol.* **11:**219.

Ransley, P. G., and Risdon, R. A., 1975a, Renal papillary morphology and intrarenal reflux in the young pig, *Urol. Res.* **3:**105.

Ransley, P. G., and Risdon, R. A., 1975b, Renal papillary morphology in infants and young children, *Urol. Res.* **3:**111.

Roberts, J. A., 1974, Vesicoureteral reflux in the primate, *Invest. Urol.* **12:**88.

Roberts, J. A., 1975, Experimental pyelonephritis in the monkey. III. Pathophysiology of ureteral malfunction induced by bacteria, *Invest. Urol.* **13:**117.

Roberts, J. A., and Riopelle, A. J., 1977, Vesicoureteral reflux in the primate: II. Maturation of the ureterovesical junction, *Pediatrics* **59:**566.

Roberts, J. A., and Riopelle, A. J., 1978, Vesicoureteral reflux in the primate: III. Effect of urinary tract infection on maturation of the ureterovesical junction, *Pediatrics* **61:**853.

Roberts, J. A., Kaack, B., Källenius, G., Möllby, R., and Winberg, J., 1984, Receptors for pyelonephritogenic *Escherichia coli* in primates, *J. Urol.* **131:**163.

Rolleston, G. L., Maling, T. M. J., and Hodson, C. J., 1974, Intrarenal reflux and the scarred kidney, *Arch. Dis. Child.* **49:**531.

Smellie, J. M., and Normand, I. C. S., 1975, Bacteriuria, reflux and renal scarring, *Arch. Dis. Child.* **50:**581.

Svanborg-Edén, C., and Jodal, U., 1979, Attachment of *Escherichia coli* to urinary sediment epithelial cells from urinary tract infection-prone and healthy children, *Infect Immunol.* **26:**837.

Svanborg-Edén, C., Hanson, L. Å., Jodal, U., Lindberg, U., and Sohl Åkerlund, A., 1976, Variable adherence to normal human urinary-tract epithelial cells of *Escherichia coli* strains associated with various forms of urinary-tract infection, *Lancet* **2:**490.

Winberg, J., Andersen, H. J., Bergström, T., Jacobsson, B., Larson, H., and Lincoln, K., 1974, Epidemiology of symptomatic urinary tract infection in childhood, *Acta Paediatr. Scand.* (suppl. 252)**:**1.

Winberg, J., Bergström, T., and Jacobsson, B., 1975, Morbidity, age and sex distribution, recurrences and renal scarring in symptomatic urinary tract infection in childhood, *Kidney Int.* **8:**101.

30

Nutritional Requirements for Growth in Children with Renal Insufficiency

Malcolm A. Holliday

Optimum requirements for growth in normal children are defined by the Recommended Dietary Allowances (RDAs) (National Research Council, Food and Nutrition Board, 1980). Given access to adequate food, it is assumed that normal children will have an appetite that assures an adequate intake of energy. Requirements for specific nutrients other than energy are usually met when children satisfy appetite for calories with customary foods. Specific nutrients are taken well in excess of RDA and, in many instances, the excess is excreted in urine. Dietary tolerances are generous in normal children (Holliday, 1976).

Children with renal insufficiency or uremia lose tolerance roughly in proportion to loss of kidney function (Holliday, 1976). They also often lose appetite and eat less. The loss of tolerance may impose dietary restraint. This and the inherent anorexia of uremia are causes for poor intake of energy and potential deficiency of specific nutrients.

Uremia changes metabolism so that some nutrients, e.g., calcium and vitamin D, must be supplied in quantities that exceed the RDA for normals. We monitor the diet and use a minilist of food composition (Pennington, 1976) to derive a pattern of nutrient intake. Where we sense deficiency, either from clinical signs or from dietary analysis, we recommend supplements.

Loss of tolerance, because of loss of excretory function, is especially notable in the case of sodium and phosphorus. In some cases, recommending sodium restrictions is easier now than it has been because public education relating salt intake to hypertension has been extensive. It is more difficult in other cases because prepared foods, fast foods, and fad foods—often high

Malcolm A. Holliday • Department of Pediatrics, School of Medicine, University of California, San Francisco 94110.

in sodium—are more widely used, especially by adolescents. Sodium restriction is achieved in some patients by counseling, teaching food tradeoffs, and demonstrating a relation between sodium intake and hypertension. In others, diuretics or antihypertensive drugs are used. Hypertension *per se* may inhibit growth (Caliguire *et al.*, 1963).

Control of phosphorus absorption commonly is achieved by using phosphate-binding gels. They are not very palatable and depress appetite. Children often will not take them. Consequently, selecting out high-phosphorus foods can be useful. This advice is given to children and families as part of nutrition counseling. Hyperphosphatemia contributes to osteodystrophy, and osteodystrophy impairs growth. Hypocalcemia and vitamin D resistance are other nutritional factors that contribute to osteodystrophy and poor growth (Chesney *et al.*, 1978).

Hyperchloremic acidosis, which occurs in renal tubular acidosis (RTA), inhibits growth. Where this is a single defect as occurs in type I RTA, correcting acidosis leads to accelerated growth (McSherry, 1978). Metabolic acidosis associated with chronic renal failure is influenced by dietary protein and mineral content. To the extent that acid–base status can be corrected by diet and intake of alkali, growth may improve. However, alkali therapy in uremic children with growth retardation has not restored stature to normal.

We have little information on requirements of vitamins and trace minerals in uremia in relation to their effect on growth (Holliday *et al.*, 1979).

We have focused our efforts over the past decade on the question of energy metabolism. The initial question was whether dietary energy deficiency contributed to poor growth and whether calorie supplements should be used. Two other questions that concern energy metabolism and which may affect growth have been the subject of recent work by several groups. These are whether the state of uremia is associated with an exaggerated catabolic response to stress with increased need for supplemental calories, protein, or carbohydrate and whether the sedentary state—characteristic of uremia—contributes to disordered metabolism which can be corrected by regular physical activity. The question should be raised: should we encourage exercise?

The question of inadequate intake of calories as a cause of poor growth in children with kidney disease was first raised by West and Smith (1956) in a review of their clinical experience. We demonstrated low energy intake in children on chronic hemodialysis and found energy intake correlated with growth rate. Giving supplements of carbohydrate was associated with improved growth (Simmons *et al.*, 1971). Others have confirmed that energy intake is low and the level of intake correlated with growth in children with renal failure, including those on dialysis (Betts and Magrath, 1974; Chantler *et al.*, 1976). The value of caloric supplements in clinical practice is less well documented both by report (Kleinknecht *et al.*, 1980; Betts *et al.*, 1977) and by personal comments from other physicians.

Table 1. Characteristics of Children with Chronic Renal Failure at the Beginning of a 1-Year Period in Which Diet Was Unsupplemented (U) with Carbohydrate and at the Beginning of a 1-Year Period When They Took a Supplement (S)

	n	U	S
Age (years)	16	5.1	5.9
Renal function (ml/min per 1.73 m^2)	16	21.0	21.0
Growth retardation[a]	16	−3.0	−3.5

[a] Standard deviations below the mean height for age.

We recently completed a study of 16 children who had renal insufficiency and who were being followed in a special clinic (Arnold and Holliday, 1979a). The purpose of the study was to evaluate energy intake in relation to growth rate and other nutritional indices and to determine whether calorie supplements were beneficial. Fourteen children were followed an average of 1 year during which management and counseling were done in accordance with our practice. They were then followed a second year during which time they were given a carbohydrate supplement as well. Two children received a supplement during the first year of the study and stopped taking the supplement during the second year.

We evaluated results by comparing growth and other indices over the year in which no supplements were given—unsupplemented (U)—and again in which the supplement was given (S). The paired t test was used for statistical evaluation.

Some of the results are listed in Table 1. The average age was greater during the S period because of the design of the study. Renal function evaluated at the end of each study year had not changed significantly. The children were an average of −3.0 standard deviations (S.D.) below mean height for age at the beginning of the U period and, because they did not grow at a normal rate during the U period, were an average of −3.5 S.D. below mean height for age at the beginning of the S period; i.e., they were severely growth retarded, and the degree of retardation progressed.

During the U period food intake as percent of normal was low (74% normal); with supplementation it reached normal (102%). Carbohydrate, as a fraction of the total calories, was 47% in the U period and increased to 53% in the S period. Growth rate increased from 4.4 to 6.1 cm/yr with supplementation or from 60% to 89% normal for height. The degree of growth retardation, which had increased during the period, remained unchanged during the S period (Table 2). In other words, supplementation improved growth from below normal to normal but did not support catch-up growth in these children with severe growth retardation. Somatomedin levels, which we have shown to be elevated in children with renal failure (Spencer *et al.*, 1979) despite the low growth rate, were higher at the end of

Table 2. Dietary Intake and Growth Responses of Children at the End of the Unsupplemented (U) and Supplemented (S) Periods of Study

	n	U	S
Duration of study (years)	16	0.98	1.02
Energy intake (% of normal)	16	74.0	102[a]
Carbohydrate content (% total calories)	12	47.0	53[b]
Growth rate (cm/year)	16	4.4	6.1[a]
Relative growth rate (% of normal)	16	60.0	89.[a]
S.D. score at end of study	16	−3.7	−3.7
Change in S.D. score during study	16	−0.7	−0.2[b]
Somatomedin level (units/ml plasma)	8	2.6	3.8[a]

[a] Difference significant at $p<0.01$.
[b] Difference significant at $p<0.05$.

supplementation corresponding with the higher food intake and growth rate observed over that period (Table 2).

We observed a significant correlation ($r = 0.68$) between growth rate and energy intake, both expressed as percent normal, during the U period. There was no correlation between these variables ($r = 0.07$) during the S period.

We believe that these findings support the hypothesis that simple dietary energy deficiency is common in children with renal insufficiency and that calorie supplement corrects the deficiency. The deficiency inhibits growth, but correcting the deficiency has only a modest impact on growth rate—no catch-up growth occurred. The absence of a correlation between food intake and growth rate in the S period contrasts with the correlation found in the U period. We interpret this difference as evidence that further supplementation would have been pointless.

Two other observations in our study support these conclusions. Serum albumin concentrations rose to normal and skinfold thickness, a measure of adipose tissue, increased to average values found in normal children over the period of supplementation. Other support comes from a study of lysine flux in uremic children. Total body lysine flux, a measure of protein synthesis, is depressed in children with renal failure (Conley *et al.*, 1980), and the degree of depression correlated with the level of energy and protein intake.

Our ability to gain acceptance by the children of a supplement was limited. Children do resist taking carbohydrate supplements or, accepting them, become tired and often stop taking them. We believe our success, where others have failed, is due to the emphasis we place on nutrition support services and the fact that a nutritionist has time to work with children rather than simply to advise. Now that supplements are integrated unobtrusively into nutrition education, their use is less an issue.

Conventional widsom has it that the catabolic response to stress is exaggerated in uremia. The stress of infection in dialysis patients is associated with large losses of body protein nitrogen (Grodstein *et al.*, 1980). We reported that uremic rats fasted 36 hr had an increased in net urea synthesis or appearance over the last 12 hr compared with fasted controls. Correlated with this was a reduction in muscle protein synthesis. The difference was abolished if carbohydrate was given (Holliday *et al.*, 1977). Plasma and intracellular leucine values rose with fasting in uremic rats whereas they declined in controls. We interpreted these findings as evidence that catabolic stress of fasting as measured both by net loss of body protein and by degree of depression of muscle protein synthesis was increased. Rubenfeld and Garber (1978) have reported alanine turnover in uremic humans fasted overnight to be 2–3 times control values, and glucose derived from alanine also was increased. These are stress responses that are augmented in uremia.

Although overnight fasting is a short event, the differences in response brought on by uremia may act cumulatively to affect growth. This was inferred from a study where uremic and control rats were pair-fed over a period of 21 days. Uremic rats grew less in length, gained less weight, and had a carcass lipid and protein contents below their pair fed controls (Mehls *et al.*, 1980). Some process in uremia impaired conversion of dietary energy and protein to body mass. Urinary area nitrogen excretion was increased in uremic rats.

Resistance to insulin-mediated carbohydrate uptake is characteristic of infection and injury—classical models of exaggerated catabolic stress. Resistance to insulin-mediated carbohydrate (Westervelt, 1969; DeFronzo *et al.*, 1978) and amino acid (Arnold and Holliday, 1979b) uptake by peripheral tissue is characteristic in uremia. Whether the insulin resistance in uremia is directly related to the exaggerated catabolic responses seen in uremia is not known.

The cumulative evidence implicates an altered metabolic response to the common stress of short fasting in which loss of body nitrogen and inefficient use of dietary energy may contribute to the poor nutritional state and to poor growth. These effects of uremia contrast with the effects of simple energy deficiency. Malnutrition results in a decline in basal metabolism, a sparing of body protein nitrogen loss in response to fasting, a lower rate of gluconeogenesis from amino acids, and more efficient use of fatty acids (Keys *et al.*, 1950; Kerr *et al.*, 1978a,b). Sensitivity to insulin-induced hypoglycemia is increased (Beeker *et al.*, 1975). However, lysine flux in malnutrition is reduced (Picou and Taylor-Robert, 1969) as it is in uremia (Conley *et al.*, 1980). When abundant food is provided to malnourished infants, energy intake and growth rate exceed normal by 1–2 times (Spady *et al.*, 1976). This contrasts with findings in our study.

Hyperlipidemia is a feature of uremia in adults (Bagdade *et al.*, 1968) and children (Bishti *et al.*, 1977). Its presence in adult dialysis patients increases the risk for myocardial infarction (Brunzell, 1980). We found in a small number of children given supplements in whom we followed plasma lipids that lipid levels increased (Table 3). This increase parallels the increase that follows a switch to a higher-carbohydrate diet in normal (Ginsberg *et al.*, 1976) and in uremic (Sanfelippo *et al.*, 1977) individuals. An increase in

Table 3. Differences in Nutritional Status of Children after 1 Year of an Unsupplemented (U) Diet and after 1 Year of a Diet Supplemented (S) with Carbohydrate

	n	U	S
Weight (% of ideal wt/ht)	16	92	95
Skinfold thickness (% normal)	16	77	101[a]
Plasma albumin (g/dl)	15	4.2	4.5[a]
Plasma cholesterol (mg/dl)	10	220	252[a]
Plasma triglycerides (mg/dl)	5	174	275[a]

[a] Difference significant at $p<0.05$.

plasma lipids occurs in patients undergoing continuous ambulatory peritoneal dialysis (CAPD) (Moncrief *et al.*, 1979). Of seven children followed on CAPD who were fed a glucose supplement that averaged 65 g/day or 260 kcal/day, plasma triglycerides rose in two. Definitive information about whether total energy intake or growth improves in children on CAPD is not available (Potter *et al.*, 1980).

We are confronted with a dilemma. Carbohydrate provided as a supplement increases energy intake. The added carbohydrate may correct a deficiency in dietary energy and may improve growth. It also causes a further increase in plasma lipids.

It is not clear that carbohydrate supplements will increase the risk of early coronary disease, but the possibility is sufficient that one must look for remedies. Hyperlipidemia is related to insulin resistance in both normal (Oleskfy *et al.*, 1974) and uremic (Reavan *et al.*, 1980) subjects. One means of lowering plasma lipids and increasing insulin sensitivity is aerobic exercise.

A recent report describes the effect of aerobic exercise training on plasma lipids and insulin sensitivity in uremic adults. Plasma lipids decreased and insulin sensitivity improved (Goldberg *et al.*, 1980). This observation poses an interesting question. Can exercise that increases energy demand be beneficial to uremic patients? It can if, associated with the increased demand, there is an improvement in appetite so that energy intake increased to match or exceed demand. If this occurs, then we have the physiological basis for encouraging an activity regimen that increases energy demand and a diet that will increase supply. This study needs to be initiated. An underlying question is whether changes in life-style that improve the individual's adaptation to uremia are acceptable and practical for patients. In children, there is the further question of whether these maneuvers will improve growth.

References

Arnold, W. C., and Holliday, M. A., 1979a, Assessment of nutritional status in children with chronic renal failure, *Kidney Int.* **16:**950.

Arnold, W. C., and Holliday, M. A., 1979b, Tissue resistance to insulin stimulation of amino acid uptake in acutely uremia rats, *Kidney Int.* **16:**124–129.

Bagdade, J. D., Porte, D., and Blerman, E. L., 1968, Hypertriglyceridemia: A metabolic consequence of chronic renal failure, *N. Engl. J. Med.* **279:**181.

Beeker, D. J., Pimstone, B. L., and Hausen, J. D. L., 1975, The relation between insulin secretion glucose tolerance, growth hormone and serum proteins in protein calorie malnutrition, *Pediatr. Res.* **9:**35–39.

Betts, P. R., and Magrath, G., 1974, Growth pattern and dietary intake of children with chronic renal insufficiency, *Br. Med. J.* **2:**189.

Betts, P. R., Magrath, G., and White, R. H. R., 1977, Role of dietary energy supplementation in growth of children with chronic renal insufficiency, *Br. Med. J.* **1:**416.

Bishti, M. M., Counahan, R., Stimmler, L., Jarrett, R. J., Wass, V. J., and Chantler, C., 1977, Abnormalities in plasma lipids in children of regular hemodialysis, *Arch. Dis. Child.* **52:**932.

Brunzell, J. D., 1980, Triglycerides and coronary heart disease (letter), *N. Engl. J. Med.* **303:**1060.

Caliguire, L. A., Shapiro, A. P., and Holliday, M. A., 1963, Clinical improvement in chronic renal hypertension in children, *Pediatrics* **31:**758.

Chantler, C., El–Bishti, M. M., Counahan, R., Wass, V. J., and Cox, B. D., 1976, Growth in children with renal failure, *Melsunger Med. Mitteilungen* **50**(11)**:**557.

Chesney, R. W., Moorthy, V., Eisman, J. A., Jax, D. K., Mazess, R. B., and DeLuca, H. F., 1978, Increased growth after long term oral 1,25-vitamin D_3 in childhood renal osteodystrophy, *N. Engl. J. Med.* **298:**238–242.

Conley, S. B., Rose, G. M., Robson, A. M., and Bier, D. M., 1980, Effects of dietary intake and hemodialysis on protein turnover in uremic children, *Kidney Int.* **17:**837–846.

DeFronzo, R. A., Tobin, J. D., Rowe, J. W., and Andres, R., 1978, Glucose intolerance in uremia, *J. Clin. Invest.* **62:**425–435.

Ginsberg, H., Olefsky, J., Kimmerling, G., Crapo, P., and Reavan, G. M., 1976, Induction of hypertriglyceridemia by a low fat diet, *J. Clin. Endocrinol. Metab.* **42:**729.

Goldberg, A. O., Hagberg, J., Delmez, J. A., Carney, R. M., McKevitt, P. M., Ehsaru, A. A., and Harter, H. R., 1980, The metabolic and psychological effects of exercise training in hemodialysis patients, *Am. J. Clin. Nutr.* **33:**1620–1628.

Grodstein, G. P., Blumenkrantz, M. J., and Kopple, J. D., 1980, Nutritional and metabolic response to stress, *Am. J. Clin. Nutr.* **33:**1411–1416.

Holliday, M. A., 1976, Management of the child with renal insufficiency, in: *Clinical Pediatric Nephrology* (E. Lieberman, ed.), Lippincott, Philadelphia.

Holliday, M. A., Chantler, C., MacDonnell, R., and Keitges, J., 1977, Effect of uremia in nutritionally-induced variations in protein metabolism, *Kidney Int.* **11:**236–245.

Holliday, M. A., McHenry, K., and Portale, A., 1979, Nutritional management of chronic renal disease, *Med. Clin. North Am.* **63:**945.

Kerr, D. S., Stevens, M. C. G., and Robinson, H. M., 1978a, Fasting metabolism in infants: I. Effect of severe undernutrition in energy and protein utilization, *Metabolism* **27:**411–435.

Kerr, D. S., Stevens, M. C. G., and Picou, D. I. M., 1978b, Fasting metabolism in infants: II. The effect of severe undernutrition and infusion of alanine on glucose production estimated with U^{13} glucose, *Metabolism* **27:**831–847.

Keys, A., Brozek, J., Henschel, A., Michelson, O., and Taylor, H. I., 1950, *The Biology of Human Starvation*, University of Minnesota Press, Minneapolis.

Kleinknect, C., Broyer, M., Gagnadoux, M., Marte–Henneberg, C., Dartois, A. M., Kermanach, C., Pouliguen, M., Degoulet, P., Usbert, M., and Roy, M. P., 1980, Growth in children treated with long-term dialysis. A study of 76 patients, *Adv. Nephrol.* **9:**133–163.

McSherry, E., 1978, Acidosis and growth in nonuremic renal disease, *Kidney Int.* **14:**349–354.

Mehls, O., Ritz, E., Gilli, G., Bartholome, K., BeiBbarth, H., Hohenegger, M., and Schafnitzel, W., 1980, Nitrogen metabolism and growth in experimental uremia, *Int. J. Pediatr. Nephrol.* **1**(1)**:**34–41.

Moncrief, J. W., Popuvich, R. P., Holph, K. D., Rubin, J., Robson, M., Dombros, N., deVeber, G. A., and Oreopoulos, D. G., 1979, Clinical experience with continuous ambulatory peritoneal dialysis, *ASAIO Journal* **2:**114–118.

National Research Council, Food and Nutrition Board, 1980, *Recommended Dietary Allowances*, 9th ed., National Academy of Science, Washington, D.C.

Olefsky, J. M., Farquhar, J. W., and Reavan, G. M., 1974, Reappraisal of the role of insulin in hypertriglyceridemia, *Am. J. Med.* **57:**551.

Pennington, J. A., 1976, *Dietary Nutrient Guide*, Avi, Westport, Connecticut.

Picou, D., and Taylor-Robert, T., 1969, The measurement of total protein synthesis and catabolism and nitrogen turnover in infants in different nutritional states and receiving different amounts of dietary protein, *Clin. Sci.* **35:**283.

Potter, D. E., McDaid, T. K., and Ramirez, J. A., 1980, Peritoneal dialysis in children, in: *Proceedings of the Pan Pacific Symposium on Peritoneal Dialysis* (R. Atkins, ed.), Churchill Livingstone, New York.

Reavan, G. M., Swenson, R. S., and Sanfelippo, M. D., 1980, An inquiry into the mechanism of hypertriglyceridemia in patients with chronic renal failure, *Am. J. Clin. Nutr.* **33:**1476–1484.

Rubenfeld, S., and Garber, A. J., 1978, Abnormal CHO metabolism in CRF. The potential role of accelerated glucose production, increased gluconeogenesis and impaired glucose disposal. *J. Clin. Invest.* **62**(1)**:**20–28.

Sanfelippo, M. L., Swenson, R. S., and Reaven, G. M., 1977, Reduction of plasma triglycerides by diet in subjects with chronic renal failure, *Kidney Int.* **11:**54–61.

Simmons, J. M., Wilson, C. J., Potter, D. E., and Holliday, M. A., 1971, Relation of calorie deficiency to growth failure in children on hemodialysis and the growth response to calorie supplementation, *N. Engl. J. Med.* **285:**653–656.

Spady, D. W., Payne, P. R., Picou, D., and Waterlow, J. C., 1976, Energy balance during recovery from malnutrition, *Am. J. Clin. Nurs.* **29:**1073–1078.

Spencer, E. M., Uthne, K. O., and Arnold, W. C., 1979, Growth impairment with elevated somatomedin levels in children with chronic renal insufficiency, *Acta Endocrinol.* **91:**36–48.

West, C. D., and Smith, W. C., 1956, An attempt to elucidate the cause of growth retardation in renal disease, *Am. J. Dis. Child.* **91:**460.

Westervelt, F. B., 1969, Insulin effect in uremia, *J. Lab Clin. Med.* **74:**79–84.

31

Protein Utilization in Chronic Renal Insufficiency in Children

Warren E. Grupe, Nancy S. Spinozzi, and William E. Harmon

It is obvious that at least some of the toxic compounds responsible for uremia are metabolic products of protein catabolism. There is also ample evidence that protein metabolism is significantly altered in children with chronic renal insufficiency (Delaporte *et al.*, 1976, 1978; Conley *et al.*, 1980; Holliday *et al.*, 1970; Grupe, 1981b). These studies, coupled with the empiric demonstration that low-protein diets alleviate many of the symptoms of uremia, have led to a precept that has now become axiomatic: stipulating low-protein intake in chronic renal insufficiency. There is, however, the rational goal of reducing the main dietary sources of hydrogen ion, phosphate, potassium, and sulfate to the lowest possible level commensurate with the patient's renal function.

For the child, in whom the attainment of growth demands an excess of protein and energy, the level of protein intake deemed low enough for uremic limitations, yet adequate for growth, remains to be resolved. There appears little question that too much protein is bad. In this respect, uremia appears almost unique in that minimal intakes are perceived as advantageous (Hegsted, 1978). However, it is justly inconceivable that growth could progress in the absence of sufficient nitrogen for nitrogen retention. With adequate dialysis, and with better means to measure and assure adequate dialysis (Harmon *et al.*, 1981; Flückiger *et al.*, 1981), it seems reasonable to challenge whether low-protein intake *per se* is still valid, particularly for the potentially growing child.

There are multiple known aberrations of protein metabolism in renal insufficiency. Separation of malnutrition from altered metabolism, however, is difficult since significant interdependence exists (Conly *et al.*, 1980;

Warren E. Grupe, Nancy S. Spinozzi, and William E. Harmon • Division of Nephrology, The Children's Hospital, Boston, Massachusetts 02115.

Table 1. Abnormal Protein Metabolism in Renal Failure[a]

A. Altered intake
   1. Decreased serum and muscle protein concentration
   2. Decreased EAA[b] concentration
   3. Decreased EEA/non-EEA ratio
   4. Decreased valine/glycine ratio
B. Altered synthesis
   1. Increased muscle EAA pool, while plasma EAA pool decreased
   2. Decreased muscle EAA/non-EAA ratio
   3. Alteration of specific amino acid concentrations
   4. Intracellular abnormalities intensified by EAA supplements
   5. Hyperammonemia with EAA supplements
   6. Decreased intracellular citrulline/arginine ratio
   7. Reduced protein flux ([^{15}N]lysine enrichment)
C. Altered utilization
   1. Decreased plasma tyrosine/diphenylalanine
   2. Abnormal turnover of specific amino acids
   3. Increased release of muscle amino acids
   4. Inhibited cellular uptake of amino acids

[a] Data extracted from Giordano *et al.*, 1970; Counahan *et al.*, 1976; Delaporte *et al.*, 1976, 1978; Kopple, 1978; Holliday *et al.*, 1978; Alvestrand *et al.*, 1978; Garber, 1978; Broyer *et al.*, 1980; Arnold and Holliday, 1980; Conley *et al.*, 1980; Motil *et al.*, 1980.
[b] EAA, essential amino acids.

Counahan *et al.*, 1976). Several known alterations previously noted in children are outlined in Table 1. Some of the alterations are consistent with malnutrition (Holliday *et al.*, 1977; Abitbol and Holliday, 1978; Holliday and Chantler, 1978). The decrease in both serum and muscle protein concentration appears to be greatest in children who are on low-protein diets and have either poor or insignificant growth (Delaporte *et al.*, 1976). Although variable results have been reported, plasma essential amino acid levels are often decreased whereas nonessential amino acids have generally increased or remained unchanged (Delaporte *et al.*, 1978; Broyer *et al.*, 1980; Counahan *et al.*, 1976). This becomes more significant the more advanced the renal failure (Broyer *et al.*, 1980). The total free-amino-acid pool is increased in both plasma and muscle when severe renal insufficiency develops, however (Delaporte *et al.*, 1978; Broyer *et al.*, 1980). The ratio of valine to glycine is also decreased in both plasma and muscle and more drastically reduced in patients on lower protein intakes (Delaporte *et al.*, 1978).

Other alterations are not consistent with simple protein malnutrition. The essential-amino-acid pool in muscle is increased during periods when the plasma essential-amino-acid pool is decreased (Delaporte *et al.*, 1978). This suggests a problem of either transport or incorporation rather than of diminished excretion. The rise in muscle essential amino acids is also disproportionate relative to nonessential amino acids (Delaporte *et al.*, 1978). Since these essential amino acids are by definition exogenous in origin, such a disproportionate rise further suggests an incorporation defect; excessive catabolism of protein would be expected to produce a proportionate rise in both. This tendency occurs early in renal insufficiency (Broyer *et al.*, 1980), even in the face of adequate nutrition and during periods of normal or catch-up growth, but reaches significance at glomerular filtration rates less than 10% (Delaporte *et al.*, 1978).

Alterations of specific amino acids also have been noted, especially an increase in the plasma concentrations of hydroxyproline, citrulline, and 1- and 3-methylhistidine (Delaporte *et al.*, 1978; Counahan *et al.*, 1976). Such changes are not fully explained on the basis of excessive intake. In muscle, there is generally an increase of most essential amino acids. However, the muscle concentrations of threonine, valine, and tyrosine are commonly decreased in severe renal insufficiency (Delaporte *et al.*, 1978). Amino acid supplements can intensify intracellular amino acid abnormalities (Alvestrand *et al.*, 1978), which are more noticeable after prolonged administration of supplements with essential amino acids. Chiefly, a decrease in the muscle concentrations of phenylalanine and tyrosine and an increase in lysine, histidine, ornithine, and citrulline have been found (Alvestrand *et al.*, 1978). This suggests interference with either transport or synthesis. Should changes in the proportions of amino acids used in supplemental mixtures abolish these intracellular effects, it would not obviate the importance of the incorporation defect.

Hyperammonemia occurs in children changed from supplementation with complete amino acid mixtures to isonitrogenous and isocaloric amounts as essential-amino-acid mixtures (Motil *et al.*, 1980). This was accompanied by a decrease in urea generation at a stage when intracellular arginine should have been adequate or normal. In both children and adults there is a disproportionate rise in intracellular citrulline, relative to arginine, with a decrease in the citrulline-to-arginine ratio. In children, citrulline can increase 256% at a time when arginine has risen only 144% (Delaporte *et al.*, 1978; Broyer *et al.*, 1980). Using [^{15}N]lysine enrichment, protein flux has been noted to be decreased in children with renal insufficiency (Conley *et al.*, 1980). This returned toward normal with dialysis, suggesting a role for abnormal excretion. However, a similar improvement was produced in both dialyzed and nondialyzed children by increasing both energy and nitrogen intake, suggesting that inadequate substrate may also play a role.

Other evidences of altered utilization include a decrease in the plasma tyrosine : diphenylalanine ratio, because of either impaired synthesis of tyrosine from diphenylalanine or a defect in tyrosine uptake or distribution (Giordano *et al.*, 1970; Young and Parsons, 1973). Abnormal turnover of specific amino acids, increased release of muscle amino acids, inhibited cellular uptake of amino acids, including insulin-stimulated amino acid uptake, and abnormal incorporation of specific amino acids also have been described in renal insufficiency (Alvestrand *et al.*, 1978; Counahan *et al.*, 1976; Kopple *et al.*, 1978; Garber, 1978; Arnold and Holliday, 1980).

Despite all that is known about protein metabolism in uremic children, several ambiguities persist. The quantitative requirements for both energy and protein remain unclear. Attempts to calculate requirements on the basis of normal infant growth, recommended daily allowances, or percentages of normal child intake have been proposed (Holliday *et al.*, 1978; Broyer, 1974; Jones *et al.*, 1980; Betts *et al.*, 1977; Chantler *et al.*, 1980). The actual requirements for the uremic child on regular hemodialysis have not been completely determined. The optimal quantitative relationship between protein and energy has not been established, if, in fact, one exists. The effect that excessive energy intake has on the interpretation of protein requirement data is unknown. The potential relationship between the efficiency of protein utilization and the relative level of energy intake is uncertain. Finally, it is not known whether the current protein recommendations are appropriate to the needs of the uremic child to build lean body mass rather than fat.

Even if it is presumed that positive protein balance is a desirable goal in uremic children as a prerequisite for growth, there is no universally accepted way to measure definitely whether the goal has been reached (Munro, 1978; Hegsted, 1978). Several errors inherent in the standard nitrogen balance technique have been well addressed, relative to the uremic individual (Hegsted, 1978; Munro, 1978). The amount of energy available directly influences nitrogen balances, with excess energy leading to positive nitrogen balance. Protein needs are higher when energy intakes are marginal, and inadequate protein can thwart the nitrogen-retention effect of energy (Munro, 1978; Calloway, 1975; Garza *et al.*, 1976). Therefore, the determination of protein needs and nitrogen balance has a marked dependence on the energy status of the individual.

Apparently humans can adapt to conserve amino acids that are in short supply (Hegsted, 1978). Therefore, previous restriction of the diet will lead to an underestimation of the true protein need by nitrogen balance techniques if an insufficient time is allowed to adapt to a more suitable level. Also, the apparent retention measured can be exorbitant, bearing no relation to reasonable expectations. The accuracy of standard nitrogen balance measurements is insufficient to distinguish between the needs of the growing child and of the stable adult man (Hegsted, 1978). Thus, nitrogen balance results may be qualitatively directive, but not quantitatively accurate. Finally, any measure of nitrogen balance reflects the net change in the entire individual and, thus, may not be reflective of all tissues. It is conceivable that a particularly critical tissue may be depleted of nitrogen, even though the measured nitrogen balance is positive.

The design of the experimental conditions can have significant impact on the results of protein requirements determined by balance techniques. Most studies in both normal and uremic individuals that have been designed to determine nitrogen utilization, protein requirements, or the influence of protein quality have been constructed to maximize energy in an effort to assure full utilization of the protein presented (Garza *et al.*, 1976). The reason for this in the uremic individual is evident. Nevertheless, high energy, either absolute or relative to protein, can maintain or increase body weight, even for those in negative nitrogen balance (Garza *et al.*, 1977). Therefore, the results of long- or short-term studies that have relied on ponderal change to define either energy or nitrogen needs may be erroneous (Giordano *et al.*, 1978). A concomitant low urea nitrogen generation rate can be perceived as nitrogen sparing, even though nitrogen retention may not be present (Holliday *et al.*, 1978). Thus, experiments that have been designated to maximize nitrogen utilization through high energy intake have promoted the inaccurate precept that only insufficient, and not excessive, energy intake can affect the interpretation of nitrogen balance results (Garza *et al.*, 1976). In this light, high energy intake, coupled with protein restriction, could generate seriously misleading information when aimed at the quantitation of nitrogen requirements, the value of nitrogen quality, the effectiveness of amino acids, or the benefit from keto acids in the uremic child.

Of further importance for the depleted uremic child, the additional nitrogen retained as a result of high energy intake does not appear to be distributed in the same fashion as nitrogen retained through an increase in nitrogen intake (Garza *et al.*, 1977; Elwyn *et al.*, 1979). High energy intake produces an increase in fat deposition. Obesity does not appear to be a valid goal in the therapy of uremic children. Studies in overfed adults have shown that no more than 25–37% of weight gain represents lean body mass (Keys *et al.*, 1955; Calloway, 1975). The increase in nitrogen retention that results from excess energy appears to be used mainly for the support of the increased fat stored. In the depleted uremic child, as in other depleted patients (Olson, 1975; Garza *et al.*, 1977; Elwyn *et al.*, 1979), an increase predominantly in energy would be expected to replete only that one quarter of lean body mass lost in association with fat. The other three fourths, or the major share of the depletion, cannot be expected to be affected by changes in energy intake alone. Restoration of that remainder occurs only with changes in nitrogen intake independent of any changes in energy intake (Elwyn *et al.*, 1979). In addition, the nitrogen retained by adding excessive calories is deposited in a less labile pool, which is poorly recoverable if or when energy intake becomes suboptimal (Munro, 1964). Nitrogen retained as the result of higher protein intake, however, becomes readily available when nitrogen intake is reduced (Garza *et al.*, 1977). In the normal situation, nitrogen retention is responsive to changes in energy in a linear relationship. Nitrogen balance responds at the same rate to energy change at both submaintenance and at excessive energy levels, suggesting that substrates other than protein, when available, are preferentially metabolized at suboptimal energy levels (Garza *et al.*, 1976). This capability would be of potential advantage to the uremic child on dialysis and suspected of an inability to adapt to periods of low energy consumption (Holliday *et al.*, 1977).

High energy intake can influence the efficiency of nitrogen retention. Nitrogen retention produced by increasing energy intake alone is only 10–40% as effective as when changes in protein intake are made. For example, increasing egg protein intake in normal adult volunteers improved nitrogen retention by as much as 10 mg of nitrogen per additional kilocalorie (Inoue *et al.*, 1974). Similar patients, however, receiving marginal protein intakes generally retained only 2–4 mg nitrogen per extra kilocalorie when nitrogen

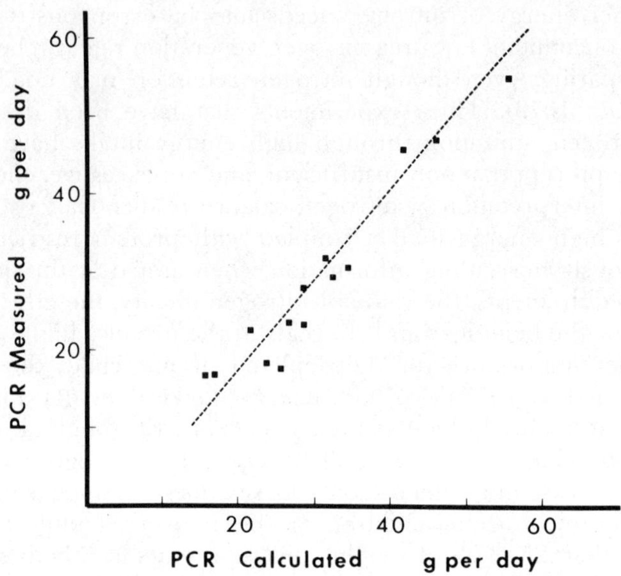

Figure 1. Net protein catabolic rate determined by standard nitrogen balance techniques (PCR measured) compared to net protein catabolic rate determined by urea kinetics (PCR calculated) ($r = 0.97$; $p = 0.94$).

balance was produced through increasing energy intake alone (Garza *et al.*, 1976). It also has been shown by Garza *et al.* (1976, 1977) that the amount of additional energy required to maintain positive nitrogen balance at borderline protein intake is 10–20% above the estimated requirements based on nitrogen balance data and weight change. The concern is that the introduction of inefficiency may force energy requirements to levels of intake beyond the already reduced appetite capabilities of uremic children, simply by limiting the amount of nitrogen to that which has been felt to be both safe and effective.

Nitrogen balance has been measured in uremic children on dialysis (Harmon *et al.*, 1979) using urea kinetics to determine urea generation rates and net protein catabolic rates (PCR). This method of net PCR estimation appears to be as valid in the child as it is in the adult (Sargent *et al.*, 1978), when appropriate correction for size is included. In one study (Harmon *et al.*, 1981) of 14 balance periods in dialyzed children (weight range 9–37 kg), a comparison between measured net PCR determined by standard balance techniques and calculated net PCR determined by urea kinetics showed excellent correlation ($p = 0.94$), as in Fig. 1. In addition, responses to dietary change seemed both quantitatively and qualitatively appropriate. An increase in energy intake reduced net PCR 32% and increased net nitrogen balance >200% whereas an increase in both protein and energy increased net PCR by 43% and net nitrogen balance 78% (Harmon *et al.*, 1981). Thus, urea

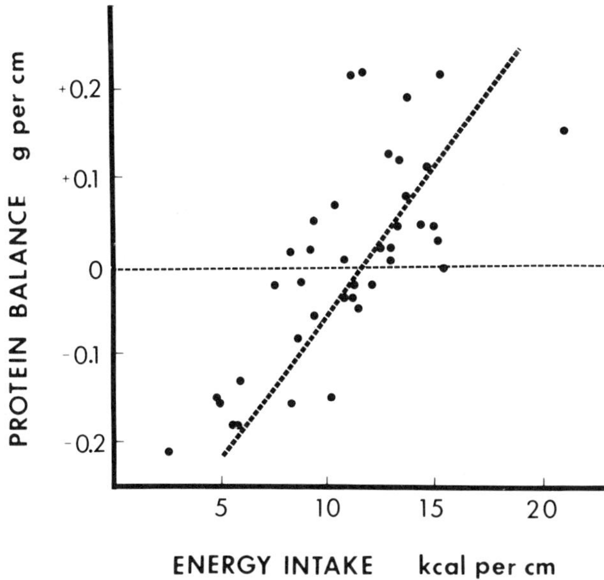

Figure 2. Protein balance as a function of daily energy intake in children on regular hemodialysis. Neutral protein balance occurs at a daily intake of 11.6 kcal/cm of height. The interrupted regression line ($r = 0.84$; $p < 0.005$) delineates a slope of 5.4 mg nitrogen retained per kilocalorie ingested.

kinetics would appear to be a convenient and accurate tool to monitor protein metabolism and to derive nitrogen balance in the uremic child on dialysis.

Extending this methodology to another group of diet-adapted children on chronic hemodialysis (Figs. 2 and 3), our unit has demonstrated a linear relationship between nitrogen balance and the intake of either energy or protein. Under the conditions used, neutral nitrogen balance appeared to occur at daily intakes of 11.6 kcal/cm of height and at 0.33 g protein per centimeter of height. In addition, the slope of the regression demonstrated a retention of 5.4 mg of nitrogen for each additional kilocalorie ingested. This retention is considerably greater than the 2–4 mg nitrogen per kilocalorie noted in normal adults receiving excess energy and marginal protein intakes (Garza *et al.*, 1976, 1977; Calloway, 1975), which is a diet more comparable to that usually given to uremic patients. Further examination of the children disclosed that 0.7 g nitrogen was retained for each additional gram of nitrogen ingested, suggesting that the highly efficient retention was related to previous nitrogen depletion. Nitrogen balance in the children was inversely related to net PCR, as previously noted in adults (Sargent *et al.*, 1978). However, the net PCR was not invariably related to either energy or protein intake, although at comparable intakes, net PCR was always lower in the patients in positive nitrogen balance.

The characteristics of the patients in positive nitrogen balance were revealing. The mean daily caloric intake of 12.1 kcal/cm of height was above

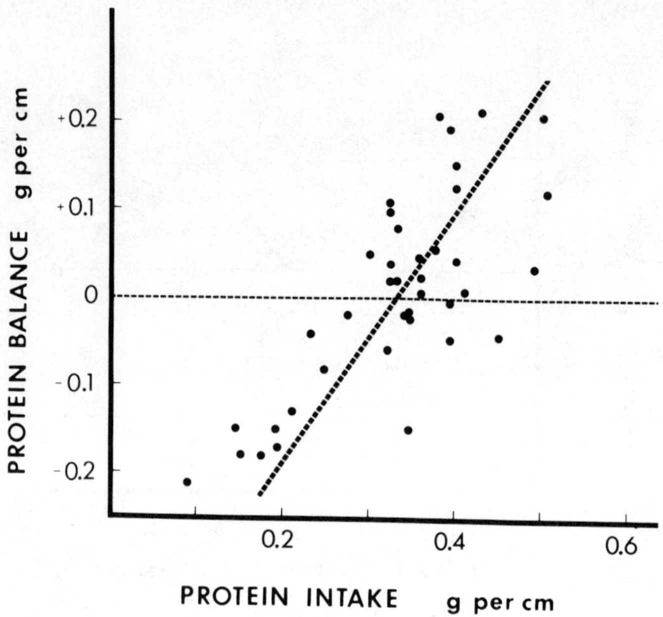

Figure 3. Protein balance as a function of daily protein intake in children on regular hemodialysis. Neutral protein balance occurs at a daily protein intake of 0.33 g/cm of height. The interrupted regression line ($r = 0.78$; $p < 0.005$) delineates a retention of 0.21 g protein per 0.3 g protein ingested.

the tenth percentile for statural age. The mean daily protein intake was 0.35 g/cm, and protein represented a normal mean for statural age of 12.4% of the total energy intake. This is higher than has been previously thought necessary (Holliday *et al.*, 1978; Chantler *et al.*, 1980; Broyer, 1974). Protein intakes as high as 0.51 g/cm per day and protein/energy ratios as high as 19.6% of total energy were well tolerated, with measurable positive nitrogen balance and acceptable levels of pre- and postdialysis blood urea and serum creatinine levels.

Other studies have used similar high protein-to-energy ratios in dialyzed and nondialyzed uremic children (Conley *et al.*, 1980; Betts *et al.*, 1977). In the Conley *et al.* (1980) study, the three patients whose protein flux was in the near-normal range had daily protein intakes above 0.4 g/cm and respective energy intakes of 8.2, 12.8, and 14.9 kcal/cm. Holliday and Chantler (1978) have reviewed the theoretical dietary protein-to-energy requirements for children with renal failure. They suggest that protein representing 6% of total energy probably will support body mass in the uremic child, if energy intake is adequate. However, the repair of malnutrition in these children may require that protein represent 8–10% of the total caloric intake. These studies imply that children with uremia probably require relatively normal protein-to-energy ratios and little, if any, protein restriction when energy levels are maintained in the 12-kcal/cm range.

Betts *et al.* (1977) studied 17 nondialyzed children with renal insufficiency. Their daily spontaneous intake averaged 14.2 kcal/cm and 0.37 g protein per centimeter with protein representing an average of 10.8% of the total energy. When these children were fed a carbohydrate supplement that contributed an average of 19% of their total caloric requirements, their total energy intake increased only 3%. Thus, the spontaneous ingestion of conventional foods declined, reducing their total protein intake by an average of 8% and their protein-to-energy ratio to only 8.6%. This raises the distinct prospect that energy supplements alone may actually be counterproductive to protein nutrition.

The implications of these studies for the nutritional management of children with renal insufficiency suggest that exogenous nitrogen, along with energy, should probably be maintained at higher levels than previously suggested (Holliday and Chantler, 1978; Chantler *et al.*, 1980; Holliday *et al.*, 1978). When caloric intake is above 12 kcal/cm per day and protein intake represents approximately 12% of the total energy intake, nitrogen balance is positive and protein turnover improved. The obvious aim would be to maintain exogenous protein intake at a level at which exogenous nitrogen excesses can be eliminated by either the remaining renal function and dialysis or incorporated into lean body mass. For some, this may require an earlier institution of dialysis than might occur if protein intake were severely restricted and urea generation reduced by excessive energy consumption. The evidence suggests that excess energy, relative to protein, is a less efficient way to promote nitrogen retention (Garza *et al.*, 1976) and likely to promote obesity rather than growth or replenishment of lean body mass (Elwyn *et al.*, 1979). In that light, and with the known anorexia that accompanies renal insufficiency (Grupe, 1981a; Spinozzi *et al.*, 1978), earlier institution of dialysis may have benefits for some patients if it facilitates adequate nutrition.

It remains to be determined whether positive nitrogen balance and improved protein synthesis are synonymous. It is questionable whether balance can be maintained sufficiently to stimulate growth. It is not known whether long-term nitrogen toxicity can be avoided. It is not clear whether the other abnormalities of protein metabolism can be alleviated. It is not evident to what degree the uremic child can adapt to changes in either energy or protein intake. What appears adequate by short-term analysis in the chronically depleted child may underestimate the long-term need in the repleted child. The importance previously placed on protein quality may not be valid (Hegsted, 1978), particularly in the presence of adequate protein intakes; nevertheless, appropriate data are not yet available.

The composition of the protein in the diet has received considerable attention. However, no study has shown that variations in the form or quality of the protein source have any advantage over an adequately designed conventional diet (Grupe, 1981b; Counahan *et al.*, 1978; Jones *et al.*, 1980; Hegsted, 1978). There is no question that children can utilize essential amino acids, complete-amino-acid mixtures, and keto acid analogues of amino acids effectively, but the effectiveness is not sustained and growth does not regularly ensue (Abitbol and Holliday, 1976; Counahan *et al.*, 1978; Jones *et al.*, 1980; Giordano *et al.*, 1978). Some evidence, using short-term changes in weight, suggests that complete amino acids are better utilized than keto acids in children (Giordano *et al.*, 1978; Giordano, 1980). Likewise, complete-amino-acid mixtures appear more beneficial than essential-amino-acid supplements (Holliday *et al.*, 1978; Motil *et al.*, 1980). The potential for enhanced toxicity and the absence of growth would suggest that low-protein diets supplemented with amino acids are of limited value in the treatment of uremic children (Alvestrand *et al.*, 1978; Motil *et al.*, 1980; Jones *et al.*, 1980; Counahan *et al.*, 1978).

However, if protein is allowed in the diet, the spontaneous intake approaches levels that are consistent with positive nitrogen balance (Spinozzi and Grupe, 1977) with the average intake approaching the ninetieth percentile for age (Grupe, 1981a; Betts and Magrath, 1974; Betts *et al.*, 1977). It is routinely difficult or impossible to persuade children to remain on prescribed low-protein intakes (Chantler *et al.*, 1980; Jones *et al.*, 1980; Betts *et al.*, 1977). Such diets have been successful only when spontaneous intake has been bypassed through nasogastric or parenteral feeding (Chantler *et al.*, 1980; Abitol and Holliday, 1976; Holliday *et al.*, 1978). Diets using conventional protein sources and protein-to-energy ratios closer to normal for age seem more palatable to the children and, therefore, more likely to maintain protein nutrition over the longer term (Betts *et al.*, 1977; Holliday and Chantler, 1978; Broyer, 1974).

Attempts to maintain adequate and appropriate protein nutrition remain reasonable. Recognizing the limitations of current quantitative techniques, the rates and the direction of change with dietary and dialytic manipulation may provide more rapid and more accurate definition of whether the management of the patient is offering any potential for long-term benefit.

References

Abitbol, C. L., and Holliday, M. A., 1976, Total parenteral nutrition in anuric children, *Clin. Nephrol.* **5:**153–158.

Abitbol, C. L., and Holliday, M. A., 1978, Effect of energy and nitrogen intake upon urea production in children with uremia and undernutrition, *Clin. Nephrol.* **10:**9–15.

Alvestrand, A., Bergström, J., Fürst, P., Germais, G., and Widstam, U., 1978, Effect of essential amino acid supplementation on muscle and plasma free amino acids in chronic uremia, *Kidney Int.* **14:**323–329.

Arnold, W. C., and Holliday, M. A., 1980, *In vitro* suppression of insulin-mediated amino acid uptake in uremic skeletal muscle, *Am. J. Clin. Nutr.* **33:**1428–1432.

Betts, P. R., and Magrath, G., 1974, Growth pattern and dietary intake of children with chronic renal insufficiency, *Br. Med. J.* **2:**189–193.

Betts, P. R., Magrath, G., and White, R. H. R., 1977, Role of dietary energy supplementation in growth of children with chronic renal insufficiency, *Br. Med. J.* **1:**416–418.

Broyer, M., 1974, Chronic renal failure, in: *Pediatric Nephrology* (P. Royer, R. Habib, H. Mathieu, M. Broyer, and A. Walsh, eds.), pp. 358–394, Saunders, Philadelphia.

Broyer, M., Jean, G., Dartois, A., and Kleinknecht, C., 1980, Plasma and muscle free amino acids in children at the early stages of renal failure, *Am. J. Clin. Nutr.* **33:**1396–1401.

Calloway, D. H., 1975, Nitrogen balance of men with marginal intakes of protein and energy, *J. Nutr.* **105:**914–923.

Chantler, C., ElBishti, M., and Counahan, R., 1980, Nutritional therapy in children with chronic renal failure, *Am. J. Clin. Nutr.* **33:**1682–1689.

Conley, S. B., Rose, G. M., Robson, A. M., and Bier, D. M., 1980, Effects of dietary intake and hemodialysis on protein turnover in uremic children, *Kidney Int.* **17:**837–846.

Counahan, R., ElBishti, M., Cox, B. D., Ogg, C. S., and Chantler, C., 1976, Plasma amino acids in children and adolescents on hemodialysis, *Kidney Int.* **10:**471–477.

Counahan, R., ElBishti, M., and Chantler, C., 1978, Oral essential amino acids in children on regular hemodialysis, *Clin. Nephrol.* **9:**11–14.

Delaporte, C., Bergstrom, J., and Broyer, M., 1976, Variations in muscle cell protein of severely uremic children, *Kidney Int.* **10:**239–245.

Delaporte, C., Geneviève, J., and Broyer, M., 1978, Free plasma and muscle amino acids in uremic children, *Am. J. Clin. Nutr.* **31:**1647–1651.

Elwyn, D. H., Gump, F. E., Munro, H. N., Iles, M., and Kinney, J. M., 1979, Changes in nitrogen balance of depleted patients with increasing infusions of glucose, *Am. J. Clin. Nutr.* **32:**1597–1611.

Flückiger, R., Harmon, W., Meier, W., Loo, S., and Gabbay, K. H., 1981, Hemoglobin carbamylation in uremia, *N. Engl. J. Med.* **304:**823–827.

Garber, A. J., 1978, Skeletal muscle protein and amino acid metabolism in experimental uremia in the rat. Accelerated alanine and glutamine formation and release, *J. Clin. Invest.* **62:**623–632.

Garza, C., Scrimshaw, N. S., and Young, V. R., 1976, Human protein requirements: The effect of variations in energy intake within the maintenance range, *Am. J. Clin. Nutr.* **29:**280–287.

Garza, C., Scrimshaw, N. S., and Young, V. R., 1977, Human protein requirements: Evaluation of the 1973 FAO/WHO safe level of protein intake for young men at high energy intakes, *Br. J. Nutr.* **37:**403–420.

Giordano, C., 1980, Amino acids and ketoacids—advantages and pitfalls, *Am. J. Clin. Nutr.* **33:**1649–1653.

Giordano, C., DePascale, C., DeSanto, N. G., Esposito, R., Cirillo, D., and Standherlin, P., 1970, Disorder in the metabolism of some amino acids in uremia, in: *Proceedings of the IVth International Congress of Nephrology*, pp. 296–302, Karger, Basel.

Giordano, C., DeSanto, N. G., DiToro, R., Pluvio, M., and Perrone, L., 1978, The imbalance effect of amino acid and keto acid diet for growth of the uremic infant, in: *Proceedings of the VIIth International Congress of Nephrology*, pp. 477–482, Karger, Basel.

Grupe, W. E., 1981a, Nutritional considerations in the prognosis and treatment of children with renal disease, in: *Textbook of Pediatric Nutrition* (R. A. Suskind, ed.), pp. 527–536, Raven Press, New York.

Grupe, W. E., 1981b, Perinatal nutrition related to renal function, in: *Gastroenterology and Nutrition in Infancy* (E. Lebenthal, ed.), pp. 837–852, Raven Press, New York.

Harmon, W. E., Spinozzi, N. S., Sargent, J. R., and Grupe, W. E., 1979, Determination of protein catabolic rate (PCR) in children on hemodialysis by urea kinetic modeling, *Pediatr. Res.* **13:**513.

Harmon, W. E., Spinozzi, N. S., Meyer, A., and Grupe, W. E., 1981, The use of protein catabolic rate to monitor pediatric hemodialysis, *Dial. Transpl.* **10:**324–330.

Hegsted, D. M., 1978, Assessment of nitrogen requirements, *Am. J. Clin. Nutr.* **31:**1669–1677.

Holliday, M. A., and Chantler, C., 1978, Metabolic and nutritional factors in children with renal insufficiency, *Kidney Int.* **14:**306–312.

Holliday, M. A., Chantler, C., MacDonnell, R., and Keitges, J., 1977, Effect of uremia on nutritionally induced variations in protein metabolism, *Kidney Int.* **11:**236–245.

Holliday, M. A., Wassner, S., and Ramirez, J., 1978, Intravenous nutrition in uremic children with protein-energy malnutrition, *Am. J. Clin. Nutr.* **31:**1854–1860.

Inoue, G., Fugita, Y., Kishi, K., Yamamoto, S., and Niiyama, Y., 1974. Nutritive value of egg protein and wheat gluten in young men, *Nutr. Rep. Intern.* **10:**201–207.

Jones, R. W. A., Dalton, N., Start, K., ElBishti, M. M., and Chantler, C., 1980, Oral essential amino acid supplements in children with advanced chronic renal failure, *Am. J. Clin. Nutr.* **33:**1696–1702.

Keys, A. J., Andersen, J. T., and Brozek, J., 1955, Weight gain from simple overeating. I. Character of tissue gained, *Metabolism* **4:**427–432.

Kopple, J. D., 1978, Abnormal amino acid and protein metabolism in uremia, *Kidney Int.* **14:**340–348

Motil, K. J., Harmon, W. E., and Grupe, W. E., 1980, Complications of essential amino acid hyperalimentation in children with acute renal failure, *J. Parent. Enteral. Nutr.* **4:**32–35.

Munro, H. N., 1964, General aspects of the regulation of protein metabolism by diet and by hormones, in: *Mammalian Protein Metabolism* (H. N. Munro and J. B. Allison, eds.), pp. 381–481, Academic Press, New York.

Munro, H. N., 1978, Energy and protein intakes as determinants of nitrogen balance, *Kidney Int.* **14:**313–316.

Olson, R. E., 1975, The effect of variations in protein and calorie intake upon rate of recovery and selected physiologic response in Thai children with PCM, in: *Protein–Calorie Malnutrition* (R. E. Olson, ed.), p. 275, Academic Press, New York.

Sargent, J., Gotch, F., Borah, M., Piercy, L., Spinozzi, N., Schoenfeld, P., and Humphreys, M., 1978, Urea kinetics: A guide to nutritional management of renal failure, *Am. J. Clin. Nutr.* **31:**1696–1702.

Spinozzi, N. S., and Grupe, W. E., 1977, Nutritional implications of renal disease, *J. Am. Diet. Assoc.* **70:**493–497.

Spinozzi, N. S., Murray, C. L., and Grupe, W. E., 1978, Altered taste acuity in children with end-stage renal disease (ESRD), *Pediatr. Res.* **12:**442.

Young, G. A., and Parsons, F. M., 1973, Impairment of phenylalanine hydroxylation in chronic renal insufficiency, *Clin. Sci. Mol. Med.* **45:**89–97.

32

Renal Osteodystrophy in Children

Russell W. Chesney

The association between renal insufficiency and bone disease has been recognized for more than 100 years since Lucas, in 1883, described anemia, dwarfism, and "late form of rickets" in children with chronic renal failure.[1] Although the term *renal rickets* has been used to describe this bone disorder, the clinical and histologic differences between vitamin D deficiency and juvenile renal osteodystrophy are sizable. Advanced osteodystrophy consists of bone pain, metaphyseal fractures, osteitis fibrosa cystica, delayed bone age, linear growth failure, severe bowing, and slipped epiphyses.[2] Mehls *et al.*[3] have made the point that childhood uremic bone disease has a unique epiphyseal lesion, largely related to secondary hyperparathyroidism, that is histologically distinct from D deficiency and which accounts for the widened growth plate and for retardation in bone age (Fig. 1). Childhood uremic osteodystrophy has certain real differences from adult renal bone disease (Table 1) that are often dramatically highlighted.[3–5]

The same pathogenic sequence probably accounts for bone disease in children as well as in adults. With the reduction in nephron mass, both phosphate (PO_4) retention and reduced 1,25-dihydroxyvitamin D synthesis occur, and this leads to intestinal calcium malabsorption and secondary hyperparathyroidism.[6–7] With the decline in glomerular filtration rate and, presumably, in functional nephron mass, progressive parathyroid hormone (PTH) gland hyperplasia and PTH secretion ensue, solubilizing the mineral portion of bone. An added feature in childhood is that uremia *per se*, as well as inadequate dietary intake, particularly of protein, results in a reduction in the usually high bone turnover and remodeling rate of bone in childhood, the extent of which is difficult to assess.

The discovery during the past decade that the kidney is the site for the production of two important vitamin D metabolites—namely, 1,25-dihy-

Russell W. Chesney • Department of Pediatrics, University of Wisconsin Center for the Health Sciences, Madison, Wisconsin 53792.

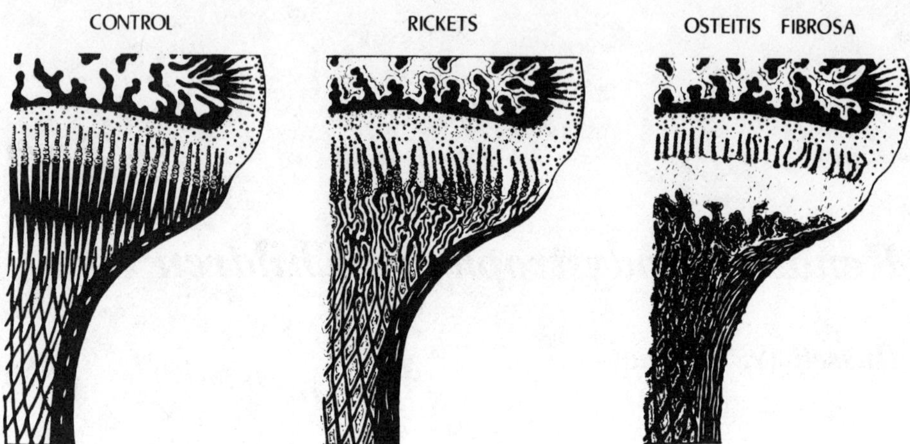

Figure 1. The growth zone in bone from a normal child, a rachitic child, and a child with osteitis fibrosa. In the normal child, the zone of provisional calcification mineralizes normally to ultimately form bone trabeculae. In the rachitic child, mineralization in the zone of provisional calcification is delayed, leading to a broad zone of poorly ossified chondroosteoid. In osteitis fibrosa, the growth cartilage is narrow and the longitudinal orientation of trabeculae is lost. (Reprinted from ref. 3, with permission.)

droxyvitamin D and 24,25-dihydroxyvitamin D [24,25$(OH)_2$D][10,11]—helps to explain the apparent resistance of uremic subjects to the biologic actions of vitamin D given in usual doses.[12] Early studies demonstrated the biologic potency of 1,25-dihydroxyvitamin D (calcitriol) in blunting iPTH secretion and in overcoming the classical features of vitamin D resistance—intestinal malabsorption and hypocalcemia.[13,14] 1,25-$(OH)_2$-vitamin D appears to be the hormonally active form of vitamin D which is both feedback inhibited and accounts for most of the biologic effects of vitamin D—increased gut calcium and phosphate absorption and increased bone resorption to maintain normal plasma calcium levels.[11] 1,25-$(OH)_2$ vitamin D does not directly

Table 1. Distinctive Features of Osteodystrophy in Childhood

Bone turnover and remodeling rates are higher in children than in adults.
Radiologic abnormalities are more common.
Slipped epiphyses and sharp angulation of bones are seen.
Renal hypoplasia/dysplasia or congenital obstructive uropathy develops *in utero,* contributing to lifelong renal disease.
Tubulointerstitial disease is more common, which may impair 1,25$(OH)_2$-vitamin D synthesis.
Bone linear growth requires adequate supply of calcium and phosphate.
Bone growth and maturation are impaired.
Chronic acidosis is often related to reduced renal tubular bicarbonate reabsorption.
Vascular and extraosseous calcification is seldom seen despite abnormal calcium × phosphate solubility product.

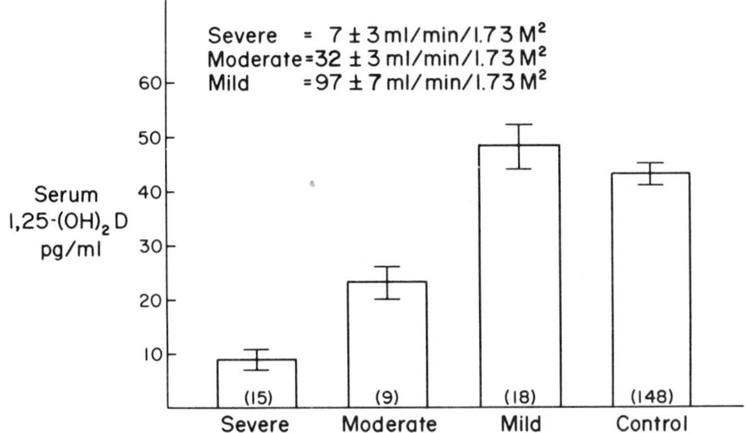

Figure 2. Shown are the serum 1,25-dihydroxyvitamin D levels in patients with severe, moderate, and mild renal failure and in control subjects.

mineralize bone, and, possibly, 24,25$(OH)_2$D or 25-hydroxyvitamin D [25(OH)D] is more active in promoting skeletal mineralization.[15,16]

The aims of this chapter are to review the evidence that childhood uremia is a 1,25-$(OH)_2$-vitamin D-deficient state, to discuss a rational therapeutic approach to childhood osteodystrophy, and to comment briefly on the controversy as to whether or not treatment with vitamin D analogues will result in a decline in renal function in nondialyzed patients with stable renal function.

Indirect indicators of abnormal vitamin D metabolism are the high incidence of elevated iPTH concentrations in sera and the abnormalities of bone evident on biopsy and histomorphometric analysis.[3,5,17] Norman *et al.*[5] in an analysis of 29 patients, provide evidence that at clearances below 45 ml/min per 1.73 m^2 iPTH is elevated and abnormal bone histology is evident, whereas abnormalities of serum chemical values or radiological appearance occur only at very low clearance values. Mehls *et al.*[3] point out that children with congenital renal diseases tend to have more severe growth retardation since their renal impairment began *in utero,* and that dietary calcium intake is often inadequate in these children. Reduced calcium intake only enhanced negative calcium balance and augments iPTH secretion. Using the technique of photon absorptiometry, Chesney *et al.*[18] have also demonstrated that children with congenital tubulointerstitial disease have a higher rate of bone undermineralization than children with other renal disorders. Demineralization in these children was correlated with higher serum creatinine levels and decreased creatinine clearance values.

Both Portale *et al.*[8] and Chesney *et al.*[9] have directly examined the circulating values of vitamin D metabolites in children with renal disease using the precise assay of Shepard *et al.*[19] Shown in Fig. 2 are the

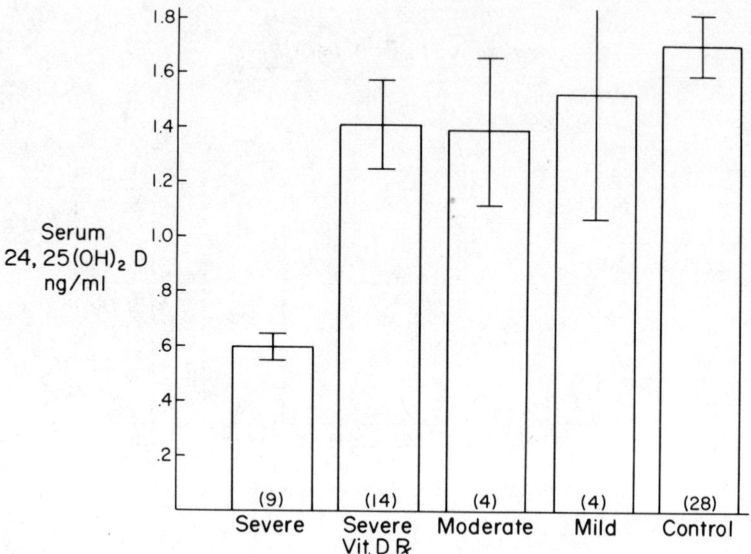

Figure 3. Serum 24,25-dihydroxyvitamin D levels in patients with severe, moderate, and mild renal failure and in control patients. Also shown are the values in patients with severe renal failure, treated wtih ergocalciferol at 10–50,000 units/day.

concentrations of 1,25-$(OH)_2$-vitamin D at various clearance values; no decline in 1,25-$(OH)_2$-vitamin D concentration is evident until clearance values fall below 48 ml/min per 1.73 m^2. In the Chesney study, almost all patients with a decreased 1,25-$(OH)_2$-vitamin D level had tubulointerstitial disease, usually on a congenital or hereditary basis. A direct relationship between creatinine clearance and serum 1,25-$(OH)_2$-vitamin D concentration was found (r + 0.683, $p < 0.001$). The study of Portale *et al.*[(8)] yielded comparable results.

In Chesney's study,[(9)] the serum values for 25(OH)-vitamin D did not vary with degree of renal failure, and no single value below 16 ng/ml was found. The only elevations of 25(OH)-vitamin D were in those patients with prior ergocalciferol (vitamin D_2) therapy where the concentrations of 25(OH)-vitamin D rose to a level of 176 ng/ml—6 times higher than the normal level of 30 ± 10 ng/ml (S.D.).

The circulating levels of 24,25$(OH)_2$-vitamin D are shown in Fig. 3, and only in severely affected patients are the concentrations of 24,25$(OH)_2$-vitamin D reduced to values significantly below control values—0.6 ± 1.4 ng/ml (S.D.) vs. 1.70 ± 0.47 ng/ml, $p < 0.01$. Prior ergocalciferol treatment was associated with a higher 24,25$(OH)_2$-vitamin D level of 1.41 ± 0.36 ng/ml, despite a marked reduction in clearance in these patients. A direct correlation was found between 1,25$(OH)_2$-vitamin D levels in sera and those of 24,25$(OH)_2$-vitamin D, $r = 0.668$, $p < 0.001$.[(9)] As in Norman's[(5)] study, hypocalcemia, hyperphosphatemia, and increased alkaline phosphatase activity were found only in patients with clearance values of less than 13 ml/

min per 1.73 m^2. Accordingly, there is evidence of reduced circulating levels of 1,25$(OH)_2$-vitamin D and 24,25$(OH)_2$-vitamin D in childhood renal failure.

The treatment of uremic bone disease in childhood is rather complex.[4] First, it is evident from childhood growth charts that children grow most during the first 24 months of life, and this is a critical period for optimizing care. Chantler *et al.*[20] have reviewed the evidence that children, and especially younger children, require more calories and greater protein intake than adults in order to maintain any growth. Again, the child with congenital obstructive uropathy, renal dysplasia, or hypoplasia is at the greatest risk for poor nutrition and subnormal protein synthesis.

Second, chronic metabolic acidosis also can contribute to bone demineralization and hypercalciuria, particularly if the calcium carbonate, which comprises 10% of bone mineral calcium content, is used as a buffer of excessive extracellular protons.[21,22] Again, the child with congenital tubular disease is at greatest risk for developing renal tubular acidosis and excessive bicarbonaturia.[23] Therapy should include correction of acidosis with sodium bicarbonate or some anion that liberates bicarbonate. Since uremic subjects require increased oral calcium intake, it is convenient to provide bicarbonate as calcium lactate or carbonate.

Third, although 1,25$(OH)_2$-vitamin D and possibly pharmacologic doses of 25(OH)-vitamin D regulate the active transport of calcium by the upper intestine, the passive transport of calcium by lower intestinal segments is directly dependent on the intake of this divalent cation.[24] Studies 60 years ago demonstrated the value of increased calcium intake in uremic children in terms of calcium balance.[25] Phosphate intake must be limited either by decreased dietary phosphate or by the use of phosphate-binding agents. Obviously, phosphate restriction is not indicated in those tubular disorders where renal phosphaturia is common.[26] It should also be recalled that severe phosphate restriction may result in osteomalacia,[27,28] and that the circulating concentrations of phosphate during childhood are higher than those found in adults—5.8 $\pm$ 0.2 mg/dl vs. 3.6 $\pm$ 0.2 mg/dl in one series.[29]

The cautious use of vitamin D compounds is indicated to augment intestinal calcium absorption, suppress iPTH secretion, and, hopefully, improve skeletal mineralization. Currently, four "active" vitamin D compounds are in use: dihydrotachysterol (DHT), 25(OH)-vitamin D, 1,25$(OH)_2$-vitamin D, and its synthetic cousin 1α-hydroxyvitamin D or "1-alpha." It has been known since 1943 that rather small doses of DHT could improve intestinal calcium absorption.[30]

The newer 1α-hydroxylated vitamin D compounds have been employed in several childhood studies.[14,31–37] Findings have included increased serum calcium levels, suppression of PTH secretion, a reduction in alkaline phosphatase activity, and relief of bone pain. Dramatic improvement in the myopathy of uremia and in gait disturbances has been noted.

Chesney *et al.*[4,34,37] have employed a dose of 10–15 ng/kg per day, given as a daily divided dose if possible, and this appears to achieve plasma levels of 1,25$(OH)_2$-vitamin D that are in the normal range when examined

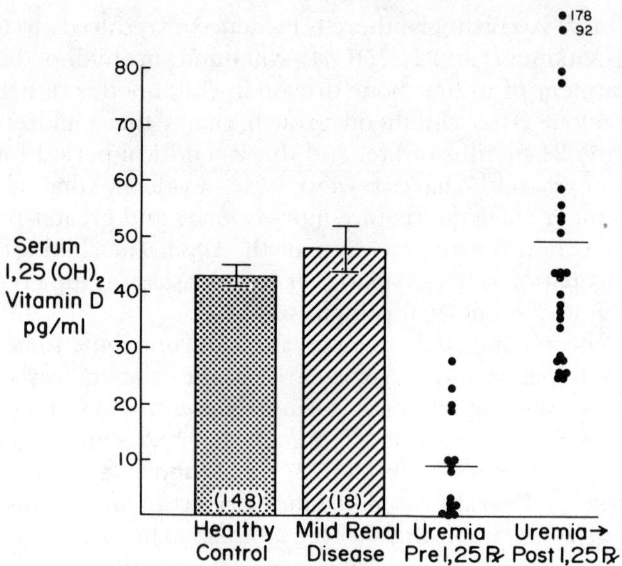

Figure 4. The serum concentrations of 1,25-dihydroxyvitamin D in controlled subjects and in patients with renal failure and creatinine clearances between 75 and 150 ml/min per 1.73 m^2. To the right are shown the 1,25-dihydroxyvitamin D levels in patients with clearances below 13 ml/min per 1.73 m^2 before and after treatment with calcitriol at 10 to 15 ng/kg per day.

4 hr after a dose (Fig. 4). The half-life of these 1α-hydroxy metabolites in plasma is a few hours, so that a level taken at 4 hr will represent the peak plasma value achieved.[38] The biologic half-life of 1,25(OH)$_2$-vitamin D is a few days,[7] so that hypercalcemia can be rapidly reversed by discontinuing the agent or lowering the agent for a few days. This short half-life is an advantage of these compounds, but it can also pose a problem in poorly compliant patients. The child who is given his medicines infrequently may have long periods of relative D deficiency that can be avoided using compounds with a longer half-life.

The serum 1,25(OH)$_2$-vitamin D values achieved will suppress iPTH secretion by raising serum calcium level.[11] We have used the PTH-to-1,25(OH)$_2$-vitamin D ratio in order to evaluate the effect of therapy in a dynamic fashion (Fig. 5). C-terminal or intact PTH molecule antibody assays do not accurately measure gland secretion, since the reduced renal mass leads to decreased degradation of the carboxy portion of the molecule.[39] By examining the ratio iPTH to 1,25(OH)$_2$D, it can be seen that therapy causes a 90% fall in this ratio, but that the ratio is still higher than that found in healthy control subjects, $p < 0.001$. Further, an examination of this ratio reveals that 1,25(OH)$_2$-vitamin D production by the diseased kidney is inappropriately reduced for the circulating PTH level.

We had noted improved growth velocity in children receiving 1,25(OH)$_2$-vitamin D over a period of 12–24 months.[34] When a group of 10 children

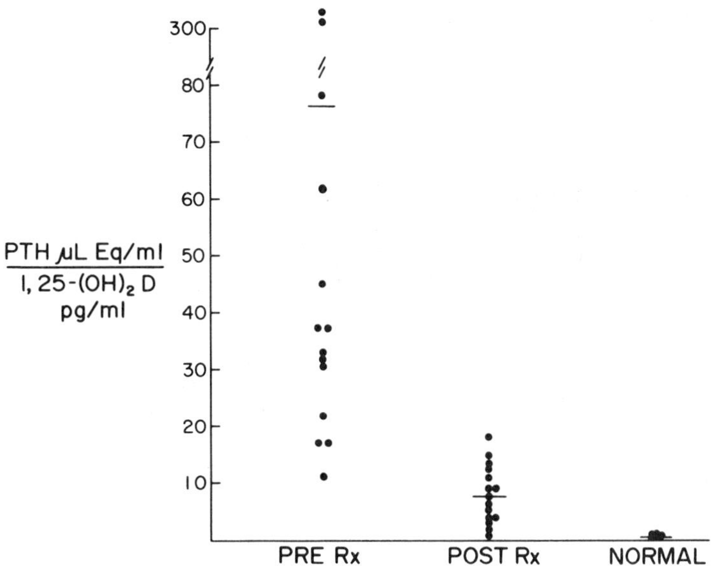

Figure 5. The ratio of PTH to 1,25-dihydroxyvitamin D in patients with creatinine clearances below 13 ml/min per 1.73 m^2 before initiation of treatment with calcitriol and after calcitriol therapy. Also shown by comparison is the ratio in normal subjects.

was followed for periods up to 51 months, the mean height velocity increased from 4.2 ± 1.1 cm/year (SE) while receiving vitamin D_2 or DHT to 7.2 ± 0.9 cm/year on $1,25(OH)_2$-vitamin D, $p < 0.001$.[37] These data indicate that long-term growth patterns parallel the usual growth percentile lines from growth charts. When length is expressed as standard deviation from control mean for chronologic age (Fig. 6), one can see that there is a marked decline in height during the initial period of observation (at least 12 months) while patients are receiving vitamin D_2 or DHT, and that $1,25(OH)_2$-vitamin D therapy will improve, but not completely reverse, this trend. Several recent studies have shown that children on chronic dialysis therapy do not have an increase in height velocity after starting $1,25(OH)_2$-vitamin D.[40] The reasons for this latter observation are unclear.

25-Hydroxyvitamin D has proven efficacious in two childhood studies. Witmer *et al.*[41] found this agent to be superior to vitamin D_2 in terms of healing osteomalacia and osteitis fibrosa cystica and in correcting hypocalcemia. Baron *et al.*[42] described a correction of hypocalcemia and a decline in alkaline phosphatase activity and PTH level. Histomorphometric analysis of bone showed improvement in the abnormal osteoblastic surface and in osteoid volume measurements after 2 years of therapy. Hypercalcemia was infrequent at a dose of 1.6 μg/kg per day.

Recent evidence suggests that 1α-hydroxyvitamin D or $1,25(OH)_2$-vitamin D therapy may result in a decline in creatinine clearance in nondialyzed subjects with uremia associated with hypercalcuria.[43–45] By contrast,

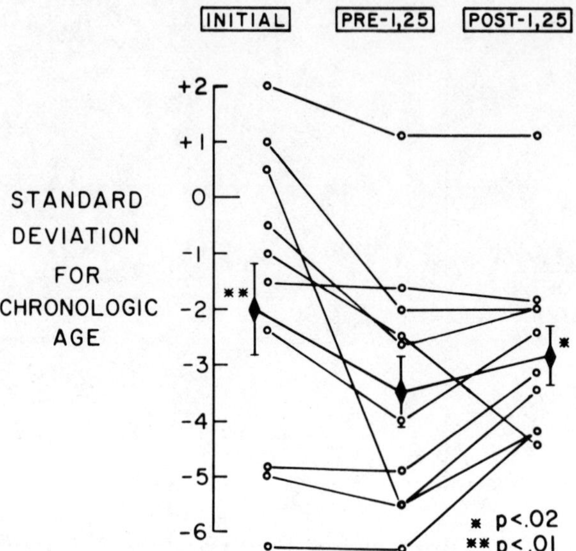

Figure 6. Changes in growth after calcitriol therapy, expressed as standard deviation for chronologic age; ♦ indicates mean ± S.E.

Healy *et al.*[46] found no change in creatinine clearance in patients treated with lower doses of 1,25$(OH)_2$-vitamin D and who did not develop hypercalcuria. Chesney *et al.*[4] found no change in the slope of the rise in serum creatinine with time during observation for 24 months before and up to 51 months after 1,25$(OH)_2$-vitamin D therapy (Fig. 7). Urinary calcium excretion

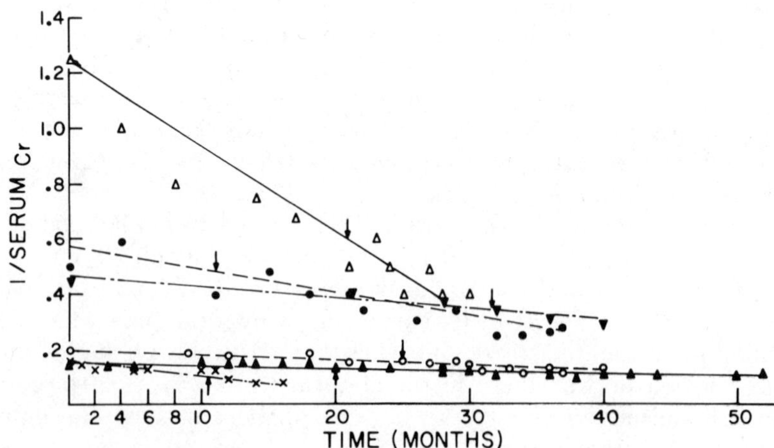

Figure 7. The ratio of 1/serum creatinine versus time in patients treated with calcitriol. The arrow on each line denotes the initiation of calcitriol therapy. Note that there is no break in the slope of the line after calcitriol therapy.

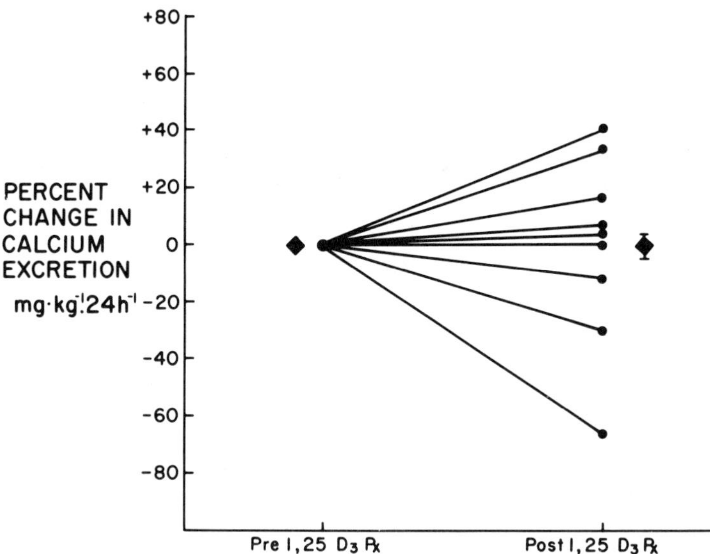

Figure 8. Change in calcium excretion expressed as a percent before and after therapy with calcitriol; ♦ indicates mean ± S.E.

did not change in these patients (Fig. 8). Lund *et al.*[47] and Nordin[48] have made the point that treatment with any vitamin D analogue can result in a fall in GFR if the patient becomes hypercalcemia. Obviously, it is imperative to prevent patients from becoming hyperphosphatemic as well so as to avoid calcium phosphate deposition in the tubules.[49] A well-designed controlled study of the prophylactic efficacy of 1,25$(OH)_2$-vitamin D therapy in patients with moderate reduction is indicated to establish whether this agent is beneficial in preventing osteodystrophy or harmful in terms of renal function.

References

1. Lucas, R. C., 1883, On a form of late rickets associated with albuminuria, rickets of adolescents, *Lancet* **1:**993.
2. Avioli, L. V., and Teitelbaum, S. L., 1978, Renal osteodystrophy, in: *Pediatric Kidney Disease* (C. M. Edelmann Jr., ed.), pp. 366–401, Little, Brown, Boston.
3. Mehls, O., Ritz, E., Kreusser, W., and Krempien, B., 1980, Renal osteodystrophy in uraemic children, *Clin. Endocrinol. Metab.* **9:**151–176.
4. Chesney, R. W., 1983, Treatment of calcium and phosphorus abnormalities in childhood renal osteodystrophy, *Dialy. Transpl.* **12:**270–279.
5. Norman, M. E., Mazur, A. T., Borden, S., Gruskin, A., Anast, C., Baron, R., and Rasmussen, H., 1980, Early diagnosis of juvenile renal osteodystrophy, *J. Pediatr.* **97:**226–232.
6. Slatopolsky, E., Gray, R., Adams, N. D., and Lemann, J., 1978, Low serum levels of 1,25$(OH)_2D_3$ are not responsible for the development of secondary hyperparathyroidism in early renal failure, *Kidney Int.* **14:**733.
7. Coburn, J. W., and Massry, S. G., 1980, Uses and actions of 1,25-dihydroxyvitamin D_3 in uremia, *Contrib. Nephrol.* **18:**1–245.

8. Portale, A. A., Booth, B. E., Tsai, H. C., and Morris, R. C. Jr., 1982, Reduced plasma concentration of $1,25(OH)_2D$ in children with moderate renal insufficiency, *Kidney Int.* **21:**627–632.
9. Chesney, R. W., Hamstra, A. J., Mazess, R. B., Rose, P., and DeLuca, H. F., 1982, Circulating vitamin D metabolite concentrations in childhood renal diseases: Relationship to varying degrees of renal failure, *Kidney Int.* **21:**65–69.
10. Fraser, D. R., and Kodicek, E., 1970, Unique biosynthesis by kidney of a biologically active vitamin D metabolite, *Nature* **228:**764–766.
11. DeLuca, H. F., 1979, The vitamin D system in the regulation of calcium and phosphorus metabolism, W. O. Atwater Memorial Lecture, *Nutr. Rev.* **37:**161–193.
12. Lumb, G. A., Mawer, E. B., and Stanbury, S. W., 1971, The apparent vitamin D resistance of chronic renal failure: A study of the physiology of vitamin D in man, *Am. J. Med.* **50:**421.
13. Brickman, A. S., Coburn, J. W., and Norman, A. W., 1972, Effect of 1,25-dihydroxycholecalciferol in uremic man, *N. Engl. J. Med.* **287:**891–895.
14. Henderson, R. G., Russell, R. G. G., Ledinghan, J. G. G., Smith, R., Oliver, D. O., Walton, R. J., Small, D. G., Preston, C., Warner, G. T., and Norman, A. W., 1974, Effects of 1,25-dihydroxycholecalciferol on calcium absorption, muscle weakness and bone disease in chronic renal failure, *Lancet* **1:**279–384.
15. Bordier, P., Zingraff, J., Gueris, J., Jungers, P., Marie, P., Pechet, M., and Rasmussen, H., 1978, The effect of $1\alpha(OH)D_3$ and $1,25(OH)_2D_3$ on the bone in patients with renal osteodystrophy, *Am. J. Med.* **64:**101–107.
16. Rasmussen, H., and Bordier, P., 1980, Evidence that different vitamin D sterols have qualitatively different effects in man, *Contr. Nephrol.* **18:**184–191.
17. Roof, B. S., Piel, C. F., and Rames, L., 1974, Parathyroid function in uremic children with and without osteodystrophy, *Pediatrics* **53:**404.
18. Chesney, R. W., Mazess, R. B., Rose, P., and Jax, D. K., 1977, Bone mineral status measured by direct photon absorptiometry in childhood renal disease, *Pediatrics* **60:**864–872.
19. Shepard, R. M., Horst, R. L., Hamstra, A. J., and DeLuca, H. F., 1979, Determination of vitamin D and its metabolites in plasma from normal and anaphric man, *Biochem. J.* **182:**55–69.
20. Chantler, C., El Bishti, M., and Counahan, R., 1980, Nutritional therapy in children with chronic renal failure, *Am. J. Clin. Nutr.* **33:**1682–1689.
21. West, C. D., and Smith, W. C., 1956, An attempt to elucidate the cause of growth retardation in renal disease, *Am. J. Dis. Child.* **91:**460.
22. Cooke, R. E., and Kleeman, C. R., 1950, Distal tubular dysfunction with renal calcification, *Yale J. Biol. Med.* **23:**199.
23. Gur, A., Siegel, N. J., Davis, C. A., Kashgarian, M., and Hayslett, J. P., 1975, Clinical aspects of bilateral renal dysplasia in children, *Nephron* **15:**50–61.
24. Coburn, J. W., Hartenbower, D. L., and Massry, S. G., 1973, Intestinal absorption of calcium and the effect of renal insufficiency, *Kidney Int.* **4:**96.
25. Boyd, G. L., Courtney, A. M., and MacLachlan, I. F., 1923, The metabolism of salts in nephritis: I. Calcium and phosphorus, *Am. J. Dis. Child.* **32:**29–39.
26. Chesney, R. W., 1981, Etiology and pathogenesis of the Fanconi syndrome, *Mineral Electrolyte Metab.* **4:**303–316.
27. Dent, C. E., and Winter, C. S., 1974, Osteomalacia due to phosphate depletion from excessive aluminum hydroxide ingestion, *Br. Med. J.* **1:**551.
28. Chesney, R. W., 1980, Tubular defects in phosphate reabsorption in clinical medicine, in: *Renal Handling of Phosphate* (S. G. Massry and H. Fleisch, eds.), pp. 321–365, Plenum Press, New York.
29. Harrison, H. E., and Harrison, H. C., 1979, *Disorders of Calcium and Phosphate Metabolism in Childhood and Adolescence*, pp. 181–193, Saunders, Philadelphia.
30. Liu, S. H., and Chu, H. I., 1943, Studies of calcium and phosphorus metabolism with special reference to pathogenesis and effect of dihydrotachysterol (A.T. 10), *Medicine (Baltimore)* **22:**103–132.

31. Chan, J. C. M., Oldham, S. B., Holick, M. F., and DeLuca, H. F., 1975, 1α-hydroxyvitamin D_3 in chronic renal failure: A potent analog of the kidney hormone, 1,25-dihydroxycholecalciferol, *JAMA* **234:**47–52.
32. Pierides, A. M., Ellis, H. A., Dellagrammatikas, H., Scott, J. E., and Norman, A. W., 1977, 1,25-Dihydroxycholecalciferol in renal osteodystrophy: Epiphysiolysis anticonvulsant therapy, *Arch. Dis. Child.* **52:**464–472, 1977.
33. Postlewaithe, R. J., and Houston, I. B., 1977, 1α-Hydroxycholecalciferol in children with renal osteodystrophy, *Calcif. Tissue Res.* **22**(suppl):371–375.
34. Chesney, R. W., Moorthy, A. V., Jax, D. K., Eisman, J. A., Mazess, R. B., and DeLuca, H. F., 1978, Increased linear growth after long-term oral $1,25(OH)_2$-vitamin D therapy in childhood renal osteodystrophy, *N. Engl. J. Med.* **298:**238–242.
35. Balsan, S., Garabedian, M., and Sorgniard, R., 1975, 1,25-Dihydroxyvitamin D_3 and 1α-hydroxyvitamin D_3 in children: Biologic and therapeutic effects of nutritional rickets and different types of vitamin D resistance, *Pediatr. Res.* **9:**586.
36. Chan, J. C. M., and DeLuca, H. F., 1977, Growth velocity in a child on prolonged hemodialysis: Beneficial effect of 1α-hydroxyvitamin D_3, *JAMA* **238:**2053.
37. Chesney, R. W., Mazess, R. B., and DeLuca, H. F., 1980, The long-term influence of calcitriol on growth patterns in childhood renal osteodystrophy, in: *A Clinical Review of Calcitriol* (J. W. Coburn, ed.), pp. 17–28, Excerpta Medica, Princeton, New Jersey.
38. Mason, R. S., Lissner, D., Posen, S., and Norman, A. W., 1980, Blood concentrations of dihydroxyvitamin D metabolites after an oral dose, *Br. Med. J.* **1:**449.
39. Freitag, J., Martin, K. J., and Hruska, K. A., 1978, Impaired parathyroid hormone metabolism in people with chronic renal failure, *N. Engl. J. Med.* **298:**29.
40. Bulla, M., Delling, G., Offermann, G., and Ziegler, R., 1980, Renal osteodystrophy in children: Therapy with vitamin D_3 or 1,25-dihydroxycholecalciferol, *Pediatr. Res.* **14:**990.
41. Witmer, G., Margolis, A., Fontaine, O., Fritsch, J., Lenoir, G., Droyer, M., and Balsan, S., 1976, Effects of 25-hydroxycholecalciferol on bone lesions of children with terminal renal failure, *Kidney Int.* **10:**395–408.
42. Baron, R., Norman, M., Mazur, A., Gruskin, A., and Rasmussen, H., 1979, Bone histomorphometry in children with early chronic renal failure treated with $25(OH)D_3$, in: *Vitamin D: Basic Research and Its Clinical Applications* (A. W. Norman, K. Schaefer, and D. V. Herrath, eds.), pp. 847–852, de Gruyter, Berlin.
43. Christiansen, C., Rodbro, P., and Christensen, M. S., 1978, Deterioration of renal function during treatment of chronic renal failure with 1,25-dihydroxycholecalciferol, *Lancet* **2:**700–702.
44. Christiansen, C., Christensen, M. S., and Rodbro, P., 1981, Calcitriol and renal function, *JAMA* **245:**463–464.
45. Winterbourne, M. H., Mace, P. T., Heath, D. A., and White, R. H. R., 1978, Impairment of renal function in patients on 1α-hydroxycholecalciferol, *Lancet* **2:**150–151.
46. Healy, M. D., Malluche, H. H., Goldstein, D. A., Singer, F. R. and Massry, S. G., 1980, Effects of long-term therapy with $1,25(OH)_2D_3$ in patients with moderate renal failure, *Arch. Intern. Med.* **140:**1030–1033.
47. Lund, B., Sorensen, O. H., and Lund, B., 1978, 1α-hydroxycholecalciferol and renal function, *Lancet* **2:**731.
48. Nordin, B. E. C., 1978, Vitamin D analogs and renal function, *Lancet* **2:**1259.
49. Massry, S. G., and Goldstein, D. A., 1979, Is calcitriol ($1,25(OH)_2D_3$) harmful to renal function?, *JAMA* **242:**1875–1876.

33

Renal Transplantation in Children Aged 1–5 Years

Review of the University of Minnesota Experience

S. Michael Mauer, Robert L. Vernier, Thomas E. Nevins, Jon I. Scheinman, David S. Fryd, and John S. Najarian

1. Introduction

The chapters of Dr. T. M. Barratt and colleagues (Chapter 36) and Dr. M. Broyer *et al.* (Chapter 35) in this book admirably set the background for the presentation of our experience in the transplantation of children age 5 years and under. In this chapter we will compare our experience with that of Barratt and Broyer to support our view that renal transplantation is feasible and is the preferred therapy for end-stage renal failure in the young child.

The causes of chronic renal failure (CRF) in our population of young children are similar to those described at other centers (Table 1). The notably different lesions causing CRF in this population, as compared to older children and adults, include hypoplasia–dysplasia, obstructive uropathy (38%), and congenital nephrotic syndrome (29%). Since these disorders do not recur in the transplanted kidney, one of the concerns commonly faced after transplantation in older children and adults is obviated.

Dr. Barratt emphasized the difficulty of achieving acceptable growth in young children with CRF, despite aggressive efforts to provide optimal

S. Michael Mauer • Department of Pediatric Nephrology, University of Minnesota Health Sciences Center, Minneapolis, Minnesota 55455. ***Robert L. Vernier and Thomas E. Nevins*** • Department of Pediatrics, University of Minnesota Health Sciences Center, Minneapolis, Minnesota 55455. ***Jon I. Scheinman*** • Department of Pediatric Nephrology, Duke University Medical Center, Durham, North Carolina 27710. ***David S. Fryd and John S. Najarian*** • Department of Surgery, University of Minnesota Health Sciences Center, Minneapolis, Minnesota 55455.

Table 1. Causes of Renal Disease in 42 Transplanted Children Aged 1–5 Years

Hypoplastic–dysplastic kidneys	16
Congenital nephrotic syndrome	12
Oxalosis	2
Hemolytic uremic syndrome	2
Infantile polycystic kidneys	1
Cystinosis	1
Rapidly progressive glomerulonephritis	1
Steroid-resistant nephrotic syndrome with focal segmental sclerosis	1
Steroid-sensitive nephrotic syndrome and interstitial nephritis	1
Jeune's syndrome	1
Gonadal dysgenesis and glomerulonephritis	1
Wilms' tumor	1
Birth asphyxia: cortical necrosis	1
Chronic glomerulonephritis, type unknown	1

nutrition, to maintain acid–base balance, and to prevent bone disease. Our parallel experience has led us to conclude that if, despite optimal management, growth does not occur for 6–12 months, transplantation may be warranted. Further procrastination and delay are unlikely to result in a larger or stronger kidney transplant recipient.

The results of long-term dialysis treatment in small children from the European Dialysis and Transplant Association registry and the Hôpital des Enfants Malades (Chapter 35) also parallel our own and are discouraging for these small patients, their families, and health care teams. Mortality is high, growth is generally poor, vascular access is technically difficult, and bone disease is frequent and often severe.

Although not discussed in detail by Dr. Broyer (Chapter 35), it is our experience that the emotional stresses of chronic dialysis on the small child and their families are enormous, and the costs of dialysis, nursing care being more intensive, are extraordinarily high. In discussions with Dr. Broyer (personal communication) it is clear that, given more abundant cadavers or living relative donors, his group would greatly prefer transplantation to long-term dialysis in these young children.

Dr. Barratt's data have demonstrated a steep downward slope of survival for children with congenital disorders in the first year of life and a continuing considerable loss of life over the next 4 years. Although there is little evidence of success in the transplantation of children much less than 1 year of age, our experience with children aged 1–5 years is encouraging. The remainder of this chapter will review that experience which we believe supports our view that early transplantation is appropriate therapy for CRF in the young child.

2. *Patients*

We have transplanted 42 children (26 boys, 16 girls) aged 1–5 years ($\bar{X}$ = 3.3 years, range = 0.9–5.9 years, median 2.9 years) between 1970 and

1981. The original diseases are listed in Table 1. All children but two were growth retarded (more than 2 S.D. below mean for chronologic age) at the time of transplant. Most had mild to severely delayed psychomotor development. One child with hypoplastic–dysplastic kidneys developed severe deterioration in neurologic function despite only moderate uremia and was transplanted in an effort to reverse this process. All failed on conservative management. All but three children received hemodialysis for an average of 2 months prior to transplant. In no case was transplantation performed because of an inability to maintain the child on dialysis.

3. *Donor Source*

Thirty-five patients initially received living related donor (LRD) grafts, 34 from parents (21 mothers and 13 fathers) and one from a grandmother. The remaining seven, with no suitable family donor, received cadaver donor (CD) grafts which, for the last 5 years, have been matched for at least two of four HLA A and B antigens. All children but one received adult donor kidneys. One received two kidneys from a 5-year-old donor. No effort was made to search for pediatric cadaver donors, since such donors are rare and waiting for a well-matched pediatric donor would greatly prolong dialysis. The advances in transplantation techniques (see Section 4) have permitted transplantation of adult kidneys into children as small as 5400 g without great technical problems.

4. *Surgical Strategies*

Since the kidneys were all placed intraabdominally in these small children,[1,2] every attempt was made to perform a one-stage procedure including nephrectomy (where necessary), splenectomy (performed in all but one child), and transplant in order to avoid two major intraabdominal operations. Exceptions included two children requiring urgent nephrectomy for malignant hypertension and children with congenital nephrotic syndrome (CNS) and anasarca. In the latter situation 6–10 weeks were allowed following nephrectomy for recovery from hypoproteinemia, hyperlipidemia, hypogammaglobulinemia, hypercoagulability, and malnutrition. Three children, two with CNS and one with steroid-resistant nephrotic syndrome, became anuric with vigorous ultrafiltration on hemodialysis, thus undergoing spontaneous reversal of nephrotic syndrome and avoiding a two-stage procedure. In the past all children with external urinary diversions underwent a two-stage procedure with removal of the kidneys and ureters in order to eliminate infectious foci and to avoid the risk of sepsis after the institution of high-dose immunosuppression. More recently we have begun to take down-loop cutaneous ureterostomies to reestablish a normal urine flow prior to transplantation in children who have been relatively free of recurrent infections.

This reconstruction substitutes a relatively minor procedure for a major intraabdominal procedure (nephrectomy), allows distention of any unused bladder, decreases the difficulty of ureteroneocystostomy at transplant, and allows the child a period of bladder control training which simplifies the posttransplant management period.

5. *Intraoperative Management*

These small children are monitored intraoperatively for central venous pressure (CVP) using lines placed via jugular veins at surgery or Hickman catheters which were previously placed as dialysis access devices. The arterial limb of modified Scribner shunts or percutaneously placed arterial lines are used to monitor blood pressure and arterial blood gases. Great care is taken to maintain normothermia by warming the operating room, the patient, and all abdominal lavage solutions and wet packs. Kidneys are perfused with warm solutions prior to clamp release. The vascular anastomoses (end to side) are made between donor renal artery and vein and the recipient aorta and vena cava, respectively. Before the vascular clamps are released, the CVP is acutely raised to 10–12 cm H_2O in order to ensure adequacy of the vascular volume needed to fill the new kidney.

The ureteral reimplantation is a standard Ledbetter–Politano tunneling technique. The large bowel is tacked to the upper pole of the kidney in order to provide access to the lower pole for percutaneous graft biopsy, should this become necessary. The kidney may appear hypoperfused during abdominal closure and may require repositioning to avoid vascular kinking and compromise of renal blood flow.

6. *Postoperative Care*

Urine output may be low in these small patients for the first few postoperative hours but usually increases spontaneously. It is important to avoid severe hypertension and fluid overload during this critical period. The CVP alone is a wholly inadequate monitoring technique in these tiny patients, and other parameters, including blood pressure, pulse, frequent chest X rays, and arterial blood gases, must be followed in addition to CVP in order to avoid fluid overload. These children may be severely hypertensive and in pulmonary edema with CVPs in the 2- to 5-cm-H_2O range. Large urine outputs are frequent in the first 24 hr postoperatively, and monitoring of urine and plasma glucose is important to avoid hyperglycmia and consequent osmotic diuresis. We switch from a 5% to a 1% glucose urine replacement solution if the urine glucose becomes positive and/or hyperglycemia develops. Immunosuppressive management and treatment of rejection episodes routine to our institution have previously been described.[2,3]

Table 2. Causes of Death in 42 Transplanted Children Aged 1–5 Years

Overwhelming pneumococcal sepsis	2
Abdominal sepsis following graft artery stenosis repair, recurrent Wilms' tumor at autopsy	1
Disseminated chickenpox	1
Iatrogenic fluid overload	1
Withdrawal of active therapy following graft rejection	1

7. Patient Surivival

We have lost six children in this series. The causes of death have been varied (Table 2) and theoretically preventable in most patients. Two splenectomized children who were receiving sulfonamide prophylaxis died of overwhelming pneumococcal sepsis. All children are now maintained on once-daily penicillin.[4] One child died of disseminated chickenpox 3 years posttransplant. A recent review of this disease disclosed that the continuation of Imuran during the course of this child's illness was probably responsible for his death.[5] One child with urine leak died of inappropriate fluid administration and unrecognized pulmonary edema. One child had treatment withdrawn at parental request after acutely rejecting a graft. In retrospect, our handling of this intrafamilial emotional crisis following graft rejection was less than ideal. Thus, the child with Wilms' tumor dying of intraabdominal postoperative sepsis (Table 2) probably represents the only inevitable death in this group since he had advanced metastatic disease at autopsy.

Deaths in these children may be further minimized by experience and consistent application of sound principles of medical and surgical care. Nonetheless, the overall risk of death is not higher for these young children than for older children or adults (Fig. 1). Although the number of patients (six) is too small for statistical comparison, the patient survival of recipients with cadaver grafts was essentially identical to that of recipients of parental grafts. These data support our view that patient survival rates after transplantation in infants and young children are comparable to those in older children and adults.

8. Graft Survival

Graft loss is no more frequent in these young children than in older children or adults (Figs. 2 and 3), and comparison of these figures indicates that parental and cadaver graft survival rates were almost identical. As expected, the dominant cause of graft loss was rejection. Acute rejection in these small children frequently presents as a picture of rapidly progressive renal failure which, despite aggressive antirejection treatment, is unremitting leading to total destruction of the graft within a few days to a few weeks. Six of the eleven first grafts lost in our series followed this dramatic clinical

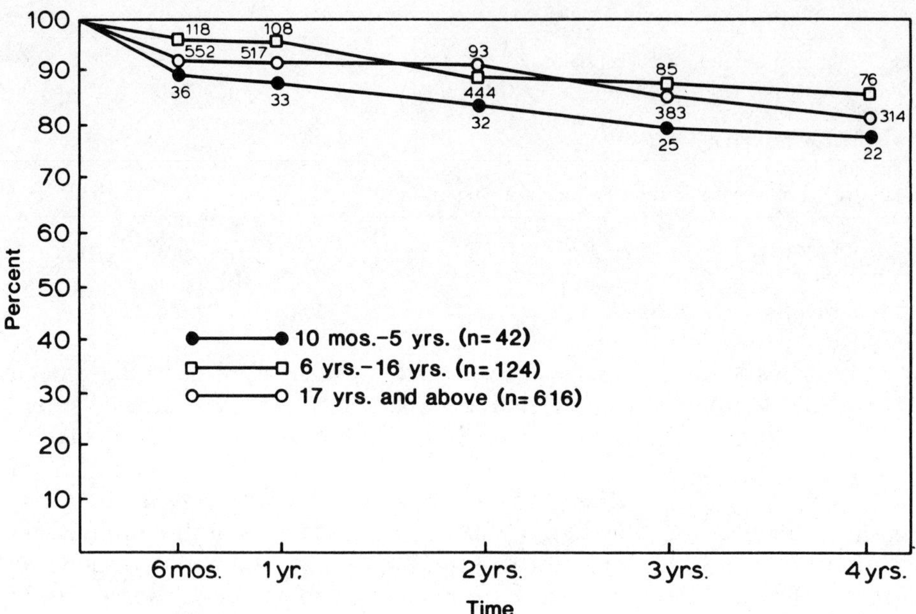

Figure 1. Actuarial patient survival curves for patients in three age groups. Numbers above data points indicate number of patients at risk at that time and numbers in parentheses (*n*) equal number of patients entered into each group in Figs. 1–3. Data describe patient survival from the initial point of all first transplants in nondiabetic patients. There are no significant differences between these curves.

pattern. Although this relatively violent rejection, in our experience, is more common in small children than in adults, it does not influence the *frequency* of graft loss (Fig. 2 and 3).

Seven children have received second grafts and two have received third grafts. Of these nine children with multiple grafts, seven are alive with functioning grafts and two are dead. Only one child in this group remains on dialysis because of 100% cytotoxic antibodies following rejection of a maternal graft. Thus, the commitment to provide aggressive care to these 42 young children has generated only a single child who is lingering on dialysis.

Recently the important influence of graft source on graft survival was shown by our associates.[6] The data derived mainly from parental grafts showed that male (paternal) donors provided statistically significantly better graft survival (73%) than female (maternal) donors (52%) at 5 years post-transplant.[6] This may represent subtle sensitization of children to maternal antigens *in utero*. Whatever the explanation, the tendency toward more frequent maternal donation (21 mothers versus 13 fathers) represents both societal maternal role expectations and our previously held *incorrect* belief that maternal kidneys, being slightly smaller, would "fit" better in the

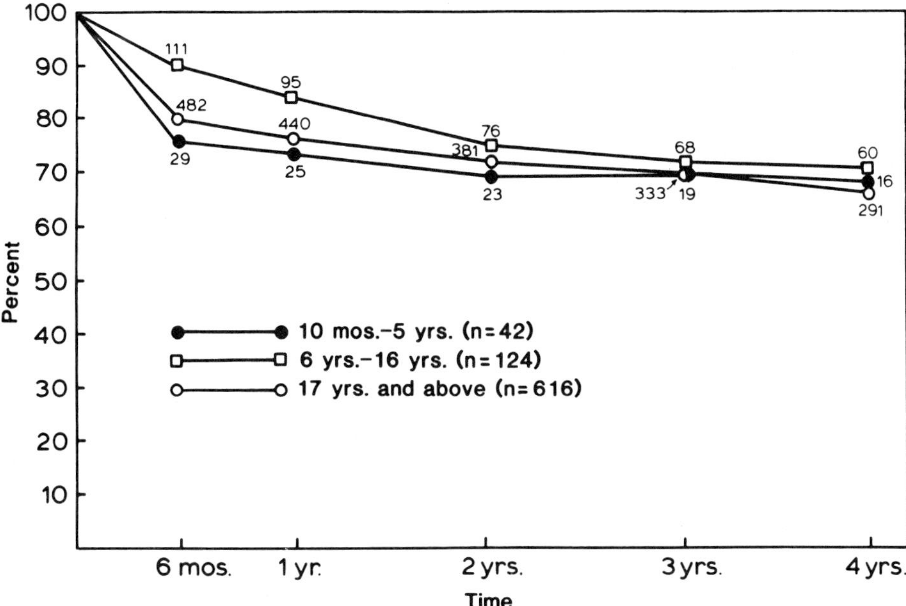

Figure 2. Actuarial graft survival for all first transplants, regardless of donor source in nondiabetic patients. There are no significant differences between these curves.

abdomen of these small children. In the future we will encourage families toward initial paternal graft donation.

In summary, it is clear from Figs. 2 and 3 that, in terms of functional graft survival, infants and small children are excellent transplant candidates.

9. Growth

The growth patterns of these children after transplantation are now quite well defined.[1,7] Given a successful graft and the presence of significant (less than fifth percentile) growth retardation prior to transplantation, all but one of these children showed catch-up growth for the first 1 or 2 posttransplant years followed by normal growth rates. The one exception grew at almost a normal rate (88% of expected growth) in the first 5 posttransplant years. Achievement of normal height for age for these profoundly growth-retarded children is unusual (20%), but most approach this goal. Children with multiple severe rejection episodes requiring repeated treatment with high-dose steroids and leading to renal insufficiency or multiple transplants grow poorly.[1,7] Recently, we have shown that low-dose once-daily prednisone ($\bar{X}$ = 0.3 mg/kg per day) does not inhibit catch-up growth and provides only a small growth disadvantage over alternate-day prednisone therapy.[8] However, a significant risk of rejection resulted from

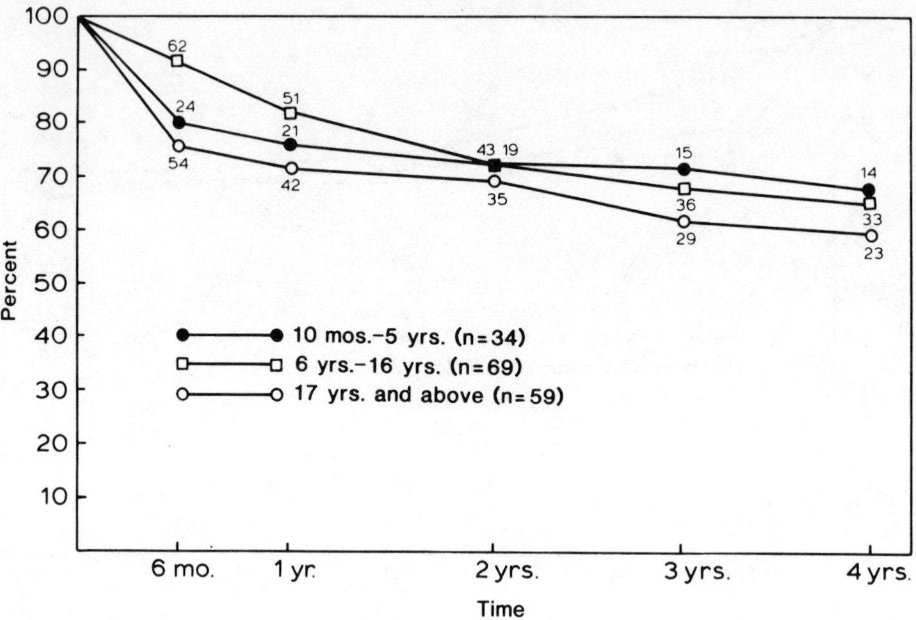

Figure 3. Actuarial graft survival for all first transplants from parental donors in nondiabetic patients. There are no significant differences between these curves.

switching to alternate-day therapy in children who had rejection episodes in the early posttransplant period.[8] Thus, we recommend alternate-day prednisone only for those children with retarded posttransplant growth who have had no history of transplant rejection.

In summary, growth in most transplanted young children is satisfactory and may be extremely good. Our experience does not support, *a priori*, that young severely growth-retarded uremic children should be excluded from consideration for transplantation because of the fear that they will remain renal dwarfs.

10. Development

Most small children with uremia or congenital nephrotic syndrome have mild to moderate delay in psychomotor development (see Chapter 60).[9] One child who developed rapid decline in global central nervous system function prior to transplant remains profoundly retarded after transplant. One child requires special education for retardation which developed posttransplant and was associated with intractable petit-mal seizures. One child with Jeune's syndrome and multiple perceptual problems and seizures remains on dialysis 4 years after loss of her maternal graft and requires special education, although her IQ is close to normal. An additional child's verbal learning has been markedly delayed by severe hearing loss which developed after her second transplant. All other successfully transplanted children have shown catchup in psychomotor development and, with the exceptions mentioned, all of school age attended regular school, and most are in their appropriate grade.

In summary, the intellectual outcome of successfully transplanted young children has been one of the most gratifying aspects of our experience in the care of the small transplant recipient.

11. General Thoughts

Clearly, the care of the very small child requiring dialysis and transplantation is highly complex. Experience is a necessary ingredient for success. Since renal failure in childhood is rare and children 5 years of age and under make up only 10–15% of the pediatric renal failure population (Chapter 35), it would be difficult for any center to gain the experience and maintain the high level of skill necessary if many centers undertake to care for these patients. It is thus our view that specialized centers should be developed and that referral patterns should be established which will foster the maintenance of an effective patient care team. This team should operate in centers with a broad base in pediatrics, including subspecialty interests in nephrology, infectious disease, cardiology, neurology, nutrition, child psychiatry, and social work. Broad-based surgical representation in transplantation surgery, vascular access surgery, urology, and orthopedics is at least of equal importance. Skilled dialysis and transplant nurses and technical personnel are essential team components. Information that we have received through personal communication indicates that many centers have been discouraged in their early efforts in this area because the requisite team approach was not established and early failures were thus predictable. It is our estimate that five or six centers in the United States concentrating on transplantation of small children would be sufficient to meet the national needs.

Many problems remain unresolved. The very long-term outcome of most of these children remains shrouded in the future as few have been transplanted for a sufficient length of time to reach puberty. The problem of graft rejection, yet to be satisfactorily solved, has much greater impact on the small child who does relatively poorly on long-term dialysis. New immunosuppressive treatments such as Cyclosporin A[10] and total lymphoid irradiation[11] are still experimental and pose ethical dilemmas, especially in young children who cannot give meaningful consent. Recent evidence that uremia in the first year of life may have a significant negative impact on the developing brain[9] (see Chapter 60) needs careful examination and may indicate that earlier transplantation may be desirable for maximal developmental potential. Despite the extra effort involved, our results indicate that discrimination against aggressive treatment of the small uremic child on the basis of age or size alone is unwarranted.

References

1. Miller LC, Lum CT, Bock GH, Simmons RL, Najarian JS, Mauer SM: Transplantation of the adult kidney into the very small child: Technical considerations. *Am J Surg* 145:243, 1983.
2. Mauer SM, Howard RJ: Renal transplantation in children, in Edelmann CM Jr (ed): *Pediatric Kidney Disease*, Boston, Little Brown, 1978, p 503.
3. Sommer BG, Sutherland DER, Kjellstrand CM, Howard RJ, Mauer SM, Simmons RL, Najarian JS: 1000 transplants at the University of Minnesota, 1963–1977. *Minnesota Med* 62:861, 1979.
4. Krivit W: Overwhelming post-splenectomy infection. *Am J Hematol* 2:193, 1977.
5. Feldhoff CM, Balfour HH Jr, Simmons RL, Najarian JS, Mauer SM: Varicella in children with renal transplants. *J Pediatr* 98:25, 1981.
6. Lum CT, Fryd DS, Najarian JS: Renal transplantation in children 0–10 years of age. *Curr Surg* 39:27, 1982.
7. Ingelfinger JR, Grupe WE, Harmon WE, Fernbach SK, Levey RH: Growth acceleration following renal transplantation in children less than 7 years of age. *Pediatrics* 68:255, 1981.
8. Feldhoff CM, Goldman AI, Najarian JS, Mauer SM: A comparison of alternate day and daily steroid therapy in children following renal transplantation. *Int J Pediatr Nephrol* 5:11, 1984.
9. Miller LC, Bock GH, Lum CT, Najarian JS, Mauer SM: Transplantation of the adult kidney into the very small child: Long-term outcome. *J Pediatr* 100:675, 1982.
10. Starzl TE, Klintmalm GBG, Weil R III, Porter KA, Iwatsuki S, Schroter GPJ, Gernandez–Bueno C, MacHugh N: Cyclosporin A and steroid therapy in sixty-six cadaver kidney recipients. *Surg Gynecol Obstet* 153:486, 1981.
11. Najarian JS, Sutherland DFR, Ferguson RM, Kersey J, Mauer SM, Slavin S, Kim TH: Total lymphoid irradiation and kidney transplantation. A clinical experience. *Transpl Proc* 13:417, 1981.

34

Experience with End-Stage Renal Disease Treatment of Young Children

A Brief Note

Richard N. Fine

The optimal treatment of young children with irreversible renal insufficiency remains controversial, and there is a paucity of data about end-stage renal disease (ESRD) therapy in this age group. Once ESRD develops, the technical capability exists to initiate either hemodialysis or peritoneal dialysis. Although there are minimal data validating the efficacy of long-term intermittent peritoneal dialysis (IPD) or continuous ambulatory peritoneal dialysis (CAPD) in young children, it would seem advantageous to consider IPD preferentially in young children. This preference should be considered because of the minimal amount of technical expertise required to implement IPD and the paucity of technical problems, especially problems related to access devices. It must be emphasized that limited data are available about the course of dialysis in young children.

Similarly, limited data are available regarding the long-term outcome of renal transplantation in young children. Rizzoni *et al.* (1980) recently reviewed the literature concerning renal transplantation in children less than 5 years of age and added the experience at Children's Hospital of Los Angeles (CHLA) over a 10-year period. The CHLA experience differed from that of the group from Minnesota (Hodson *et al.*, 1978) in that the outcome of transplants in young children was poorer than the overall CHLA results, whereas the Minnesota group reported similar results in both young and older children. It should be noted that most of the allografts were from cadaver donors in Los Angeles and from living related donors in Minnesota. These data indicate that current information requires dissemination if parents

Richard N. Fine • Division of Pediatric Nephrology, UCLA Center for Health Sciences, Los Angeles, California 90024.

of young children with ESRD are to be given a dispassionate assessment of the potential outcome from various treatment modalities.

The current status of all children less than 5 years of age at the initiation of ESRD treatment who were treated initially at CHLA, and more recently at the University of California, Los Angeles, Center for Health Sciences, during the past 14 years, is reviewed here.

The characteristics of the children are listed below:

1. Patient material: During the 14-year period February 1967 to February 1981, 29 children less than 5 years of age received ESRD care. Of the 29 children, 13 were female and 16 were male.
2. Age: At the initiation of treatment, the children were 7/12 to 4-8/12 years of age; three were less than 1 year old.
3. Primary disease: The following is the distribution of primary diseases among the 29 ESRD children: obstructive uropathy, seven; hypoplasia/dysplasia, seven; focal segmental glomerulosclerosis, five; hemolytic uremic syndrome, four; cortical necrosis/acute tubular necrosis, two; oligomeganephronia, membranoproliferative glomerulonephritis, antitubular basement antibody glomerulonephritis, bilateral Wilms' Tumor (one each).
4. Initial ESRD treatment modality: Hemodialysis was the initial modality in 20 children; IPD in seven; CAPD in one; and one child received an initial cadaver donor transplant without prior dialysis.
5. Transplantation: Of the 29 children, 23 received 40 renal allografts from five live related and 35 cadaver donors. All the living related donor transplants were initial allografts, whereas 18 of the cadaver donor allografts were first, 12 were second, four were third, and one was a fourth allograft. Currently, two of the five living related and 9 of 35 (three first, four second, and two third) cadaver donor allografts are functioning.

   The etiology of the 29 allograft failures was as follows: acute rejection, 16; chronic rejection, three; technical failure, four; recurrence of original disease one; and five children died with a functioning allograft. The incidence of technical failures and of patient deaths in this group of young recipients is higher than that observed in older children. Some of the patient deaths were attributable to overzealous attempts to salvage a rejecting allograft in a recipient who tolerated hemodialysis poorly.
6. Current status: Of the 29 children, 23 received one or more renal allografts and six received dialysis only. Two died on dialysis and four are currently undergoing dialysis therapy. Of the 23 allograft recipients, 11 currently have a functioning allograft, ten have died, and two are undergoing dialysis. All six patients currently undergoing dialysis are receiving peritoneal dialysis (IPD four and CAPD two).
7. Patient deaths: Of the 12 patients who died, the interval between initiation of ESRD treatment and death was as follows: less than 6

months, four; 6–12 months, one; 1–2 years, three; 3–4 years, two; 5–6 years, one; 10–11 years, one.

Summary

Twenty-nine children, 7 months to 4⅔ years of age, received ESRD treatment over a 14-year period. Currently, 11 of 23 (48%) allograft recipients have functioning allografts, six patients are undergoing dialysis, and 12 (41%) have died. These data indicate that the outcome of ESRD care in young children is poorer than that of older children.

References

Hodson, E. M., Najarian, J. S., Kjellstrand, C. M., Simmons, R. L., and Mauer, S. M., 1978, Renal transplantation in children ages 1 to 5 years, *Pediatrics* **61:**458.

Rizzoni, G., Malekzadeh, M. H., Pennisi, A.J., Ettenger, R. B., Uittenbogaart, C. H., and Fine, R. N., 1980, Renal transplantation in children less than 5 years of age, *Arch. Dis. Child.* **55:**532.

35

The European Experience with Treatment of End-Stage Renal Disease in Young Children

Michel Broyer, Raymond Donckervolke, Felix Brunner, Hans Brynger, Claude Jacobs, Peter Kramer, Neville Selwood, and Antony Wing

In developed countries children with terminal renal failure are accepted in dialysis–transplant programs. There is nevertheless an age limit under which these programs are not currently applied. For arbitrary reasons this limit has been fixed at 5 years in some countries, but not in others, where the treatments have been applied more broadly when feasible. This chapter deals with the European experience in treating children less than 5 years of age by dialysis and transplantation through two sources: (1) European Dialysis and Transplant Association registry—for general information; (2) Hôpital des Enfants Malades (Paris)—to provide more details on some points.

1. European Dialysis and Transplant Association (EDTA) Registry

1.1. Number of Patients

At review (December 31, 1979), 128 children less than 5 years of age were listed on the EDTA registry out of 2175 patients less than 15 years of age, that is, 5.8%. In fact, the number of young patients varied markedly from 1.7% in the United Kingdom to 12% in Israel (Table 1), the highest figures probably giving a more exact description of the patient population.

Michel Broyer • Hôpital des Enfants Malades, 75730 Paris 15, France. *Raymond Donckervolke, Felix Brunner, Hans Brynger, Claude Jacobs, Peter Kramer, Neville Selwood, and Antony Wing* • Registry Committee of the EDTA, St. Thomas Hospital, London SE1 7EH, England.
Supported in part by a grant from AURA, Paris.

Table 1. European Pediatric Registry, December 31, 1979[a]

	Total number	<5 years at onset	Percent
Belgium	74	6	8
Denmark	43	4	9.3
France	441	50	11.5
DDR	63	2	3.1
GFR	289	11	3.8
Israel	49	6	12
Italy	248	13	5.2
Netherlands	112	8	7.1
Spain	115	10	8.6
Sweden	47	1	2.1
Switzerland	52	3	5.7
UK	401	7	1.7
Others	95	6	
Total	2175	128	5.8

[a] From Donckervolke *et al.* (1980).

The number of new patients less than 15 years of age accepted each year increased regularly in Europe from 100 in 1970 to 300 in 1977 and then seemed to reach a plateau. The progression of the annual number of new patients less than 5 years is much more irregular, probably indicating the absence of a definite policy for patients of this age group.

The sex ratio of children less than 5 years at the start was 0.63 with an excess of males as contrasted to a sex ratio of 0.50 for all children on the registry.

1.2. Age at Start of Treatment

Age at start of treatment varied from 1 year to 4 years 11 months, with the following distribution:

1–2 years: 17
2–3 years: 30
3–4 years: 37
4–5 years: 44

1.3. Primary Renal Disease

The primary causes of renal failure were glomerular disease, 28% (36/128); hemolytic–uremic syndrome and/or cortical necrosis, 21% (28/128); and a group including hypoplastic kidney, dysplastic kidney, uropathy, and pyelonephritis, 21% (27/128). Some rare causes are also represented such as nephronophthisis, 7% (9/128); Wilms' tumor, 5% (6/128); polycystic disease, 2% (3/128); and oxalosis, 2% (3/128).

Table 2. Survival Rates

Age (years)	*n*	1 year	2 years
0–4	109	84%	73%
5–9	481	87%	74%
10–14	1285	88%	81%

1.4. Mode of Treatment

The majority of patients were treated by intermittent hospital hemodialysis (HD). Peritoneal dialysis (PD) was used as an alternative to HD. Thus 66 children were treated by HD alone, 40 children by both HD and PD, and seven by PD alone. In addition, eight patients were treated at home, three by HD and five by PD. Finally, seven children were transplanted directly without a preliminary period of hemodialysis.

Fifty-seven patients received kidney transplantation, 45 from a cadaver donor and 12 from a living related donor.

On December 31, 1979, 86 patients were alive; 36 were treated by HD in hospital and one at home; three were treated by PD at hospital and two at home; and 44 had a functioning renal transplant.

1.5. Survival

The overall survival of all patients less than 5 years of age was 68% (86/128). Mortality was higher on dialysis 28% (34/121) than after transplantation 17% (8/44).

Actuarial survival was lower in the age group 0–4 than in the other pediatric age groups for hospital hemodialysis (Donckervolke *et al.*, 1980) (Table 2).

1.6. Causes of Death

The causes of 15 deaths on dialysis (three on PD) and seven deaths after transplantation are documented. Infection was more frequent cause of death in this age group than in the whole pediatric group: respectively, 4/15 (26%) on dialysis and 3/7 (42%) after transplantation versus 11% and 28% of all deaths of children on the registry (Schärer *et al.*, 1976). Vascular causes of death were less frequent: respectively, 5/15 (33%) on dialysis and 1/7 (16%) after transplantation versus 63% and 32% of all deaths of children on the registry. In two cases death was due to voluntary interruption of dialysis treatment. Seven patients less than 5 years of age were lost to follow-up in specialized centers. They probably died after withdrawal from the dialysis center.

1.7. *Transplantation*

Fifty-seven transplantations had been performed in these patients, 45 from a cadaver donor. Twenty-nine of the cadaver grafts were achieved before age 5 (2–5 years) and 16 afterward (5½–9 years). The graft survival was 53% at 1 year for children 1–5 years and 67% for children more than 5 years of age. Seven children died after cadaver kidney transplantation: six of them belong to the group of children who had been transplanted at less than 5 years of age and one to the group of older children.

The mean waiting time for transplanting these young children was 16 months. In fact, this time was very variable from one country to another (1 month in the United Kingdom to 28 months in France).

Twelve patients received a live related kidney, eight before age 5 and four after this age. At the last recording all these grafts were functioning except in one patient who died at age 21-8/12 years.

2. *Data from the Hôpital des Enfants Malades*

2.1. *Number of Patients*

Thirty-three children less than 5 years and more than 16 months of age had been accepted on a dialysis–transplant (DT) program from 1969 to 1981 in this center, that is, 17% of the total number of children and adolescents less than 16 years accepted during the same period of time for the same reason ($n = 190$). The sex distribution was even more asymmetric than in the European registry with seven girls versus 26 boys (sex ratio: boys = 0.78 versus 0.63 in the EDTA).

2.2. *Etiology of Renal Failure*

Etiology was as follows: glomerular disease (12), hemolytic–uremic syndrome (4), hypoplastic kidney, dysplastic kidneys, ± urinary tract abnormalities (10), and others (7). In these young patients some special glomerular diseases were found: diffuse mesangial sclerosis (7), congenital nephrotic syndrome (Finnish type) (2), focal and segmental sclerosis (1), anti-GBM nephropathy (2).

2.3. *General Approach and Mode of Treatment*

These evolved with time. The difficulty of maintaining a permanent blood access with external bypass techniques explains the frequent and repeated use of intermittent peritoneal dialysis (IPD) during the first years. Since 1973 internal fistulas were systematically created. Improvement of surgical techniques (use of microscope) and availability of adapted artificial vessels allowed continuation of hemodialysis without the need of PD periods. Recently home continuous ambulatory peritoneal dialysis (CAPD) was applied preferentially in three cases instead of HD.

The present status of this group of patients (n = 33) is as follows: on hemodialysis—13, on CAPD—four, with a functional transplant—nine, and deceased—seven.

The seven deaths occurred—except one—before 1975, six on HD and one on PD. All children were registered as soon as possible on the cadaver transplantation program.

2.4. *HD*

2.4.1. *Dialysis Schedule*

The children initially received two dialysis sessions per week. A better approach has been applied during the last years since it was found that three sessions per week were needed to avoid mineral and water overload in these young patients (taking into account their food intake). Time on dialysis was usually 9–15 hr/week according to residual diuresis and compliance to dietary recommendations.

2.4.2. *Dialyzers*

The dialyzers used were related to the size of patients according to several principles:

1. Dialyzer surface area/body surface area ratio around 1
2. Dialysis or urea at the rate of about 3 ml/kg body weight and no higher than 5 ml/kg body weight
3. Extracorporeal blood volume less than 10 ml/kg body weight

Precise monitoring was applied during the sessions using control of weight and permanent control of ultrafiltration (Rhodial, or special module) with special procedures for the first sessions (e.g., mannitol, diazepam, phenobarbital).

2.4.3. *Vascular Access*

Internal fistulas using the humeral artery and a cephalic vein in children less than 8–12 kg of body weight were systematically created since 1973 even in very young patients. The radial artery was used in children above this weight. Of 19 children accepted after 1973 on the DT program, (1) six had no complications of vascular access and were treated for periods up to 3 years; (2) nine had thrombosis of the fistula either immediately or after 2–20 months leading to the need for creation of another fistula; among these nine children, four were submitted to several operations including vascular grafts and had recurrent thrombosis; (3) in four other patients other complications were observed: two infections, one stenosis with surgical revision, and one hand ischemia which is improving progressively. Cardiac failure was observed in one case and was attributed at least partly to a high-flow humeral fistula, since cardiac symptoms disappeared after partial ligation. Four children received one or two vascular grafts after thrombosis of radial or humeral fistulas. These grafts remained functional in two cases but were rapidly thrombosed in two others.

2.4.4. *Complications*

Anemia was not more severe than in older children. Mean hematocrit was the same in the two populations in 1980: 19.2%. Bone disease was more frequent in young patients: seven children of this series developed signs of renal rickets and hyperparathyroidism in spite of vitamin D preventive therapy, that is, 23% of patients versus 14% in the whole series of the Hôpital des Enfants Malades. Five of these children improved with medical treatment, but two patients had to be submitted to parathyroidectomy.

Seizures developed in two patients (no more frequently than in older children) and were controlled by phenobarbital.

Except for one child who died after coming back to dialysis following a transplantation failure at 13 years, all deaths occurred before 5 years of age. The causes of these deaths were pulmonary edema (two), myocardial ischemia (one), Wilms' tumor (one), anaphylactoid shock (one), and voluntary interruption of the treatment in a severely brain-damaged child (one).

2.5. *IPD*

IPD was used as the only treatment in four cases, and sequentially or alternately with hemodialysis in nine cases, especially before 1975. Two patients were treated at home for periods exceeding 2 and 3 years, respectively, and the others were treated in hospital. In all the cases dialysis was performed through a Tenckoff catheter with an automatic cycling machine (LKB) using sterile dialysate. The children were generally treated 2 × 24 hr/week.

Obstruction of the catheter was observed 14 times in seven patients, leaks three times in two patients, and evisceration twice in one patient. Peritonitis occurred 15 times in seven patients out of the 11 treated at the hospital and only once in the two patients treated at home (one episode per 5.5 months in hospital and one per 63 months at home). One patient treated at the hospital died from peritonitis. These complications explain why hospital intermittent PD was practically abandoned after 1975.

2.6. *CAPD*

Four patients aged 2½ to 5 years have been treated by CAPD for periods of 6–20 months. One of them who was switched from IPD to CAPD had four episodes of peritonitis. One catheter obstruction and one leak were observed in one other patient at the start of this treatment. At the present time these four patients continue to be treated by CAPD with satisfactory results. CAPD results seem similar in young patients and in older children, with the exception that leakage of peritoneal protein is more marked in younger children.

2.7. *Transplantation*

In the Enfants Malades series, only two patients were transplanted under 5 years of age. As a matter of fact, the mean waiting time on dialysis was 28 months because of shortage of cadaver kidneys in France and availability of living related donors. A total of 11 children with onset of renal failure prior to 5 years of age have been transplanted with cadaver kidneys. None have died. At the present time two kidneys have been rejected after 6 and 2 years, respectively, and the nine others remain functionning for periods of 5 months to 7 years. No special complication related to the young age of the patients could be recorded. The high level of graft survival could be related to the number of transfusions during the dialysis period.

2.8. *Body Growth*

On hemodialysis, 20 cases are well documented: 11 had a negative standard deviation score (SDS), three continued to grow on the same standard deviation (SD) line (SDS = 0), and six had some catchup growth. The mean SDS for these 20 patients since the start of hemodialysis and eventually up to 5 years of age was −0.26/year, and if the analysis is limited to the 14 patients referred during the last 5 years, the mean SDS was −0.05/year. These figures are clearly above the mean SDS of −0.36/year recently described in a large prepubertal population (Kleinknecht *et al.*, 1980).

On peritoneal dialysis and CAPD the data are too limited to deserve a report. They do not seem different from hemodialysis; the two patients on CAPD for the longest period, 20 and 8 months, respectively, continued to grow on their line.

2.9. *Psychologic Factors and Schooling*

Tolerance to venipuncture was generally accepted, except for two patients. Between dialysis these children looked like other children. Their psychomotor development remained in the normal range.

At the present time 26 (26/33) patients who started the DT program before 5 years are alive. Eleven remain less than 5 years old and are in kindergarten. Fifteen are aged 6–13 years; ten are in school full time at an appropriate level, three are in school part time, and two have medical problems preventing normal schooling.

2.10. *Hyperconservative Treatment*

In very small children both HD and PD may be impractical. In this situation survival remains possible in spite of a creatinine clearance less than

3 ml/min per 1.73 m^2 with a special diet using α-keto and OH analogues of amino acids and strictly calculated intakes of water and minerals. This approach was applied to three patients 6–10 months of age weighing 4–6 kg at the start and who survived up to 9 months in spite of terminal uremia. Two of these children belong to the present series and were started on hemodialysis as their urine output fell below 10 ml/kg per day and vascular access became possible.

3. Conclusion

Long-term dialysis is often more difficult to apply in young children than in older ones for technical reasons. Vascular access could vanish or become impracticable, but in these cases peritoneal dialysis could be used to allow survival.

The relatively high mortality rate observed in this series was more related to initial inexperience than to special difficulty with this age group. Finally, there is no reason to select the limit of 5 years for refusing children on DT programs, and if a limit has to be drawn, it would be rather between 1 and 2 years with the possibility to extend this limit using the "hyperconservative" approach.

References

Donckervolke, R., Chantler, C., Broyer, M., Brunner, F. P., Brynger, H., Jacobs, C., Kramer, P., Selwood, N. H., and Wing, A. J., 1980, Combined report on regular dialysis and transplantation of children in Europe, 1979, in: *Proceedings of the European Dialysis and Transplant Association,* Volume 17 (B. H. B. Robinson and J. B. Hawkins, eds.), pp. 87–115, Pitman, London.

Kleinknecht, C., Broyer, M., Gagnadoux, M. F., Marti Henneberg, C., Dartois, A. M., Kermanach, C., Pouliquen, M., Degoulet, P., Usberti, M., and Roy, M. P., 1980, Growth in children treated with long term dialysis. A study of 76 patients, in: *Advances in Nephrology,* Volume 9 (J. Hamburger, J. Crosnier, and J. P. Grunfeld, eds.), pp. 133–163, Year Book, Chicago.

Schärer, K., Chantler, C., Brunner, F. P., Gurland, H. J., Jacobs, C., Selwood, N. H., Spies, G., and Wing, A. J., 1976, Combined report on regular dialysis and transplantation of children in Europe, 1975, in: *Dialysis Transplantation Nephrology,* Volume 13 (B. H. B. Robinson, P. Vereerstaeten, and J. B. Hawkins, eds.), p. 76, Pitman, Tunbridge Wells.

36

Prognosis of Renal Disease in Infancy

T. M. Barratt, J. Fay, and S. P. A. Rigden

1. *Introduction*

Although it is generally agreed that renal transplantion should be available for children over 5 years of age, there is less certainty about the correct policy for younger children with end-stage renal failure, particularly those in the first year of life, in whom the results of transplantation are less good than at other ages (Hodson *et al.*, 1978). In order to formulate the appropriate policy for this age group, however, a prerequisite is an accurate knowledge of the natural history of renal disease presenting in the first year of life. Such knowledge is also important for the pediatricians responsible for the care of these babies in the first instance, and it has been our experience that an inappropriate air of pessimism at the time of initial diagnosis has interfered with mother–child bonding and with the institution of the detailed medical care necessary in the first months of life to obtain best results. We have reviewed the 711 infants admitted to the Nephrology and Urology Departments of the Hospital for Sick Children, Great Ormond Street, London, during 1971–1980 with this problem in mind (Barratt *et al.*, 1982).

2. *Survival*

The principal causes of death from chronic renal disease in the first year of life in infants who have actually passed urine after birth are the congenital nephrotic syndrome, infantile polycystic disease, and renal hypoplasia/dysplasia. Survival in these groups is illustrated in Fig. 1.

T. M. Barratt and J. Fay • Department of Nephrology, Institute of Child Health, London WC1N 1EH, England. ***S. P. A. Rigden*** • Department of Paediatrics, Guy's Hospital, London SE1 9RT, England. J. Fay and S. P. A. Rigden were supported by the Kidney Research Aid Fund and the National Kidney Research Fund of Great Britain.

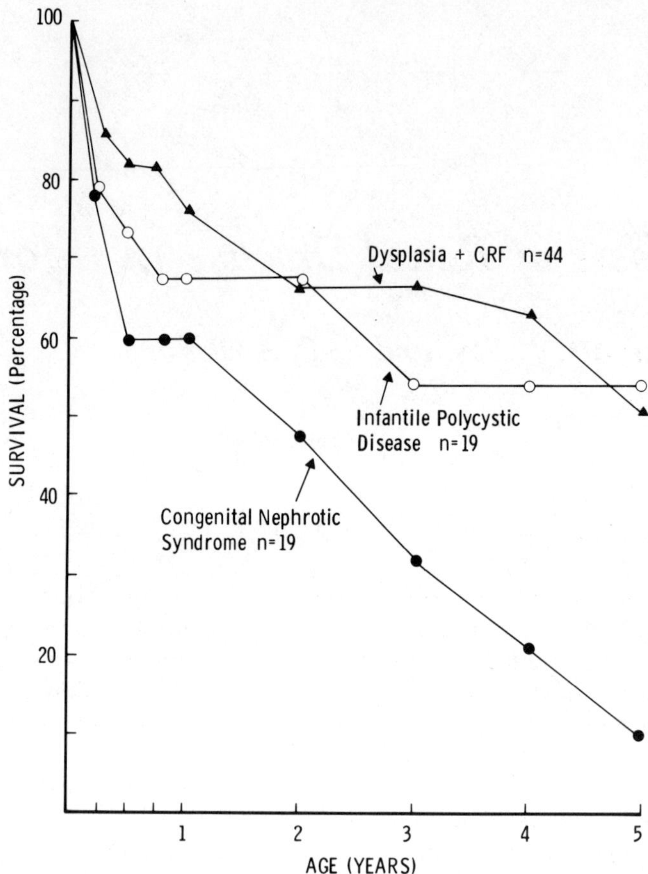

Figure 1. Survival of neonates with congenital nephrotic syndrome, or with infantile polycystic disease, and of infants with renal dysplasia and chronic renal failure (discharge plasma creatinine > 150 μmoles/liter).

2.1. *Congenital Nephrotic Syndrome*

Nephrotic syndrome appearing in the first months of life is heterogeneous, but the group as a whole has a deservedly bad reputation. However, 6 of the 19 children survived to 2 years, and although most were dead by 5 years of age, one boy (with mesangial proliferative glomerulonephritis on biopsy) was still alive at 9½ years of age.

2.2. *Infantile Polycystic Disease*

Infantile polycystic disease presenting in the neonatal period also is generally assumed to carry a poor prognosis, but in fact more than half such patients will still be living at the age of 5 years, and it is very difficult to offer at presentation an accurate prediction of outcome.

Table 1. Infants with Renal Dysplasia and Chronic Renal Failure,[a] Hospital for Sick Children, Great Ormond Street, 1971–1980

	n	CRF (Pc > 150 μmoles/liter)
Isolated dysplasia	19	12
Reflux	82	17
Urethral valves	89	9
Absent abdominal muscles	24	6

[a] Plasma creatinine > 150 μmoles/liter.

2.3. Renal Dysplasia

In this chapter we use the term *renal dysplasia* in a loose sense, encompassing all small misshapen kidneys presumed abnormal at birth, and we have not restricted it to strict histological usage. There is a clear association of such kidneys with urological problems, and insofar as our hospital has had a strong tradition of urological surgery in infants, these cases are well represented in the present series. These babies can be subdivided into four main groups: those without urological abnormality, and those with vesicoureteric reflux, with posterior urethral valves, and with absent abdominal musculature. We have further identified a subgroup with chronic renal failure on the basis of a sustained plasma creatinine concentration above 150 μmol/liter after discharge from their first hospital admission, problems of salt depletion, infection, and urinary obstruction having been corrected (Table 1).

Half of such children are living at 5 years of age; the majority of deaths have occurred in the first month of life ("deaths" include regular dialysis or transplantation) (Fig. 1). The current status of the 44 children with renal

Table 2. Status at 2 Years of Infants with Renal Dysplasia and Chronic Renal Failure

	Discharge plasma creatinine (μmoles/liter)	
	150–300	>300
Alive	17	5
Dead	6	7
Age < 2 years	5	4
Total	28	16

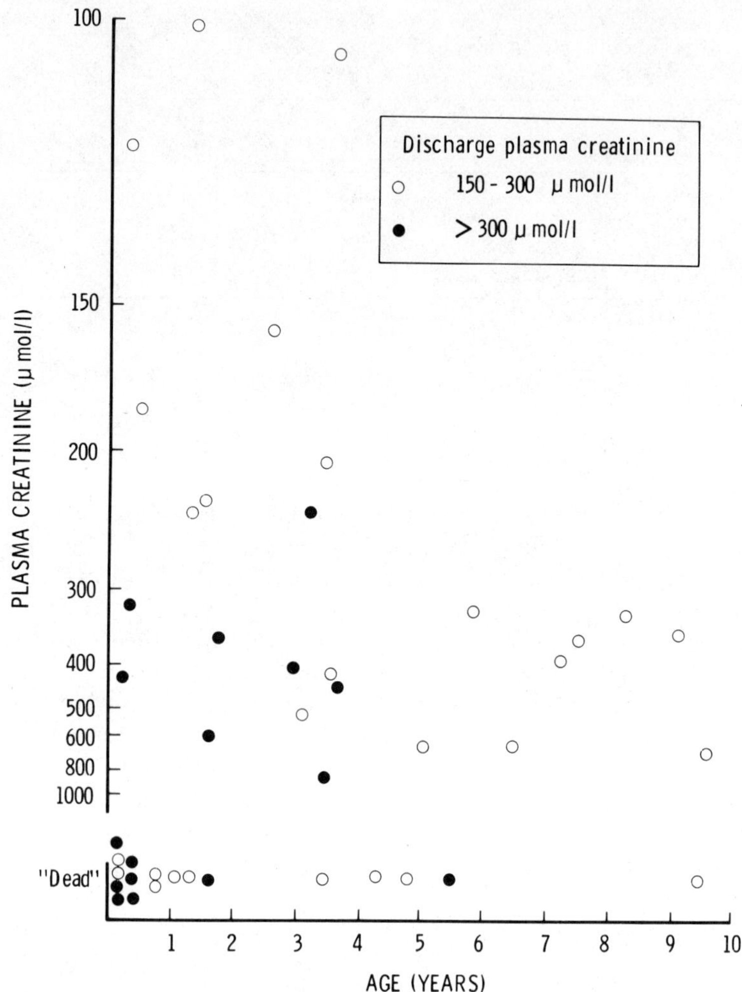

Figure 2. Current status of infants with renal dysplasia and chronic renal failure (discharge plasma creatinine > 150 μmoles/liter).

dysplasia and chronic renal failure is shown in Fig. 2. Six (21%) of the 28 children with a discharge plasma creatinine concentration between 150 and 300 μmoles/liter died under the age of 2 years, in contrast to seven (44%) of the 16 with discharge plasma creatinine concentration above 300 μmoles/liter (Table 2). There is apparently a decline in reciprocal plasma creatinine concentration with increasing age in the survivors, but this does not necessarily imply a decline in glomerular filtration rate (GFR), which is more closely related to the height/creatinine ratio (Counahan *et al.*, 1976).

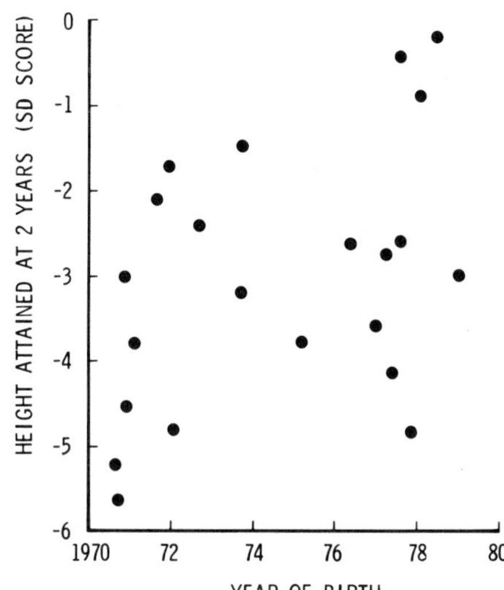

Figure 3. Height SD score for chronological age (Tanner *et al.*, 1966) at 2 years of age for infants with chronic renal failure (discharge plasma creatinine > 150μmoles/liter): there is a significant positive correlation with the year of birth (r_s + 0.42, $p < 0.05$).

3. Growth

Impaired growth of the infant with chronic renal insufficiency is a well-known phenomenon and is a major factor in the overall outcome of later dialysis and transplantation in the survivors. Many factors have been identified, particularly calorie deprivation, osteodystrophy, and acidosis, and undoubtedly the metabolic disturbance in the uremic infant is complex (Jones *et al.*, 1980). The evidence points to growth in the first year of life as the principal determinant for subsequent growth, and it is indeed difficult to recoup ground lost at that age (Betts and McGrath, 1974). As an overall measure of success in the management of these infants we have therefore taken the height standard deviation (S.D.) score at the chronological age of 2 years (Tanner *et al.*, 1966). The data on the 22 available infants are shown in Fig. 3; it is well to remember, however, that there may be other causes for growth failure in addition to renal failure, for 7 of these 22 infants had abnormalities in other systems than the urinary tract, some being already small for dates at birth. Nevertheless, the data are disturbing, with only five (23%) being within 2 S.D. of their expected height for chronological age.

Since 1977 we have run a special clinic for uremic infants, allocating to it a research fellow, dietitian, and social worker and paying special attention to calorie intake, salt and acid–base balance, and the prophylactic use of 1α-hydroxycholecalciferol (Rigden *et al.*, 1980). If such detailed attention were worthwhile, it should be discernible in an improvement in the 2-year height SD scores. There is indeed a correlation between the 2-year height SD score and the year of birth (Spearman rank correlation coefficient +0.42, $p <$

0.05), but, in our hands at least, the growth of these infants is still far from satisfactory.

4. Conclusions

Infants with infantile polycystic disease or with renal dysplasia and chronic renal failure (plasma creatinine > 150 μmoles/liter) have an approximately 50% chance of survival to the age of 5 years, but growth in the latter group is poor and has improved only slightly during the past decade.

References

Barratt, T. M., Dillon, M. J., Fay, J., Ransley, P. G., and Williams, D. I., 1982, Renal disease in the first year of life, in: *Recent Advances in Renal Disease*, 2nd edition (N. F. Jones and D. K. Peters, eds.), p. 197, Churchill, London.

Betts, P. R., and McGrath, G., 1974, Growth patterns and dietary intake of children with chronic renal insufficiency, *Br. Med. J.* **2**:189.

Counahan, R., Chantler, C., Ghazali, S., Kirkwood, B., Rose, F., and Barratt, T. M., 1976, Estimation of glomerular filtration rate from plasma creatinine concentration in children, *Arch. Dis. Child.* **51**:875.

Hodson, E. M., Najarian, J. S., Kjellstrand, C. M., Simmons, R. L., and Mauer, S. M., 1978, Renal transplantation in children aged 1 to 5 years, *Pediatrics* **61**:458.

Jones, R. W. A., El Bishti, M. M., and Chantler, C., 1980, The promotion of anabolism in children with chronic renal failure, in: *Topics in Paediatrics*, Volume 2 (B. Wharton, ed.), pp. 900–1009, Pitman, London.

Rigden, S. P. A., Jones, R. W. A., Preece, M. A., Cameron, N., and Barratt, T. M., 1980, Renal osteodystrophy in young children: A double blind trial of 1 alpha-hydroxycholecalciferol. *Pediatr. Res.* **16**:991.

Tanner, J. M., Whitehouse, R. H., and Takaishi, M., 1966, Standards from birth to maturity for height, weight, height velocity: British Children, 1965, *Arch. Dis. Child.* **41**:454–471, 613–635.

IV

SELECTED ASPECTS OF THERAPY

Drugs and Renal Failure and Acute Problems during Hemodialysis

37

Drug-Induced Nephrotoxicity

Mark H. Gardenswartz, Jan P. Goldberg, and Robert W. Schrier

Physicians have become increasingly aware that the promise and potential of the current pharmacopeia is but one blade of a double-edged sword. Drug-induced disease is an alarming problem in every area of medical endeavor and indeed has had a major impact on the incidence, nature, and natural history of commonly encountered renal disease (Table 1). The broad array of modern nephrotoxins includes, among others, the penicillin homologues and antifungal, antiinflammatory, and antineoplastic agents. However, this introduction will concentrate on the two classes of drugs of greatest epidemiologic importance, i.e., radioiodinated contrast materials and aminoglycoside antibiotics.

1. Radioiodinated Contrast Materials

Since the introduction of contrast media over 50 years ago, their use has become indispensable in routine diagnostic evaluation. A variety of procedures, including urography, cholecystography and cholangiography, angiography, and computed tomography, are widely employed, and the contrast agents utilized are generally well tolerated. However, in a small percentage of all patients undergoing such examinations, acute deterioration of renal function occurs (Table 2). The recognition that in some patients the risk of renal injury is considerably greater has led to numerous case reports and series[1–4] and to reviews[1] and editorial comment.[5,6] Part of our purpose here is to review selected aspects of this entity and to identify questions that merit investigation. The proposed pathogenetic mechanisms are several, and as they will be discussed in depth by Dr. Cronin in Chapter

Mark H. Gardenswartz, Jan P. Goldberg, and Robert W. Schrier • Department of Medicine, University of Colorado Health Sciences Center, Denver, Colorado 80262.

Table 1. *Etiology of Acute Renal Failure*[a]

Source	Years	*n*	Percent acute renal failure: Toxin	Trauma	Surgery	Medical problems and sepsis	Misc.
Levinsky and Alexander[51]	1959–1972	2200	9	9	43	26	13
McMurray *et al.*[52]	1967–1975	276	11	18	42	23	5
Anderson *et al.*[28]	1975–1976	92	21	—	24	50	5
Galpin *et al.*[53]	1978	43	33	5	21	40	2

[a] Overall toxins: 261 out of 2611 = 10%. From ref. 50.

39, they will not be considered here. Therefore, the following remarks will summarize the clinical state of the art of contrast nephrotoxicity.

1.1. Risk Factors

Historically, the first patient subgroup to highlight the potential risk of contrast procedures was that of patients with multiple myeloma.[7,8] Subsequently, as hydration was demonstrated to ameliorate the nephrotoxic risk in this group of patients,[9–11] other risk factors became evident (Table 3). In an extensive recent review by Byrd and Sherman,[1] the accumulated experience from several recent series was collated, as shown in Table 4. A constellation of apparent risk factors has emerged, though in several cases the independent contribution of one factor to the patient's risk is difficult to discern.

Table 2. *Incidence of Acute Renal Failure after Contrast Procedures*[a]

Source	Year		No. studied	Cases of acute renal failure: No.	Percent
Metys *et al.*[54]	1971	Angiogram	110	0	0
Reiss *et al.*[55]	1972	Angiogram	2,710	8	0.29
Port *et al.*[56]	1974	Angiogram	7,400	8	0.1
Older *et al.*[57]	1976	Angiogram	90	9	10
Swartz *et al.*[58]	1977	Angiogram	109	14	13
Byrd and Sherman[1]	1978	IVP, angiogram, CAT, OCG	12,000	18	0.15
Krumlovsky[17]	1978	IVP, angiogram, OCG, IVC	7,125	8	0.11

[a] From ref. 1.

Table 3. Frequency of Known and Suspected Risk Factors[a]

1.	Advanced age (mean = 70 years, range = 28–87) 60 years or older	18/23	(78%)
2.	Prior renal insufficiency (S_{cr} 1.6 mg/dl or over)	16/24	(67%)
3.	Dehydration (examination, I/O, weights)	14/24	(58%)
4.	Hyperuricemia (8.0 mg/dl or over)	12/24	(50%)
5.	Diabetes mellitus	9/24	(37%)
6.	Multiple-contrast exposure within 24 hr	8/24	(33%)
7.	Proteinuria (over 1 g/24 hr)	5/24	(21%)
8.	Hypoalbuminemia	4/24	(17%)
9.	Multiple myeloma	1/24	(4%)

[a] From ref. 1.

1.1.1. *Prior Renal Insufficiency*

Prior renal insufficiency is now well accepted as a factor predisposing to radiocontrast nephrotoxicity. Early reports that urography in azotemic patients was not particularly hazardous[(12,13)] have been contradicted in several more recent series, in which the incidence of preexisting renal insufficiency ranged from 50% to 76% percent.[(1,14–17)] In one series[(1)] the only risk factor that occurred by itself was prior renal insufficiency. In a recent prospective survey by Shafi *et al.*[(2)] pre- and posturographic renal function was analyzed in 40 patients with chronic renal insufficiency. A 25% loss of renal function was observed in 11 of 12 diabetic patients (92%) (Fig. 1) and in 17 of 28 nondiabetic patients (61%) (Fig. 2). This incidence in nondiabetic azotemic

Table 4. Clinical Course and Risk Factors in Recent Series of Heterogeneous Patient Populations[a]

	Byrd and Sherman[(1)] (n = 24)	Alexander *et al.*[(14)] (n = 7)	Krumlovsky *et al.*[(17)] (n = 14)	Ansari and Baldwin[(15)] (n = 25)
Advanced age (mean)	70	63	64	62
· age 60 or over	80%	72%	64%	76%
Prior renal insufficiency	67%	72%	50%	76%
· S_{cr} (predye)	2.0	2.9	2.4	2.4
Dehydration	58%	57%	"Frequent"	36%
Diabetes mellitus	37%	43%	21%	44%
Hyperuricemia	50%	40%	29%	—
Hypertension	—	86%	—	—
S_{cr} (mg/dl)				
Range	2.0–8.8	2.5–12.0	1.5–7.2	2.6–11.6
Mean	4.0	6.8	4.2	5.6
Return to predye S_{cr}	80%	72%	79%	64%
Dialysis required	0%	43%	7%	8%
Mortality	4%[b]	0%	0%	20%

[a] From ref. 1.
[b] Death not directly caused by renal failure.

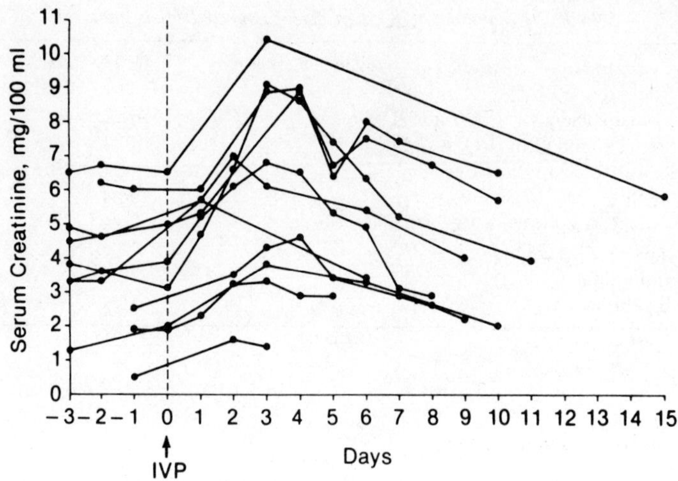

Figure 1. Radiocontrast nephrotoxicity in diabetic patients with chronic renal insufficiency. Serial serum creatinine levels from before and after excretory urography. (From ref. 2.)

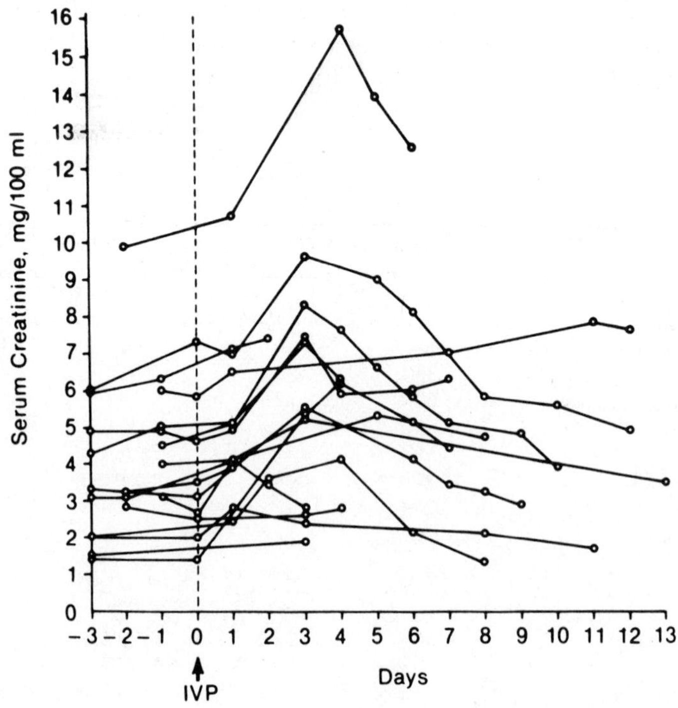

Figure 2. Radiocontrast nephrotoxicity in nondiabetic patients with chronic renal insufficiency. Serial serum creatinine levels from before and after excretory urography. (From ref. 2.)

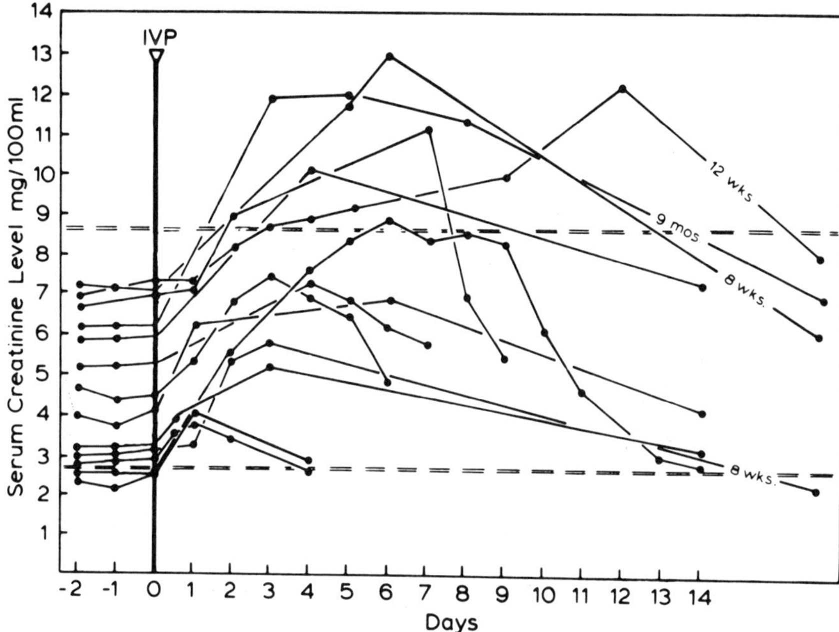

Figure 3. Reversible radiocontrast-induced renal deterioration in diabetic patients with chronic renal insufficiency. Serial serum creatinine levels from before and after excretory urography. (From ref. 19.)

patients was somewhat unexpected, but underscores the risk of urography in this group of patients.

1.1.2. *Diabetes Mellitus*

Diabetes mellitus has been recognized recently as a major risk factor, particularly in patients with diabetic nephropathy and prior renal insufficiency. Although several series have documented a predictable, alarming risk of acute renal deterioration in azotemic diabetics,[1,2,15,18–21] (Figs. 3–5), 11% of the diabetic patients with contrast nephrotoxicity in the literature did not have preexisting renal insufficiency.[1] The increased risk of contrast radiography in diabetics is particularly unfortunate in view of their incidence of generalized and coronary vascular disease and of renal and urologic disease which often necessitates such examinations.

1.1.3. *Advanced Age*

Advanced age has been a prevalent finding in a number of series reporting contrast nephrotoxicity. Whether this reflects merely the older age of patients examined with contrast media or actually represents an increased susceptibility to toxic renal injury in the aged is unclear. The latter possibility

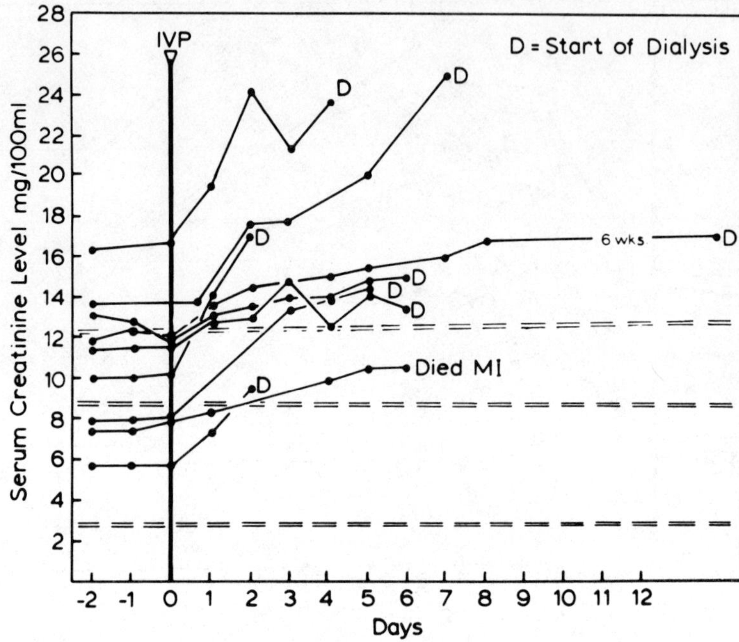

Figure 4. Irreversible radiocontrast-induced renal deterioration in diabetic patients with chronic renal insufficiency. Serial serum creatinine levels from before and after excretory urography. D represents the starting of dialysis. (From ref. 19.)

could result from underlying vascular disease in the elderly, or from an age-associated decrease in renal function. That vascular disease may contribute to the risk of contrast radiography has been suggested by Shafi *et al.*(2) and Heneghan(5) and is supported by the prominence of hypertension and diabetes in the profile of patients affected with contrast nephrotoxicity.

1.1.4. Other Factors

Other factors have been suggested as contributing to the risk of contrast nephrotoxicity, including hypertension, dehydration, and hyperuricemia. Hypertension has been considered a prominent risk factor,(2,20) but its common occurrence with renal insufficiency and/or diabetes precludes quantitation of its role. Dehydration is thought to compound the existing risks in susceptible patients, though this also is unproven,(19) and adequate hydration does not necessarily protect against renal failure.(2,15,18,20,22) Hyperuricemia generally occurs against a background of renal insufficiency and/or dehydration, and the case for its independent contribution to radiocontrast-induced acute renal failure is similarly tenuous. Other risk factors which have been proposed, but whose independent contribution is probably negligible, include high dose of contrast, impaired hepatic function, congestive heart failure, and hypoalbuminemia.

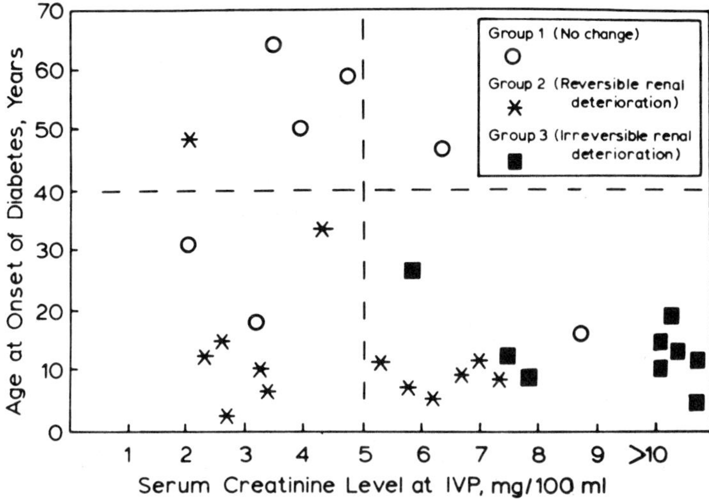

Figure 5. The distribution of patients in the three groups plotted versus age at onset of diabetes and serum creatinine levels at time of intravenous pyelography. Age at onset of diabetes of below 40 years is associated with a high incidence of renal failure. If the creatinine level is also above 5 mg/100 ml, the risk of sustaining irreversible renal failure increases considerably. All patients who sustained irreversible damage had the onset of diabetes at less than 40 years of age and had a creatinine level of 5 mg/100 ml or more. (From ref. 19.)

1.2. Clinical Features

Whatever the clinical setting, radiocontrast-induced acute renal failure generally presents with oliguria, though a nonoliguric presentation is not rare (Table 5). In fact, the proportion of affected patients whose urine output remains adequate may depend somewhat on the vigor with which evidence of decreased renal function is sought. In the prospective survey of Shafi *et al.*[(2)] in which patients with preexisting renal insufficiency were studied closely for evidence of renal failure, the affected group nevertheless maintained a urine output of approximately 1200 ml/day. This series supports the contention that many episodes of nonoliguric radiocontrast-induced acute renal failure escape our clinical recognition. Whether oliguric or

Table 5. Clinical Characteristics of Radiocontrast-Induced Acute Renal Failure

1. Oliguric more often than nonoliguric
2. Rapid onset—within 24 hr
3. May have low U_{Na}, FE_{Na}
4. Serum creatinine peaks within 1 week
5. Moderate severity—usually self-limited
6. Return to baseline serum creatinine in greater than 75%
7. Mortality—less than 5–10%

nonoliguric, radiocontrast-induced acute renal failure occurs soon after the examination and generally peaks within the first week thereafter. Though the clinical syndrome is generally that of "acute tubular necrosis (ATN)," some oliguric patients have been reported with urine sodium concentrations of less than 20 meq/liter[16] and a persistently low fractional excretion of sodium.[23]

The serum creatinine eventually returns to baseline in more than 75% of cases, though permanent renal injury, and the need for acute and chronic dialysis, are well documented.[1,19,21] The management of radiocontrast-induced acute renal failure is identical to that of acute renal failure of any other cause, though this syndrome tends to be of mild to moderate severity and is usually self-limited. Its mortality is less than 5–10% in most centers. Clearly the best approach lies in the attempt to avert this problem though an appreciation of its clinical setting, minimization of pertinent risk factors, and abstemious use of radiocontrast procedures unless the information gained is clearly necessary for the patient's best interest.

2. *Aminoglycoside Antibiotics*

The other class of nephrotoxic agents that is of compelling epidemiologic importance is that of the aminoglycoside antibiotics. Aminoglycosides have formed the cornerstone of therapy in the treatment of gram-negative infection over the past two decades. Now that gram-negative organisms account for the majority of hospital-acquired infections, there is little doubt that the use of these agents will increase. Current evidence suggests that aminoglycosides are indeed nephrotoxic in therapeutic doses.[24,25] At present, 16–30% of acute renal failure is due to nephrotoxic medications, and aminoglycosides account for the majority of these agents.[26–28]

2.1. *Incidence*

The incidence of aminoglycoside nephrotoxicity appears to be increasing.[29] In Fig. 6 the incidence of nephrotoxicity is presented from several papers and abstracts over the last 10 years. This evident increase in the incidence of nephrotoxicity probably relates to several factors. First, the more prevalent usage of these drugs and a higher dosage and longer duration of therapy have resulted in an increased incidence. In addition, our recognition of the problem has been facilitated by more frequent monitoring of renal function.

2.2. *Histology*

The histologic lesion of aminoglycoside nephrotoxicity affects the proximal tubule primarily, with occurrence of cellular necrosis, and the earlier ultrastructural appearance of myeloid bodies.[25,27] These "myelinlike"

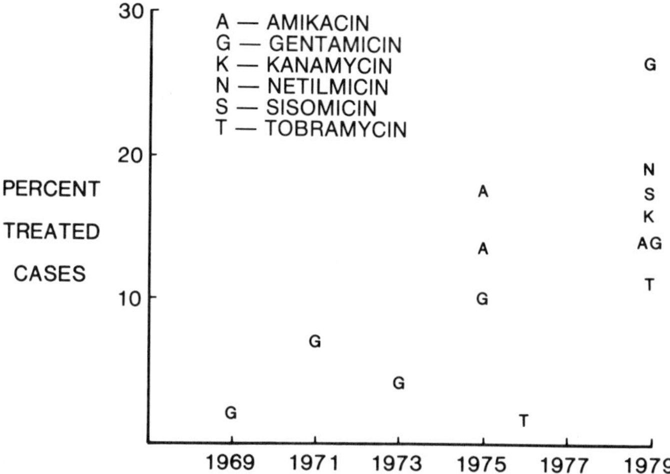

Figure 6. Aminoglycoside nephrotoxicity—incidence during the past decade. Data from several papers and abstracts covering this period. (With permission from R. Gronin.)

whorls, which represent the lysosomal ingestion of phospholipid membranes, are believed to be a histologic marker of drug administration and tissue uptake but do not necessarily correlate with the degree of toxicity.[25] Study of the glomeruli, even with electron microscopy, has failed to show glomerular histologic damage, despite the physiologic finding of a decreased glomerular capillary ultrafiltration coefficient in this entity.[30]

2.3. *Renal Tissue Binding*

The extent of aminoglycoside nephrotoxicity has been correlated with both the number of free amino groups on the antibiotic molecule[31,32] and the degree of renal cortical tissue binding of the drug. This latter correlation, though imperfect (netilmicin appears to be less nephrotoxic than gentamicin despite comparable tissue binding),[33,34] has important clinical implications. As a result of tissue binding, parenchymal drug levels may be concentrated 20-fold over serum levels.[35] After a single injection, the half-life of gentamicin in serum is 30 min, but in renal tissue it is 109 hr.[32] The observation that acute renal failure can occur after discontinuation of the aminoglycoside, and that recent exposure to aminoglycosides is a risk factor for nephrotoxicity, can be explained by the long tissue half-life of these drugs.

2.4. *Clinical Features*

Aminoglycoside nephrotoxicity presents as renal insufficiency with other characteristic abnormalities (Table 6). The urinalysis may demonstrate cylindruria, proteinuria, glycosuria, and enzymuria.[36] Urinary concentrating

Table 6. Aminoglycoside Nephrotoxicity

1. Reduce glomerular filtration rate
2. Impair urinary concentration
3. Enzymuria
4. Proteinuria
5. Glycosuria
6. Electrolyte abnormalities

ability is also impaired.[29] Azotemia ensues, and characteristic electrolyte abnormalities, including hypokalemia, may occur. In a more chronic setting, hypomagnesemia, hypocalcemia, and metabolic alkalosis have been demonstrated.[37,38]

Two clinical patterns of nephrotoxicity have been observed.[39] The first pattern is usually gradual in onset, with a transient rise in the serum creatinine, which rapidly reverses with cessation of the drug. This type may occur in the absence of predisposing risk factors and may result from inadvertent overdosage. Its incidence is 5–10% of the patients so treated.[39] The second pattern is characterized by the acute loss of renal function, often with oliguria, which occurs in the setting of concomitant risk factors. Experience with this syndrome suggests that the entity is generally self-limited and of moderate severity, with a mortality of 15–20%.[28,40]

2.5. *Risk Factors*

2.5.1. *Drug Dose and Age*

Factors known to predispose patients to the development of aminoglycoside toxicity are listed in (Table 7).[26] The dose and duration of the aminoglycoside probably are most important in determining nephrotoxicity.[29] The incidence of nephrotoxicity significantly increases with amikacin with advancing age. Lane *et al.*[41] found a 7% incidence of nephrotoxicity in patients aged 16–30 years, whereas in patients older than age 75 years there was an incidence of 20% (Fig. 7).[41] Failure to decrease drug dosage

Table 7. Risk Factors for Aminoglycoside Nephrotoxicity

1. Dose and duration of aminoglycoside
2. Renal insufficiency
3. Advancing age
4. Recent exposure to other nephrotoxins
   a. Prior aminoglycosides
   b. X-ray contrast
   c. Anesthetic agents
   d. Diuretic agents
5. Combined use of aminoglycoside and cephalosporin
6. Potassium depletion

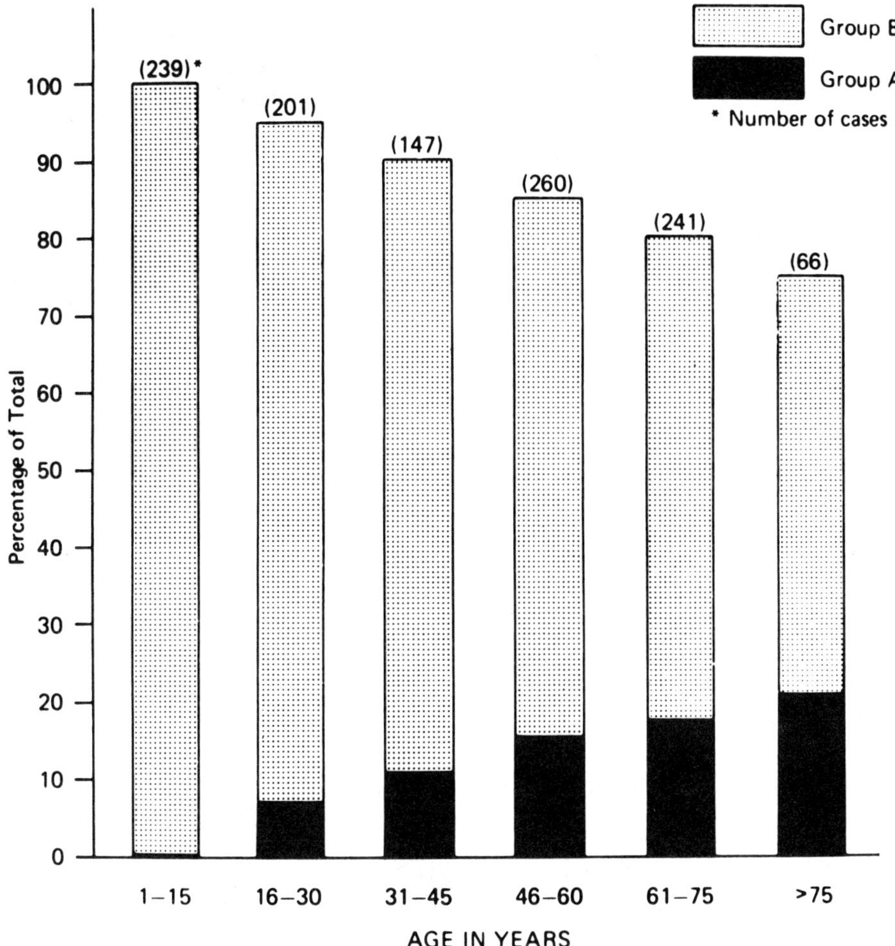

Figure 7. Amikacin nephrotoxicity—importance of age as a risk factor. Shown are percentage of each age bracket in which renal functional deterioration developed (group A) or did not develop (group B). (From ref. 41.)

in proportion to the reduced glomerular filtration rate seen with advancing age is believed to be responsible, at least partially, for this problem.

2.5.2. *Renal Impairment*

Prior renal insufficiency is another factor predisposing to aminoglycoside nephrotoxicity. A 20% incidence of nephrotoxicity was seen in patients with a serum creatinine of 2.0 mg% prior to antibiotic administration compared to an 8% incidence of nephrotoxicity in patients with an initial serum creatinine less than 1.3 mg% (Fig. 8).[41]

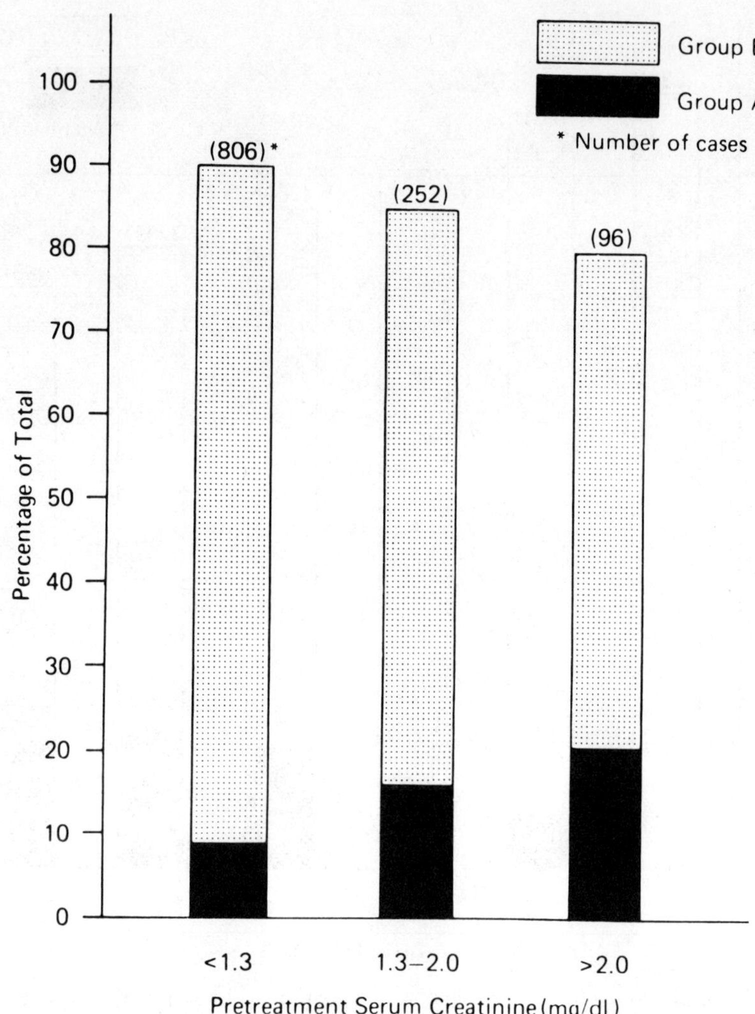

Figure 8. Amikacin nephrotoxicity—importance of prior renal insufficiency as a risk factor. Shown are percentage of patients, arranged by pretreatment serum creatinine, whose renal function deteriorated (group A) or did not deteriorate (group B). (From ref. 41.)

2.5.3. *Volume Depletion and Furosemide*

Sodium restriction and volume depletion, which have been shown to increase cortical parenchymal drug concentration, are associated with an increased incidence of aminoglycoside toxicity.[35] By extension, furosemide is thought to enhance kanamycin nephrotoxicity through its volume-depletion effection, though direct toxicity cannot be excluded.[42] Antecedent exposure to other nephrotoxic agents such as anesthetics, contrast media, and other aminoglycosides was shown to increase the incidence of amikacin nephro-

Table 8. Prospective Studies of Aminoglycoside–Cephalosporin Nephrotoxicity

	Aminoglycoside + cephalosporin (%)	Aminoglycoside + penicillin (%)
Klastersky *et al.*[46]	21	6[a]
EORTC[59]	16	6[a]
Wade *et al.*[45]	26	7[a]

[a] $p < 0.05$; EORTC, European Organization for Research and Treatment of Cancer.

toxicity from 7% in amikacin-treated patients without other toxic exposure to 22% in patients so exposed.[41]

2.5.4. *Cephalosporins*

The issue of whether cephalosporins enhance or diminish aminoglycoside nephrotoxicity is not settled. Animal studies suggest that cephalosporins may protect against aminoglycoside toxicity by decreasing aminoglycoside renal cortical tissue concentration.[43,44] Although previous clinical data had been controversial, a recent prospective, randomized, double-blind clinical trial comparing cephalothin plus an aminoglycoside to methicillin plus an aminoglycoside has clearly demonstrated a highly significant increase in aminoglycoside nephrotoxicity, 25.5% versus 7%.[45] This is in agreement with previous clinical studies (Table 8).[46] Recent animal evidence indicates that not only is hypokalemia a consequence of gentamicin nephrotoxicity, but that potassium depletion itself may enhance aminoglycoside toxicity.[29]

2.6. Monitoring for Nephrotoxicity

The widespread use of aminoglycosides, with their potential for good and harm, makes the monitoring of a marker of toxicity necessary and desirable. Though the routine measurement of serum antibiotic levels has been advocated,[27,36,39,47] the true value of such determinations has been questioned.[26,48] This skepticism has resulted, in part, from the dissociation of peak serum levels of gentamicin from nephrotoxicity in rats.[48] In addition, since the aminoglycosides primarily are filtered and excreted, much as is creatinine, a case has been made for the measurement of serum creatinine rather than following rising serum through drug levels for nephrotoxicity.[26] The actual clinical value of serum antibiotic levels thus awaits appropriate clinical study.

Other means of predicting nephrotoxicity have been sought. One animal study has demonstrated that early in the course of gentamicin nephrotoxicity the urinary excretion of α_2-microglobulin, β-glucuronidase, and other proximal tubular enzymes often preceded azotemia by several days.[29,49]

Table 9. Guidelines for Aminoglycoside Administration[a]

1. Maintain an expanded extracellular fluid volume
2. Adjust dose to glomerular filtration rate, especially in elderly, before and during therapy
3. Use with caution when an aminoglycoside has been given recently or in the presence of other nephrotoxic agents (antibiotics, anesthetics, X-ray contrast)
4. Using culture results, establish clear guidelines for continuation or discontinuation of aminoglycoside when therapy was begun empirically

[a] From ref. 26.

Though this technique may be too sensitive to be practical, it holds promise for future investigation.

Since prevention is always the best form of clinical management, reasonable guidelines to minimize aminoglycoside nephrotoxicity are presented in Table 9.

3. Summary

The previous discussion has summarized the clinical aspects of two types of common nephrotoxins. Our understanding of these entities is based, in large part, on empiric and retrospective observations. Though valuable, the instruction from this kind of experience is inherently limited. Though considerable progress has resulted from decades of disciplined clinical and laboratory investigation, the state of our ignorance remains profound. There is a sense of challenge in identifying the necessary questions and promoting their resolution about such examples of nephrotoxicity.

References

1. Byrd L, Sherman RL: Radiocontrast-induced acute renal failure: A clinical and pathophysiologic review. *Medicine* 58:270, 1979.
2. Shafi T, Chan SY, Porush JG, Shapiro W: Infusion intravenous pyelography and renal function. Effects in patients with chronic renal insufficiency. *Arch Intern Med* 138:1218, 1978.
3. Vesely DL, Mintz DH: Acute renal failure in insulin-dependent diabetics. Episodes secondary to intravenous pyelography. *Arch Intern Med* 138:1858, 1978.
4. Meeker TC, Ludwig S, Glimp R: Computerized axial tomography and acute renal failure. *JAMA* 240:2247, 1978.
5. Heneghan M: Contrast-induced acute renal failure. *Am J Roentgenol* 131:1113, 1978.
6. Wagoner RD: Acute renal failure associated with contrast agents. *Arch Intern Med* 138:353, 1978.
7. Brown M, Battle JD: Effect of urography on renal function in patients with multiple myeloma. *Canad Med Assoc J* 91:786, 1964.
8. Rees E, Waugh WH: Factors in renal failure in multiple myeloma. *Arch Intern Med* 116:400, 1965.
9. Vix VA: Intravenous pyelography in multiple myeloma: A review of 52 studies in 40 patients. *Radiology* 87:896, 1966.

10. Morgan C Jr, Hammack WJ: Intravenous urography in multiple myeloma. *N Engl J Med* 275:77, 1966.
11. Myers GH, Witten DM: Acute renal failure after excretory urography in multiple myeloma. *Am J Roentgenol* 113:583, 1971.
12. Schwartz WB, Hurwit A, Ettinger A: Intravenous urography in the patient with renal insufficiency. *N Engl J Med* 269:277, 1963.
13. Ensor RD, Anderson EE, Robinson RR: Drip infusion urography in patients with renal disease. *J Urol* 103:267, 1970.
14. Alexander RD, Beckes SL, Abuelo JG: Contrast media-induced oliguric renal failure. *Arch Intern Med* 138:381, 1978.
15. Ansari Z, Baldwin DS: Acute renal failure due to radiocontrast agents. *Nephron* 17:28, 1976.
16. Carvallo A, Rakowski TA, Argy WP, Schreiner GE: Acute renal failure during drip infusion pyelography. *Am J Med* 65:38, 1975.
17. Krumlovsky FA, Simon N, Santhanam S, de Greco F, Roxe D, Pomaranc MM: Acute renal failure—association with administration of radiographic contrast material. *JAMA* 239:125, 1978.
18. Diaz–Buxo JA, Wagoner RD, Hattery RR, Palumbo PJ: Acute renal failure after excretory urography in diabetic patients. *Ann Intern Med* 83:155, 1975.
19. Harkonen S, Kjellstrand CM: Exacerbation of diabetic renal failure following intravenous pyelography. *Am J Med* 63:939, 1977.
20. VanZee BE, Hay WE, Talley TE, Jaenike JR: Renal injury associated with intravenous pyelography in nondiabetic and diabetic patients. *Ann Intern Med* 89:51, 1978.
21. Weinrauch LA, Healy RW, Leland OS, Goldstein HH, Kassissieh SD, Libertino JA, Takacs FJ, D'Elia JA: Coronary angiography and acute renal failure in diabetic azotemic nephropathy. *Ann Intern Med* 86:56, 1977.
22. Pillary VKG, Robbins PC, Schwartz FD, Kark RM: Acute renal failure following intravenous urography in patients with long-standing diabetes mellitus and azotemia. *Radiology* 95:633, 1970.
23. Coggins C: Nephrotoxicity of radiographic contrast media in acute renal failure due to common pharmacologic agents in: *American Society of Nephrology Symposium*, Boston, 1979.
24. Gary NE, Buzzio L, Salaki J, Eisinger RP: Gentamicin-associated acute renal failure. *Arch Intern Med* 136:1101, 1976.
25. Kosek JC, Mazze RI, Cousins MJ: Nephrotoxicity of gentamicin. *Lab Invest* 30:48, 1974.
26. Cronin RE: Aminoglycoside nephrotoxicity: Pathogenesis and prevention. *Clin Nephrol* 11:251, 1979.
27. Bennett WM, Plomp C, Porter GA: Drug-related syndromes. *Ann Intern Med* 87:582, 1977.
28. Anderson RJ, Linas SL, Berns AS, Henrich WL, Miller TR, Gabow PA, Schrier RW: Nonoliguric acute renal failure. *N Engl J Med* 296:1134, 1977.
29. Brinker K, Cronin R, Bulger R, Southern P, Henrich W: Potassium (K) depletion: Risk factor for and consequence of gentamicin (G) nephrotoxicity in: *American Society of Nephrology Symposium*, Boston, 1979. p 79A (abstract).
30. Baylis C, Rennke HR, Brenner BM: Mechanisms of the defect in glomerular ultrafiltration associated with gentamicin administration. *Kidney Int* 12:344, 1977.
31. Kunin CM: Binding of antibiotics to tissue homogenates. *J Infect Dis* 121:55, 1970.
32. Luft FC, Kleit SA: Renal parenchymal accumulation of aminoglycoside antibiotics in rats. *J Infect Dis* 130:656, 1974.
33. Luft FC, Yum MN, Kleit SA: Comparative nephrotoxicities of netilmicin and gentamicin in rats. *Antimicrob Agents Chemother* 10:845, 1976.
34. Kaloyanides GJ, Bowman R, Silverblatt F: Effect of gentamicin and netilmicin on renal function in the rat. *Clin Res* 25:138A, 1977 (abstract).
35. Bennett WM, Hartnett MN, Gilbert D, Houghton D, Porter GA: Effect of sodium intake on gentamicin nephrotoxicity in the rat. *Proc Soc Exp Biol Med* 151:736, 1976.
36. Appel GB, Neu HC: The nephrotoxicity of antimicrobial agents. *N Engl J Med* 296:722, 1977 (second of three parts).

37. Bar RS, Wilson HE, Mazzafein EL: Hypomagnesemic hypocalcemia secondary to renal magnesium wasting: A possible consequence of high dose gentamicin therapy. *Ann Intern Med* 82:646, 1975.
38. Holmes AM, Hesling CM, Wilson TM: Drug induced secondary hyperaldosteronism in patients with pulmonary tuberculosis. *Quart J Med* 39:299, 1970.
39. Hewlitt WL: Gentamicin: Toxicity in perspective. *Postgrad Med J* 50(suppl 7):55, 1974.
40. Schrier RW: Acute renal failure. *Kidney Int* 15:205, 1979.
41. Lane AZ, Wright GE, Blair DC: Ototoxicity and nephrotoxicity of amikacin, in: Proceedings of the U.S. Amikacin Symposium, University of California Medical School, Los Angeles, Nov. 9–10, 1976. *Am J Med* 62:911, 1977.
42. Lawson DH, Macadam RF, Singh H, Gavras H, Hartz S, Turnbull D, Linton AL: Effect of furosemide on antibiotic-induced renal damage in rats. *J Infect Dis* 126:593, 1972.
43. Dellinger P, Murphy T, Pinn V, Barza M, Weinstein L: The protective effect of cephalothin against gentamicin-induced nephrotoxicity in rats. *Antimicrob Agents Chemother* 9:172, 1976.
44. Harrison WO, Silverblatt FJ, Turck M: Gentamicin nephrotoxicity: Failure of three cephalosporins to potentiate injury in rats. *Antimicrob Agents Chemother* 8:209, 1975.
45. Wade JC, Petty BG, Conrad G, Smith CR, Wade JC, Petty BG, Conrad G, Smith CR, Lipsky JJ, Ellner J, and Leitman P: Cephalothin plus an aminoglycoside is more nephrotoxic than methicillin plus an aminoglycoside. *Lancet* 2:604, 1978.
46. Klastersky J, Hensgens C, Debusscher L: Empiric therapy for cancer patients: Comparative study of ticarcillin–tobramycin, ticarcillin–cephalothin, and cephalothin–tobramycin. *Antimicrob Agents Chemother* 7:640, 1975.
47. Dahlgren JG, Anderson ET, Hewitt WL: Gentamicin blood levels: A guide to nephrotoxicity. *Antimicrob Agents Chemother* 8:58, 1975.
48. Plomp C, Bennett W, Gilbert D, Porter G: The effect of dosage regimen on experimental gentamicin nephrotoxicity: Dissociation of peak serum levels from renal failure. *Clin Res* 26:125A, 1978 (abstract).
49. Adelman RD, Counzelman G, Spangle W, Ishizaki G: Enzymes: An early sign of gentamicin nephrotoxicity. *Kidney Int* 10:493A, 1976.
50. Bennett WM: *American Society of Nephrology Symposium*, Boston, 1979.
51. Levinsky NG, Alexander EA: Acute renal failure, in: Brenner BM, Rector FC (eds): *The Kidney*, Vol 2. Philadelphia, W. B. Saunders, 1976, p 806.
52. McMurray SD, Luft FC, Maxwell DR, Hamburger RJ, *et al*: Prevailing patterns and predictor variables in patients with acute tubular necrosis. *Arch Intern Med* 138:950, 1978.
53. Galpin JE, Shinaberger JH, Stankey TM, Blumenkrantz MJ, *et al*: Acute interstitial nephritis due to methicillen. *Am J Med* 65:756, 1978.
54. Metys R, Hornych A, Burianova B, Jirka J: Influence of triiodinated contrast media on renal function. *Nephron* 8:559, 1971.
55. Reiss MD, Bookstein JJ, Bleifer KH: Radiology aspects of renovascular hypertension. *JAMA* 221:375, 1972.
56. Port FK, Wagoner RD, Fulton RE: Acute renal failure after angiography. *Am J Roentgenol* 121:544, 1974.
57. Older RA, Miller JP, Jackson DC, Johnsrude IS, Thompson, WM: Angiographically induced renal failure and its radiographic detection. *Am J Roentgenol* 126:1039, 1976.
58. Swartz R, Rubin J, Leeming B, Silva P: Renal failure following major angiography. *Am J Med* 65:31, 1978.
59. European Organization for Research on Treatment of Cancer (EORTC): Three antibiotic regimens in the treatment of infection in febrile granulocytopenic patients with cancer. *J Inf Dis* 137:14, 1978.

38

Antibiotic Management of Urinary Tract Infection in the Chronic Renal Failure Patient

William M. Bennett

Preservation of renal function in patients with established renal failure is an important goal in overall management, even in patients who require maintenance dialysis. Although hypertension and obstruction have been identified as reversible causes of deterioration in renal function, urinary tract infection has received little attention. In patients undergoing renal transplantation, the native kidneys might serve as a source of sepsis for the immunosuppressed recipient. In addition, bacterial antigens in the renal parenchyma could trigger rejection episodes. These theoretic possibilities have led to pretransplant bilateral nephrectomy in patients known to have active or remote urinary tract infection. Therapy of such patients with antibiotics has not been examined critically especially in the context of recent knowledge concerning the renal handling of antibiotics in patients with normal and impaired renal function.

Patients with polycystic kidney disease represent a special challenge since, in this patient group, residual cystic kidneys may provide the patient with enough excretory function to allow a liberal sodium intake and enough erythropoietic stimulus to avoid anemia. The management of infection in these patients can be difficult since individual cysts may harbor bacteria even when the urine is sterile and the patient is without symptoms. Renal transplantation in such a patient could prove hazardous although this point has not been conclusively established.

William M. Bennett • Division of Nephrology, Department of Medicine, Oregon Health Sciences University, Portland, Oregon 97201.

1. *Urinary Infection in the Presence of Renal Failure*

A substantial percentage of patients with urinary tract infections have involvement of the renal parenchyma, and relapse rates are high if antibiotic therapy is not prolonged.[1,2] Suboptimal concentrations of antibiotics might be present in patients such as those with advanced renal insufficiency and consequently impaired ability to filter, concentrate, or transport antimicrobials. In addition, there is considerable variability among antibiotics in the drug levels achieved in the medullary–papillary region of the kidney, which is the main site of bacterial infection.[3] In the case of systemic infection, the potential difficulties secondary to renal failure can be circumvented by careful adjustment of drug dosage when necessary to provide adequate serum and tissue levels without drug accumulation and toxicity.[4] However by adjusting dosage to prevent extrarenal toxicity, inadequate levels of drug may be present in the urine. Stamey *et al.* have shown that urinary drug concentrations showed a greater correlation with bacteriologic cure than with concomitant serum levels, even in upper-tract infection.[1,5] Furthermore, the presence of advanced renal disease may impair drug transport or diffusion from the blood to the site of infection even with therapeutic serum levels.

Kunin has outlined the characteristics an ideal drug should have to be effective in the urine of uremic patients. These include (1) lack of toxicity even at high serum levels so that no adjustment is needed with low glomerular filtration rates, (2) excretion unchanged in the urine and, thus, little metabolism or inactivation, and (3) renal handling by tubular secretion so that high levels are achieved in the urine.[6] There are few correlative studies relating such pharmacologic studies with clinical infections. Susceptibility testing and, indeed, drug measurement in urine, serum, and tissue from uremic patients have not been evaluated rigorously in comparison to similar studies in subjects without renal disease.

2. *Aminoglycoside Antibiotics*

With gentamicin prescribed in doses adjusted for renal insufficiency, Whelton *et al.*[7] and Bennett *et al.*[8] have demonstrated inconsistent urine concentrations below the minimum inhibitory concentrations of some urinary pathogens.[7,8] Subtherapeutic tissue levels were present in the kidneys of subjects undergoing surgery for kidney removal prior to transplant.[8] In some instances gentamicin therapy resulted in failure to eradicate infection despite adequate serum levels. These data are presented in Table 1. Although the urine levels achieved were above the minimum inhibitory levels of 6.25 μg/ml reported to kill 97% of 150 strains of *Pseudomonas aeruginosa*,[9] vascular disease. In normal man and experimental animals, aminoglycosides are largely excreted by glomerular filtration. Accumulation of a small percentage of drug by luminal and perhaps antiluminal active uptake results in renal

Table 1. Gentamicin Therapy for Urinary Infections in Patients with Severe Renal Failure[a]

GFR (ml/min)	n	Serum conc. (μg/ml)	Urine conc. (μg/ml)	Tissue conc. (μg/ml)		Clinical outcome (cures/treated)	
				Cortex	Medulla	Upper tract	Lower tract
3.3	10	4.1	8.7	1.2	0.7	—	—
7.6	5	3.5	21.6	—	—	2/3	1/2

[a] From ref. 8.

cortical concentrations 20-fold greater than in serum. Medullary uptake is fivefold less in normal kidney tissue and is reduced further in parenchymal disease.(3,7)

Miller and associates reported experimental evidence relating persistence of bacteria in the renal parenchyma to the concentration of gentamicin present 2 weeks after a full course of treatment in the rat. Renal cortex demonstrated bactericidal concentrations of drug while the drug concentrations were inadequate in the medulla.(10) Despite an extensive literature about aminoglycoside pharmacology in experimental animals, more work is needed in models of renal and extrarenal infection.

Since other aminoglycosides are handled similarly by the kidney, it is expected that other members of this class of antibiotic would behave in a like manner. Recently, low urinary netilmicin concentrations and treatment failures were reported in patients with complicated urinary tract infections and renal dysfunction.(11)

3. *Penicillins and Cephalosporins*

Oral penicillins and cephalosporins given in ordinary doses to uremic patients result in only modest accumulation in the serum and adequate therapeutic concentrations in the urine.(12) The peak in urinary concentration may be delayed somewhat as compared to that in patients with normal renal function. In patients with more severe renal failure, Bennett and Craven demonstrated bacteriologic cure of both upper and lower urinary tract infections with amipicillin prescribed in the same dosage as would be given to nonuremic subjects. No extra renal toxicity was noted.(13) Similar data ideally should be given for newer penicillins and cephalosporins as they are released. The beneficial therapeutic effects of these drugs may be due to active tubular secretion resulting in relatively high urinary levels. In addition, penicillins and cephalosporins concentrate in medullary–papillary regions to levels up to 10 times serum values. This concentration is enhanced by hydropenia and alkaline urine and reduced by hydration.(3)

4. *Sulfonamides and Trimethoprim–Sulfamethoxazole*

In a fashion similar to penicillins and cephalosporins, therapeutic urinary concentrations of sulfonamides can be achieved in the urine of uremic subjects, provided ordinary doses are administered. The appearance of adequate drug in the urine may be delayed until high blood concentrations are reached. In combination with trimethoprim (TMP), urine concentrations of this useful combination exceeded minimum inhibitory concentrations of urinary pathogens resulting in bacteriologic cure.[13] The sulfamethoxazole concentration rose in the serum whereas both sulfamethoxazole and TMP urinary levels were lower when compared to normal subjects.[14] Since the usual synergistic ratio of sulfamethoxazole to TMP is 20 : 1, the good clinical responses may be due largely to TMP. Trials with TMP as a single agent may be particularly useful in patients with renal failure. Systemic acidosis and low urine pH retard sulfamethoxazole excretion, which may partially explain lowered urine sulfamethoxazole levels in uremic subjects.[14] The lower urine concentrations may be offset by the high serum and possibly parenchymal levels in uremics. Toxicity due to systemic reactions to sulfonamides should be anticipated. Elevations in serum creatinine *per se*, however, may simply reflect TMP competition with creatinine for tubular secretory sites and not true decreases in glomerular filtration rate.[15]

5. *Other Drugs*

Drugs with liver metabolism such as chloramphenicol, erythromycin, and nitrofurantoin do not achieve adequate urinary concentrations in the presence of renal failure. Nalidixic acid does appear in the urine in sufficient quantities; however, rapid emergence of bacterial resistance limits its utility. Tetracyclines generally are considered to aggravate symptoms of renal failure by worsening azotemia, acidosis, and hyperphosphatemia. Whelton *et al.* reported the similarity of renal concentrations of doxycycline in human diseased kidneys and in normal canine kidneys.[16] This member of the tetracycline family seems to be relatively free of systemic side effects and could prove useful to treat urinary infections in uremic subjects.

6. *Urinary Infections in Patients with Renal Cystic Disease*

Genitourinary infection is a major cause of morbidity in patients with renal cystic disease. Despite seemingly adequate antibiotic therapy, these infections usually persist and often progress, although the patient may become afebrile and asymptomatic. One recent report suggests that perinephric abscesses may develop in 60% of polycystic patients with urinary tract infections on chronic hemodialysis.[17] This difficult diagnosis may be aided by ^{67}Gal scintigraphy. Indeed, surgical drainage or nephrectomy may be

Table 2. Antibiotic Determinations in Patients with Simple Renal Cysts

Drug	Serum	Cyst[a]	Urine	Urine/serum	Cyst/serum	Cyst to urine
Gentamicin	3.7	0.4	135	36.5	0.10	0.003
Sulfamethoxazole	69	0	—	—	0	0
Trimethoprim	2.4	0	—	—	0	0

[a] Values represent means of three cysts; concentrations in μg/ml.

necessary to treat infections in both simple renal cysts and in polycystic kidney disease.(17,18)

There are several possible reasons to explain the refractory nature of these infections to antibiotics. Bacteria present within cysts may differ from those cultured from urine, fostering ineffective antibiotic therapy. Resistant microorganisms also may exist within these cysts. In addition, poor antibiotic penetrance into the renal cysts may contribute to the poor clinical response of these patients.

To examine this latter possibility, we measured the cyst fluid levels of a variety of antibiotics in four patients with simple renal cysts and in four patients with polycystic kidney disease (PCKD). Mean glomerular filtration rate (GFR) in patients with simple cysts was 63 ml/min, whereas in the patients with PCKD it was less than 10 ml/min.

Antibiotics were started 2 days prior to routine cyst puncture in patients with simple renal cysts. All patients with PCKD had been on therapeutic doses of antibiotics adjusted for renal failure for at least 5 days. Two patients required nephrectomy for progressive renal infection not responsive to antibiotics. Cyst fluid was obtained from these patients at the time of surgery. No patient received more than two antibiotics simultaneously.

The results in patients with simple renal cysts are shown in Table 2. Gentamicin was detected in only one of three cysts punctured. Mean cyst fluid concentration of gentamicin was only 10% that of serum and 0.3% that of urinary levels. TMP/sulfamethoxazole was given to one patient. Despite adequate serum levels, neither sulfamethoxasole nor TMP was detected in the cyst fluid.

The results in patients with PCKD are shown in Table 3. From 3 to 33 individual cysts were punctured in each patient with PCKD. Aminoglycoside antibiotics were found in low concentrations in the cysts of PCKD. Tobramycin averaged only 8% of serum levels and 1% of urine levels. The cyst fluid level of gentamicin averaged approximately one half that of serum levels. Sulfamethoxasole cyst fluid levels averaged 36% of serum and 23% of urinary levels. Despite high serum and urinary levels in one patient, cephapirin was poorly concentrated in cysts of his polycystic kidneys. Levels averaged 1% that of urine. In another patient, 49% of urine concentrations were found in cyst fluid.

Proximal and distal cysts in PCKD can be distinguished by cyst : serum sodium ratios, with values greater than 1 suggesting proximal cysts.(19)

Table 3. Antibiotic Determinations in Patients with Polycystic Renal Disease

Drug	n	Serum	Cyst[a]	Urine	Ratio U:S	Ratio Cy:S	Ratio Cy:U
Tobramycin	3	3.7 ± 0.3	0.3 ± 0.1	28 ± 5	7.6	0.08	0.01
Gentamicin	1	3.1	1.4	—	—	0.45	—
Sulfamethoxazole	1	28	10	43	1.5	0.36	0.23
Trimethoprim	1	0.6	0	0.6	1.	0	0
Cephapirin	2	105	15.6	1300	12.4	0.15	0.01
		27	10.5[b]	22	0.81	0.39	0.48

[a] Values are means of all cysts punctured (3–33). Units are μg/ml.
[b] Proximal cysts only.

Aminoglycoside antibiotics were detected only in cysts with proximal tubular electrolyte patterns. Neither tobramycin nor gentamicin was detected in distal cysts. Cephapirin, on the other hand, was detected in greater absolute concentrations in the cysts of distal nephrons. However, the ratio between cyst fluid and urine decreased owing to high urinary concentrations.

Cysts in PCKD are thought to be cysts of single nephrons. The single-nephron GFR in man is at least 10^{-8} liters/min. Therefore, it would take months for a cyst to reach its usual volume (3–5 cm^3) by glomerular filtration alone. It seems unlikely that any antibiotics detected in renal cysts within 5 days could accumulate solely by filtration. Abnormal tubular function of polycystic nephrons may contribute to the poor antibiotic penetrance, particularly of drugs normally transported by the renal tubules such as the cephalosporins. Also, dilution of the drug within the cyst is almost certain to occur by the inward movement of water. Drugs could enter cysts by diffusion across abnormal cyst epithelium, although this could not account for the discrepancy of drugs detected in proximal versus distal cysts. Diffusion trapping due to the effect of pH could account for this difference. This seems not to be an important factor since distal nephron cysts, with lower pH, would be expected to have a high concentration of organic bases (i.e., aminoglycosides) and a low concentration of organic acids (i.e., cephalosporins). Our results suggest the opposite.

Thus, simultaneous determination of serum, cyst fluid, and urine concentrations of various antibiotics showed low drug levels in both simple renal cysts and polycystic kidney disease. These data help explain the poor response of infected renal cysts to antibiotic therapy. Surgical management of these patients is warranted. Study of pharmacology of drug accumulation in cysts may give insights into the pathophysiology of polycystic kidney disease and antibiotic management of urinary tract infections in patients with renal failure.

References

1. Stamey TA, Govan DE, Palmer JM: The location and treatment of urinary tract infections: The role of bacteriocidal urine levels as opposed to serum levels. *Medicine* 44:1–36, 1965.

2. Ronald AR, Cutler RE, Turck M: Effect of bacteriuria on renal concentrating mechanisms. *Ann Intern Med* 70:723–733, 1969.
3. Whelton A, Walker WG: Intrarenal antibiotic distribution in health and disease. *Kidney Int* 6:131–137, 1974.
4. Bennett WM, Singer I, Golper T, Feig P, Coggins CJ: Guidelines for drug therapy in renal failure. *Ann Intern Med* 86:754–783, 1977.
5. Stamey TA, Fair WR, Timothy MM, Millar MA, Mihara G, Lowery YC: Serum versus urinary antimicrobial concentrations in the cure of urinary tract infections. *N Engl J Med* 291:1159–1163, 1974.
6. Kunin C: *Detection, Prevention and Management of Urinary Tract Infections.* Philadelphia, Lea & Febiger, 1979, pp 263–265.
7. Whelton A, Carter G, Bryant H, Fox L, Walker WG: Therapeutic implications of gentamicin accumulation in severely diseased kidneys. *Arch Intern Med* 136:172–176, 1976.
8. Bennett WM, Hartnett MN, Craven R, Gilbert D, Porter GA: Gentamicin concentrations in blood, urine and renal tissue of patients with end stage renal disease. *J Lab Clin Med* 90:389–393, 1977.
9. Cox CE: Gentamicin sulfate, a new aminoglycoside antibiotic: Clinical and laboratory studies in urinary tract infection. *J Infect Dis* 119:486–490, 1969.
10. Miller T, Phillips S, North D: Pharmacokinetics of gentamicin in the treatment of renal infection: A therapeutic anomaly explained. *Kidney Int* 15:160–166, 1979.
11. Frimodt-Moller N, Maigaard S, Madsen PO: Netilmicin treatment of complicated urinary tract infection in patients with renal function impairment. *Antimicrob Agents Chemother* 16:406–410, 1979.
12. Kunin CM, Finkelberg Z: Oral cephalexin and ampicillin: Antimicrobial activity, recovery in the urine and persistence in the blood of uremic patients. *Ann Intern Med* 72:349–356, 1970.
13. Bennett WM, Craven RM: Urinary tract infections in patients with severe renal disease. *JAMA* 236:946–948, 1976.
14. Craig WA, Kunin CM: Trimethoprim-sulfamethoxazole: Pharmacodynamic effects of urine pH and impaired renal function. *Ann Intern Med* 78:491–497, 1973.
15. Berglund F, Killander J, Pompeius R: The effect of trimethoprim–sulfamethoxazole on renal excretion of creatinine in man. *J Urol* 114:802–808, 1975.
16. Whelton A, Nightingale S, Carter GC, Gordon LS, Bryant HH, Walker WG: Pharmacokinetic characteristics of doxycycline accumulation in normal and severely diseased kidney. *J Infect Dis* 132:467–471, 1975.
17. Sweet R, Keane WF: Perinephric abscess in patients undergoing chronic hemodialysis. *Nephron* 23:237–240, 1979.
18. Patel NP, Pitts WR, Ward JN: Solitary infected renal cyst. *Urology* 11:164–168, 1978.
19. Grantham JJ: Polycystic renal disease, in: Early LE, Gottschalk CW (eds): *Strauss and Welt's Diseases of the Kidney.* Boston, Little, Brown, 1979, p 1123.

39

Contrast Media Acute Renal Failure

Robert E. Cronin

1. Hemodynamic Changes

Several observations point to the possibility that contrast-induced vascular alterations could be the common pathway for contrast-related cases of acute renal failure. Porter and Associates[1] noted that iothalamate, when injected into the left ventricle of the dog, resulted in an increase in cardiac output and caused a 25% decrease in renal blood flow. When isoosmolar quantities of mannitol were injected, however, the same increase in cardiac output occurred, but renal blood flow increased. Transient decreases in renal plasma flow and glomerular filtration rate occur after large-dose excretory urography.[2–4] In fact, noncontrast hypertonic solutions also produce this effect.[5] The response tends to be biphasic showing initially a transient increase in renal flood flow followed by a more prolonged (10–20%) decrease in renal blood flow which may persist for up to 1 hr.

The effect on renal vascular resistance of contrast agents injected directly intraarterially may be directly related to the osmolality of the solution. Contrast agents with a high osmolality when injected into the renal circulation affect renal blood flow much more than do those of lower osmolality.[6,7] Microcirculatory changes also occur after injection of contrast material.[8–10] The mechanism for this increase in flow may involve blood sludging resulting from alterations in red cell shape[8,11,12] and vascular endothelial injury.[10] The role of osmolality in the microcirculatory changes was called into question by the demonstration that ionic and the newer nonionic contrast agents, which have a much lower osmolality, cause equal degrees of ischemia on the rabbit microcirculation.[9]

Although these studies indicate that the tonicity of contrast materials injected into the renal artery can have a major effect on renal vascular

Robert E. Cronin • Veterans Administration Medical Center, University of Texas Southwestern Medical School, Dallas, Texas 75216.

resistance, it is unclear how contrast material that is injected into the venous circulation and is substantially diluted by the time it reaches the kidney might have an effect on renal vascular resistance. More than half of the reported cases of contrast-induced acute renal failure have been reported following excretory urography in which the contrast media is injected intravenously rather than intraarterially. Clearly, other factors must be involved.

2. *Tubular Obstruction*

The histology of myeloma kidney is characterized by intratubular casts.[13,14] The associated renal functional impairment is felt to be at least partly due to tubular obstruction. Such observations have lead to the theory that contrast agents may accelerate the precipitation of Bence Jones proteins. Lasser and associates[15] demonstrated that two urographic contrast agents no longer in use because of their toxicity, iodopyracet (Diodrast) and sodium acetrizoate (Urokon), produced *in vitro* precipitates in the urine of myeloma patients in a pH range of 4.5–5.5. However, agents that have been in use for the last 15–20 years, meglumine diatrizoate (Renografin) and sodium diatrizoate (Hypaque), produced no precipitate in this pH range. However, both these agents are capable of causing acute renal failure in multiple myeloma.[16] Also, McQueen[17] demonstrated that Bence Jones proteins readily cause Tamm–Horsfall proteins to sludge *in vitro*. Whether this same phenomenon occurs *in vivo* and causes tubular obstruction, as proposed by Berdon *et al.*,[18] is still unproven.

Since contrast materials are uricosuric, the idea that intratubular obstruction might occur from uric acid crystals has been suggested.[19,20] The oral cholecystographic agents (Telepaque, Oragrafin, and Cholografin) are the most likely agents to cause uricosuria, but Hypaque to some degree also shares this property.[20] Urinary uric acid measurements before and after contrast have been reported in one patient who developed acute renal failure.[21] Acute renal failure occurred despite a 3-week course of Allopurinol and in the absence of any uricosuric effect in the 6 hr after diatrizoate injection. A recent clinical study demonstrated a prompt increase in urinary oxalate excretion in normal individuals after diatrizoate injection.[22] Whether this enhanced oxalate excretion could be a factor in tubular obstruction is unknown.

Based on these data, however, it seems unlikely that either acute urate nephropathy or enhanced oxalate excretion is a major factor in the pathogenesis of contrast-induced acute renal failure.

3. *Immunologic Reactions*

Kleinknecht *et al.*[23] detected IgM kappa-type antibodies against contrast material in one patient who developed acute renal failure after her first exposure to X-ray contrast during excretory urography. The authors speculated that circulating immune complexes may have liberated vasoactive substances capable of inducing renal cortical ischemia and anuria. Two reports raised the possibility that X-ray contrast material injected either intravenously or intraarterially was responsible in some way for renal transplant rejection.[24,25] Although X-ray contrast agents clearly can cause induction of antibodies,[26] how they might lead to acute renal failure is not known. Based on these few reports, it would be premature to suggest that X-ray contrast material is capable of triggering an immunologic reaction in the kidney. Further studies are required in this area.

4. *Direct Toxicity*

A direct nephrotoxic effect of X-ray contrast on the kidney is the theory most widely held to explain contrast-induced acute renal failure. Changes of acute tubular necrosis are associated with various X-ray contrast agents.[27] Intraarterial injection of X-ray contrast into the dog kidney[28,29] and in man[30] may result in heavy glomerular proteinuria. In addition, enzymuria, a finding indicative of injury to proximal tubular cells, has been reported.[31,32] Since hypertonic mannitol and hypertonic saline also produced enzymuria,[32] it is possible that hypertonicity rather than a direct effect of the contrast agent is the cause of the damage. However, in the dog the degree of glomerular proteinuria produced by contrast is 100-fold higher than that resulting from equally hypertonic saline.[29] This indicates that some other factor besides hypertonicity is important.

Diatrizoate and iothalamate both have been shown to alter tubular transport of sodium.[1,33] It is unclear whether the effect on sodium transport is a direct effect of the contrast agent or rather is an effect of hypertonicity.

Lasser *et al.*[27] studied the histologic effect of several contrast agents injected directly into the dog kidney. The halogen portion of the molecule appeared to represent the toxic portion, since injection of the basic nonhalogenated molecule constructed with prosthetic groups on all positions on the benzene ring caused little renal histologic damage. In humans, renal biopsies following excretory urography or renal arteriography show intense vacuolization of proximal tubular cell cytoplasm.[34] Similar changes can be seen after hypertonic mannitol, and the significance of this abnormality is unknown.

Proximal tubular injury occurs after administration of several contrast agents,[27] but whether it is the contrast molecule or iodide that is toxic is not known. Clearance studies with most of the commonly used X-ray contrast agents indicate that they are excreted by glomerular filtration with no significant tubular secretion or reabsorption.[3,35,36] However, one study shows that approximately 20% of filtered hypaque is reabsorbed.[37] Studies of the new nonionic agent metrizamide in man[38] and in dogs[39] indicate substantial reabsorption with a fractional excretion compared to inulin of

70%. However, experimentally, metrizamide has been shown to be less toxic than ionic contrast agents. The LD_{50} for mice was found to be 8.9 g of iodine per kilogram for the ionic contrast media (diatrizoate, iothalamate, metriazoate) compared with 17.5 g of iodine per kilogram for metrizoate.[40]

Little is known about the degree of inorganic iodide liberated from X-ray contrast media, but it is clear that its release occurs.[41] Clearance studies indicate that the fractional excretion of ^{131}I is 35–40%.[42] Since protein binding of ^{131}I is very small, these data indicate significant tubular reabsorption of the free iodide molecule. Older cholecystographic agents were known to cause acute renal failure commonly, and they released substantial free iodide into the circulation with levels that remained above normal for up to 5 days.[43] Protein-bound iodine remained high for many months. Thus, it is likely that with any contrast agent some free iodide is administered or released *in vivo*, and under the proper circumstances, reabsorption of the iodine in the proximal tubule could lead to cell injury. Little is known regarding renal cortical levels of X-ray contrast or free iodine after exposure to X-ray contrast. Also, little is known regarding the disappearance curves of these substances from the proximal tubular cell. Although the amount of these agents contained in the proximal tubular cells may be small in a quantitative sense, their effects on cellular function (e.g., protein synthesis, membrane transport) could be substantial. By analogy, aminoglycoside antibiotics are handled almost exclusively by glomerular filtration, but a small portion is reabsorbed by proximal tubular cells. It is this fraction that apparently is responsible for proximal tubular necrosis and nephrotoxicity. In a normal individual, the usual contrast load is probably handled with minor impairment of normal cellular function. (Enzymuria might be considered a marker of such transient tubular injury.) However, in the presence of chronic disease characterized by sublethal cellular dysfunction, the added stress of a contrast and/or iodine load might precipitate cellular death.

Many questions are left unanswered when examining the problem of X-ray contrast-induced acute renal failure. The site of action of contrast agents in causing acute renal failure remains unknown. The transient effect of X-ray contrast on renal blood flow and glomerular filtration rate does not suggest that these are primary mechanisms leading to acute renal failure. Toad bladder studies showing impairment of sodium transport[33] raise the possibility that X-ray contrast agents may impair sodium pump activity, possibly by inhibiting Na^+,K^+-ATPase.

It is even more difficult to correlate the clinical risk factors (Table 1) with the clinical and animal studies described previously. The increased incidence of radiocontrast-induced acute renal failure in older patients may reflect the increased likelihood for these patients to have vascular disease and renal impairment. There is good evidence that a progressive reduction in renal mass and renal blood flow occurs with age. Preexisting renal dysfunction appears to be the most common predisposing historical finding in patients who develop contrast-induced acute renal failure.[44] Renal insufficiency is also very prevalent in those patients with diabetes who develop

Table 1. *Risk Factors*

1.	Advanced age	7.	Hyperuricemia
2.	Generalized vascular disease	8.	Multiple contrast exposures within 24 hr
3.	Prior renal insufficiency	9.	Exposure to other nephrotoxins
4.	Diabetes mellitus	10.	Proteinuria
5.	Hepatic insufficiency	11.	Hypoalbuminemia
6.	Dehydration	12.	Multiple myeloma

X-ray contrast-induced acute renal failure and is probably the single most important risk factor for this group.[45] Dehydration has been cited as a major risk factor in patients with multiple myeloma or diabetes mellitus. Other factors, such as proteinuria, hypoalbuminemia, and hyperurcemia, are present in some patients who develop contrast-induced acute renal failure, but what role they have in the pathogenesis is unclear.

In summary, it is likely that X-ray contrast in one form or another is a nephrotoxin. However, it is likely that only in certain patients is there a high risk of development of overt nephrotoxicity. It is possible that a cell that is compromised either by ischemia, a metabolic insult (diabetes mellitus), volume depletion, or recent exposure to another nephrotoxin (e.g., an aminoglycoside antibiotic) will undergo further injury and possible necrosis in the presence of iodinated X-ray contrast material.

5. *Future Research*

Several fruitful areas for research in the area of contrast-induced acute renal failure are suggested by the preceding review. Currently there is no good animal model of contrast-induced acute renal failure comparable to that seen in man, and one should be sought. However, even in the absence of frank acute renal failure, preliminary animal studies could explore the following areas: (1) What portion of currently used urographic contrast media is reabsorbed by the nephron and at what site along the nephron is it reabsorbed? This question could be approached through tissue analysis for contrast media and by radioautography studies of radiolabeled contrast. (2) A model of diabetes mellitus in the rat or dog could be tested regarding the acute and chronic effects of X-ray contrast on renal function and tissue concentrations of contrast and/or iodine. (3) Reports indicate that X-ray contrast potentiates the toxicity of other nephrotoxins (aminoglycosides, methoxyflurane anesthesia). These possibilities could be explored since animal models already exist for these latter nephrotoxins.

References

1. Porter GA, Kloster FE, Bristow JD: Sequential effect of angiographic contrast agent on canine renal and systemic hemodynamics. *Am Heart J* 81:80, 1971.

2. Talner LB, Davidson AJ: Renal hemodynamic effects of contrast media. *Invest Rad* 3:310, 1968.
3. Donaldson IML: Comparison of the renal clearances of inulin and radioactive diatrizoate ("Hypaque") as measures of the glomerular filtration rate in man. *Clin Sci* 35:513, 1968.
4. Gup AK, Schlegel JU: Physiologic effects of high dosage excretory urography. *J Urol* 100:85, 1968.
5. Chou CC, Hook JB, Hsieh CP, Burns TD, Dabney JM: Effects of radiopaque dyes on renal vascular resistance. *J Lab Clin Med* 78:705, 1974.
6. Russel SB, Sherwood T: Monomer/dimer contrast media in the renal circulation: experimental angiography. *Br J Radiol* 47:268, 1974.
7. Morris TW, Katzberg RW, Fischer HW: A comparison of the hemodynamic responses to metrizamide and meglumine/sodium diatrizoate in canine renal angiography. *Invest Radiol* 13:74, 1978.
8. Sobin SS, Frasher WG, Johnson G: Nature of adverse reactions to radiopaque agents; preliminary report. *JAMA* 170:1546, 1959.
9. Ekeland A, Uflacker R: Effect of meglumine metrizoate and metrizamide on the microcirculation. *Acta Radiol Diag* 19:969, 1978.
10. Endrich B, Ring J, Intaglietta M: Effect of radiopaque contast media on the microcirculation of the rabbit omentum. *Diag Radiol* 132:331, 1979.
11. Bernstein EF, Evans RL, Blum JA, Avant RF: Further experimental observations concerning the protective action of low molecular weight dextran upon intravenous hypaque toxicity. *Radiology* 76:260, 1961.
12. Schiantarelli P, Peroni F, Turone P, Rosati G: Effects of iodinated contrast media on erythrocytes. *Invest Radiol* 8:199, 1973.
13. Healy JK: Acute oliguric renal failure associated with multiple myeloma: Report of three cases. *Br Med J* 1:1126, 1963.
14. Rees ED, Waugh WH: Factors in renal failure in multiple myeloma. *Arch Intern Med* 116:400, 1965.
15. Lasser EC, Lang JH, Zawadski ZA: Contrast media: myeloma protein precipitates in urography. *JAMA* 198:945, 1966.
16. Myers GH, Witten DM: Acute renal failure after excretory urography in multiple myeloma. *Am J Roentgenol* 113:583, 1971.
17. McQueen EG: The nature of urinary casts. *J Clin Pathol* 15:367, 1962.
18. Berdon WE, Schwartz RH, Becker J, Baker DH: Tamm–Horsfall proteinuria. *Radiology* 92:714, 1969.
19. Mudge GH: Uricosuric action of cholangiographic agents: A possible factor in nephrotoxicity. *N Engl J Med* 284:929, 1971.
20. Postlethwaite AE, Kelley WN: Uricosuric effect of radiocontrast agents: Study in man of four commonly used preparations. *Ann Intern Med* 74:845, 1971.
21. Feldman MA, Goldfarb S, McCurdy DK: Recurrent radiography dye-induced acute renal failure. *JAMA* 229:72, 1974.
22. Gelman ML, Rowe JW, Coggins CH, Athanasoulis C: Effects of an angiographic contrast agent on renal function. *Cardiovascular Med* 4:313, 1979.
23. Kleinknecht D, Deloux J, Homberg JC: Acute renal failure after intravenous urography: Detection of antibodies against contrast media. *Clin Nephrol* 2:116, 1974.
24. Light JA, Perloff LJ, Etheredge EE, Hill G, Spees EK: Adverse effects of meglumine diatrizoate on renal function in the early post-transplant period. *Transplantation* 20:404, 1975.
25. Heidemann M, Claes G, Nilson AE: The risk of renal allograft rejection following angiography. *Transplantation* 21:289, 1976.
26. Brasch RC, Caldwell JL, Fundenberg HH: Antibodies to radiographic contrast agents. Induction and characterization of rabbit antibody. *Invest Radiol* 11:1, 1976.
27. Lasser EC, Lee SH, Fisher E, Fisher B: Some further pertinent considerations regarding the comparative toxicity of contrast materials for the dog kidney. *Radiology* 78:240, 1962.

28. Holtas S, Almen T, Tejler L: Proteinuria following nephroangiography. II. Influence of contrast medium and catheterization in dogs. *Acta Radiol Diag* 19:33, 1978.
29. Holtas S, Tejler L: Proteinuria following nephroangiography. IV. Comparison in dogs between ionic and non-ionic contrast media. *Acta Radiol Diag* 20:13, 1979.
30. Teljer L, Almen T, Holtas S: Proteinuria following nephroangiography. I. Clinical experiences. *Acta Radiol Diag* 18:634, 1977.
31. Goldstein EJ, Feinfeld DA, Fleischner GM, Elkin M: Enzymatic evidence of renal tubular damage following renal angiography. *Radiology* 121:167, 1976.
32. Talner LB, Rushman HN, Coel MN: The effect of renal artery injection of contrast material on urinary enzyme excretion. *Invest Radiol* 7:311, 1972.
33. Ziegler TW, Ladens JH, Fanestil DD, Talner LB: Inhibition of active sodium transport by radiographic contrast media. *Kidney Int* 7:68, 1975.
34. Moreau JF, Diaz D, Sabato J, Jungers P, Kleinknecht D, Hinglais N, Michel JR: Osmotic nephrosis induced by water soluble triiodinated contrast media in man. *Radiology* 115:329, 1975.
35. Blaufox MD, Sanderson DR, Tauxe WN, Wakim KG, Orvis AL, Owen CA Jr: Plasmatic Diatrizoate I^{131} and glomerular filtration in the dog. *Am J Physiol* 204:536, 1963.
36. Denneberg T: Clinical studies of kidney function with radioactive sodium diatrizoate (Hypaque). *Acta Med Scand* 179(suppl 442):1, 1966.
37. Stokes JM, Conklin JW, Huntley HC: Measurement of glomerular filtration rate by contrast media containing I^{131} isotopes. *J Urol* 87:630, 1962.
38. Golman K, Denneberg T, Nosslin B: Metrizamide in urography. II. A comparison of ^{51}Cr EDTA clearance and metrizamide clearance in man. *Invest Radiol* 12:353, 1977.
39. Golman K, Scient C: Metrizamide in experimental urography. V. Renal excretion mechanism of a non-ionic contrast medium in rabbit and cat. *Invest Radiol* 11:187, 1976.
40. Golman K, Almen T: Metrizamide in experimental urography. VI. Effect of renal contrast media on urinary solutes. *Acta Pharmacol Toxicol* 38:120, 1976.
41. McChesney EW: The biotransformation of iodinated radiocontrast agents, in Knoefel PK (ed): *International Encyclopedia of Pharmacology and Therapeutics.* Section 76. *Radio contrast agents.* New York, Pergamon Press, Vol 1, 1971, pp 147–163.
42. Bricker NS, Hlad CJ. Observations on the mechanism of the renal clearance of I^{131}. *J Clin Invest* 34:1057, 1955.
43. Cassidy CE: The duration of increased serum iodine concentration after ingestion of Bunamiodyl (Orabilex). *J Clin Endocrinol* 20:1034, 1960.
44. Swartz RD, Rubin JE, Lemming BW, Silva P: Renal failure following major angiography. *Am J Med* 65:31, 1978.
45. Harkonen S, Kjellstrand CM: Exacerbation of diabetic renal failure following intravenous pyelography. *Am J Med* 63:939, 1977.

40

Effect of Renal Disease on Pharmacokinetics and Bioavailability

Thomas P. Gibson

Therapeutically it is of vital importance to understand the pharmacokinetics and bioavailability of drugs, especially of those handled by the kidney. It would seem logical that with declining renal function, these functions might alter.

A major assumption of the approach delineated by the equations listed in this chapter is that the processes of absorption, distribution, and nonrenal elimination of a drug are the same in patients with end-stage renal failure as they are in patients with normal renal function.[1] It also assumes that the metabolites found are inactive or nontoxic and do not accumulate in patients with renal failure.

It is the purpose of this chapter to examine the validity of these assumptions using procainamide and D-xylose as model compounds.

The total body clearance (Cl_T) of a drug is defined as

$$Cl_T = Cl_R + Cl_{NR} \qquad (1)$$

where Cl_R and Cl_{NR} are the renal and nonrenal clearance of the drug. Cl_T is also defined as

$$Cl_T = V_d \cdot k_e \qquad (2)$$

where V_d is the volume of distribution. k_e is the overall elimination rate

Thomas P. Gibson • Section of Nephrology/Hypertension and Department of Medicine, Northwestern University Medical School, Northwestern Memorial Hospital, and Veterans Administration Lakeside Medical Center, Chicago, Illinois 60611. Supported by the Research and Development Service of the Veterans Administration and the Clinical Research Center of Northwestern University, RR-48, Division of Research Resources, National Institutes of Health.

constant for any drug and is inversely related to the biologic half-life ($t_{1/2}$) of that drug:

$$k_e = 0.693/t_{1/2} \tag{3}$$

k_e is also equal to the sum of the renal (k_r) and nonrenal (k_{nr}) elimination rate constants:

$$k_e = k_r + k_{nr} \tag{4}$$

For most drugs dependent on renal function for elimination k_e is linearly related to some function (f) of creatinine clearance (C_{cr}) such that

$$k_e = f \cdot C_{cr} + k_{nr} \tag{5}$$

If k_{nr} and $f \cdot C_{cr}$ of a drug are known then the new k_e, and hence $t_{1/2}$, can be established for any degree of renal function.[2,3] If k_{nr} is not known, it can be estimated as

$$k_{nr} = k_e(1 - A_u^\infty) \tag{6}$$

where A_u^∞ is the fraction of the systemically available drug ultimately excreted unchanged in the urine.

1. *Procainamide*

Approximately 50% of an oral or intravenous dose of procainamide (PA) is eliminated unchanged in the urine, and the average $t_{1/2}$ is 3 hr.[4–7] On the basis of this alone, it would be predicted (from equation 4) that the $t_{1/2}$ of PA in renal failure would be approximately 6 hr. However, we found that the apparent $t_{1/2}$ of PA elimination in renal failure was variable and could range from 5.3 to 20.7 hr after an oral dose.[8] Since the patients in that study were either physiologically or surgically anephric, those data suggested that the metabolic transformation of PA was impaired by renal failure.

Dreyfuss *et al.* identified *N*-acetylprocainamide (NAPA) as a metabolite of procainamide in 1972.[9] Additional studies have shown that the acetylation of PA is under genetic control and that phenotypic rapid acetylators of PA are rapid acetylators of isonicotinic acid hydrazide (INH).[6,7,10]

The pharmacokinetics of intravenous procainamide was studied in four subjects with normal renal function and in four patients with anuric end-stage renal failure.[11] Two members of each group were fast INH acetylators with an INH $t_{1/2}$ of less than 2.0 hr, and two were slow acetylators with an INH $t_{1/2}$ greater than 3.0 hr[12] (Table 1).

Table 1. Data on Normal Subjects and on Patients with End-Stage Renal Failure[a]

	Body wt (kg)	Sex	Age (years)	INH $t_{1/2}$ (hr)	C_{cr} (ml/min)
Normal subjects					
1	86.4	M	34	3.6	115
2	87.5	M	36	3.7	120
3	81.8	M	32	1.6	125
4	85.0	M	33	1.3	110
Mean	85.2 ± 2.5		33.7 ± 1.7		117.5 ± 6.5
Patients with end-stage renal failure					
1	72.5	M	51	1.6	SAN
2	80.5	M	56	1.2	PAN
3	78.0	M	56	3.8	PAN
4	59.0	F	45	3.0	SAN
Mean	72.5 ± 9.6		52.0 ± 5.2		

[a] INH, isonicotinic acid hydrazide; C_{cr}, creatinine clearance; SAN, surgically anephric; PAN, physiologically anephric.

All subjects were given procainamide hydrochloride, 6.5 mg/kg, intravenously over 20–25 min. At the conclusion of the infusion blood and urine were sampled for 8 hr in normal subjects and blood alone for 24 hr in the patients with renal failure. Concentrations of PA and NAPA in serum were determined by spectrophotofluorometry.[13] Urine concentrations of PA and NAPA were determined by gas liquid chromatography.[6] A two-compartment system was used to model the distribution kinetics of PA.[11]

After a single PA dose, NAPA concentrations in the serum of normal subjects were undetectable. However, NAPA was detectable in the serum of all patients with renal failure.[11]

The pharmacokinetic parameters of PA in normals and in renal failure patients are given in Table 2. The volume of distribution and renal clearance of PA were similar in normal subjects regardless of acetylator phenotype. Nonrenal clearance was faster (383 versus 243 ml/min), and PA elimination

Table 2. Effects of Renal Failure on PA Pharmacokinetics

	Normals		Anephric patients	
Acetylation phenotype:	Fast	Slow	Fast	Slow
Distribution volume (liters/kg)	1.95	1.93	1.41	1.93
Amount excreted unchanged in urine (%)	52	59	0	0
Elimination half-life (hr)	2.6	3.5	10.8	17.0
Plasma clearance (ml/min)	809	600	118	94
Renal clearance (ml/min)	426	357	0	0
Nonrenal clearance (ml/min)	383	243	118	94

Table 3. Effect of Renal Failure on NAPA Pharmacokinetics

	Normals	Renal failure patients
Distribution volume (liters/kg)	1.46	1.50
Amount excreted unchanged in urine (%)	85	0
Elimination half-life (hr)	6.2	42
Plasma clearance (ml/min)	234	2.7
Renal clearance (ml/min)	200	3
Nonrenal clearance (ml/min)	34	24

$t_{1/2}$ shorter (2.6 versus 3.5 hr) in fast acetylators. In the functionally anephric patients the volume of distribution of PA was similar to that in normals. The nonrenal clearance (118 versus 94 ml/min) was again faster and PA $t_{1/2}$ shorter (10.8 versus 17.0 hr) in fast than in slow acetylators.

The nonrenal clearance of PA predominantly represents acetylation and possibly other metabolic pathways, since Giardina and associates have incompletely identified two other PA metabolites in the urine of subjects receiving PA orally.[14] PA is acetylated by *N*-acetyltransferase, the same enzyme responsible for the acetylation of INH.[6,7,10] Some investigators have reported that acetylation of INH is normal in renal failure,[15,16] whereas others have found it impaired.[17] In the present study, fast INH acetylators had a faster nonrenal (metabolic) clearance of PA than did slow acetylators (Table 2) and a shorter PA $t_{1/2}$. Half-life changes are not as accurate a reflection of altered drug elimination as are clearance changes, since $t_{1/2}$, as opposed to clearance, is not a primary pharmacokinetic parameter and is influenced by distribution volume as well as clearance rates.[18] As shown in Table 2, nonrenal elimination of PA is markedly decreased in renal failure and appears to be even less in slow than in rapid acetylators. Since acetylation accounts for 56% of the total elimination of PA in renal failure,[11] it is likely that both this route and the other pathways accounting for the remaining 44% are slowed.

These results clearly demonstrate that the nonrenal or metabolic clearance of PA is severely impaired in renal failure. Because of this, *a priori* estimation of correct PA dosage in renal failure using the Dettli nomogram or any other approach is impossible.

NAPA is an antiarrhythmically active metabolite of PA.[19,20] Strong *et al.* found that the $t_{1/2}$ of NAPA in subjects with normal renal function was 6.2 hr,[21] and 85% of the intravenous dose of NAPA was recovered unchanged in the urine (Table 3). The expected $t_{1/2}$ of NAPA in anuric renal failure would be 41 hr. Stec and associates recently reported that $t_{1/2}$ of NAPA in functionally anephric patients to be 42 hr[22] (Table 3). This indicates that the nonrenal clearance of NAPA, unlike that of PA, is unaltered in renal disease. NAPA accumulates in anephric patients and has been found to persist in the serum for over 123 hr after a single oral dose of PA.[23]

If a renal failure patient is to be treated with PA, the serum concentrations of both PA and NAPA must be monitored. Goldstein and associates have shown that if a drug is given without a loading dose, it will take 3.3 half-lives to reach 90% of the eventual steady-state level.[24] For PA this would be 48 hr on the average, but since the $t_{1/2}$ of NAPA is 42 hr, its steady-state levels would not be reached for 139 hr. The steady-state ratio of NAPA:PA in subjects with normal renal function may be as high as 6:1 in genetic fast acetylators or as low as 1:1 in genetic slow acetylators.[10,25] In renal failure the ratio may be greater than 12:1.[19]

The usual therapeutic concentration range of PA is considered to be 4–8 mcg/ml [4,26] However, Elson and associates have found that the therapeutic range is 4–30 μg/ml, representing the sum of PA and NAPA.[25] If only PA concentrations were monitored and used as the sole guide for PA dosing in a renal failure patient, NAPA concentrations could reach extremely high levels and would not reach steady state until long after PA had. In this setting continued accumulation of NAPA could result in clinical toxicity that represents a combination of PA and NAPA effects. Therefore, unless both PA and NAPA concentrations can be measured, PA should not be used in renal failure patients.

2. D-Xylose

The whole area of drug bioavailability in renal failure has been sadly neglected. In general, it has been assumed that if, after a given oral dose, the drug concentrations in renal failure are the same, or nearly the same, as in normals, drug absorption is unimpaired. This totally neglects the fact that if the volume of distribution is reduced in renal failure, drug concentrations could be similar to those in normals even if availability were reduced substantially.

Bioavailability is defined as the relative amount of an administered drug dose that reaches the systemic circulation unchanged and the rate at which this occurs.[27] The bioavailability of a given drug is determined by plotting the plasma concentration versus time after an oral dose and comparing the area under the curve (AUC) to the AUC of a reference standard. The best comparison is made with the curve after intravenous administration of a parenteral formulation since bioavailability by this route is complete. Bioavailability determined in this manner is known as the absolute bioavailability (F).

D-Xylose is a monosaccharide absorbed passively in the jejunum.[28] In normals approximately 65% of an ingested dose is absorbed.[28] When it is infused intravenously, 40% is recovered unchanged in the urine.[29,30]

Although D-xylose is only partially absorbed and partially excreted in the urine, the urinary xylose excretion is widely used as a test to assess the absorptive function of the small bowel.[29,31–33] The standard clinical test entails measuring the 5-hr urinary excretion following the ingestion of 25 g

Table 4. Pharmacokinetics of Intravenous D-Xylose in Normals and Renal Failure

	Normals	Renal failure patients
Distribution volume (liter/kg)	0.22	0.33[a]
Amount excreted unchanged in urine (%)	49	0
Elimination half-life (min)	75	388[b]
Plasma clearance (ml/min)	180	43[b]
Renal clearance (ml/min)	89	0
Nonrenal clearance (ml/min)	91	43[b]

[a] $p < 0.01$.
[b] $p < 0.005$.

of D-xylose. Alternatively, serum levels have been measured at various times after oral administration.[32] Recently the serum level obtained 1 hr after ingestion of 5 g of D-xylose has been advocated as a good discriminating test for small intestinal malabsorption.[33]

Obviously, the standard D-xylose test based on urinary excretion cannot be used in patients with diminished or absent renal function. To ascertain if D-xylose absorption was normal in renal failure, the extent of absorption, distribution, renal, and nonrenal clearance of D-xylose after oral and intravenous administration was determined in normals and renal failure patients requiring maintenance dialysis.[34]

Twelve subjects with normal renal function, endogenous creatinine clearance greater than 80 ml/min, and nine patients with end-stage renal failure were studied. All patients were studied on a nondialysis day. All participants received 10 g of D-xylose intravenously over 2 min. Blood and urine samples were obtained for 8 hr in normal subjects and blood only for 24 hr in renal failure patients. At least 1 week after the intravenous study 25 g of D-xylose was given orally. Blood and urine samples were obtained at the same intervals as in the previous study.

D-Xylose concentrations in serum and urine were determined by the spectrophotometric method of Roe and Rice.[53] Preliminary studies indicated that uremic sera did not interfere with the analytical procedure. A two-compartment mamillary system was used to model the distribution kinetics.

The percent absolute bioavailability (F) was calculated by comparing the AUC of the intravenous (IV) dose to the AUC of the oral (PO) dose as follows:

$$F = \frac{AUC_{IV}}{AUC_{PO}} \times \frac{Dose_{PO}}{Dose_{IV}} \times 100 \tag{7}$$

The pharmacokinetics of D-xylose in normals and renal failure subjects are given in Table 4. The volume of distribution of D-xylose was significantly increased in renal failure from 0.22 to 0.33 liter/kg ($p < 0.01$). Of the administered intravenous dose 49 ± 9% was recovered unchanged in the

Table 5. Absolute Bioavailability of D*-Xylose in Normals and Patients with Renal Failure*

	Normals	Renal failure patients
Half time of absorption (min)	29	64[a]
Lag time (min)	22	45[b]
Time to maximum concentration (min)	71	166[b]
Maximum concentration (mg/liter)	0.53	0.48
Absolute bioavailability	69	47[b]

[a] $p < 0.05$.
[b] $p < 0.01$.

urine. The observed $t_{1/2}$ in normals was 75 ± 11 min and would have been predicted to be approximately 150 min in renal failure. However, the observed $t_{1/2}$ in renal failure was 388 ± 137 min. This is considerably greater than expected because of the unanticipated marked reduction in the nonrenal clearance of D-xylose in renal failure, 43 ± 9 ml/min compared to 91 ± 29 ml/min, $p < 0.005$, in normals.

The mechanisms that determine the nonrenal clearance of D-xylose are still incompletely understood but probably involve hepatic metabolism and biliary excretion. Segal and Foley[(36)] have shown that 16% of ^{14}C-labeled D-xylose will be converted to $^{14}CO_2$. The disposition of the remaining D-xylose that is not cleared by the kidney, however, was not clarified. Recently four patients with biliary fistulas were found to have biliary D-xylose concentrations similar to those in serum.[(37)] However, the magnitude of the contribution of biliary excretion in D-xylose disposition is unknown.

It has already been shown that the metabolism of PA, most likely by acetylation, is impaired in renal disease. It now appears that the metabolism of the pentose D-xylose also is greatly altered in renal disease probably secondary to reduced oxidation. It has been shown recently in a uremic rat model that the oxidation of [^{14}C] glucose is significantly reduced as compared to that in control rats.[(38)]

A comparison of the factors relevant to the estimation of the absolute bioavailability of D-xylose in subjects with normal renal function and in renal failure is given in Table 5.

The absolute bioavailability of D-xylose was significantly less in patients with renal failure, 47%, as compared to 69% in normals, $p < 0.01$. It is possible that end-stage renal failure impairs the absorptive capacity of the small intestine. The absolute bioavailability of furosemide[(39)] and of pindolol[(40)] also has been reported diminished in renal failure. This suggests that defects in drug absorption may be more common than generally is believed. The reduced absorption of D-xylose could be due to bacterial overgrowth in the small intestine. The bacterial flora of the small intestine is significantly increased in some patients with chronic renal failure.[(41)] This could cause bacterial fermentation of D-xylose in the intestine and consequently its reduced absorption.[(42)]

After ingestion of a drug there is a delay before the drug appears in the systemic circulation (lag time). This delay primarily reflects mainly the time required for a drug to traverse the stomach to the small intestine.[43] The lag time in patients with renal failure was significantly longer than in normals, 45 min and 22 min, respectively ($p < 0.01$, Table 4). Impaired gastric emptying has been reported in dialysis patients[44] and could contribute to the increased lag time.

The absorption $t_{1/2}$ was also significantly prolonged in renal failure compared to normals, 64 min and 29 min respectively ($p < 0.05$, Table 4).

Even though the absorption of D-xylose is reduced in renal failure and the volume of distribution increased, it is not surprising that there was no statistical difference in the maximum concentration as compared to normals, 0.43 ± 0.19 mg/liter compared to 0.53 ± 0.10 mg/liter, respectively, Table 4. The maximum amount of a drug in the body (X_{max}) after oral administration can be determined from the following relationship:

$$X_{max} = \left[\frac{k_a}{k_e}\right]^{k_e/(k_e - k_a)} \times D \times F \times V_d^{-1} \quad (8)$$

where k_e is the absorption rate constant ($0.695/t_{1/2}$ absorption) and D is the administered dose.[24] It is obvious that X_{max} is most sensitive to changes in k_e. In renal failure patients the k_e of D-xylose is prolonged to a much greater extent than k_a, and hence, no difference in the maximum concentration of D-xylose would be anticipated. For these reasons, the measurement of maximum concentration alone as an index of the completeness of absorption must be discouraged.

Although the systemic availability of some drugs may be reduced in renal failure, it has been suggested that the first-pass metabolism of some drugs such as propoxyphene[45] may be reduced in renal failure and bioavailability increased. The first-pass metabolism of propranolol is apparently unchanged in renal failure.[46]

It should be apparent from the examples given that renal disease can alter the pharmacokinetics and absorption of drugs. Although the metabolic clearance of PA and D-xylose is reduced in renal failure, the metabolic clearance of pindolol is markedly increased.[47] D-Xylose and pindolol absorption are decreased but propoxyphene absorption may be increased.

The message is clear. The metabolism, disposition, and absorption of any drug must be shown to be unaltered in renal failure before they can be considered to be. Therefore, formal pharmacokinetic studies, utilizing intravenous dosing where possible, must be conducted on those drugs commonly used in renal failure patients. Pharmacokinetic studies utilizing oral dosage forms can only be accepted for those drugs without parenteral preparations.

References

1. Dettli L: Individualization of drug dosage in patients with renal disease. *Med Clin North Am* 58:977–985, 1974.

2. Dettli L, Spring P, Habersang R: Drug dosage in patients with impaired renal function. *Postgrad Med J* 46(suppl):32–35, 1970.
3. Dettli L: Drug dosage in renal disease. *Clin Pharmacokinet* 1:126–134, 1976.
4. Koch–Weser J: Pharmacokinetics of procainamide in man. *Ann NY Acad Sci* 179:370–382, 1971.
5. Mark LC, Kayden HJ, Steele JM, Cooper JR, Berlin I, Rovenstine EA, Brodie BB: The physiological dispostion and cardiac effects of procainamide. *J Pharmacol Exp Ther* 102:5–15, 1951.
6. Gibson TP, Matusik J, Matusik E, Nelson HA, Wilkinson J, Briggs WA: Acetylation of procainamide in man and its relationship to isonicotinic acid hydrazide acetylation phenotype. *Clin Pharmacol Ther* 17:395–399, 1975.
7. Karlsson E, Molin L: Polymorphic acetylation of procainamide in healthy subjects. *Acta Med Scand* 197:299–302, 1975.
8. Gibson TP, Lowenthal DT, Nelson HA, Briggs WA: Elimination of procainamide in end stage renal failure. *Clin Pharmacol Ther* 17:321–329, 1975.
9. Dreyfuss J, Bigger JT, Jr., Cohen AI, Schreiber EC: Metabolism of procainamide in rhesus monkey and man. *Clin Pharmacol Ther* 13:366–371, 1972.
10. Reidenberg MM, Drayer DE, Levy M, Warner H: Polymorphic acetylation of procainamide in man. *Clin Pharmacol Ther* 17:722–730, 1975.
11. Gibson TP, Atkinson AJ, Jr., Matusik E, Nelson LD, Briggs WA: Kinetics of procainamide and N-acetylprocainamide in renal failure. *Kidney Int* 12:422–429, 1977.
12. Scott Em, Wright RC: Fluorometric determination of isonicotinic acid hydrazide in serum. *J Lab Clin Med* 70:355–360, 1967.
13. Matusik E, Gibson TP: Fluorometric assay for *N*-acetylprocainamide. *Clin Chem* 21:1899–1902, 1975.
14. Giardina EV, Dreyfuss J, Bigger JT, Shaw JM, Schreiber EC: Metabolism of procainamide in normal and cardiac subjects. *Clin Pharmacol Ther* 19:339–351, 1976.
15. Bowersox DW, Winterbauer RH, Stewart GL, Orme B, Barron E: Isoniazide dosage in patients with renal failure. *N Engl J Med* 289:84–87, 1973.
16. Reidenberg MM, Shear L, Cohen RV: Elimination of isoniazide in patients with impaired renal function. *Am Rev Resp Dis* 108:1426–1428, 1973.
17. Dettli L, Spring P: in Okita GT, Acheson GH (eds): *The Modifying Effects of Physiological Variables and Disease upon Pharmacokinetics—An Introduction.* Basel, Karger, 1973, vol 3, pp 165–173.
18. Perrier D, Gibaldi M: Clearance and biologic half-life as indices of intrinsic hepatic metabolism. *J Pharmacol Exp Ther* 19:17–24, 1974.
19. Atkinson AJ, Jr., Lee W–K, Quinn ML, Cushner W, Nevin MJ, Strong JM: Dose-ranging trial of *N*-acetylprocainamide in patients with premature ventricular contractions. *Clin Pharmacol Ther* 21:575–587, 1977.
20. Lee W–K, Strong JM, Kehoe RF, Dutcher JS, Atkinson AJ, Jr.: Antiarrhythmic efficacy of *N*-acetylprocainamide in patients with premature ventricular contractions. *Clin Pharmacol Ther* 19:508–514, 1976.
21. Strong JM, Dutcher JS, Lee W–K, Atkinson AJ, Jr.: Pharmacokinetics in man of the N-acetylated metabolite of procainamide. *J Pharmacokinet Biopharm* 3:223–235, 1975.
22. Stec GP, Atkinson AJ, Jr., Nevin MJ, Thenot J–P, Ruo TI, Gibson TP, Ivanovich P, del Greco F: *N*-acetylprocainamide pharmacokinetics in functionally anephric patients before and after perturbation by hemodialysis. *Clin Pharmacol Ther* 26:618–628, 1979.
23. Gibson TP, Matusik E, Briggs WA: *N*-acetylprocainamide levels in patients with end stage renal failure. *Clin Pharmacol Ther* 19:206–212, 1976.
24. Goldstein A, Aronow L, Kalman SM: *Principles of Drug Actions: The Basis of Pharmacology.* New York, Wiley, 1975, p 324.
25. Elson J, Strong JM, Lee W–K, Atkinson AJ, Jr.: Antiarrhythmic potency of *N*-acetylprocainamide. *Clin Pharmcol Ther* 17:134–140, 1975.
26. Koch–Weser J, Klein SW: Procainamide dosage schedules, plasma concentrations, and clinical effects. *JAMA* 215:1454–1460, 1971.

27. Dittert LW, Cressman WA, Kaplan SA, Riegelman S, Wagner JG: *Guidelines for biopharmaceutical studies in man.* Washington, D.C., American Pharmaceutical Association, Academy of Pharmaceutical Sciences, 1972, p 17.
28. Fordtran JS, Soergel HR, Ingelfinger FJ: Intestinal absorption of D-xylose in man. *N Engl J Med* 267:274–279, 1962.
29. Christiansen PA, Kirsner JB, Ablaya J: D-xylose and its use in the diagnosis of malabsorptive states. *Am J Med* 27:443–453, 1959.
30. Wyngaarden JB, Segal S, Foley JB: Physiological disposition and metabolic fate of infused pentoses in man. *J Clin Invest* 36:1395–1407, 1967.
31. Butterworth CE, Perey–Santiago E, Martinez de Jesus J, Santiri R: Studies on the oral and parenteral administration of D-xylose. *N Engl J Med.* 261:157–161, 1959.
32. Finlay JM, Hogarth J, Nightman KJR: A clinical evaluation of the D-xylose tolerance test. *Ann Intern Med* 61:411–422, 1964.
33. Hoeney MR, Culank LS, Montgomery RD, Sarmmous HG: Evaluation of xylose absorption as measured in blood and urine. A one hour blood xylose screening test in malabsorption. *Gastroenterology* 75:393–400, 1978.
34. Craig RM, Murphy P, Gibson TP, Quintanilla A, Chao GC, Cochrane C, Patterson A, Athinson AJ Jr.: Kinetic analysis of D-xylose absorption in normal subjects and in patients with chronic renal failure. *J Lab Clin Med* 101:496–506, 1893.
35. Roe JH, Rice EW: A photometric method for the determination of free pentoses in animal tissues. *J Biol Chem* 173:507–512, 1948.
36. Segal S, Foley JB: The metabolism of C^{14} labeled pentoses in man. *J Clin Invest* 38:407–413, 1959.
37. Huguenin P, Cochet B, Balant L, Loizeau ED: Test d'absorption du D-xylose. *Schweiz Med Wschr* 108:206–214, 1978.
38. Quintanilla A, Craig R, Gibson T, Shambaugh G: Glucose metabolism in uremia. *Am J Clin Nutr* 33:1446–1450, 1980.
39. Tilstone WJ, Fine A: Furosemide kinetics in renal failure. *Clin Pharmacol Ther* 23:644–650, 1978.
40. Chau NP, Weiss YA, Safara ME, Lavene DE, Georges DR, Milliez PL: Pindolol availability in hypertensive patients with normal and impaired renal function. *Clin Pharmacol Ther* 22:505–510, 1977.
41. Simenhoff ML: Metabolism and toxicity of aliphatic amines. *Kidney Int* 7:5314–5317, 1975.
42. Toshes PP, King CE, Spivey JC, Lorenz E: Xylose catabolism in the experimental rat blind loop syndrome. *Gastroenterology* 74:691–697, 1978.
43. Wagner JC: Biopharmaceutics: Absorption aspects. *J Pharm Sci* 50:359–387, 1961.
44. Grodstein G, Harrison A, Roberts C, Ippoliti A, Kopple J: Impaired gastric emptying in hemodialysis patients. *Am Soc Neph* 12:182A, 1979.
45. Gibson TP, Giacomini KM, Briggs WA, Whitman W, Levy G: Pharmacokinetics of D-propoxyphine in anephric patients. *Clin Pharmacol Ther* 21:103, 1977.
46. Wood AJJ, Vestal RE, Spannath C, Stone WJ, Wilkinson GR, Shand DG: Propranolol disposition in renal failure. *Clin Res* 27:239A, 1979.
47. Galeazzi RL, Gugger M, Weidmann P: Beta blockade with pindolol: Differential cardiac and renal effects despite similar plasma kinetics in normal and uremic man. *Kidney Int* 15:661–668, 1979.

41

Pathogenesis of Aminoglycoside Nephrotoxicity

Friedrich C. Luft

The effect of aminoglycoside antibiotics on the kidneys has been the subject of considerable interest, not only because of its clinical importance,[1] but also because of the useful acute renal failure model produced by these compounds. Although the pathogenesis of aminoglycoside nephrotoxicity remains incompletely defined, the work of numerous investigators has produced much information from a variety of diverse sources. The contributions of pharmacologists, physiologists, biochemists, pathologists, and clinicians provide a framework that should encourage further investigations of aminoglycoside nephrotoxicity in particular, and the pathogenesis of acute renal failure in general.

The aminoglycosides exhibit interesting pharmacokinetic properties. On the basis of clearance studies in man[2–4] and in experimental animals,[5,6] it is apparent that aminoglycosides are excreted primarily by glomerular filtration. Since the clearance of the aminoglycoside gentamicin is slightly less than the glomerular filtration rate,[3–5] investigators have concluded that net tubular reabsorption probably occurs. The validity of this conclusion depends on the plasma protein binding of gentamicin, which remains a highly controversial issue. Some investigators[7,8] have reported no significant binding of gentamicin to plasma proteins, whereas others have reported that 20–30% of the drug is protein bound.[9]

Aminoglycosides accumulate in renal parenchyma, primarily in the cortex, where concentrations considerably greater than those in serum are attained.[10–12] In the rat, the half-lives of gentamicin and of tobramycin in renal tissue exceed those observed in serum 150-fold.[10] After a single subcutaneous injection these drugs can be detected in urine for several

Friedrich C. Luft • Renal Section, Department of Medicine, Indiana University School of Medicine, Indianapolis, Indiana 46223.

weeks. With repetitive injections, or continuous infusions, aminoglycosides achieve extremely high concentrations in renal tissue, but do not exceed peak urine concentrations.[13–15] Observations of human renal tissue concentrations are similar to those in experimental animals.[16,17]

Gentamicin and tobramycin have been identified inside tubular cells where they bind to subcellular organelles.[18,19] The mode of entry has not been entirely clarified. Tubular microinjection experiments utilizing [^{3}H]gentamicin have shown that the drug is absorbed along the proximal convoluted tubule and Henle's loop.[20] Transtubular reabsorption of [^{3}H]gentamicin was not detected in these experiments. In addition, microperfusion of peritubular capillaries failed to demonstrate transtubular secretory flux of [^{3}H]gentamicin. Significant uptake of gentamicin has been demonstrated by studies of renal cortical slices.[20–23] Thus, it is likely that gentamicin accumulation reflects transport across both the apical and basolateral epithelial cell membranes.

The bulk of gentamicin uptake appears to take place on the luminal surface. Results obtained from a nonfiltering kidney model indicate that gentamicin accumulation in renal cortex was markedly decreased compared to results obtained in filtering kidneys. Cortical concentrations of cephaloridine, a drug known to be transported from the basolateral to the luminal surface, actually were increased in nonfiltering kidneys.[24]

The renal accumulation of gentamicin is not influenced by probenecid,[20,25] *N*-methyl nicotinamide,[20] glucose, or quinine.[26] However, preliminary evidence suggests that solutions of mixed aminoglycosides may influence renal cortical aminoglycoside accumulation.[26] Evidence regarding the influence of concomitantly administered β-lactam antibiotics on aminoglycoside accumulation in renal cortex is conflicting.[26–28] Alkalinization of the urine with sodium bicarbonate causes a modest decrease in accumulation of gentamicin in renal cortex probably by changing the cationic nature of the molecule.[29] Urinary acidification has little or no effect on gentamicin accumulation. A dietary regimen low in sodium has been shown to result in increased renal cortical gentamicin accumulation as well as in increased toxicity.[30]

The mechanism by which gentamicin, and presumably other aminoglycosides, enter renal tubular cells has been studied in detail by means of autoradiography.[31–33] Electron microscopic observations of [^{3}H]gentamicin showed that the drug was associated with apical vesicles 10 min after injection.[33] The autoradiographic granules were identified subsequently within lysosomes at 1 and at 24 hr. It appears that the drug is transported into proximal tubular cells by pinocytosis and subsequently becomes sequestered within lysosomes.

Although the pathogenesis of aminoglycoside nephrotoxicity is thought to be linked to the accumulation of drug in proximal tubular epithelium and to the subsequent interaction of these agents with intracellular organelles, a good correlation between the drug concentration within renal cortex and the nephrotoxic effect has not been shown.[34–36] It is possible that the extent to which aminoglycosides accumulate in renal cortex is not the sole factor responsible for nephrotoxicity. The toxic effect of a given drug on intracellular organelles may be equally or more important. *In vitro* studies, in which increasing concentrations of aminoglycosides were added to lysosomal suspensions, have shown that at similar concentrations aminoglycosides differ considerably in their proclivity to induce release of beta-*N*-acetyl hexosaminidase.[37] Thus, it is likely that not only drug accumulation but also the intracellular toxic effect determines the nephrotoxic potential. The complexity of the relationship between nephrotoxicity and drug accumulation has been illustrated by long-term experiments in rats, in which gentamicin was given for 6 weeks.[38] In the course of these studies, the animals recovered renal function in spite of the continued administration of gentamicin. Cortical drug concentrations were not related to the development of renal failure or to recovery. In man, a computer model has been proposed to differentiate prospectively the prenephrotoxic patient from the nontoxic patient by routine monitoring of aminoglycoside serum concentrations during therapy.[39] The success of this approach has not been established. Models assuming first-order kinetics may be inappropriate since at least two mechanisms involved in the handling of aminoglycosides, namely, tubular reabsorption and tissue binding and elimination, may not occur as first-order processes.[40]

In animal models of nephrotoxicity, the repetitive administration of aminoglycosides produces polyuria, proteinuria, glycosuria, enzymuria, decreases in urinary osmolality, and, in some species, electrolyte disturbances.[15,41–45] The excretion of lysosomal acid hydrolases has been studied in detail[43] and clinically has been utilized as an early indicator of nephrotoxicity.[46] The decrease in urinary osmolality has been investigated and has been found to represent renal resistance to the effects of antidiuretic hormone.[47] Hypokalemia has been shown to develop after chronic gentamicin administration in the dog,[46] but not in the rat.[42,43] These functional changes occur prior to decreases in glomerular filtration rate.

Histologically, progressive, dose-dependent necrosis is most prominent in the convoluted portion of the proximal tubule.[42,48] Hyaline droplet degeneration is a regular feature. After approximately 10 days of gentamicin administration in the rat, areas of regeneration are observed. If the dose is such that complete necrosis does not occur, recovery progresses whether or not the drug is discontinued.[38,49] Thus, the regenerating epithelium appears resistant to the nephrotoxic insult, a feature that has been reported previously in several different models of nephrotoxicity.[50,51]

Transmission electron microscopy reveals the appearance of cytosegresomes, modified lysosomes, which contain myeloid whorls of membranous structures within the cytoplasm of proximal and occasionally distal or collecting tubular epithelial cells.[15,42,48,51] These autophagic structures appear even at low doses of gentamicin (52) and also have been observed in human tissue.[17] Cytosegresomes with myeloid bodies are not specific for aminoglycoside toxicity. They have been reported with numerous potentially toxic substances including clindamycin, chloroquine, and erythromycin in various tissues.[53,54] Paraquat is known to cause similar changes in renal tissue.[55] Cytosegresomes with myeloid bodies are modified secondary lysosomes formed by the process of cytoplasmic degradation.[56] The myeloid bodies persist because of protracted degradation of sequestered organelle membranes, possibly endoplasmic reticulum.

Although gentamicin appears to result in autophagia when injected into rats, its mode of cellular injury is not clear. Although lysosomal acid hydrolases are released from lysosomal suspensions *in vitro* when aminoglycosides are added, *in vivo* experiments have not suggested that cellular injury is related to the release of hydrolytic enzymes from lysosomes.[57] Experimental evidence suggests that gentamicin interferes with oxidative metabolism.[42,58,59] Renal cortical homogenates from rats receiving the antibiotic exhibit decreased oxygen uptake and P:O ratio in mitochondrial fractions.[42] An inhibitory effect on oxidative phosphorylation in renal cortical mitochondria has been demonstrated prior to morphological evidence of renal cell necrosis.[59] Aminoglycoside antibiotics also have been found to inhibit renal Na, K-ATPase.[60] This inhibition, as demonstrated *in vitro*, occurs at aminoglycoside concentrations well within those realized within proximal tubular cells *in vivo*. The rank order of inhibition correlates reasonably well with the nephrotoxic potential of the aminoglycosides *in vivo*.

A novel approach to the question of aminoglycoside nephrotoxicity has resulted from observations that gentamicin is incorporated into lysosomes in cultured fibroblasts.[61] Morphometric analysis of such fibroblasts showed a marked increase in the volume of lysosomes as well as a reduction in their number.[62] Chemical analyses revealed a large increase in all major phospholipids including in an ill-defined polar lipid. Lysosomal sphingomyelinase was markedly deficient. These observations suggest that in rat fibroblasts gentamicin induced a lysosomal phospholipidosis through dysfunction of sphingomyelinase and possibly other phospholipases. Conceivably, nephrotoxicity could develop by means of a similar mechanism in renal tissue.

Recently, micropuncture studies have shed new light on the mechanisms of the defect in glomerular ultrafiltration observed with gentamicin-induced nephrotoxicity. Experiments performed in Munich–Wistar rats, which have surface glomeruli suitable for micropuncture, indicate that rats given even low-dose gentamicin treatment develop reductions in single-nephron glomerular filtration rate.[63] The primary cause for this reduction was a marked decrease in glomerular capillary ultrafiltration coefficient. Transmission electron microscopic examination of glomeruli from gentamicin-treated animals revealed no abnormalities in the glomerular capillary wall, although the previously described abnormalities in tubular cells were readily identified. The results of these studies have been corroborated by experiments performed in rabbits.[64] In those studies, glomerular ultrafiltration coefficient was determined by an osmometric technique. The decreases observed were similar to those recorded by micropuncture in the rat. Mature rabbits were found to be more sensitive to the nephrotoxic effects of gentamicin than immature rabbits.

Decreases in glomerular ultrafiltration coefficient have been observed in other models of acute renal failure.[65] Transmission electron microscopy has not revealed structural causes for reductions in glomerular ultrafiltration coefficient. However, scanning electron microscopy has added a new dimension to the study of the glomerular filtration barrier. Scanning electron microscopy permits not only the assessment of qualitative changes, but also quantitative measurements of the density and size of endothelial fenestrae. The glomeruli of rats receiving gentamicin have recently been studied by means of scanning electron microscopy.[66] These experiments identified specific qualititative and quantitative abnormalities on the capillary endothelial surface. In addition to a decrease in number and size of endothelial fenestrae, endothelial cell swelling and the formation of bulbous projections were identified. At the doses employed, the epithelial surface remained normal. These studies suggest a morphological basis for the reductions in glomerular ultrafiltration coefficient described in animals given gentamicin. In addition, they support the idea that a specific glomerular aberration is at least in part responsible for the acute renal failure associated with the administration of large doses of gentamicin in experimental animals and man. Experiments in a rat model utilizing uranyl nitrate as the nephrotoxic agent [65] have demonstrated that the capillary endothelial surface is specifically involved. After the administration of uranyl nitrate, both endothelial fenestral density and size were significantly reduced. Abnormalities of the glomerular epithelial foot processes were noted as well.

Aminoglycoside antibiotics are indicated in cases of life-threatening infections involving gram-negative aerobic bacilli. Generally, the patients receiving aminoglycosides are critically ill. For this reason, aminoglycosides are frequently given in conjunction with other medications, some of which have been reported to result in increased nephrotoxicity. These agents include methoxyflurane,[67] amphotericin B,[68] cisplatin,[69] clindamycin,[70] furosemide,[71] cephaloridine,[72] and cephalothin.[73] A number of these agents have been studied specifically in combination with gentamicin in animal models.

The combination of gentamicin and methoxyflurane has been studied in the rat.[74] Rats receiving gentamicin either prior to or after methoxyflurane anesthesia for 3.5 hr developed worse renal insufficiency than rats treated with either drug alone. Renal histology revealed typical changes associated with both drug treatments. Gentamicin nephrotoxicity is enhanced by furosemide in both the rat[75] and the dog.[76] The enhanced nephrotoxicity was attributed to volume depletion, a reasonable explanation since dietary sodium intake is known to affect significantly gentamicin-induced nephrotoxicity.[30] Although a prospective, randomized, double-blind study in man has shown that the combination of aminoglycoside plus cephalothin is more nephrotoxic than the combination of aminoglycoside plus methicillin,[73] studies in experimental animals have produced conflicting results. In the rabbit, the combination of cephalothin plus gentamicin appeared more nephrotoxic than gentamicin alone.[36] However, the study addressing the question included no discrete pathological grading scale, and critical statistical analysis was not applied. In the dog, the addition of cephalothin to gentamicin produced no additive nephrotoxic effect.[35] In the rat, investigators have observed either no change[77,78] or an amelioration of gentamicin-induced nephrotoxicity.[28,79–82] Why cephalothin should ameliorate gentamicin-induced nephrotoxicity is unclear. However, several investigators have suggested that cephalothin may affect intrarenal aminoglycoside accumulation.[27,28] The ameliorative affect apparently is not confined to cephalothin but has been described in the rat when other B-lactam antibiotics are administered in conjunction with gentamicin.[83] Elucidation of this phenomenon and interpretation of its clinical significance, if any, will require additional investigation.

In summary, the aminoglycosides are complex, potentially nephrotoxic, antimicrobial agents. Their pharmacokinetics are best defined by a three-compartment, open model, with significant renal cortical accumulation. Aminoglycoside antibiotics are transported across both the apical and basolateral cell surfaces. However, the bulk of reabsorption appears to be on the apical surface of proximal renal tubular epithelium by a process involving pinocytosis. The relationship between drug accumulation and nephrotoxicity has not been entirely clarified. Aminoglycosides accumulate within lysosomes. They appear to induce cellular dysfunction and eventual necrosis by several mechanisms, including interference with sodium- and potassium-dependent ATPase, disturbances in mitochondrial respiration, and a decrease in the activity of phospholipases. Although a decrease in glomerular filtration rate eventually occurs, aminoglycosides initially induce tubular malfunction including enzymuria, glycosuria, a decrease in urinary osmolality, and electrolyte disturbances. The failure of filtration is accompanied by a decrease in the glomerular ultrafiltration coefficient which may be explained in part by recent scanning electron microscopic findings which reveal striking glomerular endothelial aberrations. Aminoglycoside nephrotoxicity potentially is enhanced by other therapeutic agents, a characteristic that warrants further investigations in experimental animals.

References

1. Appel GB, Neu HC: The nephrotoxicity of antimicrobial agents. *N Engl J Med* 296:722–728, 1977.
2. Gyselynck AM, Forrey A, Cutler R: Pharmacokinetics of gentamicin: Distribution and plasma and renal clearance. *J Infect Dis* 124(suppl):S70–S76, 1971.
3. Nedden R, Fuchs T, Schröder K, Wundt W: Die renale Ausscheidung von Gentamicin beim Menschen. *Deut Med Wochenschr* 97:1496–1503, 1972.
4. Schentag JJ, Jusko WJ: Renal clearance and tissue accumulation of gentamicin. *Clin Pharmacol Ther* 22:364–370, 1977.
5. Chiu PJ, Brown A, Miller G, Long JF: Renal extraction of gentamicin in anesthetized dogs. *Antimicrob Agents Chemother* 10:277–282, 1976.
6. Schultz RG, Winters RE, Kauffman H: Possible nephrotoxicity of gentamicin. *J Infect Dis* 124(suppl):S145–S147, 1971.

7. Gordon RC, Regamey C, Kirby WMM: Serum protein binding of the aminoglycoside antibiotics. *Antimicrob Agents Chemother* 2:214–216, 1972.
8. Ramirez-Ronda CH, Holmes RK, Sanford JP: Effects of divalent cations on binding of aminoglycoside antibiotics to human serum protein and to bacteria. *Antimicrob Agents Chemother* 7:239–245, 1975.
9. Meyers DR, DeFehr J, Bennett WM, Porter GA, Olsen GD: Gentamicin binding to serum and plasma proteins. *Clin Pharmacol Ther* 23:356–360, 1978.
10. Luft FC, Kleit SA: Renal parenchymal accumulation of aminoglycoside antibiotics in rats. *J Infect Dis* 130:656–659, 1974.
11. Fabre J, Rudhart M, Blanchard P, Regamey C: Persistence of sisomicin and gentamicin in renal cortex and medulla compared with other organs and serum of rats. *Kidney Int* 10:444–449, 1976.
12. Trottier S, Bergeron MG, Gauvreau L: Intrarenal concentration of netilmicin and gentamicin, in: Siegenthaler W, Lüthy R (eds): *Current Chemotherapy*. Washington, American Society for Microbiology, 1979, pp 953–955.
13. Reiner NE, Bloxham DD, Thompson WL: Nephrotoxicity of gentamicin and tobramycin given once daily or continuously in dogs. *J Antimicrob Chemother* 4(suppl A):85–89, 1978.
14. Whelton A, Carter GG, Craig TJ, Bryant HH, Herbst DV, Walker WG: Comparison of the intrarenal disposition of tobramycin and gentamicin: Therapeutic and toxicologic answers. *J Antimicrob Chemother* 4(suppl A):13–16, 1978.
15. Luft FC, Patel V, Yum MN, Patel B, Kleit SA: Experimental aminoglycoside nephrotoxicity. *J Lab Clin Med* 86:213–220, 1975.
16. Edwards CQ, Smith CR, Baughman KL, Rogers JF, Lietman PS: Concentrations of gentamicin and amikacin in human kidneys. *Antimicrob Agents Chemother* 9:925–927, 1976.
17. Luft FC, Yum MN, Walker PD, Kleit SA: Gentamicin gradient patterns and morphologic changes in human kidneys. *Nephron* 18:167–174, 1977.
18. Lietman PS: Aminoglycoside nephrotoxicity: Transport and subcellular aspects, in: *Symposium: Mechanics of Toxicity. 17th Interscience Conference on Antimicrobial Agents and Chemotherapy*. 12–14 Oct 1977, New York.
19. Mahon WA, Ezer JI, Inaba T: Renal binding of aminoglycosides, in: *Assessment of Aminoglycoside Toxicity*. Switzerland, Bürgenstock, 1978, p 14.
20. Pastoriza–Muñoz E, Bowman RL, Kaloyanides GJ: Renal tubular transport of gentamicin in the rat. *Kidney Int* 16:440–450, 1979.
21. Hsu CH, Kurtz TW, Weller JM: *In vitro* uptake of gentamicin by rat renal cortical tissue. *Antimicrob Agents Chemother* 12:192–194, 1977.
22. Bennett WM, Plamp CE, Parter RA, Gilbert DN, Houghton DC, Porter GA: Renal transport of organic acids and bases in aminoglycoside nephrotoxicity. *Antimicrob Agents Chemother* 16:231–233, 1979.
23. Kluwe WM, Hook JB: Analysis of gentamicin uptake by rat renal cortical slices. *Toxicol Appl Pharmacol* 45:513–539, 1978.
24. Collier VU, Lietman PS, Mitch WE: Evidence for luminal uptake of gentamicin in the perfused rat kidney. *J Pharmacol Exp Ther* 210:247–251, 1979.
25. Bergan T, Westlie L, Brodwall EK: Influence of probenecid on gentamicin pharmacokinetics. *Acta Med Scand* 191:221–224, 1972.
26. Whelton A, Carter GG, Bryant HH, Cody TS, Craig TJ, Walker WG: Intrarenal distribution of aminoglycosides; nephrotoxicity of aminoglycosides and cephalosporins, in: Siegenthaler W, Lüthy R (eds): *Current Chemotherapy*. Washington, American Society for Microbiology, 1979, pp 951–953.
27. Dellinger P, Murphy T, Barza M, Pinn V, Weinstein L: Effects of cephalothin on renal cortical concentrations of gentamicin in rats. *Antimicrob Agents Chemother* 9:587–588, 1976.
28. Roos R, Jackson GG: Protective effect of cephalothin on gentamicin nephrotoxicity: effect of cephalothin anion, not sodium cation, in: Siegenthaler W, Lüthy R (eds): *Current Chemotherapy*. Washington, American Society for Microbiology, 1979, pp 962–964.
29. Chiu PJS, Miller GH, Long JF, Waitz JA: Renal uptake and nephrotoxicity of gentamicin during urinary alkalinization in rats. *Clin Exp Pharmacol Physiol* 6:317–326, 1979.

30. Bennett WM, Hartnett MN, Gilbert D, Houghton D, Porter GA: Effect of sodium intake on gentamicin nephrotoxicity in the rat. *Proc Soc Exp Biol Med* 151:736–738, 1976.
31. Just M, Erdmann G, Habermann E: The renal handling of poly basic drugs: 1. Gentamicin and aprotinin in intact animals. *Naunyn-Schmiedebergs Arch Pharmakol* 300:57–66, 1977.
32. Kuhar MJ, Mak LL, Lietman PS: Autoradiographic localization of [^{3}H]gentamicin in the proximal renal tubules of mice. *Antimicrob Agents Chemother* 15:131–133, 1979.
33. Silverblatt FJ, Kuehn C: Autoradiography of gentamicin uptake by the rat proximal tubule cell. *Kidney Int* 15:335–345, 1979.
34. Soberon L, Bowman RL, Pastoriza-Muñoz E, Kaloyanides GL: Comparative nephrotoxicities of gentamicin, netilmicin and tobramycin in the rat. *J Pharmacol Exp Ther* 210:334–339, 1979.
35. Bloxham DD, Meliere CC, Thompson WL: Aminoglycoside nephrotoxicity: Effects of dosage regimen and cephalothin. *Clin Res* 26:286A, 1978.
36. Luft FC, Bloch R, Sloan RS, Yum MN, Costello R, Maxwell DR: Comparative nephrotoxicity of aminoglycoside antibiotics in rats. *J Infect Dis* 138:541–545, 1978.
37. Morin JD, Fillastre JP, Vaillant R: Prediction of aminoglycoside cephalosporin nephrotoxicity, in: Siegenthaler W, Lüthy R (eds): *Current Chemotherapy*. Washington, American Society for Microbiology, 1979, pp 960–962.
38. Gilbert DN, Houghton DC, Bennett WM, Plamp CE, Roger K, Porter GA: Reversibility of gentamicin nephrotoxicity in rats: Recovery during continuous drug administration. *Proc Soc Exp Biol Med* 160:99–103, 1979.
39. Colburn WA, Schentag JJ, Jusko WJ, Gibaldi M: A model for the prospective identification of the pre nephrotoxic state during gentamicin therapy. *J Pharmacokinetics Biopharm* 6:179–186, 1978.
40. Kahlmeter G: Gentamicin and tobramycin clinical pharmacokinetic and nephrotoxicity aspects on assay techniques. Lund, Sweden Berlings, 1979, p 29.
41. Cohen L, Lapkin R, Kaloyanides GJ: Effect of gentamicin on renal function in the rat. *J Pharmacol Exp Ther* 193:264–273, 1975.
42. Cuppage FE, Setter K, Sullivan LP, Reitzes EJ, Melnykovych AO: Gentamicin nephrotoxicity. II. Physiological, biochemical and morphological effects of prolonged administration to rats. *Virchows Arch B Cell Path* 24:121–138, 1977.
43. Patel V, Luft FC, Yum MN, Patel B, Zeman W, Kleit SA: Enzymuria in gentamicin-induced kidney damage. *Antimicrob Agents Chemother* 7:364–369, 1975.
44. Ginsburg DS, Quintanilla AP, Levin M: Renal glycosuria due to gentamicin in rabbits. *J Infect Dis* 134:119–122, 1976.
45. Cronin RE, Bulger RE, Southern P, Henrich WL: Natural history of aminoglycoside nephrotoxicity in the dog. *J Lab Clin Med* 95:463–474, 1980.
46. Benner EJ: Comparison of the renal toxicity of gentamicin and tobramycin in humans during clinical therapy of infections, in: Siegenthaler W, Lüthy R (eds): *Current Chemotherapy*. Washington, American Society for Microbiology, 1979, pp 949–950.
47. Bennett WM, Plamp C, Reger K, McClung M, Porter GA: The concentrating defect in experimental gentamicin nephrotoxicity. *Clin Res* 26:540A, 1978.
48. Houghton DC, Hartnett M, Campbell–Boswell M, Porter G, Bennett W: A light and microscopic analysis of gentamicin nephrotoxicity in rats. *Am J Pathol* 82:589–599, 1976.
49. Luft FC, Rankin LI, Sloan RS, Yum MN: Recovery during aminoglycoside administration. *Antimicrob Agents Chemother* 14:284–287, 1978.
50. MacNider WdeB: The functional and pathological response of the kidney in dogs subjected to a second subcutaneous injection of uranium nitrate. *J Exp Med* 49:411–431, 1929.
51. Luft FC, Yum MN, Kleit SA: The effect of concomitant mercuric chloride and gentamicin on kidney function and structure in the rat. *J Lab Clin Med* 89:622–631, 1977.
52. Kosek JD, Mazze RI, Cousins MJ: Nephrotoxicity of gentamicin. *Lab Invest* 30:48–57, 1974.
53. Fedorko ME: Effect of chloroquin on morphology of leukocytes and pancreatic exocrine cells in the rat. *Lab Invest* 18:27–37, 1968.
54. Gray JE, Purmalis A, Purmalis B, Mathews JJ: Ultrastructural studies of the hepatic changes brought about by clindamycin and erythromycin in animals. *Toxicol Appl Pharmacol* 19:217–227, 1971.

55. Fowler BA, Brooks RE: Effects of the herbicide paraquat on the ultrastructure of mouse kidney. *Am J Pathol* 63:62–70, 1971.
56. Hruban F, Slesers A, Hopkins E: Drug induced and naturally occurring myeloid bodies. *Lab Invest* 27:62–70, 1972.
57. Vera-Roman J, Krishnakantha TP, Cuppage FE: Gentamicin nephrotoxicity in rats. I. Acute biochemical and structural effects. *Lab Invest* 33:412–417, 1975.
58. Bendirdjian JP, Foucher B, Fillastre JP: Influence des aminoglycosides sur le metabolisme respiratoire des mitochondries isolees de foie et de rein de rat, in: Fillastre JP (ed): *Nephrotoxicity Interaction of Drugs with Membranes Systems Mitochondria–Lysosomes.* Paris, Masson, 1978, pp 315–332.
59. Simons CF, Bogusky RT, Humes HD: Inhibitory effects of gentamicin on renal cortical mitochondrial oxidation phosphorylation. A primary pathogenetic event in gentamicin nephrotoxicity. *Proc Am Soc Nephrol* 12:6A, 1979.
60. Lietman PS: Aminoglycoside inhibition of a renal sodium-potassium ATP-ase. A possible model for nephrotoxicity. *Antimicrob Agents Chemother* 18:328, 1978.
61. Tulkens P, Trouet A: Uptake and intracellular localization of kanamycin and gentamicin in the lysosomes of cultured fibroblasts. *Arch Int Physiol Biochim* 82:1018–1019, 1974.
62. Aubert-Tulkens G, VanHoof F, Tulkens P: Gentamicin-induced lysosomal phospholipidosis in cultured rat fibroblasts. *Lab Invest* 40:481–491, 1979.
63. Baylis C, Rennke HR, Brenner BM: Mechanisms of the defect in glomerular ultrafiltration associated with gentamicin administration. *Kidney Int* 12:344–348, 1977.
64. Chonko A, Savin V, Stewart R, Karniski L, Cuppage F, Hodges G: The effects of gentamicin on renal function of gentamicin on renal function in the mature vs. immature rabbit. *Clin Res* 27:664A, 1979.
65. Avasthi PS, Evan AP, Hay D: Glomerular endothelial cells in uranyl nitrate-induced acute renal failure in rats. *J Clin Invest* 65:121–127, 1980.
66. Evan AP, Huser J, Avasthi PS, Rankin LI, Luft FC: Gentamicin induced glomerular injury. *Proc Intersci Conf Antimicrob Agents Chemother* 19:933, 1979.
67. Mazze RI, Cousins M: Combined nephrotoxicity of gentamicin and methoxyflurane anaesthesia in man. *Br. J Anaesth* 45:394–397, 1973.
68. Churchill DN, Seely J: Nephrotoxicity associated with combined gentamicin–amphotericin B therapy. *Nephron* 19:176–181, 1977.
69. Dentino ME, Luft FC, Yum MN, Einhorn LH: Long term effect of *cis*-diamminedichloride platinum on renal function and structure in man. *Cancer* 41:1274–1281, 1978.
70. Butkus DE, de Torrente A, Terman DS: Renal failure following gentamicin in combination with clindamycin. *Nephron* 17:307–313, 1976.
71. Noël P, Levy VG: Toxicité rénale de l'association gentamicin–furosemide. *Nouv Presse Med* 7:351–353, 1978.
72. Barza M: The nephrotoxicity of cephalosporins: an overview. *J Infect Dis* 130:S60–S73, 1978.
73. Wade JC, Smith CR, Petty BG, Lipsky JJ, Conrad G, Ellner J, Lietman PS: Cephalothin plus an aminoglycoside is more nephrotoxic than methicillin plus an aminoglycoside. *Lancet* 3:604–606, 1978.
74. Barr GA, Mazze RI, Cousins MJ, Kosek JC: An animal model for combined methoxy flurane and gentamicin nephrotoxicity. *Br J Anaesth* 45:306–311, 1973.
75. Chiu PJS, Long JF: Effect of hydration on gentamicin excretion and renal accumulation in furosemide treated rats. *Antimicrob Agents Chemother* 14:214–217.
76. Adelman RD, Spangler WL, Beason F, Isizaki G, Conzelman GM: Furosemide enhancement of experimental gentamicin nephrotoxicity: A comparison of functional and morphological changes with urinary enzyme activities. *J Infect Dis* 140:342–352, 1979.
77. Harrison WO, Silverblatt FJ, Turck M: Gentamicin nephrotoxicity: Failure of three cephalosporins to potentiate injury in rats. *Antimicrob Agents Chemother* 8:209–215, 1975.
78. Hagstrom GL, Luft FC, Yum MN, Sloan RS, Maxwell DR: Nephrotoxicity of netilmicin in combination with nonaminoglycoside antibiotics. *Antimicrob Agents Chemother* 13:490–493, 1978.

79. Dellinger P, Murphy T, Pinn V, Barza M, Weinstein L: The protective effect of cephalothin against gentamicin-induced nephrotoxicity in rats. *Antimicrob Agents Chemother* 9:172–178, 1976.
80. Luft FC, Patel V, Yum MN, Kleit SA: The nephrotoxicity of cephalosporin-gentamicin combinations in rats. *Antimicrob Agents Chemother* 9:831–839, 1976.
81. Sugarman A, Brown RS, Rosen S: Gentamicin nephrotoxicity and the beneficial effect of simultaneous administration of cephalothin or other sodium salts. *Proc Am Soc Nephrol* 10:80A, 1976.
82. Barza M, Pinn V, Tanguay P, Murray T: Comparative nephrotoxicity of newer cephalosporins and aminoglycosides alone and in combination in a rat model, in: Sigenthaler W, Lüthy R (eds): *Current Chemotherapy*. Washington, American Society for Microbiology, 1978, pp 964–966.
83. Bloch R, Luft FC, Rankin LI, Sloan RS, Yum MN, Maxwell DR: Protection from gentamicin nephrotoxicity by cephalothin and carbenicillin. *Antimicrob Agents Chemother* 15:46–49, 1979.

42

Acute Problems during Hemodialysis

C. M. Kjellstrand

The outcomes of chronic hemodialysis have improved greatly during the last 15 years. This improvement has taken place without any real "breakthrough" in our understanding of performance of dialysis. It seems to represent the cumulative results of small technical improvements, the "shuffling of details," and the tendency to increase the frequency of dialysis from 2 to 3 times weekly. The improvement is very real. The first-year mortality has decreased from 50% to 14% (Table 1). This is astounding, particularly as mean patient age has increased markedly and the percentage of patients with systemic complicated diseases has increased markedly.

Most research efforts in chronic dialysis have gone into solving chronic pathophysiologic complications such as anemia, bone disease, neuropathy, accelerated arterial sclerosis, and the organic brain syndrome.

It is generally believed that chronic hemodialysis is a reasonably comfortable procedure for the patients once they are stabilized. However, close scrutiny does not bear this out. When we reviewed the effects and problems of changing dialysis schedules, two things became clear.(1) First, many side effects such as vomiting, cramps, and shock were common, and with increasing efficiency of dialysis those complications got much worse. Secondly, both staff and patients seemed to prefer shortening the dialysis time in spite of increasing problems with each dialysis run. Obviously patients fear and dislike the time spent on hemodialysis, and the less time spent on dialysis, the more pleased is the patient (Fig. 1).

1. Incidence of Acute Side Effects of Dialysis

We therefore undertook a study to see how common acute problems during dialysis were.(2) During the first 40 dialyses in 21 patients accepted

C. M. Kjellstrand • Division of Nephrology, Department of Medicine, Hennepin County Medical Center, Minneapolis, Minnesota 55415.

Table 1. First Year Cumulated Survival Ratios of Chronic Hemodialysis Reported by the European Dialysis and Transplant Association

Year dialysis started	Percent patients alive at 1 year after start	Number of patients observed
1965	50	232
1966	53	516
1968	64	1,767
1970	83	1,611
1975	86	17,288
1978	86	56,083

for chronic hemodialysis at the University of Minnesota, we studied the incidence of hypotension, nausea, vomiting, muscle cramps, and headache. Overall, three complications tended to occur during the first dialysis. Thereafter, a decrease occurred and the patient seemed to stabilize after 13–20 dialyses. However, even after this number of dialyses, as a mean, one of these complications usually occurred with each dialysis. Most common were problems with hypotension (blood pressure fall > 25% of initial pressure) occurring about every other dialysis. Second most common was an increase in blood pressure or nausea occurring every sixth dialysis, headache every tenth dialysis, vomiting occurring every fifteenth dialysis, and muscle cramps every twenty-fifth dialysis. The incidence of side effects of dialysis decreased approximately 50% from the incidence during the initial introductory phase until the patient had stabilized on dialysis at about 1 month. Other studies have not been designed to study the occurrence of side effects directly but mainly to describe how they change when dialysis therapies are varied.

A literature review of such studies suggests that findings are not unique but are fairly representative.[1–9] The largest study comes from France and basically confirms our observations.[9] Thus, dialysis is a procedure accom-

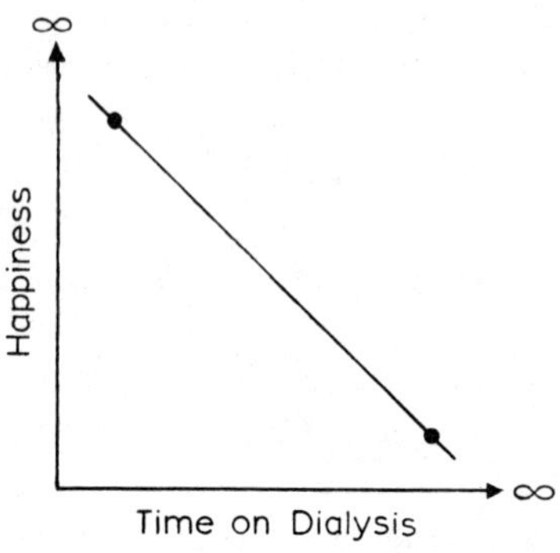

Figure 1. The relationship between shortening of dialysis sessions and happiness in patients.

Table 2. Factors Causing or Contributing to Hypotension during Dialysis

Pathogenesis	Mediators	Underlying pathology	Pathophysiology
Ultrafiltration Osmolality fall Dialysis removal of vasoactive substances (epinephrine, norepinephrine) Dialysis into patient of destabilizing factors (acetate) Failure to remove destabilizing factor ("middle molecules") Damage to white cells or platelets Protein changes (complement activation)	Hypovolemia Decrease in vasoactive amines, vasopressin Osmostat turned off Endothelial or blood cell damage with release of prostacyclin	Autonomous dysfunction Endocrine dysfunction (adrenal medulla, adrenal cortex) Juxtaglomerular app. Vessel dysfunction, peripheral "stiffness," peripheral "sluggishness," capacitance compliance Myocardiopathy Drugs Infections, pain	Decrease in cardiac output, peripheral resistance, or both; or a decrease in one not compensated by enough increase in the other

panied by considerable morbidity and by a marked discomfort for the patients. It is no wonder that patients eagerly grasp at the reduction in time they need to spend on dialysis. Paradoxically, the incidence of side effects has increased as dialysis efficiency is increased.[1]

2. *Causes of Acute Side Effects*

When discussing the causes of side effects of hemodialysis, it is important to differentiate the pathogenesis, the pathophysiology, the mediators, and underlying aggravating pathology. Under each heading it is easy to list five or six different factors; all exist to different degrees in different patients, and all are interrelated in a complicated manner. Unless these two facts are understood, much confusion and contradiction will occur. To exemplify, in one article it was claimed that autonomic nervous system insufficiency in uremia caused hemodialysis-induced hypotension.[10] Another study reached the conclusion that hemodialysis hypotension was not the result of uremic autonomic neuropathy.[11] It is obvious that the autonomic dysfunction that some patients have *per se* is not a cause of hypotension during dialysis. It is an underlying pathologic factor that interferes with a patient's ability to deal with hypotension that is somehow triggered by dialysis.

In Table 2 several known factors are listed.

2.1. Pathogenetic Factors

Hypovolemia secondary to ultrafiltration may cause hypotension. However, there is unanimity in the literature that volume reduction alone is rarely responsible for dialysis-induced hypotension.[12–14] Some other factor induced by the dialysis procedure must be responsible for the patient's inability to defend himself against ultrafiltration-induced hypovolemia or in itself can trigger a decrease in peripheral resistance or cardiac output.

The osmolality fall that occurs during dialysis seems to be one important factor. Thus, we have shown that mannitol infusion will decrease both the fall in blood pressure and the number of mild and severe hypotensive episodes occurring during dialysis.[4,12] A whole series of low versus a high dialysate sodium confirm this observation. Whenever dialysate sodium concentration is increased, hypotensive episodes and other side effects occur less frequently.[15–27]

The dialysis procedure also may deplete some patients of vasoactive amines,[28–31] although opinions differ about this.[32–34]

Acetate also has been thought to be the culprit of many problems arising during dialysis, particularly hypotensive episodes and fatigue.[35,36] Wehle and co-workers, however, as well as Raja and associates suggest that this is of much less importance than is osmolality. Bicarbonate seems superior to acetate only when hyponatremic dialysate is used.[3,25]

We have found in a double-blind crossover study of 30 patients receiving 130 dialyses for acute renal failure that the mean blood pressure fall during acetate dialysis was 17.5 mm Hg versus 20.5 mm Hg for bicarbonate. The number of episodes when the blood pressure fell more than 25% of the initial value was 11.6% during acetate dialysis and 19.1% during dialysis with bicarbonate dialysate. None of these differences are statistically significant. It is obvious that our studies performed in acute patients cannot be extrapolated to chronic ones.

One of the most puzzling aspects of dialysis-induced hypotension is the claim that hemofiltration causes fewer blood pressure problems than does hemodialysis. Part of this may be explained by the fact that hemofiltration usually is less efficient in small-molecule removal than is hemodialysis, and the observation that very rapid dialysis is more likely to cause hypotension.[1] However, Shaldon and co-workers note that when small-molecule removal during hemofiltration was set carefully, it was as efficient as that occurring during hemodialysis, and they could show that in some patients prone to hypotension, hemofiltration was better tolerated.[37] There may be two explanations for this. First, hemofiltration, which physically removes higher molecular substances more efficiently, could remove a substance that destabilizes the cardiovascular system of these patients. This substance would be retained during hemodialysis. Second, the membranes used for hemofiltration seem to induce fewer changes in white cell count and in serum proteins as evident by less complement activation and neutropenia.[38]

2.2. *Mediators*

Possible mediators of some of the side effects of dialysis are listed in Table 2. Hypovolemia *per se* does not seem to be an important mediator alone.

One possible consequence of hemodialysis is that some of the small molecules are vasoactive and may be removed.[28–34] It also has been shown that vasopressin occurring at a higher-than-normal concentration in dialyzed patients decreases if hypotonic dialysate is used.[39] Therefore, one of the mediators could be a decrease in vasopressin secretion secondary to the pathogenesis of osmolality fall.[40] It has been shown that increasing sodium in the dialysate maintains vasopressin concentration in blood.[39]

It is also possible that the osmolality fall could cause acute autonomous dysfunction by leading to cell edema directly. The result could be that the body is not able to mobilize norepineprine or epinephrine during dialysis as well as during isolated ultrafiltration.[28] Theoretically, the same could apply to the renin–angiotensin system, but Zucchelli and co-workers' findings contradict this as an explanation.[28]

One of our speculations is that release of prostacyclin during dialysis may cause hypotension. Raij and Wrigley have previously shown that during dialysis converting enzyme is released into circulation from the lungs.[41] It also is known that prostacyclin occurs in much higher concentrations in blood vessels of patients with uremia.[42,43] Finally, the infusion of prostacyclins into patients causes a decrease in blood pressure[44,45] comparable to that occurring in most hemodialyses.[3,12] Therefore, one hypothetical mechanism is that during hemodialysis, acute blood changes take place during the blood passage through the dialyzer. This could damage white cells or platelets, both known to decrease during dialysis.[38,46] Thus, these cells could release prostacyclin which would lead to hypotension. An alternate explanation is that endothelial damage that seems to take place in the lungs during dialysis[41] also could result in the release of prostacyclin, and this in turn could decrease the blood pressure. Obviously, this hypothesis needs testing.

2.3. *Underlying Pathology*

A whole series of subtle organ damages exist in patients on dialysis. Many suffer from autonomic dysfunction.[10,11] Myocardial dysfunction also has been described.[47] Finally, it is known that peripheral vessels seem to undergo accelerated degeneration as evident by the arteriosclerosis that such patients have.[48,49] All these factors obviously would not in themselves cause hypotension but could make a patient unable to defend himself against many of the pathogenetic factors working over a variety of mediators as discussed previously. Also, some drugs used by patients will cause them to have difficulties in defending themselves. Thus, for example, the usage of Aldomet is known to almost triple the incidence of hypotensive episodes during dialysis,[50] and the decrease in phosphorus may be another factor.[51] Finally, individual susceptibility will enter into the confusing picture, possibly by working over vasovagal effector mechanisms. One clinical observation we have made is that patients in pain or those with infections seem to be much more likely to develop hypotension than when they are not infected or not in pain.

2.4. Long-Term Consequence of Acute Side Effects

It is obvious that the acute side effects that occur during dialysis are frightening and dismaying to patients, and these alone necessitate their vigorous study.

The side effects make patients push eagerly for shorter dialysis. The time spent on dialysis therefore has decreased over the last years.[9,52] This in turn actually has led to an increase in the number of side effects.[1,9] Thus, the number of hypotensive episodes as well as of muscle cramps has approximately doubled from 1973 to 1975 in France, as the weekly time on dialysis has decreased from 20 to 17 hr. However, in spite of more side effects, the patients continue to push vigorously for shorter dialysis sessions.[1]

Entirely speculative is that many acute side effects may have a slow cumulative effect and give rise to some of the chronic mortal side effects of dialysis. We feel it may be possible that repeated hypo- or hypertensive episodes may contribute to the vascular degeneration and to increased deaths in cardiovascular catastrophes that occur in these patients. A possible contributing factor to dialysis encephalopathy would be the intermittent brain edema that is one of the consequences and one of the acute causes of side effects in dialysis. It is obviously naive to believe that either vascular degeneration or dialysis encephalopathy has a single cause. Figures 2 and 3 illustrate how many potential causes might be added in causing these long-term complications.

3. Conclusion

Acute side effects of dialysis are very common and on an average occur every other dialysis even after patients have undergone dialysis for months. Most common seems to be sudden drops in blood pressure.

In order to understand and to carry out research on these problems it is important to keep pathogenetic factors, pathophysiology, mediators, and underlying pathology separate. It is also important to understand that many pathogenetic factors may work over many different or in the same mechanisms and may have different expressions in patients whose underlying pathology is different. The side effects in themselves are worthy of study to make dialysis more pleasant and safe for the patients, and potentially repeated acute side effects may cause some of the very long-term ill effects of dialysis.

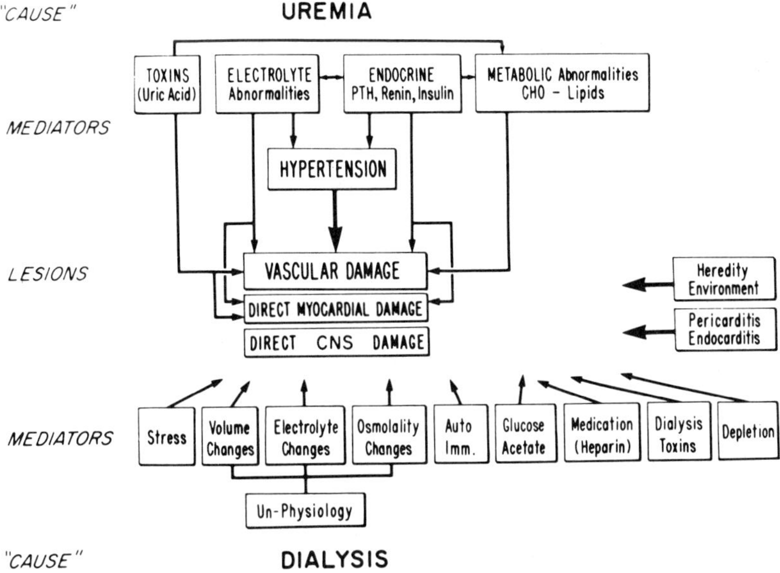

Figure 2. A scheme of the multifactorial etiology of vascular damage in patients on chronic hemodialysis. Unphysiology of dialysis increases acute side effects. Thus, it seems reasonable to speculate that repeated episodes of acute problems may lead to chronic problems or vascular damage. (Figure from ref. 53, with permission of the American Society for Artificial Internal Organs.)

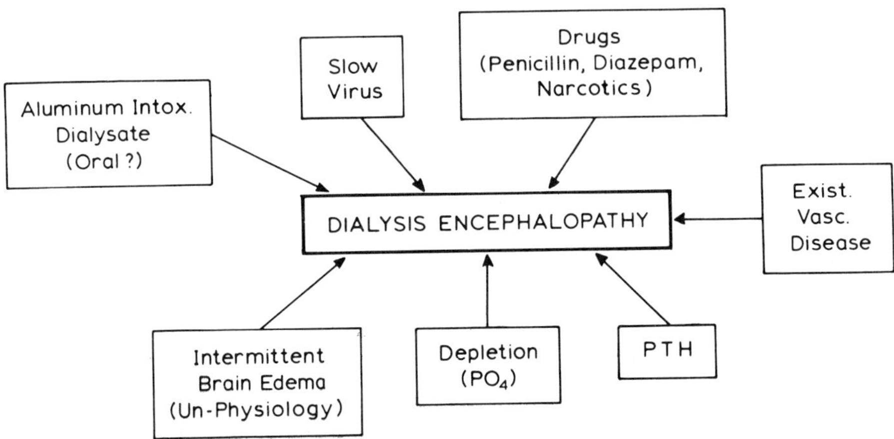

Figure 3. A scheme of multifactorial etiology of dialysis encephalopathy. Intermittent brain edema is an acute side effect of dialysis that may contribute to a chronic one, dialysis encephalopathy. (Figure from ref. 54, with permission of the First Asian Pacific Congress of Nephrology.)

References

1. Kjellstrand CM, Evans RL: Considerations of new dialysis schedules: Theoretical evaluation and review of literature, in: Maiorca R, Lindholm T (eds): *Gardia Meeting on Short Dialysis.* Lund, Sweden, Rahmus, 1975, pp 26–37.
2. Rosa A, Fryd DS, Kjellstrand CM: Dialysis symptoms and stabilization on chronic dialysis—practical application of the Cusum plot. *Arch Intern Med* 140:804–807, 1980.
3. Wehle B, Asaba H, Castenfors J, Furst P, Grahn A, Gunnarsson B, Shaldon S, Bergstrom J: The influence of dialysis fluid composition on the blood pressure response during dialysis. *Clin Nephrol* 10:62–66, 1978.
4. Rodrigo F, Shideman J, McHugh R, Buselmeier T, Kjellstrand C: Osmolality changes during hemodialysis—natural history, clinical correlations, and influence of dialysate glucose and intravenous mannitol. *Ann Intern Med* 86:554–561, 1977.
5. Graefe U, Milutinovich J, Follette WC, Vizzo JE, Babb AL, Scribner BH: Less dialysis-induced morbidity and vascular instability with bicarbonate in dialysate. *Ann Intern Med* 88:332–336, 1978.
6. Hagstam KE, Lindergord B, Tabbling G: Mannitol influence in regular hemodialysis. Treatment for chronic renal insufficiency. *Scand J Urol Nephrol* 3:257–263, 1969.
7. Wilkinson R, Barber SG, Robson V: Cramps, thirst and hypertension in hemodialysis patients—the influence of dialysate sodium concentration. *Clin Nephrol* 7:101–105, 1977.
8. Uriarte AL, Gamez CL, Valenzuela SL: Hypotension arterial durante hemodialisis con sodio bajo en ninos, in: *Abstracts Sociedad Mexicana de Nefrologia—XI Annual Meeting, 1977.*
9. Degoulet P, Roulx J–P, Aime F, Berger C, Bloch P, Goupy F, Legrain M: Programme dialyse—informatique III. Donnees epidemiologiques strategies de dialyse et resultats biologiques. *J Urol Nephrol* 82:1001–1042, 1976.
10. Kersh ES, Kronfield SJ, Unger A, Popper RW, Cantor S, Cohn K: Autonomic insufficiency in uremia as a cause of hemodialysis-induced hypotension. *N Engl J Med* 290:650–653, 1974.
11. Nies AS, Robertson D, Stone WJ: Hemodialysis hypotension is not the result of uremic peripheral autonomic neuropathy. *J Lab Clin Med* 94:395–402, 1979.
12. Kjellstrand CM, Rosa AA, Shideman JR: Hypotension during hemodialysis—osmolality fall is an important pathogenetic factor. *ASAIO J* 3:11–19, 1980.
13. Ing TS, Ashbach DL, Kanter A, Oyama JH, Armbruster KFW, Merkel FK: Fluid removal with negative-pressure hydrostatic ultrafiltration using a partial vacuum. *Nephron* 14:451–455, 1975.
14. Bergstrom J, Asaba H, Furst P, Oules R: Dialysis, ultrafiltration, and blood pressure, in Robinson B (ed): *Dialysis and Renal Transplantation.* London, Pitman Press, 1977, vol 13.
15. Levine J, Falk B, Henriquez M, Raja RM, Kramer MS, Rosenbaum JL: Effects of varying dialysate sodium using large surface area dialyzers. *Tr Am Soc Artif Intern Organs* 24:139–141, 1978.
16. Boquin E, Parnell S, Grondin G, Wollard C, Leonard D, Michales R, Levin NW: Crossover study of the effects of different dialysate sodium concentrations in large surface area, short-term dialysis. *Proc Clin Dial Transpl Forum* 7:48–52, 1977.
17. Gurich W, Mann H, Stiller S, Hacke W: Sodium elimination and alterations of the EEG during dialysis. *Artif Organs* 3(A):15, 1979.
18. Van Stone JC, Cook J: Decreased postdialysis fatigue with increased dialysate sodium concentration. *Proc Clin Dial Transpl Forum* 8:152–156, 1978.
19. Ogden DA: A double blind crossover comparison of high and low sodium dialysis. *Proc Clin Dial Transpl Forum* 8:157–165, 1978.
20. Raja R, Henriquez M, Kramer M, Rosenbaum JL: Hypertonic glucose, mannitol and saline infusion in hemodialysis. *Artif Organs* 3(A):37, 1979.
21. Locatelli F, Costanzo R, Di Filippo S, Pedrini L, Marai P, Pozzi C, Ponti R, Sforzini S, Redaelli B: Ultrafiltration and high sodium concentration dialysis: Pathophysiological correlation. *Proc Eur Dial Transpl Assoc* 15:253–259, 1978.

22. Robson M, Oren A, Ravid M: Dialysate sodium concentration, hypertension, and pulmonary edema in hemodialysis patients. *Dial Transpl* 7:678–679, 1978.
23. Stewart WK, Fleming LW, Manuel MA: Benefits obtained by the use of high sodium dialysate during maintenance haemodialysis. *Proc Eur Dial Transpl Assoc* 9:111–116, 1972.
24. Locatelli F, Costanzo R, Di Filippo S: High sodium dialysate. *Int J Artif Organs* 2:171, 1979.
25. Raja R, Henriquez M, Kramer M, Rosenbaum JL: Intradialytic hypotension—role of osmolar changes and acetate influx. *Tr Am Soc Artif Intern Organs* 25:419–421, 1979.
26. Dumler F, Grondin G, Levin NW: Sequential high/low sodium hemodialysis: An alternative to ultrafiltration. *Tr Am Soc Artif Intern Organs* 25:351–353, 1979.
27. Leski M, Niethammer T, Wyss T: Glucose-enriched dialysate and tolerance to maintenance hemodialysis. *Nephron* 24:271–273, 1979.
28. Zucchelli P, Catizone L, Esposti ED, Fusaroli M, Ligabue A, Zuccala A: Influence of ultrafiltration on plasma renin activity and adrenergic system. *Nephron* 21:317–324, 1978.
29. Cannella G, Picotti GB, Mioni G, Cristinelli L, Maiorca R: Blood pressure behaviors during dialysis and ultrafiltration. A pathogenic hypothesis on hemodialysis-induced hypotension. *Int J Artif Organs* 1:69–75, 1978.
30. Brecht HM, Ernst W, Koch KM: Plasma noradrenaline levels in regular hemodialysis patients. *Proc Eur Dial Transpl Assoc* 12:281–290, 1976.
31. Hamp H: Hemodialysis induced hypotension. *Int J Artif Organs* 2:43–44, 1979.
32. Korchik WP, Brown DC, DeMaster EG: Hemodialysis induced hypotension. *Int J Artif Organs* 1:151, 1978.
33. Korchik WP, DeMaster EG, Brown DC: Plasma norepinephrine and hemodialysis. *Kidney Int* 12:484, 1977 (abstract).
34. Ksiqzek A: Dopamine-beta-hydroxylase activity and catecholamine levels in the plasma of patients with renal failure. *Nephron* 24:170–173, 1979.
35. Graefe U, Milutinovich J Follette WC, Babb AL, Scribner BH: Improved tolerance to rapid ultrafiltration with the use of bicarbonate in dialysate. *Proc Eur Dial Transpl Assoc* 14:153–159, 1977.
36. Van Stone JC, Cook J: The effect of replacing acetate with bicarbonate in the dialysate of stable chronic hemodialysis patients. *Proc Clin Dial Transpl Forum* 8:103–105, 1978.
37. Shaldon S, Deschodt G, Beau MC, Claret G, Mion H, Mion C: Vascular resistance and stability during high flux haemofiltration compared to haemodialysis. *Abstr Am Soc Nephrol* 12:129A, 1979.
38. Aljama P, Bird PAE, Ward MK, Feest TG, Walker W, Tanboga H, Sussman M, Kerr DNS: Haemodialysis-induced leucopenia and activation of complement: Effects of different membranes. *Proc Eur Dial Transpl Assoc* 15:144–153, 1978.
39. Nord E, Danovitch GM: Vasopressin response in hemodialysis patients. *Kidney Int* 16:234, 1979.
40. Schrier RW, Berl T, Anderson RJ: Osmotic and nonosmotic control of vasopressin release. *Am J Physiol* 236:F321–F332, 1979.
41. Raij L, Wrigley B: Increase in angiotensin converting enzyme during hemodialysis. *Abstr Am Soc Nephrol* 11:49A, 1978.
42. Remuzzi G, Cavenaghi AE, Mecca G, Donati MB, de Gaetano G: Prostacyclin-like activity and bleeding in renal failure. *Lancet* 2:1195, 1977.
43. Remuzzi G, Marchesi D, Cavenaghi AE, Livio M, Conati MB, de Gaetano G, Mecca G: Bleeding in renal failure: A possible role of vascular prostacyclin. *Clin Nephrol* 12:127–131, 1979.
44. Szczeklik A, Nizankowski R, Skawinski S, Sczceklik J, Gluszko P, Gryglewski RJ: Successful therapy of advanced arteriosclerosis obliterans with prostacyclin. *Lancet* 1:1111, 1979.
45. Casals–Stenzel J, Morton JJ: The vasodepressor action of prostacyclin and its effect on plasma angiotensin II and vasopressin in unanaesthetized normotensive and hypertensive rats. *Clin Exp Hypertension* 1:577–596, 1979.
46. Lynch RE, Bosl RH, Streifel AJ, Ebben JP, Ehlers SM, Kjellstrand CM: Dialysis thrombocytopenia: Parallel plate vs hollow fiber dialyzers. *Tr Am Soc Artif Intern Organs* 24:704–708, 1978.

47. Prosser D, Parsons V: The case for a specific uraemic myocardiopathy. *Nephron* 15:4–7, 1975.
48. Ejerblad S, Eriksson I, Johansson H: Uraemic arterial disease. *Scand J Urol Nephrol* 13:161–169, 1979.
49. Ibels LS, Alfrey AC, Huffer WE, Craswell PW, Anderson JT, Weil R: Arterial calcification and pathology in uremic patients undergoing dialysis. *Am J Med* 66:790–796, 1979.
50. de Fremont JF, Coevoet B, Andrejak M, Makdassi R, Quichaud J, Lambrey G, Gueris J, Caillens C, Harichaux P, Alexandre JM, Fournier A: Effects of antihypertensive drugs on dialysis-resistant hypertension, plasma renin and dopamine betahydroxylase activities, metabolic risk factors and calcium phosphate homeostasis: Comparison of metoprolol, alphamethylodopa and clonidine in a cross-over trial. *Clin Nephrol* 12:198–205, 1979.
51. Lentz RD, Brown DM, Kjellstrand CM: Treatment of severe hypophosphatemia. *Ann Intern Med* 89:941–944, 1978.
52. Wing AJ, Brunner FP, Brynger H, Chantler C, Donckerwolcke RA, Gurland HJ, Hathway RA, Jacobs CJ, Selwood NH: Combined report on regular dialysis and transplantation in Europe, VIII, 1977. *Proc Eur Dial Transpl Assoc* 15:4–76, 1978.
53. Kjellstrand CM, Arieff AI, Friedman EA, Furst P, Henderson LW, Massry SG: Inadequacy of dialysis: Why patients are not well. *Tr Am Soc Artif Intern Organs* 25:518–520, 1979.
54. Kjellstrand CM: Current problems in long-term hemodialysis, in: *Proceedings of the First Asian Pacific Congress of Nephrology*, pp 169–183, 1979.

Control of Treatment Morbidity and Uremic Toxicity with Hemodialysis and Hemofiltration Therapy

43

The Role of Net Na and H_2O Flux in the Morbidity of Hemodialysis and Hemofiltration

Frank A. Gotch

The most objective and serious morbidity associated with hemodialysis (HD) and with hemofiltration (HF) is symptomatic hypotension, which is still reported to occur in 30% of HD treatments.[1] The cause undoubtedly is multifactorial and, as recently reviewed by Henderson,[2] may include (1) osmotic and ultrafiltration-induced changes in extracellular fluid volume (V_E); (2) autonomic neuropathy; (3) toxicity of acetate and acute changes in acid–base equilibrium; (4) membrane toxicity; and (5) other as yet undefined factors. The purpose of this chapter is consideration of the relationship of net Na and H_2O flux and changes in V_E to morbidity.

The extracellular fluid volume is very precisely regulated in normal man through multiple feedback control mechanisms. It is well established that the primary determinant of V_E is the quantity of Na present, whereas the magnitude of total body water (V_T) has a smaller influence on V_E.[3] in HD and HF rapid changes are induced in the quantity of Na both in V_E (Na_E) and in V_T. The amount of H_2O removal is individualized for each treatment and matched to the interdialytic weight gain. With the current state of the art there is no attempt to match Na removal precisely to interdialytic Na loading. It has long been considered that Na was loaded isotonically and removed primarily by convection with water and that small diffusive Na gradients were of little consequence in net Na removal or morbidity. Over the past 5 years it has become clear from clinical studies that diffusive Na gradients markedly affect morbidity, which can be greatly reduced by increasing dialysate Na.[4–6] However, quantitative definition of this relationship is essential since there may be a significant risk of excessive Na and

Frank A. Gotch • Franklin Hospital Hemodialysis Center, San Francisco, California 94114.

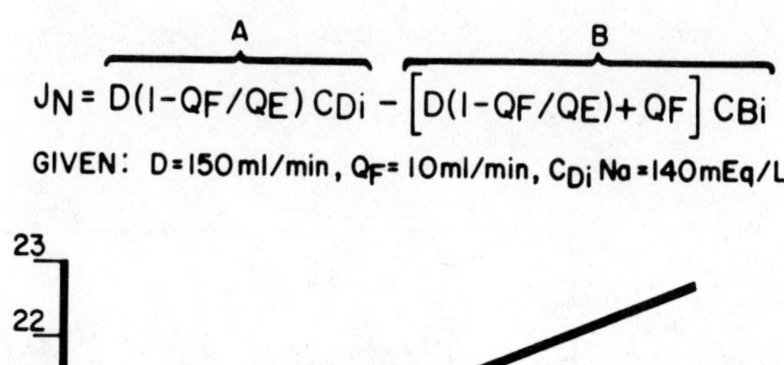

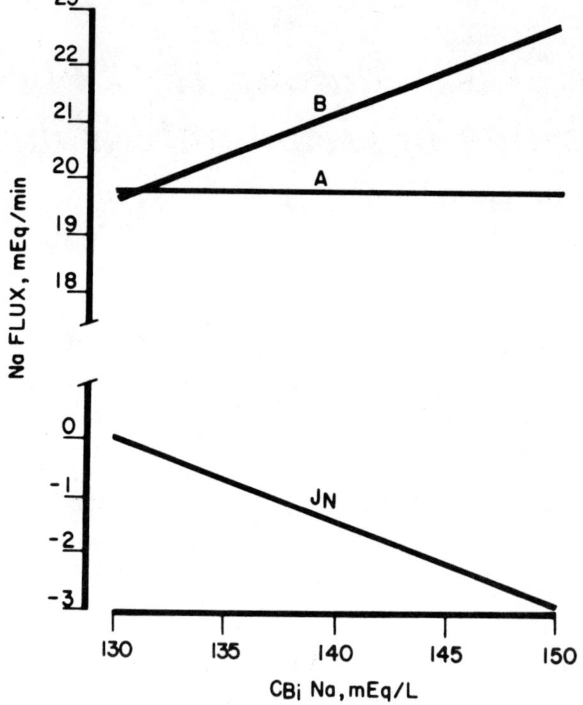

Figure 1. Effect of diffusive Na gradients on net Na flux (J_N) at fixed Q_F = 10 ml/min.

H_2O loading by uniform, empiric increase in dialysate Na until morbidity is minimized in a sizable population of dialysis patients.

The quantitative effect of modest diffusive Na gradients on net Na removal is illustrated in Fig. 1 for a dialyzer with Na dialysance (D) of 150 ml/min operated with a Na concentration of 140 mEq/liter in the dialysate (C_{Di}Na) and flow (Q_f) of 10 ml/min or 600 ml/hr. The standard flux equation[(7)] is shown at the top where term A describes Na flux from dialysate to blood and is constant at 19.8 mEq/min. Term B describes the combined diffusive and convective Na flux from blood to dialysate and can be seen to increase from 19.7 to 22.8 mEq/liter as the concentration of C_{Bi} Na in the blood increases from 130 to 150 mEq/liter. The net Na removal is given by (A − B) as shown in the bottom plot where this value changes from +0.1 to −3.0 mEq/min at a constant Q_F of 10 ml/min. The Na content of ultrafiltrate can readily be calculated to range from essentially zero at C_{Bi} Na = 130 to 300 mEq/liter at C_{Bi} Na = 150 mEq/liter. Thus, the composition of ultrafiltrate

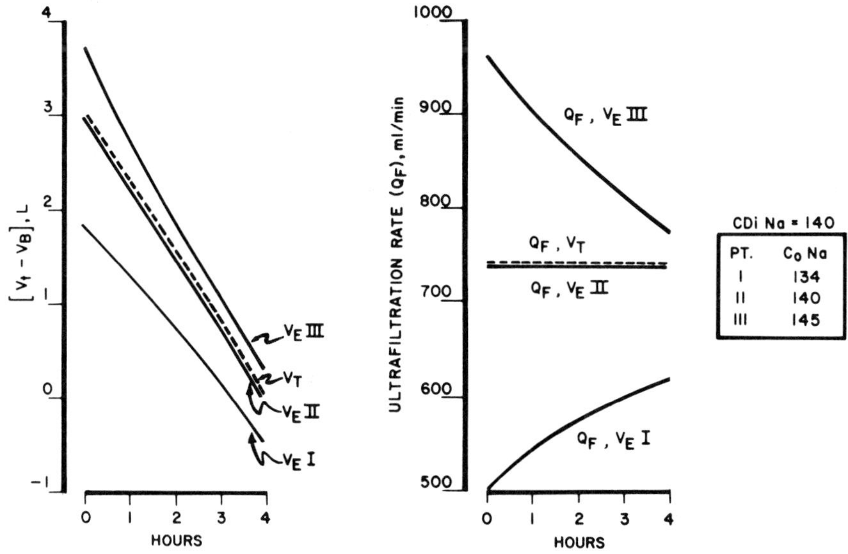

Figure 2. Effect of diffusive Na gradient on ultrafiltration rate from extracellular fluid (V_E) relative to total body weight (V_T).

removed varies from pure water to a very hypertonic solution over a diffusive gradient from blood to dialysate of ± 10 mEq/liter.

The rate at which V_E is changing relative to Q_F can also be expected to vary markedly as a function of the Na concentration of the ultrafiltrate. We have recently described a kinetic model to quantify interdialytic Na and H_2O loading and removal during the subsequent dialysis.[8] The model is based on osmotic distribution of Na equal to V_T (determined from urea kinetic analysis) and permits calculation of Na balance between and during treatments from calculated changes in osmotically active cation present in V_T.[8] The model can readily be adapted to estimation of interdialytic changes in V_E relative to a specified normalized or baseline value of V_E for the patient. In the following calculations of ΔV_E, it is assumed that the baseline serum Na is 140 mEq/liter and the baseline V_E is one third of V_T at "dry body weight."

In Fig. 2 calculated changes in V_E are shown for an average-sized patient who presents for dialysis with a 3.0-kg weight gain or 3.0-liter excess in V_T. Over a 4-hr dialysis 3.0 liters of H_2O are removed at a constant rate of 750 ml/hr (dashed lines in Fig. 2).

The changes in V_E are calculated for three different predialysis Na values of 134, 140, and 145 mEq/liter, which reflect, respectively, hypotonic, isotonic, and hypertonic interdialytic Na/H_2O loading relative to the assumed baseline Na of 140 mEq/liter. The excess of V_E relative to baseline is shown on the left, and the rate at which V_E is changing as a result of the Na content and volume of the ultrafiltrate is shown on the right. The rate of change in

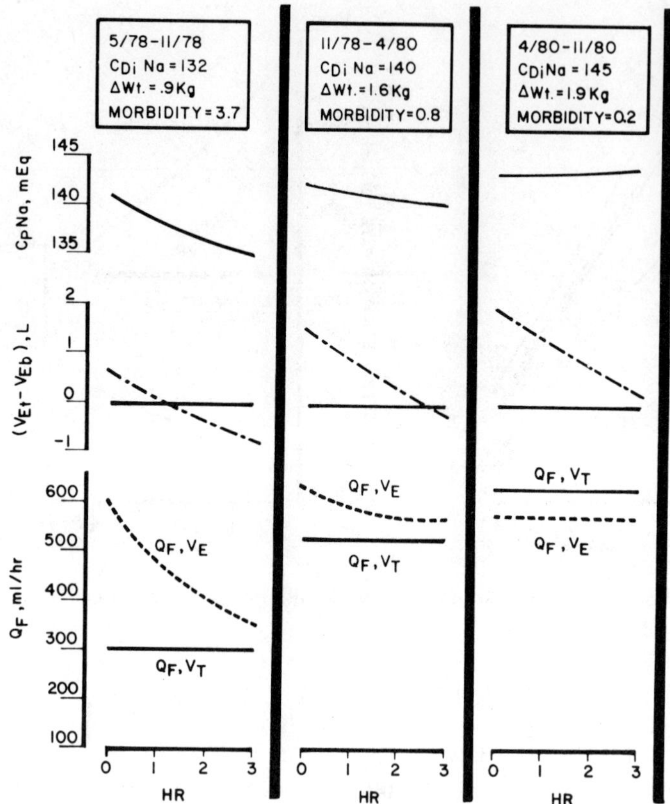

Figure 3. Effect of dialysate Na on morbidity and body H_2O and electrolyte composition.

V_E varies from 500 to 950 mg/hr at the start of dialysis as a function of predialysis serum Na concentration despite a constant Q_F of 750 ml/hr.

Similar calculations are shown in Fig. 3 for a patient in our center whose kinetic parameters have been previously reported (patient 1, ref. 8). This patient was dialyzed sequentially for extended periods with C_{Di} Na 132, 140, and 145 which resulted in end dialysis serum Na values of 135, 139, and 143, respectively. Despite variable C_t Na resulting from variable C_{Di} Na, the C_O Na was quite constant (141–143 mEq/liter). Thus, the baseline C_O Na used to model the patient was 142 mEq/liter, and calculated changes in V_T and V_E over 3-hr dialyses are depicted in Fig. 3. During the period of treatment with C_{Di} Na 132, the V_E decreased to nearly 1 liter below the baseline value, and although Q_F was only 300 ml/hr, V_E was decreasing at a rate of 600 ml/hr at the start of dialysis because of the removal of hypertonic ultrafiltrate. This was associated with 3.8 episodes of hypotension and/or severe muscle cramping per treatment.

The effects of C_{Di} Na 140 and 145 are also shown in Fig. 3. With C_{Di} Na 140 (Q_F, V_E) was only slightly greater than (Q_F, V_T), and there was much

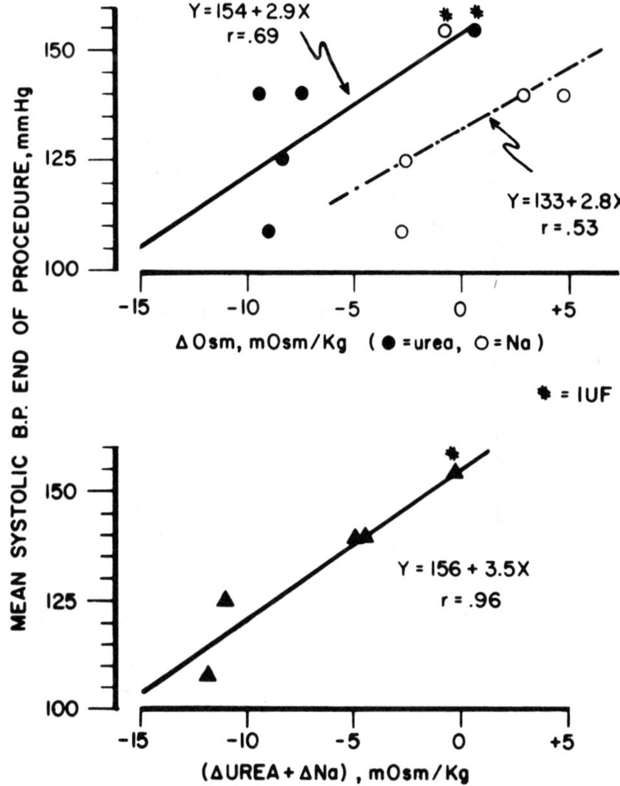

Figure 4. Relationship of systolic BP to Δosmolality with 2.0 liters ultrafiltration in 1 hr. (From Ref. 17.)

less depletion of V_E and morbidity decreased to 0.8 episode per treatment. With C_{Di} Na 145, slightly hypertonic to the predialysis serum Na (C_O), the ultrafiltrate was slightly hypotonic to plasma, (Q_F, V_E) became less than (Q_F, V_T), and there was a further substantial decrease in morbidity to 0.2 episode per treatment. The effect of increasing C_{Di} Na on V_E excess is shown in the middle plots of Fig. 3. During the period of treatment with C_{Di} Na 132 there was substantial residual urine volume of $\simeq$ 1 liter/24 hr, so that calculated expansion of V_E predialysis was minimal, 0.6 liter. Residual renal function steadily diminished to near 0 so that the increased weight gains and predialysis V_E excess with C_{Di} Na 140 compared to 132 were largely due to decreased urine volume. When C_{Di} was increased from 140 to 145, predialysis V_E increased from 1.5 to 1.9 over baseline value, and the postdialysis value increased from -0.3 to $+0.2$ liter relative to baseline. Thus the model indicates that in this patient when C_{Di} Na was increased from 140 to 145, there was an increase in V_E of 0.4 liter predialysis and an increase of 0.5 liter end dialysis.

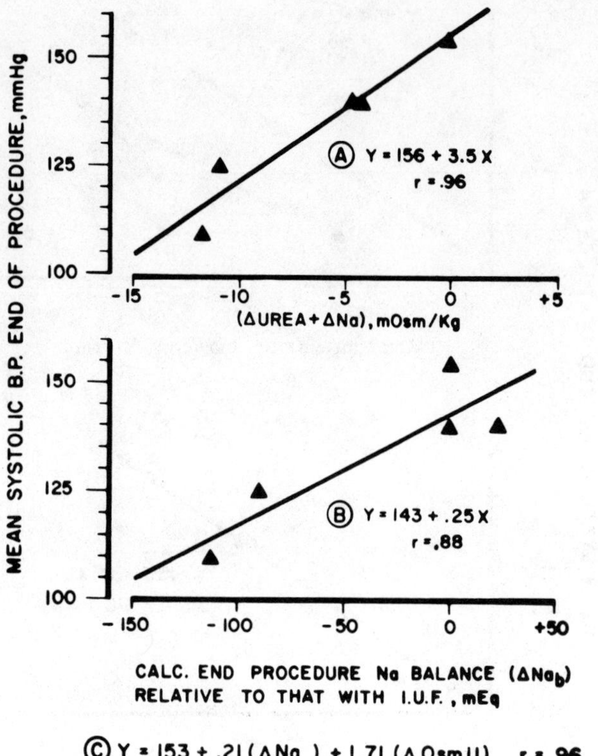

Figure 5. Relationship of systolic BP to ΔNa_b relative to IUF and Δurea + ΔNa osmolality. (From ref. 17.)

It has been suggested by several investigators that acute hypotension during dialysis is due to the rapidly decreasing total osmolality of plasma.[9–11] This implies a mechanism causing hypotension that is equally sensitive to changes in urea and Na concentration, which contribute most of the change in total plasma osmolality during dialysis. Such a mechanism intuitively seems unlikely in view of the marked difference in physiologic behavior of these solutes. Sodium ion is essentially confined to V_E and is the major determinant of volume of that compartment whereas urea freely and rapidly diffuses throughout body water.

Wehle *et al.* studied the effect of change in urea and Na concentration and total osmolality on blood pressure in carefully controlled studies with isolated ultrafiltration (IUF) and dialysis at two dialysate Na concentrations (145 and 133) with both bicarbonate and acetate but equivalent ultrafiltration rates.[9] The mean systolic blood pressure (BP) at end procedure is plotted in Fig. 4 from their data as a function of Δurea, ΔNa, and (Δurea + ΔNa). These plots suggest that BP was strongly dependent on the summed change in urea and Na osmolality and poorly correlated to either independently.

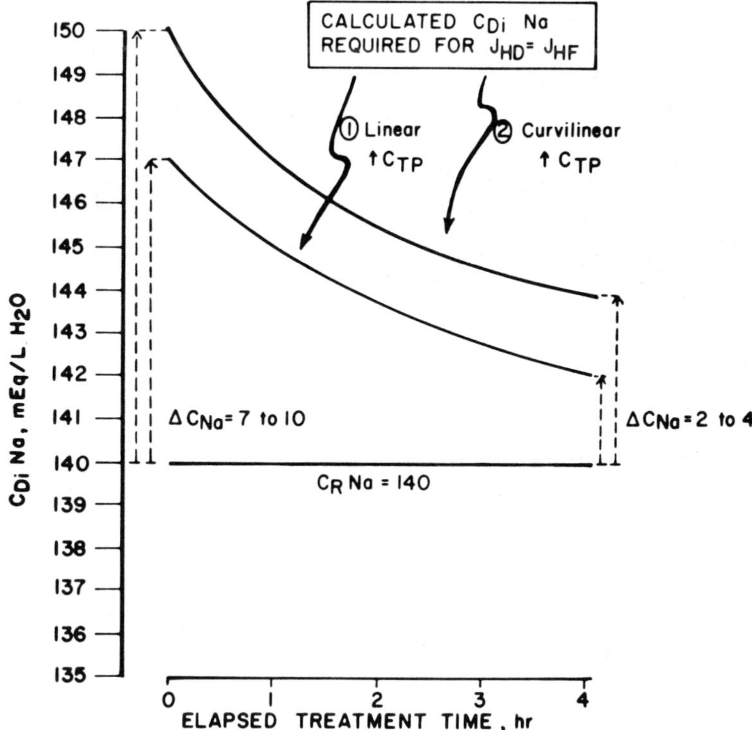

Figure 6. Calculated C_{Di} Na required for diffusive gradient equivalent to HF with FF decreasing from 0.60 to 0.40 over a 4-hr treatment with C_P = 150 mEq/liter (aqueous plasma Na).

The Na-volume model was used to analyze these data and compute Na balance with the dialysis treatments relative to that with IUF. The results in Fig. 5 indicate that BP correlated very well with ΔNa_b alone (r = 0.88). Further analysis with multiple linear regression of BP on ΔNa_b and Δurea showed r = 0.96, identical to that with (Δurea + ΔNa). The fact that BP correlates very strongly to ΔNa_b alone supports the alternative explanation that the change in BP was due largely to the magnitude of change in extracellular fluid volume resulting with the different therapies whereas change in urea concentration contributed relatively little to change in BP.

Reports from several investigators have indicated that hypotension is less with postdilution HF than with conventional HD.[12–14] Several explanations have been offered including smaller decrease in osmolality in HF due to lower urea clearance, removal of a larger-molecular-weight vascular destabilizer with HF, and better biocompatibility of HF membrane. However, none of the comparative HF studies have been designed to assure that net Na removal during HD was equivalent to that in HF.

The high filtration fraction (FF) achieved in HF results in substantially increased plasma protein concentration in the hemofilter. We have recently reported the quantitative dependence of the Donnan ratio for plasma Na/ultrafiltrate Na concentration in HD and HF as a function of mean protein concentration in these devices.[15] A linear relationship was found between the reciprocal of the Donnan ratio, α, and the mean concentration of total protein in the device. It can be further surmised that these studies, performed at relatively low FF, may underestimate the Donnan effect with high filtration fractions since the bulk of filtration occurs across the proximal membrane area in such devices.[16]The impact of the Donnan effect on Na transport in HF relative to HD is depicted in Fig. 6 where standard Na flux equations and the α values described previously were used to calculate C_{Di} Na values required to achieve Na removal in HD equal to HF with replacement fluid Na (C_R Na) of 140 mEq/liter for an average-sized patient with equal fluid removal with both treatments. The two C_{Di} Na curves are based on linear and curvilinear[16] ultrafiltration along the length of the hemofilter. It is apparent that substantially higher and declining dialysate Na concentrations are required to match net Na flux during HF with high FF devices.

In conclusion, although treatment morbidity very likely reflects multifactorial mechanisms, a major factor is likely to be rapid changes in body Na content which are not well controlled with the current state of the art. In comparison of morbidity with variously modified therapies, it is essential to design the studies so that Na removal is equal in experimental and control therapies.

References

1. Rubin LJ, Gutman RA: Hypotension during haemodialysis. *Kidney* 11:21, 1978.
2. Henderson LW: Symptomatic hypotension during hemodialysis. *Kidney Int* 17:571, 1980.
3. Skorecki KL, Brenner BM: Body fluid homeostasis in man. *Am J Med* 70:77, 1981.
4. Ogden DA: A double blind crossover comparison of high and low sodium dialysis. *Proc Clin Dial Transpl Forum* 8:157, 1978.
5. Van Stone JC, Cook J: Decreased postdialysis fatigue with increased dialysate sodium concentration. *Proc Clin Dial Transpl Forum* 8:152, 1978.
6. Levin NW, Grondin G: Dialysate sodium concentration. *Int J Artif Organs* 1:255, 1978.
7. Sargent JA, Gotch FA: Principles and biophysics of dialysis, in: Drukker W, Parsons FM, Maher JF (eds): *Replacement of Renal Function by Dialysis.* Martinus–Nijhoff, 1978, p 38.
8. Gotch FA, Lam MA, Prowitt M, Keen M: Preliminary clinical results with sodium-volume modeling of hemodialysis (HD) therapy. *Proc Clin Dial Transpl Forum* 10:10–18, 1980.
9. Wehle B, Asaba H, Castenfors J, Fürst P, Grahn A, Gunnarsson B, Shaldon S, Bergström J: The influence of dialysis fluid composition on the blood pressure response during dialysis. *Clin Nephrol* 2:62, 1978.
10. Kjellstrand CM, Rosa AA, Shideman JR: Hypotension during hemodialysis: Osmolality fall is an important pathogenetic factor. *Am Soc Artif Intern Organs J* 1:11, 1980.
11. Henrich WL, Woodard TD, Blachley JD, Gomez–Sanchez C, Pettinger W, Cronin RE: Role of osmolality in blood pressure stability after dialysis and ultrafiltration. *Kidney Int* 18:480, 1980.
12. Quellhorst E, Rieger J, Doht B, Beckmann H, Jacob I, Kraft B, Mietzsch G, Scheler F: Treatment of chronic uremia by an ultrafiltration kidney—first clinical experience. *Proc Eur Dial Transpl Assoc* 13:314, 1976.

13. Bosch JP, Albertini BV, Geronemus R: Comparison of hemofiltration and ultrafiltration plus hemodialysis to conventional hemodialysis, in: *First Annual Progress Report, Artificial Kidney–Chronic Uremia Program,* NIAMDD. Bethesda, Maryland National Institutes of Health, 1978.
14. Shaldon S, Beau MC, Deschodt G, Ramperez P, Mion C: Vascular stability during hemofiltration. *Tr Am Soc Artif Intern Organs* 26:391, 1980.
15. Gotch FA: Net sodium flux (J) in post-dilution hemofiltration (HF) and hemodialysis (HD), in: *Abstracts American Society of Nephrology*, 1980, p 39A.
16. Henderson LW: Ultrafiltration, in: Drukker W, Parsons FM, Maher JF (eds): *Replacement of Renal Function by Dialysis*. Martinus–Nijhoff, 1978, p 135.
17. Asaba H, *et al*: *Clin Nephrol* 10:62–66, 1978.

44

The Role of Small-Molecule Removal in the Control of Treatment Morbidity with Hemodialysis and Hemofiltration

Stanley Shaldon

In 1976, it was suggested that the critical factor in maintaining the blood pressure during isolated ultrafiltration (UF) was the stability of the serum osmolality, and that by inference the high incidence of symptomatic hypotension seen with efficient dialysis was due primarily to large drops in the serum osmolality.[1] A consequence of this ingenious study, limited to one series of acute experiments in only six selected patients, was the birth of the "shifters" school. The "shifters" believe that dialysis hypotension is due to hypovolemia during UF. The hypovolemia is exaggerated by the passage of extracellular fluid into the cells at the same time as it is removed from the body. Their conclusions are based on imprecise space measurements, and their results are often dubious.[2,3] I have never believed in the "shifter" school and feel that Bergström and associates' conclusions[1] could not apply in a chronic situation. To study this matter in more detail we selected six patients[4] with a high incidence of symptomatic hypotension (drop in mean arterial pressure of more than 20% together with a requirement for nursing attention ± fluid replacement) during conventional hemodialysis lasting 4 hr and employing a l-m^2 cuprophane dialyzer. The study was divided into three parts. Each part lasted for 1 month. During part 1, the dialysate flow rate (single pass) was 500 ml/min; in part 2, the dialysate flow rate was 300 ml/min; and in part 3, the dialysate flow rate was 100 ml/min. All other parameters were kept as near constant during all parts of the study. Thus, the Gambro Lundia 1-m^2 13.5-unit cuprophan dialyzer was used throughout the study for 4 hr three times per week. The dialysate electrolyte composition was kept constant at sodium 140 mEq/liter, potassium 2.0 mEq/liter, calcium

Stanley Shaldon • Department of Nephrology, University Hospital, Nîmes-Montpellier, France.

3.5 mEq/liter, and acetate 40 mEq/liter without glucose. Blood flow was kept as constant as possible at about 200 ml/min. Weight loss was kept linear by the use of an ABG Semca balancing device which kept the input and output dialysate flow to and from the dialyzer constant, while permitting ultrafiltrate (excess weight loss) to be removed by a separate pump and measured directly. Weight loss was also checked by a Datex metabolic bed scale and continuously recorded on a Kontron WW 1200 chart recorder. Blood pressure and pulse were recorded manually at 30-min intervals. Serum sodium, osmolality, urea, and hematocrit were measured before and after each dialysis in the last week of each part of the study.

The results were expressed as mean ± S.D. of all parameters measured during the last week of each part of the study. There was a progressive rise in the mean pretreatment level of serum urea from 35.0 ± 3.35 mmoles/liter during the last week of part 1 to 43.8 ± 6.79 mmoles/liter in the last week of part 3. The drop in serum urea (Δurea) was similar in all three parts (Fig. 1). Serum sodium concentrations did not alter from pre- to postdialysis or between any of the parts of the study. Serum osmolality changes paralleled those of serum urea, rising progressively from part 1 to part 3, but with a similar drop during dialysis in each part (Fig. 2).

The predialysis body weight was similar for each part of the study, and the mean weight loss in each part averaged 2.0 kg. The percentage increase in hematocrit in each part was similar—about 10%. However, there was a significant reduction in the incidence of symptomatic hypotension in part 3 compared to parts 1 and 2 (Fig. 3).

These results suggested that the critical factor in the etiology of symptomatic hypotension was not hypovolemia or changes in serum osmolality.

Thus, the fact that the use of a high dialysate sodium concentration has been associated with less hypotension and acutely with a smaller reduction in serum osmolality[5] does not necessarily mean that in a chronic study a smaller reduction of serum osmolality would be obtained. Furthermore, the mechanism by which sodium prevents hypotension is still not clear. Other osmotically active agents such as mannitol also help to reduce symptomatic hypotension.[6] However, the alleviation of a condition does not mean that the absence of the therapeutic agent was the cause of the condition.

A similar observation was also first reported in 1976,[7] when Quellhorst *et al.* described their initial clinical results with postdilution hemofiltration (HF). The similarity between the clinical response seen with UF and HF was intriguing. Subsequently hemodynamic studies have shown that the peripheral resistance increases to the same extent in both treatments,[8] and even when HF is associated with a very high urea clearance (>200 ml/min) and the reduction in serum osmolality is identical to that seen with high-efficiency hemodialysis, the phenomenon still occurs.[9] In the latter study the changes in peripheral resistance during acetate or bicarbonate hemodialysis were compared to HF with acetate or bicarbonate replacement fluid. The urea clearances were the same in hemodialysis and in hemofiltration. However, the dialysate sodium was 145 mmoles/liter whereas the replacement fluid for

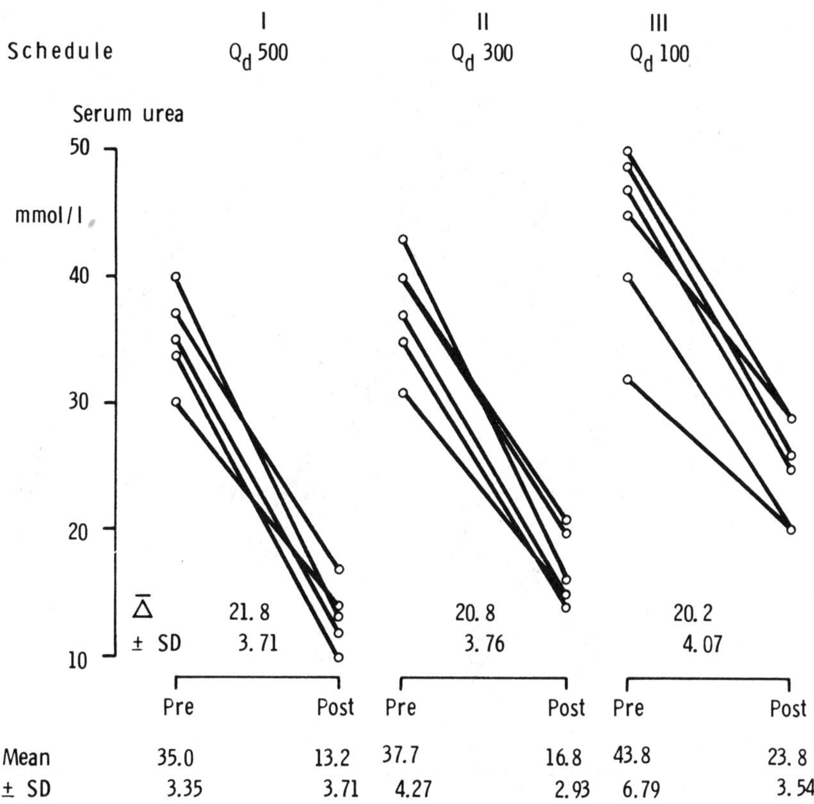

Figure 1. Reduction in serum urea during dialysis at three different dialysate flow rates. $\bar{\Delta}$, Mean pre to post change ± 1 S.D. (Reprinted from ref. 4, with permission of the editor of the American Society of Artificial Internal Organs.)

HF contained only 139 mmoles/liter. In spite of this sodium difference, the increase of peripheral resistance during HF was far more appropriate than that seen during hemodialysis (Fig. 4). In addition, this effect was independent of the use of acetate or bicarbonate. These results have been confirmed and associated with increases in circulating catecholamines during HF or UF but not during hemodialysis be it with acetate or bicarbonate (Fig. 5).[8] More recently, the peripheral resistance response seen with simultaneous hemodialysis and hemodiafiltration has been shown to be less appropriate than with HF alone.[10] In addition, it has recently been shown that the polyacrylonitrile RP6 device produces more vascular instability when it is used as a dialyzer, even with a high dialysate sodium, than when it is used as a hemofilter.[11]

The explanation of the phenomenon of improved vascular stability during HF is still unknown. It cannot be due to the removal of a large-molecular-weight substance alone, as the convective solute removal during UF is no greater than when hemodialysis is performed with conventional

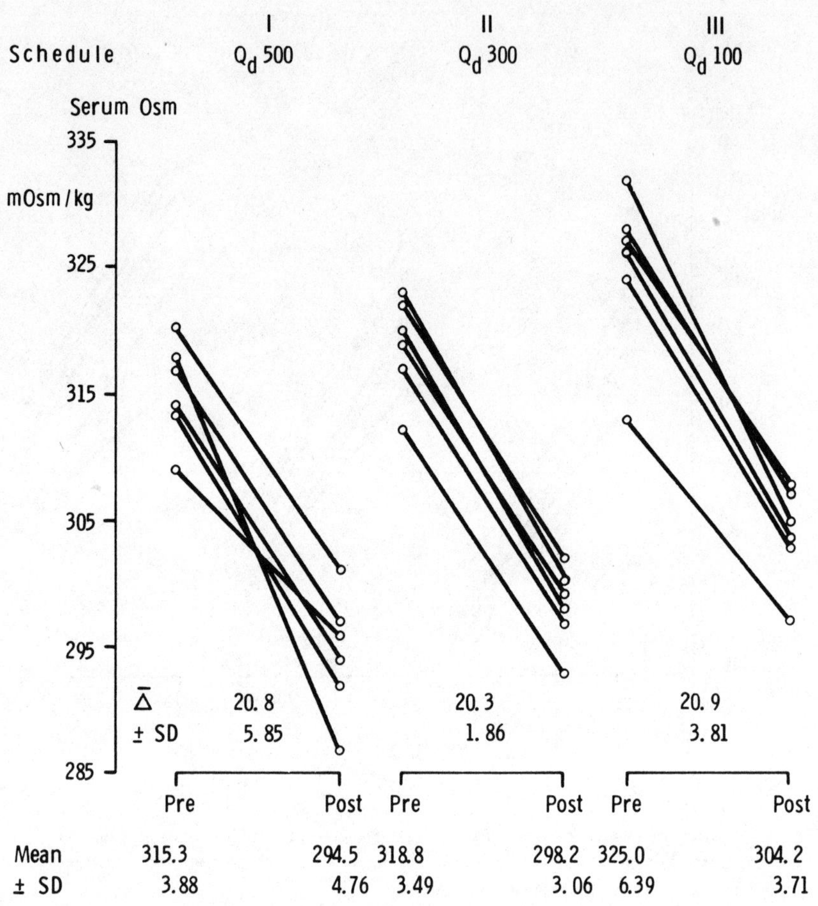

Figure 2. Reduction in serum osmolality during dialysis at three different dialysate flow rates. $\bar{\Delta}$, As in Fig. 1. (Reprinted from ref. 4, with permission of the editor of the American Society of Artificial Internal Organs.)

UF rates. Furthermore, it has recently been suggested that large molecular clearances during clinical HF are exaggerated if the clearance *in vitro* using an aqueous solution is compared to that using a protein-containing solution.(12) This suggests that the phenomenon may be related to factors other than solute removal. The possibility of protein caking causing selective sodium retention due to an increased Donnan effect is an attractive hypothesis that has recently been suggested.(13) However, the phenomenon also occurs in predilution HF(14) where this effect would be less evident. An alternative explanation might be that the protein cake seen with HF alters the biocompatibility of the membrane and prevents activation of enzymes that liberate vasodilator substances such as prostaglandins when blood normally comes in contact with cellulosic membranes in hemodialysis.(15) Thus, although symp-

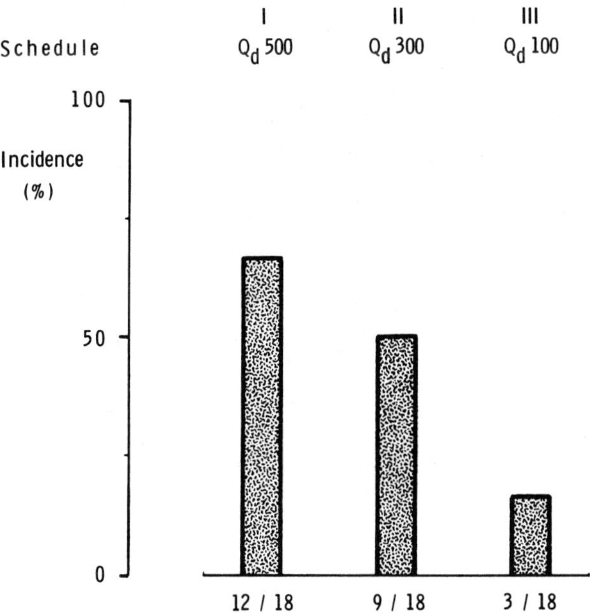

Figure 3. Incidence of symptomatic hypotension during dialysis at three different dialysate flow rates. (Reprinted from ref. 4, with permission of the editor of the American Society of Artificial Internal Organs.)

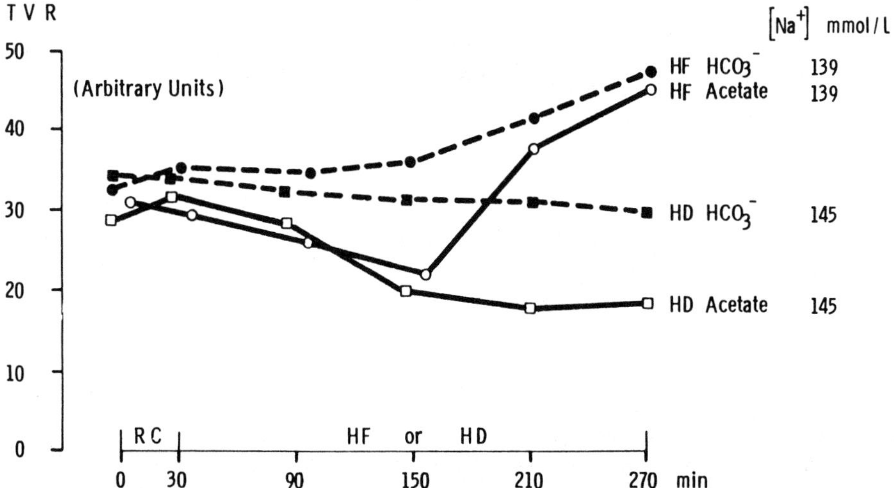

Figure 4. Mean changes in total vascular resistance expressed in arbitrary units derived from mean arterial pressure divided by cardiac index in liters per minute. RC, 30-min control period with extracorporeal recirculation of blood without net diffusion or filtration. HF, hemofiltration. HD, hemodialysis. (Reprinted from ref. 9, with permission of the editor of the American Society of Artificial Internal Organs.)

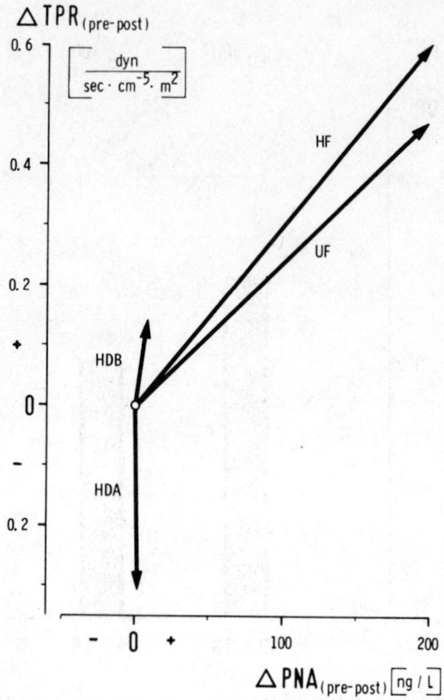

Figure 5. Correlation of volume-removal-induced mean intratreatment change of total peripheral resistance (TPR) and plasma noradrenaline (PNA) during isolated ultrafiltration (UF), postdilution hemofiltration (HF), acetate hemodialysis (HDA), and bicarbonate hemodialysis (HDB). (Derived from ref. 8.)

tomatic hypotension is clearly multifactorial in origin, biocompatibility may be a key factor which until recently has received little attention.

References

1. Bergström J, Asaba H, Fürst P, Oulès R: Dialysis, ultrafiltration and blood pressure. *Proc Eur Dial Transpl Assoc* 13:293, 1976.
2. Keshinah P, Cadwell K, Walker R, Shapiro F: Acid base changes in sequential therapy. *Proc Clin Dial Transpl Forum* 7:53, 1977.
3. Schuenemann B, Berghardt J, Falda Z, Jacob I, Kramer P, Kraft B, Quellhorst E: Reactions of blood pressure and body spaces to haemofiltration treatment. *Tr Am Soc Artif Intern Organs* 24:687, 1978.
4. Shaldon S, Deschodt G, Beau MC, Ramperez P, Mion C: The importance of serum osmotic changes in symptomatic hypotension during short hemodialysis. *Proc Clin Dial Transpl Forum* 8:184, 1978.
5. Wehle B, Asaba H, Castenfors J, Fürst P, Grann A, Gunnarsson S, Shaldon S, Bergström J: The influence of dialysis fluid composition on the blood pressure response during dialysis. *Clin Nephrol* 10:62, 1978.
6. Rosa AA, Fryd DS, Kjellstrand CM: Dialysis symptoms and stabilization in long term dialysis. Practical application of the CUSUM plot. *Arch Intern Med* 140:804, 1980.

7. Quellhorst E, Ruger J, Doht B, Beckmann H, Jacob I, Kraft B, Mietzsch G, Scheler F: Treatment of chronic uraemia by an ultrafiltration kidney—first clinical experience. *Proc Eur Dial Transpl Assoc* 13:314, 1976.
8. Baldamus CA, Ernst W, Fassbinder W, Koch KM: Differing haemodynamic stability due to differing sympathetic response: Comparison of ultrafiltration, haemodialysis and haemofiltration. *Proc Eur Dial Transpl Assoc* 17:205, 1980.
9. Shaldon S, Beau MC, Deschodt G, Ramperez P, Mion C: Vascular stability during hemofiltration. *Tr Am Soc Artif Intern Organs* 26:391, 1980.
10. Wizeman V, Sychla M, Leber HW: Simultaneous hemofiltration/hemodialysis versus hemofiltration and hemodialysis: Hemodynamic parameters. *Proc Eur Soc Artif Organs* 7:143, 1980.
11. Quellhorst E, Schuenemann B, Hildebrand U, Falda Z: Response of the vascular system to different modi membranes of hemofiltration and hemodialysis. *Proc Eur Dial Transpl Assoc* 17:197, 1980.
12. Henderson LW, Beans E, Prestidge H, Ford CA, Colton C, Frigon R: Evaluation of hemofiltration membranes. *Tr Am Soc Artif Intern Organs*, 9:48, 1980 (abstract).
13. Gotch FA, Lam MA, Prowitt M, Keen M: Preliminary clinical results with sodium-volume modeling of hemodialysis therapy. *Proc Clin Dial Transpl Forum* 10:10–18, 1980.
14. Henderson LW, San Felippo ML, Stone RA: Blood pressure control with hemodiafiltration. 12th Annual Contractors Conference, AKCUP NIAAMDD, January 1979, NIH Publication No. 81-1979. Bethesda, Md, US Government Printing Office, 1981, p 112.
15. Schimtt G, Tobin JM, Flamenbaum W: Prostaglandin E (PGE) blood levels during hemodialysis (HD): Comparison of cellulosic (CL) and polyacrylonitrile (PAN) membranes, in: *Book of Abstracts*. American Society of Nephrology, Washington, November 1980, p 51A.

45

The Role of Membrane Biocompatibility on the Clinical Effects of Hemodialysis Therapy

Edmund G. Lowrie

There has been increasing interest in biomaterials research during the past several years. This is true in a number of areas of clinical endeavor, but these comments are confined to artificial kidney systems. Figure 1 illustrates a continuum for the development of dialysis therapies from the invention of new membranes through the optimization of clinical treatment. We have been interested in and involved with clinical evaluation of new and established artificial kidneys for a number of years, as shown in the second panel of the figure. More recently, we have been privileged to participate in a clinical trial that evaluates the control of blood urea nitrogen concentration by using pharmacokinetics and the effect this may have on clinical outcome, as shown by panels 3 and 4. Recent data suggest, however, that there may be a direct link between the biomaterials used to manufacture artificial kidneys and the clinical effects of therapy. In other words, Fig. 1 should probably be redrawn to show a direct connection between panels 1 and 4.

Table 1 outlines one approach for evaluation of the biocompability of the dialysis process. Potential adverse effects may be viewed conveniently as either process or material related. For example, the pumping of blood may expose cells to abnormal forces. Similarly, disequilibrium and acid–base abnormalities may be related to the rates of transfer of various materials across dialysis membranes. The composition of dialysate, as well as the water used in the preparation of dialysate, has been reported to have clinical effects, although neither dialysate nor water contacts blood directly. Materials may be leached from the surface of blood-contacting materials, and diethylphthalate has been shown to enter the blood from various plastics used in

Edmund G. Lowrie • National Medical Care, Waltham, Massachusetts 02154.

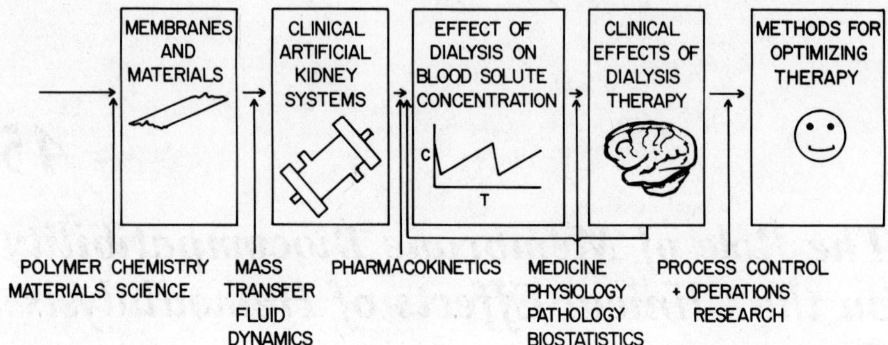

Figure 1. Schematic showing the interaction of various disciplines that combine to produce clinical dialysis therapy.

extracorporeal therapy. Attention is directed to the physical interactions between dialysis membranes and the formed or humoral elements of blood.

1. *Red Blood Cells*

The data shown in Table 2[1] suggest that the erythroid iron turnover increases in patients with chronic renal failure after hemodialysis therapy is initiated. Red blood cell survival, however, is shortened and the net effect appears to be a reduction of hematocrit. Studies by Hochmuth and coworkers[2] suggest that red blood cells attach to foreign surfaces, and the strength of this attachment depends on the nature of the surface. Cells attach more firmly to those materials which have high surface tension. Red blood cells so attached deform under the influence of shear, even at relatively low shear rates similar to those observed in artificial kidney systems. Once

Table 1. Dialysis Compatibility

1. Processes
   a. Blood pumping
   b. Mass-transfer-related
      - Dysequilibrium
      - Acid base
2. Materials—non-blood-contacting
   a. Dialysate
   b. Water
3. Materials—blood-contacting
   a. Chemical
      - Leachables
   b. Physical
      - Surface interactions

Table 2. Hematokinetics in Eight Patients before and after Starting Dialysis Therapy

	Before starting dialysis	After starting dialysis	*p*
Erythroid (mg/100 ml per day) iron turnover	0.34 ± 0.003	0.44 ± 0.05	<0.001
Red cell half-life (days)	26.4 ± 1.5	19.8 ± 1.2	<0.001
Average hematocrit (vol %)	31.8 ± 2.6	23.8 ± 3.0	<0.001

cells detach they are frequently misshapen, appearing as schistocytes. Sandza and co-workers (3) have found tha exposure of erythrocytes to low rates of shear comparable to those found in artificial kidneys shorten their survival and that sheared cells are culled from the circulation by the spleen. Taken in the aggregate, these data suggest strongly that red blood cells may be injured but not destroyed as a result of their exposure to foreign surfaces in a shear field. The effect may be to increase the rate at which red blood cells are destroyed, thus making the anemia worse. By inference, the nature of the surface to which cells are exposed may well have significant clinical effects on anemia in dialysis patients.

2. *White Blood Cells*

Studies have shown that the white blood cell count falls sharply within the first few minutes after initiation of hemodialysis therapy. The magnitude of this effect is much greater when membranes are made from regenerated cellulose than when they are noncellulosic, e.g., polyacrylonitrile or polymethylmethacrylate.[(4)] Both polymorphonuclear leukocytes and lymphocytes fall during dialysis. Similarly, the effect of reprocessed dialyzers manufactured with regenerated cellulose or Cuprophan is much less pronounced than when the same device is new and unused. The clinical consequences of this plummeting of white blood cell count are not clear. The leukocytes of dialysis patients, however, do not function normally and undergo structural changes.[(5)] Both migration and chemotaxis are impaired, and these are important functions in fighting infection. Bacterial infection is the principal cause of hospitalization in chronic dialysis patients, and the apparent injury to white blood cells may therefore contribute significantly to long-term dialysis morbidity.

3. *Complement*

Craddock and co-workers[(6)] have shown that dialysis membranes activate the alternate complement pathway. Further, serum complement falls during dialysis, and the effect appears much greater with cellulosic than with

Table 3. Symptom Score[a]

Symptom	Percent symptomatic treatments		p
	PAN	Cellulose	
Nausea	5.6	25.9	<0.01
Vomiting	3.7	3.7	NS
Headache	9.3	11.1	NS
Dizziness	5.5	35.2	<0.001
Pruritus	14.8	24.1	0.05
Cramps	13.0	18.5	NS
Fatigue	7.4	35.2	<0.001
Dyspnea	3.7	5.6	NS
Restlessness	11.1	38.9	<0.01

[a] Nine patients treated 2 weeks with polyacrylonitrile (PAN) or regenerated cellulose.

noncellulosic artificial kidneys. Further, artificial kidneys which have been reprocessed seem to activate complement less than those which are used for the first time.[7] These data suggest that there may be interactions between the humoral elements of blood and artificial kidney membranes. Again, the clinical consequences of complement activation are not clear. Nonetheless, other enzyme systems may be activated by exposure to foreign surfaces such as dialysis membranes.

Table 3 shows the fraction of symptomatic treatments experienced by nine patients who were treated with both a dialyzer manufactured from regenerated cellulose (Cordis Dow Model 3) and one manufactured from a noncellulosic material (polyacrylonitrile, Hospal RP6). The data suggest that the nature of the membrane material may affect the frequency of clinical symptoms, and it is attractive to speculate that these symptoms are reduced because polyacrylonitrile does not react with certain blood substances as much as regenerated cellulose.

The data reviewed herein suggest that artificial kidneys are not inert devices existing in an extracorporeal circuit. The materials from which they are constructed interact with the formed and humoral elements of blood in a dynamic way. As such, the nature of the material from which artificial kidneys are constructed should be considered when evaluating the effects of clinical therapy.

References

1. Yen MC, Ball JH, Lowrie EG, Lazarus JM, Hampers CL, Merrill JP: The effect of androgens and dialysis on erythropoiesis in chronic renal failure. *Proc Dial Transpl Forum* 3:33–37, 1973.
2. Hochmuth RM, Mohandas N, Spaeth EE, Williamson JR, Blackshear PL Jr, Johnson DW: Surface adhesion, deformation and detachment at low shear of red cells and white cells. *Tr Am Soc Artif Intern Organs* 18:325–332, 1972.

3. Sandza JG, Clark RD, Weldon CS, Sutera SP: Subhemolytic trauma of erythrocytes: Recognition and sequestration by the spleen as a function of shear. *Tr Am Soc Artif Intern Organs* 20:457, 1974.
4. Hakim, RL, Lowrie EG: Hemodialysis associated neutropenia and hypoxemia: The effect of dialyzer membrane materials. *Nephron* 32:32–39, 1982.
5. Bjorksten B, Mauer SM, Mills EL, Quie PG: The effect of neutrophil chemotactic responsiveness. *Acta Med Scand* 203:67, 1978.
6. Craddock PR, Fehr J, Dalmasso AP, Brigham KL, Jacob HS: Hemodialysis leukopenia: Pulmonary vascular leukostasis resulting from complement activation by dialyzer cellophane membranes. *J Clin Invest* 59:879, 1977.
7. Lowrie EG, Hakim RM: The effect on patient health of using reprocessed artificial kidneys. *Clin Dial Transplant Forum*, November 1980, pp 86–91.

46

Comparative Physiology of Acetate and Bicarbonate Alkalinization

F. John Gennari

In 1964, acetate was introduced into dialysis therapy as a substitute for bicarbonate to overcome the technical problem of precipitation of carbonate salts in the bath (Mion *et al.*, 1964). At that time, a few studies were carried out to demonstrate that acetate was indeed an effective source of alkali during dialysis, and then this organic anion rapidly replaced bicarbonate in dialysis baths. Only after a decade or more of widespread use of acetate in dialysis have physicians begun to examine in detail the implications of the substitution of acetate for bicarbonate (Kveim and Nesbakken, 1975; Tolchin *et al.*, 1977; Graefe *et al.*, 1978; Vreeman *et al.*, 1980). These investigations increased our understanding of acid–base balance in dialysis patients. At the same time, however, some controversy has arisen. Acetate has been condemned by some, but as yet no one has uncovered convincing evidence that acetate use should be discontinued altogether.

This chapter reviews the comparative physiology of alkalinization with bicarbonate or acetate. In 1949, Mudge *et al.* demonstrated that the parenteral administration of acetate to normal individuals (in a dose of 2.8 mmoles/kg body weight per hr) was as effective as bicarbonate in increasing plasma bicarbonate concentration. The authors were aware of and concerned about the possibility that acetate might cause vasodilation. Bauer and Richards (1928) had shown that the rapid infusion of sodium acetate decreased blood pressure in anesthetized dogs or cats by direct vasodilation of small blood vessels. Nonetheless, blood pressure, pulse, and electrocardiograms were unchanged in the human subjects studied by Mudge and co-workers. These investigators also gave anesthetized dogs sodium acetate in a much larger dose, 15 mmoles/kg body weight over 1 hr. Despite this massive dose, no

F. John Gennari • Department of Medicine, University of Vermont College of Medicine, Burlington, Vermont 05405.

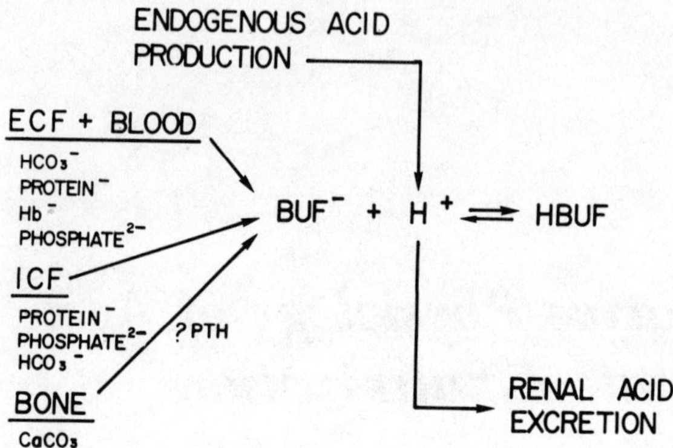

Figure 1. Schematic representation of body buffering and hydrogen ion balance.

hypotension was observed. This study and others (Lipsky *et al.*, 1954) provided evidence that acetate was a safe and rapid source for bicarbonate addition to body fluids. In the last several years, however, acetate has been implicated as a cause of hypotension during dialysis (Graefe *et al.*, 1978; Raja *et al.*, 1980). I will discuss this issue later but first will review hydrogen ion balance and the way in which it is affected by acetate or bicarbonate administration.

Hydrogen ions are added to the body fluids daily by the metabolism of ingested foods, a process termed endogenous acid production (Fig. 1). On a normal American diet, endogenous acid production yields new hydrogen ions at a rate of approximately 1 mmoles/kg body weight per day. This acid load is normally excreted by the kidney, so that no retention of acid (termed positive acid balance) occurs. Because renal acid excretion is not immediate, the hydrogen ions produced must be sequestered by body buffer stores until they are excreted or balanced by alkali administration. At a normal plasma bicarbonate concentration, extracellular bicarbonate stores account for approximately half the buffer response. When bicarbonate is the buffer, this anion is consumed since the carbonic acid formed is volatile and excreted as CO_2 via the lungs. Other body buffers can be renewed by back-titration. The extent to which the release of carbonate stores from bone contributes to the immediate buffer response to an acid load and the role of parathyroid hormone (PTH) in this response are unclear at present.

In the process of renal acid excretion, new bicarbonate ions are produced which back-titrate all buffers and replenish normal bicarbonate stores. Thus, addition of bicarbonate to the body either by renal mechanisms or by exogenous administration counterbalances acid retention and restores acid balance to zero. The renal mechanisms that regulate acid balance are quite precise but are as yet undefined. If renal mechanisms fail and acid retention continues for a sustained period of time, bone carbonate becomes an important buffer source, leading to metabolic bone disease. A clinical example of bone disease occurring as a result of acid retention is distal renal tubular acidosis (RTA) (Gennari and Cohen, 1978). Patients with distal RTA contin-

$$H_2O + CO_2 \rightarrow H_2CO_3$$

$$H_2CO_3 \rightarrow HCO_3^- + H^+$$

$$H^+ + CH_3COO^- \rightarrow \Big(\rightarrow CH_3COO^- + H^+ + HS\underline{CoA} \rightarrow CH_3COS\underline{CoA} + H_2O$$

Figure 2. Acetate entry into cells and reaction with CoA. This process generates new bicarbonate in the extracellular fluid.

ually retain acid (if untreated) and can develop severe bone disease. In patients on dialysis, renal excretory mechanisms are lost, and bone carbonate may well contribute to the buffering of acid retained between dialysis treatments. Nonetheless, sustained positive acid balance probably does not occur because alkali addition during dialysis usually matches acid production through a unique interplay between the dialysis membrane and the patient's body.

The addition of either acetate or bicarbonate to the body during dialysis provides a source of new alkali. If acetate ions are administered, new alkali is generated in the following manner. Acetate in solution is in equilibrium with the undissociated acid, acetic acid. At the pH of the body fluids, the concentration of acetate is some 500-fold higher than that of undissociated acetic acid. Administered acetate anions, therefore, combine with a small amount of hydrogen ions from carbonic acid, generating new bicarbonate ions. This reaction would be trivial if the undissociated form were not removed from the circulation and metabolized. Because the undissociated form is removed (Fig. 2), however, the process continues until all the acetate is utilized. Acetic acid enters the cell and is metabolized in both the cytosol and mitochondria, by reaction with coenzyme A (CoA). The capture of a proton by acetate and its conversion to acetyl CoA in the cell are the steps that yield a new bicarbonate ion in the circulation. What happens to the acetyl CoA after its formation is inconsequential so long as a new acid is not produced. From an acid–base point of view, it is irrelevant whether CO_2 and H_2O, neutral fat, or protein is the final destiny of the acetyl moiety. Only if acetoacetic acid is produced is the newly generated bicarbonate lost. In fact, the metabolic destiny for almost all the acetate metabolized (80–90%) is CO_2 and water, the remainder being used in the production of neutral fats (Ballard, 1972). By this metabolic process, acetate is the equimolar equivalent of bicarbonate. A major difference, however, is the generation of energy in the process of acetate metabolism. Bicarbonate ions are not a caloric source.

Although the net result is the same, transitory differences exist. The addition of bicarbonate to the extracellular fluid (ECF) immediately reduces ECF hydrogen ion concentration (increases pH) and results in hydrogen ion secretion from cells. Approximately half the alkali load is offset by hydrogen ion release from intracellular buffers. In this process sodium or potassium enters cells. Acetate anion, by contrast, has no immediate effect on buffers

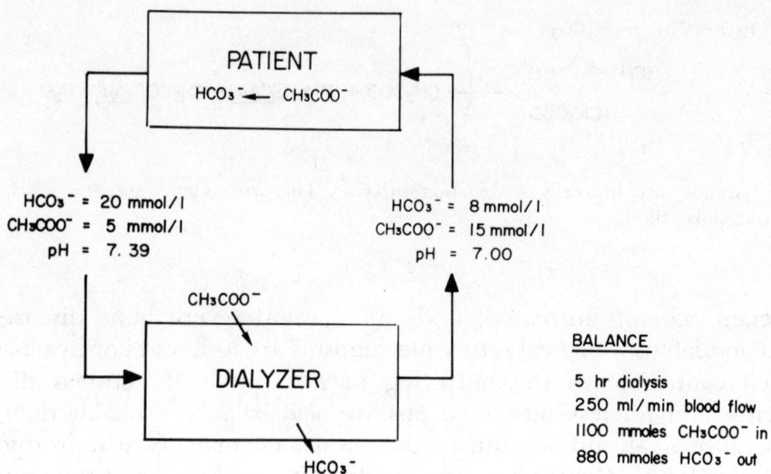

Figure 3. Changes in plasma bicarbonate and acetate concentration as the blood traverses the dialysis membrane. Total acetate entry and bicarbonate exit for a 5-hr dialysis are shown in the lower right.

or on the ambient hydrogen ion concentration. As discussed previously, its effect on hydrogen ion balance is dependent on (1) entry into cells, and (2) conversion to acetyl CoA. The rate of acetate entry into cells depends on its concentration in the ECF. Its reaction with CoA appears to be limited as well by the availability of CoA (Lundquist, 1962; Vreeman *et al.*, 1980). Although there appears to be wide patient variability, the maximal rate of bicarbonate generation from acetate ranges from 4 to 6 mmoles/kg body weight per hour. This limitation reduces the usefulness of acetate as a source of alkali acutely in some dialysis settings (Lundquist, 1962; Tolchin *et al.*, 1977; Vreeman *et al.*, 1980). Because acetate is rapidly metabolized and replaced by new bicarbonate ions, acetate administration does not affect the distribution of solutes between cells and the ECF any differently than does bicarbonate administration.

As discussed earlier, acetate given to normal individuals is equivalent to bicarbonate and appears to be nontoxic. Kirkendol *et al.* (1977) have shown a myocardial depressant effect of acetate, but in much larger acute doses than those given during dialysis. Despite its apparent nontoxicity in normal individuals, acetate has been implicated as a contributor to dialysis hypotension and symptomatology (Graefe *et al.*, 1978). A major difference between intravenous acetate administration and acetate infused during dialysis is that simultaneous bicarbonate loss occurs in the latter setting (Fig. 3). Acetate enters and bicarbonate leaves the blood as it traverses the dialysis membrane. Thus, the concentration of bicarbonate in the blood returning to the patient falls below 10 mmoles/liter, and the concentration of acetate ions rises to 15 mmoles/liter or higher. If blood P_{CO_2} did not decrease simultaneously, the pH of the blood leaving the dialysis machine would fall to 7.00. CO_2 is also

Table 1. Acid Balance in Dialysis Patients

1. Acid production
   a. From dietary protein = 60 mmoles/day
      420 mmoles/week
   b. Organic anion losses = 100 mmoles/dialysis
      300 mmoles/week

   Total: 720 mmoles/week

2. Alkali required 720 mmoles/week
   240 mmoles/dialysis (3 times/week)

3. Dialysis specifications
   a. 4-hr duration
   b. Dialysate acetate concentration = 37 mmoles/liter
   c. $D_{acetate}$ = 120 ml/min, $D_{HCO_3^-}$ = 150 ml/min

Plasma HCO_3^- (mmoles/liter)	Acetate in (mmoles)	HCO_3^- out (mmoles)	Net alkali (mmoles)	Net alkali—240 (mmoles)
16	980	576	404	164
18	980	648	332	92
20	980	720	260	20
22	980	792	188	−52
24	980	864	116	−124

removed by the dialysis process, however, so that the pH does not fall dramatically. As the blood reenters the body, the pH may fall transiently as it equilibrates with the ambient P_{CO_2}. With admixture and metabolism of acetate, the bicarbonate concentration rises to its previous levels, and the acetate concentration falls but is persistently measurable during dialysis. One can only speculate whether these dramatic and rapid compositional changes impact on vasomotor stability. Despite these changes, the pH of the blood does not change notably during dialysis (Tolchin *et al.*, 1977; Vreeman *et al.*, 1980).

The net entry of acetate and exit of bicarbonate during dialysis are determined by the dialysance of each of these anions and the transmembrane concentration gradient. For acetate, we set the concentration in the bath, and the rate of metabolism sets it in the blood. For bicarbonate, the plasma bicarbonate concentration is the sole determinant of its transmembrane concentration gradient in a single-pass system. The plasma bicarbonate concentration, however, in turn is determined by net acid balance. Therefore, the relative dialysances for bicarbonate and acetate in a given dialysis setting are the ultimate determinants of the plasma bicarbonate concentration at which acid balance is achieved. This concept is illustrated in Table 1. The values for acid production in the example shown in this table represent only estimates because no good systematic measurements have been made in this group of patients. The principle holds, however, regardless of the precise values. If one assumes a hydrogen ion production rate of 60 mmoles/day from the metabolism of proteins, the weekly production rate is 420 mmoles. Vreeman *et al.* (1980) have provided an estimate of organic acid production (actually a component of "endogenous acid production" although separately cata logued here) from the measured losses of organic anions during dialysis. Adding these values, approximately 720 mmoles of hydrogen ions are produced weekly which must be countered by an equal amount of alkali to prevent positive acid balance. For three-times-weekly dialysis, this represents 240 mmoles per dialysis. For standard hemodialysis membranes and flows used today, the dialysances of bicarbonate and acetate are approximately 150 and 120 ml/min, respectively (Vreeman *et al.*, 1980). Given a typical dialysate acetate concentration of 37 mmoles/liter and its dialysance, approximately 980 mmoles of acetate are infused during a 4-hr dialysis treatment. The amount of bicarbonate lost during dialysis, however, varies with the plasma bicarbonate concentration. If the bicarbonate concentration is less than 20 mmoles/liter, more than 240 mmoles of net alkali is gained. Because alkali intake exceeds acid production, the predialysis bicarbonate concentration will rise. By contrast, if the plasma bicarbonate level is greater than 20 mmoles/liter, insufficient net alkali is gained and the plasma bicarbonate concentration will fall. Thus, in this example, the chronic predialysis bicarbonate concentration is "regulated" at a level of approximately 20 mmoles/liter, and at that level, the patient is in acid balance.

A corollary of this observation is that, although the ambient bicarbonate concentration is maintained lower than normal, long-term positive acid balance should not occur, and therefore bone calcium salts should not be continually lost in the buffering process. The bicarbonate lost during dialysis is analogous to the defect in renal bicarbonate reabsorption seen in proximal RTA. In this disorder, the magnitude of the renal bicarbonate leak regulates the chronic steady-state plasma bicarbonate concentration at which acid balance is achieved (Gennari and Cohen, 1978). Bone disease is not a feature of the acidosis in that disorder (Brenes *et al.*, 1977). By analogy, acidosis-related bone disease should not occur in dialysis patients, unless some factor prevents regeneration of the bone carbonate salts utilized in buffering acid retained in the interdialytic period.

Table 2 reviews the same events when a large-surface-area membrane is used. If one uses the same estimate for alkali requirement in this example, it is apparent (given the higher dialysances for acetate and bicarbonate for this membrane) that sufficient net alkali is only delivered at bicarbonate concentrations less than 18 mmoles/liter. Fortunately, as shown in the lower part of Table 2, patients using a large-surface-area membrane can maintain a plasma bicarbonate concentration higher than 18 mmoles/liter between dialysis treatments because the rate of bicarbonate loss simply exceeds the rate of acetate conversion to bicarbonate early in dialysis. Thus, during dialysis, plasma bicarbonate concentration falls to a level at which bicarbonate losses are reduced. At the same time, high circulating acetate levels are achieved during dialysis, which subsequently provide the substrate for the needed alkali (Tolchin *et al.*, 1977). In these patients with high acetate and

Table 2. Acid Balance with 2.5-m² Dialysis Membrane

Dialysis specifications
a. 4-hr duration
b. Dialysate acetate concentration = 40 mmoles/liter
c. $D_{acetate}$ = 140 ml/min, $D_{HCO_3^-}$ = 208 ml/min

Plasma HCO_3^- (mmoles/liter)	Acetate in (mmoles)	HCO_3^- out (mmoles)	Net alkali (mmoles)
16	1092	800	292
18	1092	898	194
20	1092	1000	92
22	1092	1098	−6
	Kinetics—hourly		
Hours			
1 18	311	225	86
2 16	277	200	77
3 16	269	200	69
4 16	252	200	52
4-hr totals	1109	825	284

low bicarbonate levels during dialysis, hypotension and other symptoms are most likely to occur. These symptoms are probably related to both the high acetate and the low bicarbonate levels induced, but the specific mechanisms remain to be elucidated. Even in these patients, arterial pH does not fall notably during dialysis because arterial P_{CO_2} falls concomitantly with the fall in plasma bicarbonate concentration (Tolchin *et al.*, 1977).

From this analysis, it is apparent that, for a given dialysis setting, the concentration of acetate in the bath determines the plasma bicarbonate concentration at which long-term acid balance is maintained. To induce a sustained increase in plasma bicarbonate concentration using acetate dialysis, one has to increase the rate of acetate delivery relative to bicarbonate loss. However, given the dialysis membranes used at present, a higher acetate delivery results in acetate infusion faster than the rate of acetate metabolism. This will produce a fall in plasma bicarbonate concentration during dialysis, as illustrated in Table 2. Alternatively, bicarbonate can be used in the bath rather than acetate. In this case, a high bicarbonate dialysance works in our favor. Plasma bicarbonate concentration increases more for a given bath bicarbonate concentration with a larger-surface-area dialysis membrane.

The predialysis plasma bicarbonate concentration in stable chronic dialysis patients averages about 17 mmoles/liter, but ranges from 10 to 24 mmoles/liter. A question that needs answering is whether this wide scatter is a reflection of individual variations in bicarbonate and acetate dialysance, or whether other factors are responsible. The factors affecting acid balance in patients on dialysis are shown in Table 3. I have discussed the dialysis-related factors, except for dialysis time. Clearly, if there is a favorable ratio between dialysis acetate entry and bicarbonate loss, then increasing dialysis time will

Table 3. Factors Influencing Acid Balance in Dialysis Patients

Endogenous acid production
Renal HCO_3^- wasting
Organic anion loss during dialysis
Dialysis factors
Discrepancy between $D_{HCO_3^-}$ and $D_{acetate}$
Dialysis time
Bath acetate/HCO_3^- concentration

increase plasma bicarbonate concentration. Turning to the production side, endogenous acid production and organic anion loss are part of the same process, except that dialysis (either with acetate or bicarbonate) may actually stimulate organic acid production. Little is known about the effect of dialysis on this metabolic process. Variations in endogenous acid production will certainly affect plasma bicarbonate concentration. Finally, if residual renal function results in the loss of sufficient bicarbonate in the urine, this factor also will influence plasma bicarbonate concentration. Only by understanding the roles of all these factors can we provide the necessary therapeutic approaches to regulation of bicarbonate concentration in patients on dialysis. We must examine our goals. In patients with proximal RTA, the only cost of a low bicarbonate concentration when acid balance is maintained is stunting of growth. If patients on dialysis are in acid balance, then continued bone carbonate loss should not occur unless, as noted earlier, some factor prevents replenishing the bone carbonate losses sustained in the interdialytic period. If restoration of bone carbonate is impaired, increasing plasma bicarbonate concentration to normal or above normal may or may not correct this defect. A clear case can be made for attempting to maintain a normal bicarbonate concentration in pediatric patients, but in adults further studies are needed to evaluate whether such a goal is necessary. A quite separate issue is acute dialysis-related morbidity. If, indeed, the replacement of acetate with bicarbonate in the dialysis bath can be shown to reduce such morbidity in some patients, then bicarbonate should be used if our goal is to increase the rate of rehabilitation of dialysis patients to active and useful lives.

References

Ballard, F. J., 1972, Supply and utilization of acetate in mammals, *Am. J. Clin. Nutr.* **25:**773.

Bauer, W., and Richards, D. W., 1928. A vasodilator action of acetates, *J. Physiol.* **66:**371.

Brenes, L. G., Brenes, J. N., Rodrigues, V. M., and Hernandez, M. M., 1977, Familial proximal renal tubular acidosis. A distinct clinical entity, *Am. J. Med.* **63:**244.

Gennari, F. J., and Cohen, J. J., 1978, Renal tubular acidosis, *Annu. Rev. Med.* **29:**521.

Graefe, U., Milutinovich, J., Follette, W. C., Vizzo, J. E., Babb, A. L., and Scribner, B. H., 1978, Less dialysis-induced morbidity and vascular instability with bicarbonate in dialysate, *Ann. Intern. Med* **88:**332.

Kirkendol, P. L., Devia, C. J., Bower, J. D., and R. D. Holbert, 1977, A comparison of the cardiovascular effects of sodium acetate, sodium bicarbonate and other potential sources of fixed base in hemodialysate solutions, *Tr. Am. Soc. Artif. Intern. Organs* **23:**399.

Kveim, M., and Nesbakken, R., 1975, Utilization of exogenous acetate during hemodialysis, *Tr. Am. Soc. Artif. Intern. Organs* **21:**138.

Lipsky, S., Alper, B., Rubini, M., Van Eck, W., and Gordon, M., 1954, The effects of alkalosis upon ketone body production and carbohydrate metabolism in man, *J. Clin. Invest.* **33:**1269.

Lundquist, F., 1962, Production and utilization of free acetate in man, *Nature* **193:**579.

Mion, C. M., Hegstrom, R. M., Boen, S. T., and Scribner, H. B., 1964, Substitution of sodium acetate for sodium bicarbonate in the bath fluid for hemodialysis, *Tr. Am. Soc. Artif. Intern. Organs* **10:**110.

Mudge, G. H., Manning, J. A., and Gilman, A., 1949. Sodium acetate as a source of fixed base, *Proc. Soc. Exp. Biol. Med.* **71:**136.

Raja, R., Kramer, M., Rosenbaum, J. L., Bolisay, C. and Krug, M., 1980, Prevention of hypotension during iso-osmolar hemodialysis with bicarbonate dialysate, *Tr. Am. Soc. Artif. Intern. Organs* **26:**375.

Tolchin, N., Roberts, J. L., Hayashi, J. and Lewis, E. J., 1977, Metabolic consequences of high mass-transfer hemodialysis, *Kidney Int.* **11:**366

Vreeman, H. J., Assomull, V. M., Kaiser, B. A., Blaschke, T. F., and Weiner, M. W., 1980, Acetate metabolism and acid-base homeostasis during hemodialysis: Influence of dialyzer efficiency and rate of acetate metabolism, *Kidney Int.* **18**(suppl. 10)**:** S62.

Transplantation and Immunosuppression

47

The State of the Art

John S. Najarian

End-stage kidney disease reached several important anniversaries in 1980. It was the 30-year anniversary of the first successful clinical hemodialysis and the 25-year anniversary of the first successful kidney transplant between identical twins. In addition, it was 20 years after the first successful non-identical twin transplant—approximately 35,000 people have received kidney transplants in the United States.

Kidney transplantation is the most effective means of treatment of patients with end-stage kidney disease. Actually, it is the only cure for the disease because chronic dialysis is only a form of treatment of the underlying condition. In addition, during 1983 the Social Security Administration will spend almost two billion dollars in the treatment of patients with chronic renal disease. This figure continues to rise at a precipitous rate, almost double the estimated amount.

Renal transplantation is the most financially efficient means of management because it involves a single expenditure for a successful transplant. If the transplant fails, the patient can go back on dialysis and be considered again for a kidney transplant. The current cost for a renal transplant is approximately $20,000, essentially the same as it was 20 years ago. The reason for this stablized cost is the decreased number of days required for hospitalization after transplantation. Thus, it appears that the government funding agencies should accept transplantation as the most effective and cost-efficient method of treating patients with end-stage kidney disease. Unfortunately, only four to five thousand people are transplanted each year, and more than 15,000 are placed on chronic hemodialysis. The major reason for this difference is that the 5- and 10-year kidney survival results have not improved appreciably in the past 10 years.

John S. Najarian • Departments of Surgery and Therapeutic Radiology, University of Minnesota, Minneapolis, Minnesota 55455.

The current national 5-year kidney survival results are approximately 50% for related-kidney transplants and 40% for cadaveric-kidney transplants. The 10-year results are approximately 10% less than this. It is apparent that the next advance in kidney transplantation should be made in trying to improve recipients' acceptance of donor kidneys. This subpart focuses on new techniques and therapies of immunosuppression; the possible development of techniques of acquired immunologic tolerance; and better methods of tissue typing to obtain closer genetic donor–recipient matching.

In new methods of immunosuppression the four areas to be covered will include total lymphoid irradiation (TLI), the use of cyclosporin A, thoracic duct drainage, and, finally, the more widespread use of antilymphocyte globulin (ALG). All these techniques of immunosuppression initially offer some hope that kidney, and thus patient, survival can be remarkably improved.

Dr. Anthony Monaco's chapter discusses progress in developing acquired immunologic tolerance, either with the use of total-body irradiation and bone marrow transplantation or with the use of ALG and bone marrow transplantation. Finally, Dr. Fritz Bach's chapter focuses on the newer techniques used in tissue matching, with primary emphasis on the HLA-D locus or DR typing. He will address the possibility of adding this newer modality to conventional serologic typing for HLA-A and HLA-B.

These chapters identify practical avenues of approach for treatment and for further research. It is hoped that kidney transplant survival statistics will improve as better methods are applied. We need a much more cost-efficient method of management of the catastrophic illness of chronic end-stage kidney disease.

48

Use of Total Lymphoid Irradiation in Organ Transplantation

S. Strober, M. S. Gottlieb, R. T. Hoppe, C. P. Bieber, D. P. (King) Paulnock, B. L. Kotzin, S. H. Koretz, B. A. Reitz, and H. S. Kaplan

1. Immunosuppressive Effects of TLI in Humans

In the course of investigating the cellular basis of the immunodeficiency of patients with Hodgkin's disease, we examined the number and function of T lymphocytes in the peripheral blood before and after treatment with total lymphoid irradiation (TLI).[1] Treated patients received a total of 4400 rads to the lymph nodes, thymus, and spleen (if not removed previously), in fractions of 200–250 rads to the subdiaphragmatic tissues. A similar schedule of radiation was given subsequently to the supradiaphragmatic tissues. The skull, lungs, kidneys, pelvis, and long bones were shielded with lead.

In patients with Hodgkin's disease, TLI produced a reduction in T cells and an increase in B cells in the blood for at least 10 years in patients with no recurrence. In addition to the numerical deficit, TLI reduced the *in vitro* immune (MLR) response of peripheral blood T lymphocytes to allogeneic cells for approximately 2 years. A gradual recovery was noted thereafter,

S. Strober • Division of Immunology, Department of Medicine, Stanford University Medical Center, Stanford, California 94305. ***M. S. Gottlieb*** • Division of Clinical Immunology (CIA), Department of Medicine, UCLA Center for the Health Sciences, Los Angeles, California 90024. ***R. T. Hoppe and H. S. Kaplan*** (deceased) • Department of Radiology, Stanford University Medical Center, Stanford, California 94305. ***C. P. Bieber*** • Los Altos Hills, California 94022. ***D. P. (King) Paulnock*** • Department of Medical Microbiology, University of Wisconsin Medical School, Madison, Wisconsin 53706. ***B. L. Kotzin*** • Division of Rheumatology, Department of Internal Medicine, Medical Center, Denver, Colorado 80220. ***S. H. Koretz*** • Institute of Clinical Medicine, Syntex Research, Palo Alto, California 94304. ***B. A. Reitz*** • Department of Surgery, Johns Hopkins Medical School, Baltimore, Maryland 21218.

until the response returned to normal levels by 5–10 years after treatment. In addition, untreated patients who showed intact cell-mediated immunity, as judged by normal skin reactivity to bacterial and fungal antigens, lost their skin reactivity for at least 18 months after radiotherapy. Despite this intense and prolonged immunosuppression, less than 1% of patients developed serious systemic infections.[2]

2. *Immunosuppressive Effects of TLI in Mice*

In view of the potent immunosuppression in humans without severe side effects, we investigated the use of TLI in tissue transplantation in mice.[3] Adult (6-month-old) BALB/c mice were given high-dose, fractionated lymphoid irradiation. The lymph nodes, as well as the spleen and thymus, were exposed to radiation. The skull, long bones, tail, and lungs were shielded with lead. Each animal was given 17 fractions of 200 rads each to achieve a total dose of 3400 rads within approximately 3 weeks. Mice were anesthetized with pentobarbital during each treatment.

TLI prolonged the survival of C57BL/Ka skin grafts in BALB/c recipients about 5 times (mean 50 days) longer than nonirradiated controls (mean 10 days). Inclusion of the thymus in the radiation field was essential for full immunosuppression, since shielding of this organ during TLI resulted in only minor prolongation of graft survival. However, thymic irradiation alone had little effect. Irradiation of both the thymus and the peripheral lymphoid tissues is required for optimal suppression of graft rejection.

3. *BM Transplantation without GVHD Using TLI*

In several experiments, BALB/c mice were given TLI, and an intravenous injection of bone marrow (BM) cells from C57BL/Ka donors 1 day later.[4] Twenty-four of twenty-seven recipients given BM cells were chimeras as judged by the presence of donor-type lymphocytes in the peripheral blood more than 100 days after BM transplantation. The majority of lymphocytes in the lymph nodes, spleen, and bone marrow (exposed to irradiation) were donor type, and chimerism was found also in the erythrocytes.

Although allogeneic BM engraftment was achieved in this strain combination, no clinical evidence of graft-versus-host disease (GVHD) was observed in the recipients. BALB/c mice lost up to one third of their body weight during TLI but regained their normal weight within a few weeks after BM transplantation. There was no hair loss, diarrhea, hunched back, or skin rash usually associated with GVHD. To determine whether vigorous GVHD can occur in this strain combination, BALB/c mice were given a single, lethal dose of whole-body irradiation (1000 rads), and 1 day later were injected intravenously with C57BL/Ka BM cells. All mice given whole-body irradiation without marrow replacement were dead within 11 days.

Control mice given syngeneic (BALB/c) BM cells survived for more than 250 days. The majority of mice given allogeneic (C57BL/Ka) BM cells died within 2 weeks, and 95% died within 60 days. The latter animals showed the typical clinical changes of GVHD. On the other hand, more than 80% of BALB/c mice given TLI and allogeneic BM cells survived at least 110 days, which approximated the survival of animals given TLI alone. These findings show that TLI prevents the development of GVHD ordinarily observed following allogeneic marrow transplantation.

4. *Transplantation Tolerance after TLI*

BALB/c mice given both TLI and allogeneic BM cells also received a skin graft from the BM donors on the day of BM transplantation.[3,4] All recipients shown to be chimeric maintained the skin grafts with full hair growth for at least 250 days. To determine whether animals with long-standing skin grafts were specifically tolerant to donor-type tissues, six of the latter recipients were given skin grafts from C3H (H-2^k) donors more than 100 days after BM transplantation. All C3H grafts were rejected by 13 days, whereas the C57BL/Ka grafts remained intact. Specific tolerance was also shown by the ability of PBL from chimeric recipients to respond *in vitro* to stimulator lymphocytes from C3H, but not C57BL/Ka or BALB/c, donors.

5. *Bone Marrow Transplantation and Tolerance in Rats after TLI*

Adult Lewis rats were given TLI using lead shields and a radiation protocol similar to that used in mice.[5] One day after the completion of TLI, animals were given an intravenous injection of ACI BM cells. An ACI skin graft was placed on the anterior chest wall 1 day later. All the recipients given BM cells were chimeric and maintained their skin grafts more than 100 days after BM transplantation. Permanent survival of ACI heart allografts directly sutured to the abdominal aorta and inferior vena cava was observed in four out of five recipients given TLI and ACI BM cells.

As in the experiments with mice, none of the chimeric rats showed clinical evidence of GVHD. In addition, chimeras were found to be specifically tolerant to donor-type tissues, since they rejected third-party BN skin grafts and responded *in vitro* to stimulator lymphocytes from BN but not ACI or Lewis donors.

6. *Transplantation of Allogeneic BM in Dogs Using TLI*

The use of TLI in BM transplantation in mongrel dogs was examined to determine the applicability of this technique to large outbred animals. Unrelated mongrels were paired so that they differed by sex and blood group types. Our initial group of recipients was given between 3600 and 4800 rads to the lymphoid tissues in 100- to 150-rad fractions over a period of 3–4 months using a 5-MeV linear accelerator as the radiation source. The majority of fractions were administered to the supra- and subdiaphragmatic fields separately.[6]

Two of three recipients given at least 1×10^9 BM cells per kilogram body weight 1 day after radiotherapy were stable chimeras for at least 9 months, as judged by the presence of donor-type sex chromosomes in BM samples from these recipients. Donor-type cells were also found in the peripheral blood—there were donor-type blood group antigens on the red blood cells. Although these recipients accepted the allogeneic BM grafts, they showed neither clinical signs of GVHD nor evidence of liver dysfunction usually accompanying GVHD during an 18-month observation period. These findings show that TLI allows for allogeneic BM engraftment without GVHD in large outbred animals.

In further experiments 12 dogs were given 18 fractions of 100 rads each to the supra- and subdiaphragmatic tissues simultaneously.[7,8] The regimen was completed in about 3 weeks, and allogeneic bone marrow was transplanted within 48 hr after the completion of TLI. All dogs with and without prior blood transfusions accepted the marrow grafts and became stable chimeras as judged by karyotype and blood group analysis (Tables 1 and 2). These dogs are now 8–24 months post-marrow transplantation and have no clinical signs of GVHD. At the end of TLI all animals developed a mild leukopenia (WBC $\simeq 3\text{–}5 \times 10^3/\text{mm}^3$) and thrombocytopenia (platelet count 50–150,000/mm^3); there was no evidence of infection or spontaneous bleeding.

7. *Combined Organ and Bone Marrow Transplantation in Dogs*

We attempted to transplant skin, kidney, or heart allografts to mongrel dogs given TLI and allogeneic bone marrow cells. Organ grafts were obtained from the marrow donor in all cases. Pilot experiments were performed with two dogs shown to be chimeric at least 8–12 months after BM transplantation. Both recipients received approximately 4000 rads to the abdomen and chest separately in fractions of 100–200 rads.[6] Skin grafts transplanted several months after BM transplantation were rejected within 21 days. A heart allograft anastomosed to the abdominal aorta and inferior vena cava 8 months after BM transplantation was rejected within 2 weeks (Table 3, dog no. 27).

In further experiments, seven dogs were given 18 fractions of 100 rads each, and allogeneic BM was injected intravenously, as described in the previous section. Within 2 days after the BM infusion, heart or kidney grafts from the marrow donor were transplanted to the recipient. Anastomosis of the heart or kidney grafts to the abdominal aorta and inferior vena cava resulted in bowel intussusception and death within 10 days in all seven dogs. The high frequency of intussusception appeared to be due to a combination

Table 1. Erythrocyte Antigen and Karyotype Analysis of Bone Marrow Recipients Not Given Prior Blood Transfusions

Recipient number	Months after transplantation	Karyotype analysis (% donor type)	Blood group analysis (DEA)[a]
826	0		—, 3, 4, —, 6, —
	1	36 (♀)	$\underline{1.1}$, 3, 4, —, 6, $\underline{8}$
	2		$\underline{1.1}$, n, n, —, n, —
	3		$\underline{1.1}$, n, n, —, n, —
	5	33 (♀)	$\underline{1.1}$, 3, 4, —, 6, —
	8		$\underline{1.1}$, 3, 4, —, 6, —
	10	32 (♀)	$\underline{1.1}$, 3, 4, —, 6, $\underline{8}$
38	0		1.1, —, 4, —, 6, —
	1	44 (♂)	1.1, —, 4, $\underline{5}$, 6, —
	2		1.1, —, n, —, 6, —
	3		1.1, —, n, $\underline{5}$, n, —
	5	44 (♂)	1.1, —, n, $\underline{5}$, n, —
	8		1.1, —, n, $\underline{5}$, n, —
	10	40 (♂)	1.1, —, 4, $\underline{5}$, 6, —
806	0		1.1, —, 4, —, 6
	1	50 (♂)	1.1, —, 4, —, 6
	2		n, —, n, $\underline{5}$, 6
	3		n, —, n, —, n
	5	47 (♂)	n, —, n, —, n
	8		1.1, —, 4, $\underline{5}$, 6
	10	40 (♂)	1.1, —, 4, $\underline{5}$, 6

[a] DEA types of donors of 826 and 38 1.1, 4, 5, 6, 8 and 4, 5, 6 respectively. Donor of 806 was 1.1, 4, 5, 6. Donor-type antigens detected in recipients are underlined. DEA typing of pretransplant recipient blood samples was confirmed on at least three occasions. —, Not detected. n, Not tested.

of radiotherapy and abdominal operation because intussusception was not observed in animals given TLI without operation or in control animals given abdominal grafts without TLI. A similar problem has not been observed in monkeys or reported in humans.[(2)]

Subsequently, dogs given TLI and BM transplants received heart allografts which were directly anastomosed to the thoracic aorta and the superior vena cava using an approach through the right chest wall.

The preliminary experimental results are summarized in Table 3. Dogs given 1800 rads and BM and heart transplants from the same donor rejected their heart grafts within 84 days. Microscopic examination of the hearts showed severe acellular rejection patterns with necrosis and hemorrhage in the myocardium. One of the three dogs in the latter group was evaluated for chimerism shortly after rejection of the graft. Approximately 25% of karyotypes in spontaneous metaphase preparations of the femoral bone marrow of the recipient carried the sex chromosome marker of the donor. Thus in two dogs (no. 22 and no. 27), heart allografts were rejected even though chimerism was evident. This suggests that organ-specific antigens may play an important role in organ graft rejection in these highly outbred mongrel dogs.

Table 2. Erythrocyte Antigen and Karyotype Analysis of Bone Marrow Recipients Given Random Blood Transfusions during TLI

Recipient number		Months after transplantation	Karyotype analysis (% donor type)	Blood group analysis (DEA)[a]
Group 1	348	2	37 (♀)	MNA
		8	25 (♀)	
	484	2	29 (♀)	1.1, —, —, —, 6, 8
		8	45 (♀)	1.1, —, 4, —, 6, 8
		10		1.1, —, 4, —, 6, 8
	480	2	40 (♀)	MNA
		8	43 (♀)	
Group 2	517	0		1.1, —, 4, —, 6, 8
		1		1.1, —, 4, 5, 6, 8
		2	20 (♀)	
		3		1.1, —, 4, 5, 6, 8
		7	31 (♀)	1.1, —, 4, 5, 6, 8
	508	2	40 (♂)	MNA
		7	26 (♂)	
	513	2	33 (♂)	MNA
Group 3	515	0		—, —, 4, 5, 6, 8
		1		1.1, —, 4, 5, 6, 8
		2	25 (♀)	1.1, —, 4, 5, 6, 8
		4		1.1, —, 4, 5, 6, 8
		5		1.1, —, 4, 5, 6, 8

Two groups of dogs were given TLI, BM cells, and antithymocyte globulin (ATG) alone or in combination with azathioprine to prevent the rejection of subsequent heart transplants. The TLI and BM infusion procedures were carried out as described previously. Within 2 days heart allografts were transplanted, and recipients received rabbit antidog thymocyte globulin (4 mg/kg, intramuscularly) on postoperative days 0, 2, 4,6, 8, and 10. Azathioprine (0.5–1 mg/kg intramuscularly) was given to one of the two groups on a daily basis (for 90 days) as long as the total white blood cell count was >5000 cells/mm^3. Recipients given ATG alone rejected their heart grafts between 29 and 121 days after transplantation (Table 3). Microscopic examination of the grafts showed moderate to severe rejection involving the myocardium and arterial vessels.

Dogs given a combination of ATG and azathioprine were to receive the latter drug for 90 days. Graft survival was monitored thereafter in the absence of all drugs to determine whether permanent graft survival could be achieved after a brief course of these immunosuppressive agents. Thus far, only one dog in this group has survived the 90-day period (Table 3). One dog each died because of infection (following leukopenia) and of polyarthritis of unknown etiology. There has been no evidence of rejection by electrocardiogram (EKG) or biopsy criteria between 20 and 104 days after heart transplantation (Table 3). Although it is too early to determine the

Table 3. Survival of Heart Transplants Obtained from Donors of Allogeneic Bone Marrow[a]

Dog no.	Treatment	EKG evaluation	Biopsy evaluation	Death
27	TLI, BM[b] (8-month delay)	Arrest, <14 days	Acellular rejection	—
41	TLI, BM	Arrest, <14 days	Acellular rejection	—
28	TLI, BM	Arrest, <14 days	Acellular rejection	—
22	TLI, BM[b]	Fibrillation	Cellular rejection	—
389	TLI, BM, ATG	Fibrillation, 121 days	Cellular rejection, day 90	—
365	TLI, BM, ATG	Decreased voltage, 39 days	Cellular rejection, day 39	Day 39, empyema
419	TLI, BM, ATG	Fibrillation, 29 days	Cellular rejection, day 29	—
515	TLI, BM, ATG, Aza	Normal, 104 days	Normal, day 90	—
520	TLI, BM, ATG, Aza	Normal, 80 days	—	—
468	TLI, BM, ATG, Aza	Normal, 68 days	Normal, day 68	Day 68, polyarthritis
524	TLI, BM, ATG, Aza	Normal, 37 days	Normal, day 37	Day 37, leukopenia
616	TLI, BM, ATG, Aza	Normal, 20 days	—	—

[a] Hearts were transplanted within 2 days after BM, except for 8-month delay in dog no. 27. TLI, BM, all dogs given 18 × 100-rad fractions in continuity (except no. 27, given ~ 4000 rads to abdomen and chest separately in 100- to 200-rad fractions) and allogeneic bone marrow intravenously 1 day later. ATG, antithymocyte globulin, 4 mg/kg IM on days 0, 2, 4, 6, 8, 10. Aza, azathioprine, 0.5–1 mg/kg IM daily until day 90.

[b] Chimerism documented by karyotype analysis of the recipient bone marrow.

efficacy of combined ATG and azathioprine therapy, biopsy results suggest that dogs maintained on low doses of azathioprine do not have the rejection pattern observed in dogs given ATG alone.

8. *Organ Transplantation in Monkeys Using TLI*

To examine the immunosuppressive effects of a combination of low-dose (600 rads) TLI and ATG, rhesus monkeys were given TLI alone (six doses of 100 rads each—total 600 rads), four doses of rabbit antimonkey thymocyte globulin alone, or TLI and ATG in combination.[(9)] Allogeneic hearts were anastomosed to the abdominal aorta and inferior vena cava to determine the effect of these regimens on prolongation of graft survival. Graft function was determined by electrocardiography and direct palpation. Graft survival in untreated animals showed a range of 10–13 days. Prolongation of 29–50 days was observed when recipients were given 600 rads, 1 day before heart transplantation. Animals given a heart transplant and four doses of ATG on alternate days showed no prolongation of survival in four out of five cases. Although only slight prolongation was observed with either low-dose TLI or ATG, the range of heart allograft survival in recipients given TLI (600 rads) and ATG in combination was 133–229 days. This extensive prolongation indicates that the immunosuppressive effects of TLI and ATG act synergistically and are effective in preventing early graft rejection.

In recent experiments, three monkeys were given 18 fractions of 100 rads each to abdominal and chest ports. A heart allograft was transplanted orthotopically after removal of the recipient heart. Six doses of ATG (4 mg/kg intramuscularly) were given during the first 12 postoperative days, and maintenance azathioprine (0.5 mg/kg intramuscularly) was given daily when the total white blood cell count was >5000 cells/mm^3. At present, all three recipients are alive 20–50 days after transplantation.

9. Conclusion

Although chimerism in mice and rats allowed for the long-term survival of organ grafts from the marrow donors, chimerism in mongrel dogs did not have the same effect. Two possible explanations for this difference are that the dose of irradiation (3400 rads) used in the rodents was considerably higher than that used in dogs (1800 rads), and that polymorphic organ-specific antigens may be more heterogeneous in highly outbred dog populations than in inbred rodent species which are initially derived from a small number of strains.

We continue to investigate the use of short-term posttransplant chemical immunosuppression to prevent organ graft rejection which may be based on organ-specific antigens. Although it is too early to assess the outcome, preliminary results using TLI in combination with ATG and daily azathioprine (without marrow transplantation) suggest that low doses of azathioprine may be sufficient to maintain long-term organ grafts in monkeys. This regimen may be preferable to those in current clinical use because it eliminates corticosteroids as the core immunosuppressive agent.

References

1. Fuks Z, Strober S, King DP, Kaplan HS: Reversal of cell surface abnormalities of T lymphocytes in Hodgkin's disease after *in vitro* incubation in fetal sera. *J Immunol* 117:1331, 1976.

2. Kaplan HS: *Hodgkin's Disease*. 2nd edition. Cambridge, Mass., Harvard University Press, 1980.
3. Slavin S, Strober S, Fuks Z, Kaplan HS: Induction of specific tissue transplantation tolerance using fractionated total lymphoid irradiation in adult mice: Long-term survival of allogeneic bone marrow and skin grafts. *J Exp Med* 146:34, 1977.
4. Slavin S, Fuks Z, Kaplan HS, Strober S: Transplantation of allogeneic bone marrow without graft vs. host disease using total lymphoid irradiation. *J Exp Med* 147:963, 1978.
5. Slavin S, Reitz B, Bieber CP, Kaplan HS, Strober S: Transplantation tolerance in adult rats using total lymphoid irradiation (TLI): Permanent survival of skin, heart, and marrow allografts. *J Exp Med* 147:700, 1978.
6. Slavin S, Gottlieb M, Bieber C, Hoppe R, Kaplan HS, Grumet FC, Strober S: Transplantation of bone marrow in outbred dogs without graft vs. host disease using total lymphoid irradiation (TLI). *Transplantation* 27:139, 1979.
7. Strober S, Slavin S, Gottlieb M, Zan-Bar I, King DP, Hoppe RT, Fuks Z, Grumet FC, Kaplan HS: Allograft tolerance after total lymphoid irradiation (TLI). *Immunol Rev* 46:87, 1979.
8. Gottlieb M, Strober S, Hoppe R, Grumet FC, Kaplan HS: Engraftment of allogeneic bone marrow without graft vs. host disease in mongrel dogs using total lymphoid irradiation (TLI). *Transplantation* 29:487, 1980.
9. Bieber CP, Jamieson A, Raney A, Burton N, Bogarty S, Hoppe R, Kaplan HS, Strober S, Stinson EB: Cardiac allograft survival in rhesus primates treated with combined total lymphoid irradiation and rabbit anti-thymocyte globulin. *Transplantation* 28:347, 1979.

49

Total Lymphoid Irradiation for Immunosuppression

Review of Animal Experiments and Results of a Clinical Trial in Renal Allograft Recipients

David E. R. Sutherland, Ronald M. Ferguson, Richard L. Simmons, Tae H. Kim, Shimon Slavin, and John S. Najarian

The therapeutic immunosuppressive effects of ionizing radiation were applied to transplant patients as long as 25 years ago by administration of full-body irradiation to prospective renal allograft recipients. The radiation dose required to prolong allograft survival produced severe bone marrow and other toxicities, and this approach was virtually abandoned by the mid-1960s.[(1)] Since then, various attempts have been made to direct radiation specifically at immunocompetent lymphoid cells,[(2)] including by local graft irradiation,[(3)] intralymphatic[(4)] or intravenous[(5)] administration of radioisotopes that focus upon lymphatic tissue, and by extracorpeal irradiation of blood[(6)] and lymph.[(7)] The radiation dose delivered by these techniques is difficult to control. The effect on allograft survival also has been variable, so that clinical application has been limited.

Total lymphoid irradiation (TLI) has been a standard treatment for Hodgkin's disease for over 20 years.[(8)] Fuks *et al.*[(9)] were the first to observe that patients so treated had a long-lasting impairment of cell-mediated immune functions. This observation was followed by the animal experiments of Slavin *et al.*[(10)] showing that TLI impaired the ability of rodents to reject organ allografts. When donor-strain bone marrow was administered after

---

David E. R. Sutherland, Ronald M. Ferguson, Richard L. Simmons, Tae H. Kim, Shimon Slavin, and John S. Najarian • Departments of Surgery and Therapeutic Radiology, University of Minnesota, Minneapolis, Minnesota 55455. Supported by NIH Grant AM13083.

TLI, chimerism without graft-versus-host disease (GVHD) was induced and allografts were permanently accepted.[11,12] Some investigators have observed GVHD in TLI-treated recipients of bone marrow.[13,14]

At the time that the Stanford group made their initial observations,[15] the stimulus to test new immunosuppressive regimens in clinical transplantation was great. Between 30 and 50% of kidneys from cadavers of mismatched related donors were rejected by recipients treated with conventional immunosuppression.[16] For patients who had to be retransplanted after rapid rejection of a previous graft, the situation was even worse—only one quarter had a satisfactory outcome.[17]

In an attempt to improve the outcome, in 1979 the Minnesota group began to treat patients who were at high risk to reject renal allografts by conventional immunosuppression with TLI.[18] They initiated this trial before cyclosporine became available. TLI was used primarily for its generalized immunosuppressive effect, but when it was logistically feasible, donor bone marrow cells were administered at the time of renal transplantation. It was not assumed that this protocol would induce tolerance, and azathioprine and prednisone were administered in order to suppress continually the immune response as the effect of TLI dissipated. Twenty patients were treated with TLI before undergoing retransplantation, and the graft survival rate was nearly double that of previous patients treated with conventional immunosuppression alone after retransplantation.[19] Although the results in the specific group of patients treated with TLI were satisfactory it was cumbersome to administer and sometimes it was difficult to procure a kidney immediately after completion of the treatment course. For these reasons, when cyclosporine became available, the ability of this new immunosuppressive drug to prevent rejection after retransplantation in patients who had rapidly rejected the previous grafts on conventional immunosuppression was tested.[20]

The Minnesota clinical experience with TLI is described in detail, and a comparison is made to the results in a separate trial in which patients undergoing retransplantation were treated with cyclosporine. First the animal experiments with TLI that provided the initial background for this clinical trial, as well as later experiments designed to help solve some of the problems encountered in the clinical situation, are summarized briefly.

1. TLI in Experimental Animals

Total lymphoid irradiation is a misnomer because not all lymphoid tissue is irradiated and some nonlymphatic tissue is always included in the radiation fields. The areas of the body that are irradiated and the precise regions that are shielded during TLI have varied depending on the animal model, but in general the long bones and skull, lungs, and lateral abdomen are shielded, and the axilla, neck and midabdomen (and spleen if present), pelvis, and groin are irradiated. Although most of the bone marrow is shielded, a large area is not, and the effect of TLI may vary considerably depending on the extent of shielding.

TLI by itself is immunosuppressive, but the effect dissipates with time. Thus, investigators either have used TLI as preparation for allogeneic bone marrow transplantation in an attempt to induce tolerance to the bone marrow donor or have combined TLI with pharmacological immunosuppression in order to have a more sustained effect. In most experiments, TLI has been administered prior to transplantation, but posttransplant TLI also has been evaluated because of the logistical advantages in relation to the timing of transplantation. Single-dose TLI has been used in some experiments, but TLI usually has been given in fractionated doses. The immunosuppressive effect and side effects depend upon the dose fraction size, the intervals between doses, and the total dose delivered. The above variations and the special problems in applying TLI to large animal models are described separately in the following subsections.

1.1. Pretransplant TLI Alone

The generalized immunosuppressive effect of TLI was first shown in animals by Slavin *et al.*[10] Balb/C mice were pretreated with 3400 rads (17 fractions of 200 rads each) of TLI and developed severe leukopenia, marked depletion of peripheral blood lymphocytes, depression of T and B cells, and allogeneic responsiveness *in vitro*. C57/B1 skin grafts were accepted for a mean of 49.1 days, as compared to a mean skin graft survival time of 10.7 days in control mice.

Since this report many investigators have shown that TLI prolongs the survival of allografts in animals. In some of the experiments, animals treated with TLI alone were controls for other groups in which TLI was used in conjunction with bone marrow transplantation in attempts to induce tolerance or with pharmacological immunosuppression as part of combination immunosuppressive therapy. Slavin *et al.*[12] also found that irradiation of Lewis rats by a protocol identical to that used in mice (200 rads × 17 doses) increased BN and ACI skin allograft survival times from a mean of 10 days in unirradiated rats to means of 39 and 41 days in treated rats, and heart allograft survival times were increased from 9–10 days to 35–300 days with TLI treatment.

Rynasiewicz *et al.*[13,21] tried various dose fraction schedules in an ACI-to-Lewis heart allograft model and found fractionated treatment more immunosuppressive than the same total dose given as a single treatment. When the total dose was 1000 rads, 200-rad fractions were optimal and resulted in a median graft survival time of 26 days. With 200-rad fractions, a progressive prolongation of allograft survival times occurred with increasing total doses; 2600 rads was the maximal total dose that resulted in no irradiation deaths, and this dose resulted in a median graft survival of 58 days. Rynasiewicz *et al.*[22] also used TLI in rat pancreas and islet allograft models and showed that a total dose of 1000 rads (200 rads × 5 doses) more than tripled graft survival times. Larger doses of TLI could not be used because of excessive toxicity in diabetic rats, a problem encountered by other investigators using diabetic animal models for islet transplantation. Britt *et al.*[23] had to deliver the TLI before the animals were made diabetic. However, Mullen and Shibukawa[24] found that the functional survival of fetal pancreas allografts transplanted across a minor barrier was more than doubled in diabetic rats treated with 2400 rads (200 rads × 12 doses). Nakajima *et al.*[25] increased the survival of hamster islet xenografts in diabetic rats more than tenfold by administration of 1200 rads (200 rads × 6 doses).

These experiments amply demonstrate the generalized immunosuppressive effective of fractionated TLI, but TLI by itself does not result, or rarely results, in indefinite allograft survival even in rodents, in which a variety of manipulations are known to do so.[26] Thus, for optimal results TLI must be combined with other treatments of the recipient.

1.2. TLI Plus Donor Bone Marrow Administration to Induce Tolerance

Induction of specific tolerance in adult recipients of organ allografts to eliminate the need for continual immunosuppression of the host is the major goal of transplantation immunobiology. An exciting aspect of the initial experiments by Slavin *et al.*[11,12] was the demonstration that TLI induced an environment in which allogenic bone marrow engrafted and produced permanent chimerism of the recipients without the development of GVHD. Skin grafts from the same donor strain were not rejected, in contrast to the results with whole-body irradiation in which graft versus host disease (GVHD) occurred or with thymus shielding in which engraftment did not occur.[11] In further experiments by Slavin and Strober,[27] mixed-lymphocyte culture (MLC) results from TLI-treated chimeric mice were interpreted as showing that splenocytes from TLI-treated chimeric mice exhibited nonspecific suppressor activity, but that long-term suppressor activity was specific for the strain. Okada and Strober[28] in the later experiments found that cells of donor origin in TLI-treated chimeric mice partially suppressed the generation of cytotoxic cells *in vitro* of the donor strain against the recipient, results consistent with the absence of GVHD in the chimeras and the specific loss of ability to produce GVHD with chimeric cells in secondarily irradiated hosts of the original but not of a third-party strain. The suppressor cells have since been characterized.[29] Waer *et al.*[30,31] have induced stable chimerism by a protocol similar to that of Slavin *et al.* and also have identified environmental and genetic conditions and protocol variations that influence the results.

Other investigators have been less successful with TLI and bone marrow transplantation in rodents. Ascher *et al.*[32] injected Balb/C bone marrow into C3H mice treated with 3400 rads fractionated TLI (200 rads × 17 doses). Although 20% of the mice became chimeric, *in vitro* work failed to demonstrate suppression in MLC over time. Instead, antihost cytotoxic cells were present in chimeric animals, an observation consistent with the failure of chimeric mice to gain weight on the basis of a chronic low-grade GVHD and also an explanation of suppression of a rejection response by the host. Kersey *et al.*[33] found that approximately 90% of Balb/C mice treated with 3400 rads fractionated TLI (200 rads × 17 doses) or with one dose of TLI (900 rads) plus cyclophosphamide became chimeric after transplantation of C57/B1 bone marrow and did not reject the C57/B1 skin grafts. There also was a 10% and 40% mortality from presumed GVHD produced with each of the respective protocols. Pierce *et al.*[14] treated Balb/C mice with 3400 rads of fractionated TLI (200 rads × 17 doses) followed by injection of C57/B1 bone marrow. Although none of the bone-marrow-treated mice rejected C57/B1 skin grafts (in contrast, TLI-alone-treated animals rejected at a mean of 22.3 days), they had progressive weight loss and died at the mean of 33.1 days, a course consistent with GVHD. Rynasiewicz *et al.*[13] observed an 83% mortality from GVHD in TLI Lewis rat recipients of ACI bone marrow. However, those who did not die of GVHD maintained heart allografts from the donor strain for more than 200 days. Mullen and Shibukawa[24] were able to achieve only a low degree of chimerism (0–23%) in standard shielded TLI-treated Lewis rats, but in those given irradiation to a larger amount of bone (greater than 50%), chimerism was achieved and fetal pancreas allografts from Balb/C donors were accepted permanently.[34] Slavin *et al.*[12] had previously shown the importance of extending the radiation fields in order to obtain chimerism after allogenic bone marrow transplantation in rats.

Why GVHD was observed by some investigators and not by others in rodents treated with TLI and bone marrow transplantation is not clear. It is known that microbial flora play a role in the development of GVHD, and the differences in environment in which the animals were maintained seems to be the most logical explanation. Bone marrow engraftment without the occurrence of GVHD also has been described in mongrel dogs treated with TLI,[35,36] but heart allografts from the donors were not permanently accepted.[37] The Minnesota group[38] and other investigators[39] have found that engraftment of bone marrow is difficult to achieve in dogs treated only with TLI, and in those in which chimerism has been demonstrated there has also been evidence of GVHD. Since GVHD is a potentially lethal complication and since it is uncertain whether TLI by itself can induce an environment in humans to obviate its occurrence without additional measures, at this time it may be more prudent to use TLI for its immunosuppressive effect rather than for its tolerance-inducing potential.

1.3. TLI Plus Pharmacological Immunosuppression

TLI has been combined with pharmacological immunosuppression in several animal allograft models in attempts to improve the therapeutic ratio of a generalized immunosuppression. Rynasiewicz *et al.*[21] used a combination of low-dose cyclosporine (1.25 mg/kg) and pretransplant TLI (1000 rads; 200 rads × 5 doses. Neither alone prolonged the survival of ACI heart allografts in Lewis rats beyond the mean of 3 weeks), but the combination had a synergistic effect with a median graft survival time of 96 days, nearly half of the grafts surviving indefinitely. In the more difficult pancreas transplant model (same donor recipient strain combination), 1000 rads of TLI pretransplant slightly prolonged the survival of grafts beyond that achieved with low-dose cyclosporine alone.[40] Sadeghi *et al.*[41] also found posttransplant fractionated TLI (200 rads per fraction) to be synergistic when combined with CsA for prevention or delay of rejection of cardiac allografts in rats. The most effective protocol was a 600-rad course of TLI completed 14 days preoperatively, followed by postoperative cyclosporine 2 mg/kg per day, and 1000 rads of TLI begun 6 days postoperatively (four of six grafts functioned more than 50 days).

Pennock *et al.*[42] combined fractionated TLI (100 rads per fraction) with cyclosporine (17 mg/kg per day intramuscularly) in a monkey orthotopic cardiac allograft model and observed mean allograft survival times with cyclosporine alone of 59 days and with cyclosporine plus TLI 600 rads or TLI 800 rads of 89 and 115 days, respectively, only a slightly additive effect. Similar experiments in a canine renal allograft model have been performed by the Minnesota group who found a mild synergism with cyclosporine (5 mg/kg per day) and pretransplant TLI (150 rads/fraction) in delaying or preventing rejection.[43] In splenectomized dogs median allograft survival times with cyclosporine alone were 8 days and with 1800 rads of TLI alone were 8 days, whereas it was 39 days with the combination. In nonsplenectomized dogs, the median survival time with cyclosporine was 12.5 days, with TLI 1800 rads it was 8.5 days, and with the combination it was 40 days. The therapeutic ratio was relatively poor compared to the results in the rat heart allograft model.

A synergistic effect of TLI with antithymocyte globulin (ATG) and azathioprine was seen in a primate heart allograft model by Bieber *et al.*[44,45] Three doses of ATG alone or of 600 rads of TLI alone resulted in mean survival times of 22 and 38 days, respectively, whereas the combination resulted in a mean survival time of 169 days. When Pennock *et al.*[42] added azathioprine to the combination, early deaths from leukopenia and infection occurred, and the mean graft survival time, with death counted as a graft loss, were approximately 7 weeks with each of the two doses of TLI used.

Mixed results have also been observed in canine allograft models testing the combinations of TLI and azathioprine or ATG. Pennock *et al.*[46] reported a mean survival time of greater than 240 days for heterotopic heart allografts in dogs receiving triple therapy (TLI 1800 rads, ATG × 6 doses and azathioprine 0.25 to 2.0 mg/kg per day given for 90 days tailored to the white count), whereas the mean survival time was only 31 days in dogs receiving ATG and azathioprine alone. Strober *et al.*[47] found that 1800 rads of TLI followed by six doses of ATG alone gave a median survival time of 170 days, and in three of eight animals whose grafts functioned for greater than 1 year, specific unresponsiveness to the donor was demonstrated. The addition of azathioprine did not improve the results.

Lewis *et al.*,[48] in a canine renal allograft model, administered azathioprine (2.5 mg/kg per day) and 2100 rads of TLI in 150-rad fractions. Graft survival times for azathioprine alone ranged from 5 to 48 days, with TLI alone from 8 to 21 days, and with the combination from 40 to 226 days, but 70% of the animals in the latter group died with functioning grafts from azathioprine-induced leukopenia. Thus, azathioprine is difficult to use in combination with TLI unless dose adjustments are made to compensate for the myelosuppressive effect of both treatments.

1.4. *TLI in Large-Animal Allograft Models*

Most of the immunosuppressive regimens in rodents that have given spectacular results in terms of allograft survival[26] have been difficult to reproduce in large-animal models and difficult to apply clinically. TLI, with or without bone marrow transplantation, is no exception. It is clear that TLI is immunosuppressive in large animals. The therapeutic ratio remains rather narrow, particularly in dogs, as evidenced by the results of the experiments of TLI in combination with pharmacological immunosuppression summarized in the preceeding subsection.[34–48] The Stanford group engrafted allogenic bone marrow without producing GVHD in mongrel dogs treated with TLI,[35,36] but even though chimerism has been detected, cardiac allografts were rejected[37] unless ATG was also given. On the other hand, two dogs treated by Howard *et al.*[49] with 2400 rads of pretransplant TLI maintained renal allografts for more than 500 days. The dogs received a low dose of bone marrow from the donor, but chimerism was not detected, and they have survived more than 3 years with functioning grafts.

Myburgh *et al.*[50,51] have observed very prolonged or indefinite survival of renal[50] and liver[51] allografts in baboons treated with 1600 rads of TLI (200 rads × 8 doses) followed by bone marrow and allotransplantation 3 weeks later. Although chimerism was demonstrated in some animals, its role in the graft prolongation is uncertain as well as that of the bone marrow injection, since control groups receiving TLI alone were not included in these experiments. Smit *et al.*[52] of the same group, showed that the lymphocyte proliferative responses *in vitro* of the treated animals were depressed and obtained preliminary data suggesting the presence of both donor-specific and -nonspecific suppression mechanisms. In further experiments Myburgh *et al.*[53] found that bone marrow transplantation in TLI-treated primates was not essential for the graft-prolonging effect. They also demonstrated that 100-rad fractions were safer than 200-rad fractions, that as little as 800 rads prevented rejection for up to 5 weeks, that with more than 1600 rads (200-rad fractions) indefinite graft survival could be achieved in some animals, that extended irradiation fields were necessary to achieve this effect, and that the effect of TLI was seen even with delays of up to 3 months before transplantation. These findings are of great potential clinical relevance, particularly if humans are able to tolerate a regimen similar to that used by Myburgh *et al.*[54] in baboons.

1.5. Posttransplant TLI

A major difficulty with the use of TLI for clinical transplantation has been the inability to always procure a donor organ soon after the completion of TLI. Rynasiewicz *et al.*[21] showed that in rats given 2600 rads of pretransplant TLI, median ACI heart allograft survival time was 57 days in those transplanted immediately versus 20 days for those in whom the transplant was delayed for 1 month. Thus, the effect of TLI dissipates with time. Further difficulties are foreseen in the clinical application of TLI for heart transplantation, in which a prolonged period of preoperative radiation might not be tolerated by a very sick patient. For this reason, Pennock *et al.*[46] and Bieber *et al.*[44,45] in the heart allograft experiments in large animals described in the preceding section, investigated the use of an abbreviated course of pretransplant TLI.

In order to avoid the difficulties with pretransplant TLI altogether, Rynasiewicz *et al.*[21] and Bentley *et al.*[55,56] performed a series of experiments designed to determine whether postoperative TLI could provide effective immunosuppression to delay or prevent rejection of heart allografts in rats. TLI in 200-rad fractions posttransplant by itself was not effective, but it was when combined with low-dose cyclosporine (1.25 mg/kg per day); median ACI heart allograft survival time in Lewis rats was 60 days, as compared to 15 days with cyclosporine alone. Bentley *et al.*[55] found that posttransplant TLI could increase rat heart allograft survival from 6 days to 25 days by using a schedule of 300-rad fractions times 3 days followed by a 2-day rest and then 200 rads times five doses. Bentley *et al.*[56] also combined perioperative ALG (two doses) with posttransplant TLI (200 rads × 7 doses) beginning on day 6 (delayed to avoid synergistic toxicities of ALG and TLI) and obtained a mean rat heart allograft survival time of 114 days as opposed to 10.7 days with ALG alone. Administration of cyclosporine (5 mg/kg per day) for just 5 days along with posttransplant TLI (200 rads × 10 doses) gave a mean graft survival time of 69.6 days, as opposed to 12.7 and 6.3 days with either treatment alone.[56] Sadeghi *et al.*[41] also used posttransplant TLI in a rat heart allograft model but did not find a regimen that significantly prolonged graft survival times except when pretransplant TLI was also given. The experiments of Rynasiewicz *et al.*[21] and Bentley *et al.*[55,56], however, show that posttransplant TLI can exert its immunosuppressive effect if the graft is protected early with pharmacological immunosuppression.

Such regimens have been subjected to very limited investigations in large-animal models. Lewis *et al.*[38] tested posttransplant TLI (150-rad fractions) in combination with azathioprine or antithymocyte globulin in dog renal allograft recipients and with 1800 rads doubled median graft survival times, but only one dog survived long-term with a functioning graft. A regimen more effective than the one tested might be found, and further experiments in large-animal models should be performed. If schedules giving therapeutic indices more favorable than those achieved with pharmacological immunosuppression alone can be developed, such an approach could be tested clinically.

2. *TLI for Clinical Renal Allotransplantation*

The clinical experience of TLI as a renal allograft recipients is, at this time, quite limited. The earliest and largest series is that of the University of Minnesota,[19,20,43] which began in February 1979 and ended in August 1981. There are, however, ongoing trials with TLI at the University of California and Pacific Medical Center in conjunction with the Radiation Therapy and Immunology groups at Stanford,[57,58] at the University of Leuven in Belgium,[59,60] and at the University of Rome.[61] In these institutions, TLI is being administered for its generalized immunosuppressive effect with adjuvant pharmacological immunosuppression as either low-dose prednisone[57–60] or cyclosporine.[61] Data from the first patients in the California trial indicate that drugs other than azathioprine are appropriate for adjunctive immunosuppression because the myelosuppressive effect of azathioprine potentiates that induced by TLI. Preliminary information (not summarized here) on these trials have been reported[57–61] and show that high graft survival rates can be achieved with minimal need for maintenance immunosuppression in recipients of first transplants. The patients in these trials differ from those in the Minnesota trial.

The University of Minnesota experience[19,20,43] is largely restricted to patients who were judged to be at high risk to reject renal allografts if treated with conventional immunosuppression. Twenty patients, who had rejected previous renal allografts less than 1 year after transplantation and treatment with ALG, azathioprine, and prednisone, received TLI in preparation for retransplantation, and two recipients of primary renal allografts from completely HLA-mismatched siblings were treated with TLI. The latter two patients were treated similarly to those undergoing retransplantation. Both patients have functioning renal allografts at 2 and 3 years after transplantation, but since the graft survival rates for kidneys from siblings mismatched for one or both haplotypes are similar at the University of Minnesota,[62] they would not have been considered at high risk to reject even if they had been treated with conventional immunosuppression. Their course has been described in previous publications,[19] and they are not included in the following summary updating the results of TLI in renal allograft recipients undergoing retransplantation at the University of Minnesota.

2.1. *Patient Population*

Twenty patients who previously rejected primary renal allografts at less than 1 year after transplantation were treated with fractionated TLI before

Table 1. Demographic Features of Patients Who Rapidly Rejected Previous Renal Allografts According to Immunosuppressive Regimen Used for Retransplantation

	TLI (n = 20)		Cyclosporine (n = 33)	
Age				
Range	4–51 yr		6–58 yr	
Mean	27 ± 13		35 ± 11	
Percent diabetic	30%		24%	
Mean time of rejection of previous allografts	5.8 ± 5.5 mo		2.6 ± 2.1 mo	
Interval between loss of previous allograft and retransplantation	2–49 mo (15.6 ± 12.8 mo)		2–57 mo (22.9 ± 15.8 mo)	
No. males/No. females (%)	15 M/5 F	(25%)	2 M/12 F	(36%)
No. 2nd/No. 3rd Txs (%)	13/7	(35%)	25/8	(24%)
No. rel/No. unrel donors (%)	1/19	(95%)	8/25	(76%)
Follow-up				
Range	22–52 mo		1–36 mo	
Median	38.5 mo		17 mo	
Mean	38.8 ± 7.8 mo		14.3 ± 9.0 mo	

retransplantation between February 1979 and August 1981. There were 13 second and seven third transplants. The grafts came from an uncle in one recipient and from unrelated donors for 19 recipients. The original kidney diseases were glomerulonephritis in ten patients, diabetes mellitus in six, and hemolytic uremic syndrome, obstructive uropathy, drug-induced nephritis, and renal tubular acidosis in one patient each. The demographic features of the TLI-treated recipients and a similar group of patients treated with cyclosporine after retransplantation[(43)] are summarized in Table 1.

2.2. *Irradiation*

The irradiation protocol was tailored for individual patients and during the course of the Minnesota experience was modified. The irradiation was delivered using either 10-MeV or 4-MeV linear accelerators to mantle and inverted Y fields simultaneously. The initial protocol entailed delivering 3200 rads total dose at 150 rads daily fraction, but several patients subjected to this regimen developed gastrointestinal symptoms or leukopenia (WBC < $2500/mm^3$), necessitating interruption of the radiation until the symptoms disappeared. Therefore, the daily fraction dose was reduced to 100 rads after the first nine patients. The total doses ranged from 1600 to 4150 rads (mean 2739 ± 718 rads), and they were delivered over periods ranging from 24 to 124 days. The intervals from completion of TLI to retransplantation ranged from 1 to 330 days. Three patients received maintenance radiation ranging from 625 to 800 rads twice weekly during the time they awaited for a compatible cadaver kidney after completion of planned radiation.

Table 2. In Vitro Assessment of T-Cell Numbers and Function in Patients Receiving Fractionated TLI

		Rads of TLI					
	Pre TLI	500	1000	1500	2000	2500	3000
Percent T	59 ± 3	58 ± 4	62 ± 4	54 ± 5	47 ± 8	46 ± 6	56 ± 9
No. T	1024 ± 81	347 ± 85	301 ± 39	254 ± 48	200 ± 49	156 ± 70	124 ± 110
Con A[a]	76 ± 27	36 ± 14	39 ± 11	28 ± 8	18 ± 10	14 ± 11	7 ± 7
PHA[a]	61 ± 13	34 ± 10	30 ± 8	29 ± 10	17 ± 7	11 ± 5	10 ± 3
MLC[a]	80 ± 9	37 ± 5	28 ± 4	22 ± 4	12 ± 2	15 ± 2	11 ± 6

[a] Con A, PHA, and MLC are expressed as relative response, or the response of the patient relative to a control normal response. Values are means ± S.E.M. of ten patients at each point up to 2000 rads. Five patients received more than 2000 rads.

2.3. *Posttransplant Immunosuppression*

The patients were treated with low dose (<1.5 mg/kg per day) azathioprine, adjusted to white blood cell count, and variable doses of prednisone (0.4–2.0 mg/kg initially, followed by a taper). Rejection episodes were treated with an increase in prednisone dose, except in one instance when ALG was used. Three patients received donor bone marrow (0.5×10^8 nucleated cells per kg) at the time of transplantation, but there was no evidence of engraftment in these patients.

2.4. *Immunological Monitoring*

T-cell levels, the response to plant mitogens, and MLC reactions were serially performed in the patients before and during irradiation (Table 2) and after transplantation. There was an 80–90% decrease in activity of all parameters by the time 1600 rads had been given. The two patients with the longest interval between completion of TLI transplantation had nearly complete recovery of responses before transplantation. In the other patients, T cells returned to normal by 6 months after transplantation. Although, T-cell numbers were normal, function usually was not normal except in three patients who had a chronic rejection process in the kidney. In 11 TLI-treated patients with normal renal allograft function followed for over 1 year, PHA, Con A, and MLC responsiveness ranged from 16 to 28% that of controls. In contrast, in the three patients undergoing chronic rejection, *in vitro* responsiveness was 77–98% that of controls. The three patients who chronically rejected their grafts had 53 ± 8% T cells in their peripheral blood (697 ± 397 total T cells/mm^3) as compared to 46 ± 7% in the 11 with normal function (346 ± 112% total T cells/mm^3). In some patients T-cell subsets were determined by the recently available commercially monoclonal OKT3, OKT4, and OKT8 antibodies, and there was a reversal in the normal ratio of helper/inducer cells (OKT4) to cytotoxic/suppressor cells (OKT8), with the latter predominating.

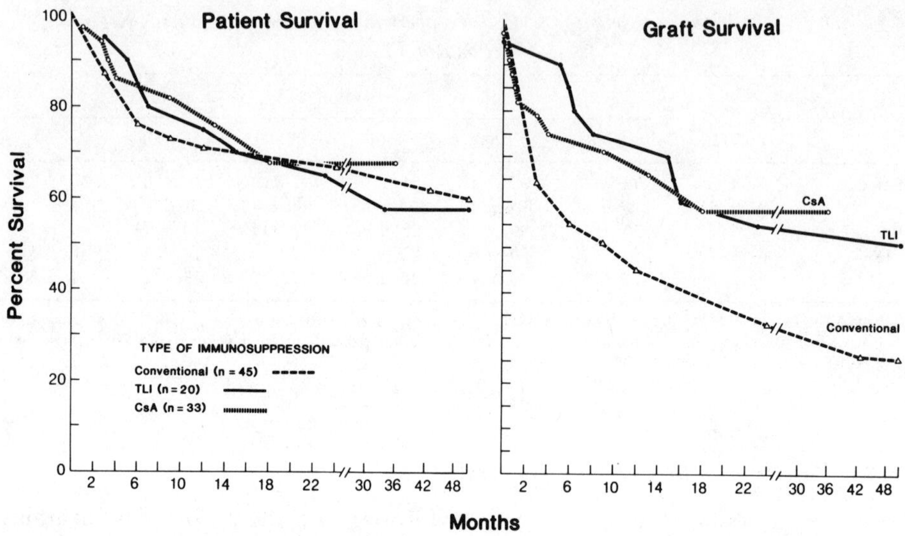

Figure 1. Actuarial patient and renal allograft survival rates according to immunosuppressive regimen after retransplantation in University of Minnesota patient who rejected previous allograft in less than 12 months. All patients in whom treatments were initiated are included in the calculations. (From Sutherland *et al.*, reference 19, with permission from Grune and Stratton, Inc., New York.)

2.5. *Patient and Graft Survival Rates*

Patient and graft survival rates were calculated May 1, 1983.[43] The overall results after transplantation in patients treated with TLI are depicted in Fig. 1. The results are compared to an historical control group treated with conventional immunosuppression for retransplantation after rapidly rejecting a previous graft.[63] Comparison also was made to a group of 33 patients who had previously rejected primary renal allografts in less than 1 year while receiving conventional immunosuppression and then were treated with cyclosporine after retransplantation.[43] The characteristics of the latter two groups in terms of mean rejection time of preceding grafts, mean interval between transplantation, and demographic features, such as age, sex, and primary renal disease, were virtually identical to the TLI group (Table 1).

The causes of graft loss included technical difficulties, rejection, or death with a functioning graft. One technical failure occurred in the TLI group and two in the cyclosporine group. In addition, two patients treated with cyclosporine initially were switched to conventional immunosuppression at 27 and 36 days, respectively, after transplantation. If the three technical failures (two TLI and one cyclosporine) and the two patients switched from cyclosporine to conventional immunosuppression are excluded, the 1-year patient survival rates were 79% in the TLI and 95% in the cyclosporine groups, and the corresponding graft survival rates were 79% and 81% (Table 3). The graft survival rates in both these subgroups were significantly higher

Table 3. Actuarial Patient and Graft Survival Rates according to Immunosuppressive Regimen Used for Retransplantation in Patients Who Rejected Previous Renal Allografts in <12 Months While on Conventional Immunosuppression[a]

	Patient survival (%)		Graft survival (%)	
Time post-Tx (mo)	TLI (n = 19)	CSA (n = 21)	TLI (n = 19)	CSA (n = 21)
1	100	86	100	86
3	100	86	100	100
6	84	81	89	95
12	79	81	79	95
18	63	76	74	90
24	58	76	68	90
36	58	76	63	90
48	58		63	

[a] Technical failures (one TLI and three CSA) and patients switched from CSA to conventional immunosuppression (n = 9) are excluded. See text for fate of excluded patients. They are included in survival rate curves of Fig. 1.

than those in the historical control group, which had a graft survival rate of 47% at 1 year.(63)

Of the original group of 20 patients treated with TLI before retransplantation, 12 are alive at this writing and 11 have functioning grafts with a serum creatinine concentration of 1.7 ± 0.5 mg/dl at 25 and 51 months posttransplant. The one patient who is alive at 31 months without graft function rejected the grafts at 15 months. Of the eight patients who died, four did so with functioning grafts, two from lymphoma at 5 and 11 months, respectively, one at 12 months from pneumococcal sepsis, and one at 5 months from cytomegalovirus infection. Four patients died after loss of graft function, one at 3 months from diabetic complications after a technical loss, another at 12 months after rejecting the graft at 8 months, another at 2 months from a perforated ulcer, and one of sepsis at 34 months after rejection at 6 months.

2.6. *Complications of TLI*

In the course of administration, TLI was associated with leukopenia in five patients and with gastrointestinal symptoms in seven patients, and the treatment had to be interrupted for 3–38 days. The patients experienced varying degrees of weight loss and anemia throughout the course of radiation. In general, radiation was tolerated less well in diabetic patients. The diabetics seemed to experience more severe weight loss and gastrointestinal symptoms than did their nondiabetic counterparts. The two patients who developed lymphoma both had Epstein–Barr virus (EBV) infections, and their course has been described previously.(64) One of the lymphoma patients received 3200 and one received 4050 rads. The latter also had a course of antilymphocyte globulin (ALG) to treat a rejection episode posttransplant. The EBV infections and lymphoma are thought to be related. They are probably a consequence of overimmunosuppression in general and not of TLI *per se* since similar courses have been seen in patients receiving different immunosuppressive regimens.[64]

2.7. *Factors Influencing Course of Patients Treated with TLI*

The variables that were associated with success or failure after retransplantation in patients treated with TLI included the dose and timing of TLI, the interval from TLI to transplantation, and the pharmacological immunosuppressive protocol employed in the immediate posttransplant period. Eleven patients had no rejection episodes. They received at least 2500 rads (mean of 2700 rads). They also received tapering prednisone dosage and maintenance azathioprine in nearly standard doses. The patients who had rejection episodes received less than 2500 rads of irradiation, or they received low doses of prednisone at the time of transplantation, or there was a long interval between transplantation and TLI. Still the rejection episodes were easily reversible in all but two patients.

In the patients who had optimal therapeutic courses, the critical factor was the dose of 2500 rads. If 2500 rads was administered, the interval between TLI and transplantation was not important. If less than 2500 rads was administered, the outcome was still good if the transplant occurred soon after completion of TLI and if a standard dose of prednisone was administered. These observations also were correlated with the immune response status of the patients at the time of transplantation. Patients who had a long interval between TLI and transplantation had a nearly normal number of T cells in the peripheral blood at the time of transplantation, and those with a short interval had low T-cell numbers. The MLC responsiveness at the time of transplantation in the subgroup of patients who received a standard taper of prednisone and who had rejection episodes was 27 ± 7% of normal, whereas in those who did not have rejection episodes the MLC response was only 14 ± 3% of normal. In a subgroup of three patients treated with a low dose of prednisone, MLC responsiveness was only 11 ± 2% of normal, but all three had rejection episodes.

These observations should be taken into account in devising future protocols. Every effort should be made to perform the transplant soon after completion of TLI. A high dose of prednisone should be administered initially, although a rapid taper is acceptable if the number of peripheral blood T cells is low and immune responsiveness *in vitro* is low at the time of transplantation. Such an aggressive immunosuppressive protocol might not be necessary for patients receiving TLI for primary transplantation,[56–61] but in the selected group of patients who have demonstrated their propensity to reject renal allografts, low-dose pharmacological immunosuppression does not appear to be sufficient to prevent rejection episodes, even with pretransplant TLI administration.[43]

The major factor precluding procurement of the kidneys soon after completion of TLI is the percentage of cyotoxic antibodies potential recipients expressed against a panel of cells from individuals representative of the potential donor pool. Cytotoxic antibodies did not decrease during TLI. In fact, the percentage of cytotoxic antibiotics often increased after the patients received blood transfusions for correction of TLI-aggravated uremic anemia. Transplantation across a positive crossmatch with either fresh or concurrent sera was not studied.

Since many of the patients who have rejected previous grafts have a high percentage of antibodies to the panel, the alternative protocol of cyclosporine was logistically easier to apply.[20,43] Since the results of retransplantation with cyclosporine appear to be as good as those achieved with TLI, cyclosporine appears to be the preferable treatment for this group of patients. TLI may still have a role for those patients who rapidly reject primary grafts while receiving cyclosporine. It should be possible to use TLI in the posttransplant period, since this has been shown to be effective in animal models.[21,38,41,55,56] Alternative TLI protocols also may prove to be more suitable for primary transplantation than the ones chosen to treat patients undergoing retransplantation at Minnesota.

3. Summary and Conclusions

TLI by itself can produce sufficient immunosuppression to prolong the survival of a variety of organ allografts in experimental animals. The degree of prolongation is dose dependent, and also is limited by the toxicity that occurs with higher doses. Pretransplant TLI is more effective than posttransplant TLI. However, the latter can be combined with pharmacological immunosuppression to achieve a positive effect.

In some animal models, TLI induces an environment in which fully allogenic bone marrow will engraft and induce permanent chimerism. The recipients are then tolerant to organ allografts from the original donor strain. If TLI is ever to have clinical applicability on a large scale, it probably will have to be under circumstances in which tolerance can be induced. However, in some animal models GVHD occurs after bone marrow transplantation. Methods to avoid GVHD probably will be needed if this approach is to be applied clinically.

In recent years, patient and graft survival rates in renal allograft recipients treated with conventional immunosuppression have improved considerably.[65,66] Thus, the need to utilize TLI for its immunosuppressive effect alone is less compelling. For example, at the University of Minnesota, the current 1-year patient and graft survival rates in recipients of kidneys from cadaver donors are, respectively, 90% and 84% in those treated with cyclosporine and 91% and 73% in those treated with conventional immunosuppression.[67] Similar results also might be achieved by protocols that use TLI as an immunosuppressant. It will be difficult to improve on the current results with cyclosporine or conventional immunosuppression, at least for primary transplantation.[68] The future of TLI would seem to lie in devising protocols in which maintenance immunosuppression can be eliminated, or nearly eliminated, altogether. Such protocols are effective in rodents. It remains to be seen whether or not they can be applied to clinical transplantation.

References

1. Hamburger J, Vaysse J, Crosnier J, Auvert J, Lalanne CM, Hopper J: Renal homotransplantation in man after radiation of the recipient. *Am J Med* 32:854–871, 1962.
2. Miller J: Immunological competence: Alterations by whole body x-irradiation and shielding of selected lymphoid tissues. *Science* 151:1395–1397, 1966.
3. Hume DM, Wolf JS: Abrogation of the immune response: Irradiation therapy and lymphocyte depletion. *Transplantation* 5:1174–91, 1967.
4. von Bekkum DW: Use of ionizing radiation in transplantation. *Transpl Proc* 6(4):59–65, 1974.
5. Hardy MA, Fawwaz RA, Oluwole S, Todd G, Nowygrod R, Reemstma K: Selective lymphoid irradiation. I. An approach to transplantation. *Surgery* 86:194–200, 1979.
6. Cronkite EP, Chanana AD, Schnappauf HP: Extracorporeal irradiation of blood and lymph in animals. *N Engl J Med* 272:456–461, 1965.
7. Joel DD, Chanana AD, Cronkite EP, Schiffer LM: Modification of skin allograft immunity by extracorporeal irradiation of lymph. *Transplantation* 5:1192–1197, 1967.
8. Kaplan HS: *Hodgkin's Disease*, 2nd ed. Cambridge, Massachusetts, Harvard University Press, 1980.
9. Fuks Z, Strober S, Bobrove AM, Sasazuki T, McMichael A, Kaplan HS: Long term effects of radiation on T and B lymphocytes in peripheral blood of patients with Hodgkin's disease. *J Clin Invest* 58:803–814, 1976.
10. Slavin S, Strober S, Fuks Z, Kaplan HS: Long term survival of skin allografts in mice treated with fractionated total lymphoid irradiation. *Science* 193:1252–1254, 1976.
11. Slavin S, Strober S, Fuks Z, Kaplan HS: Induction of specific tissue transplantation tolerance using fractionated total lymphoid irradiation in adult mice: Long-term survival of allogeneic bone marrow and skin grafts. *J Exp Med* 146:34–48, 1977.
12. Slavin S, Reitz B, Bieber CP, Kaplan HS, Strober S: Transplantation tolerance in adult rats using total lymphoid irradiation (TLI): Permanent survival of skin, heart and marrow allografts. *J Exp Med* 47:700–707, 1978.
13. Rynasiewicz JJ, Sutherland DER, Kawahara K, Kim T, Najarian JS: Total lymphoid irradiation in rat heart allografts: Dose, fractionation, and combination with cyclosporin-A. *Transpl Proc* 13:452–454, 1981.
14. Pierce GE, Wahs LM, Kinnaman ML, Thomas JH: Evidence for graft-versus-host disease in total-lymphoid-irradiated recipients of allogenic bone marrow and skin grafts. *J Surg Res* 30:398, 1981.
15. Strober S, Slavin S, Gottlief M, Zan–Bar I, King DP, Hoppe RT, Fuks Z, Grumet FC, Kaplan HS: Allograft tolerance after total lymphoid irradiation (TLI). *Immunol Rev* 46:87–112, 1979.
16. Opelz G., Mickey MR, Terasaki PI: Calculations on long term graft and patient survival in human kidney transplantation. *Transpl Proc* 9:27–30, 1977.
17. Ascher N, Ahrenholz D, Simmons RL, Najarian JS: 100 second renal allografts from a single transplantation institution. *Transplantation* 27:30–34, 1979.
18. Najarian JS, Sutherland DER, Ferguson RM, Simmons RL, Kersey J, Mauer SM, Slavin S, Kim TH: Total lymphoid irradiation and kidney transplantation: A clinical experience. *Transpl Proc* 13:417–424, 1981.

19. Najarian JS, Ferguson RM, Sutherland DER, Slavin S, Kim T, Kersey J, Simmons RL: Fractionated total lymphoid irradiation as preparative immunosuppression in high risk renal transplantation. *Ann Surg* 196:442–451, 1982.
20. Sutherland DER, Ferguson RM, Rynasiewicz JJ, Kim TH, Fryd DS, Dhein B, Slavin S, Simmons RL, Najarian JS: Total lymphoid irradiation versus cyclosporine for retransplantation in recipients at high risk to reject renal allografts. *Transpl Proc* 15(1): 460–464, 1983.
21. Rynasiewicz JJ, Sutherland DER, Kawahara K, Najarian JS: Total lymphoid irradiation: Critical timing and combination with cyclosporin A for immunosuppression in a rat heart allograft model. *J Surg Res* 30:365–371, 1981.
22. Rynasiewicz JJ, Sutherland DER, Kawahara K, Najarian JS: Total lymphoid irradiation for prolongation of pancreas and islet allograft survival in rats. *Surg Forum* 31:359–360, 1980.
23. Britt LD, Scharp DW, Lacy PE, Slavin S: Transplantation of islet cells across major histocompatibility barriers after total lymphoid irradiation and infusion of allogeneic bone marrow cells. *Diabetes* 31:63–68, 1982.
24. Mullen Y, Shibukawa RL: Use of total lymphoid irradiation in transplantation of rat fetal pancreases. *Diabetes* 31:69–74, 1982.
25. Nakajima Y, Nakano H, Nakagawa K, Segawa M, Shiratori T: Effect of total lymphoid irradiation (TLI) on pancreatic islet xenografts survival in rats. *Transplantation* 34:98–100, 1982.
26. Fabre JW: Rat kidney allograft model: Was it all too good to be true? *Transplantation* 34:223–225, 1982.
27. Slavin S, Strober S: Induction of allograft tolerance after total lymphoid irradiation (TLI): Development of suppressor cells of the mixed leukocyte reaction (MLR). *J Immunol* 123:942–946, 1979.
28. Okada S, Strober S: Spleen cells from adult mice given total lymphoid irradiation or from newborn mice have similar regulatory effects in the mixed leukocyte reaction. I. Generation of antigen-specific suppressor cells in the mixed leukocyte reaction after the addition of spleen cells from adult mice given total lymphoid irradiation. *J Exp Med* 156:522–538, 1982.
29. Weigensberg M, Morecki S, Weiss L, Fuks Z, Slavin S: Suppression of cell-mediated immune responses after total lymphoid irradiation (TLI). *J Immunol* 132:971–978, 1984.
30. Waer M, Ang KK, Van Der Schueren E, Vandeputte M: Influence of radiation field and fractionation schedule of total lymphoid irradiation (TLI) on the induction of suppressor cells and stable chimerism after bone marrow transplantation in mice. *J Immunol* 132:985–990, 1984.
31. Waer M, Ang KK, Van Der Schueren E, Vandeputte M: Allogeneic bone marrow transplantation in mice after total lymphoid irradiation: Influence of breeding conditions and strain of recipient mice. *J Immunol* 132:991–996, 1984.
32. Ascher NL, Sullivan W, Simmons RL: An alternative hypothesis for the basis of chimerism in mice receiving total lymphoid irradiation and bone marrow transplantation. *Surg Forum* 31:366–368, 1980.
33. Kersey JH, Kruger J, Sone C, Kloster G: Prolonged bone marrow and skin allograft survival after pretransplant conditioning with cyclophosphamide and total lymphoid irradiation. *Transplantation* 29:388–391, 1980.
34. Mullen Y, Gottrib M, Shibukawa RL: Reversal of diabetes in rats by foetal pancreas allografts following TLI. *Transpl Proc* 15 (1), 1983.
35. Slavin S, Gottlieb M, Strober S, Bieber C, Hoppe R, Kaplan HS, Grumet FC: Transplantation of bone marrow in outbred dogs without graft-versus-host disease using total lymphoid irradiation. *Transplantation* 27:139–142, 1979.
36. Gottlieb M, Strober S, Hoppe RT, Grumet FC, Kaplan HS: Engraftment of allogeneic bone marrow without graft-versus-host disease in mongrel dogs using total lymphoid irradiation. *Transplantation* 29:487–491, 1980.
37. Koretz SH, Gottlieb MS, Strober S, Pennock J, Bieber CP, Hoppe RT, Reitz BA, Kaplan HS: Organ transplantation in mongrel dogs using total lymphoid irradiation. *Transpl Proc* 13:443, 1981.

38. Lewis WI, Aeder MI, Sutherland DER, Kim TH, Najarian JS: Effect of pre- versus posttransplant total lymphoid irradiation in combination with azathioprine and antithymocyte globulin immunosuppression in a canine renal allogaft model. *Surg Forum* 34:393–395, 1983.
39. Raff J, Bryan M, Marsden M, Bray A, Kim JH, Chu F, Chaganti RSK, Shaw KB, Cohan A, Fortner JG: Bone marrow and renal transplantation in canine recipients prepared by total lymphoid irradiation. *Transpl Proc* 13:429, 1981.
40. Rynasiewicz JJ, Sutherland DER, Ferguson RM, Squifflet JP, Morrow CE, Goetz FC, Najarian JS: Cyclosporin A for immunosuppression: Observations in rat heart, pancreas and islet allograft models and in human renal and pancreas transplantation. *Diabetes* 31:92–107, 1982.
41. Sadeghi AM, Downing TP, Bieber CP, Reitz BA, Stinson EB, Shumway NE,: Heterotopic cardiac allograft in rats: Prolonged survival with low-dose preoperative and postoperative total lymphoid irradiation combined with low-dose cyclosporine. *Heart Transpl* 2:209–211, 1983.
42. Pennock JL, Reitz BA, Bieber CP, Aziz S, Oyer PE, Strober S, Hoppe R, Kaplan HS, Stinson EB, Shumway NE: Survival of primates following orthotopic cardiac transplantation treated with total lymphoid irradiation and chemical immune suppression. *Transplantation* 32:467–473, 1981.
43. Sutherland DER, Ferguson RM, Aeder MI, Lewis WI, Bentley FR, Ascher NL, Simmons RL, Najarian JS: Total lymphoid irradiation and cyclosporine. *Transpl Proc* 15:2881–2886, 1984.
44. Bieber CP, Jamieson S, Raney A, Burton N, Bogarty S, Hoppe R, Kaplan HS, Strober S, Stinson EB: Cardiac allograft survival in Rhesus primates treated with combined total lymphoid irradiation and rabbit antithymocyte globulin. *Transplantation* 28:347–350, 1979.
45. Bieber CP, Jamieson SW, Raney A, Burton NA, Bogarty S, Hoppe R, Kaplan HS, Strober S, Stinson EB: Cardiac allograft survival in Rhesus primates treated with total lymphoid irradiation and rabbit antithymocyte globulin. *Surg Forum* 30:284–286, 1979.
46. Pennock JL, Strober S, Reitz BA, Hoppe R, Koretz S, Bieber CP, Kaplan HS, Stinson EB, Shumway NE: Cardiac allograft survival in dogs treated with total lymphoid irradiation and chemical immune suppression. *Surg Forum* 32:362–364, 1981.
47. Strober S, Modry DL, Hoppe RT, Pennock JL, Bieber CP, Holm BI, Jamieson SW, Stinson EB, Schroder J, Suomalainen H, Kaplan HS: Induction of specific unresponsiveness to heart allografts in mongrel dogs treated with total lymphoid irradiation and antithymocyte globulin. *J Immunol* 132:1013–1018, 1984.
48. Lewis WI, Sutherland DER, Najarian JS: Total lymphoid irradiation and azathioprine combined in the canine renal allograft model. *Surg Forum* 32:365–367, 1981.
49. Howard RJ, Sutherland DER, Lum CT, Lewis WI, Kim TH, Slavin S, Najarian JS: Kidney allograft survival in dogs treated with total lymphoid irradiation. *Ann Surg* 193:196–200, 1981.
50. Myburgh JA, Smit JA, Hill RRH, Browde S: Transplantation tolerance in primates following total lymphoid irradiation and allogeneic bone marrow injection. II. Renal allografts. *Transplantation* 29:405–408, 1980.
51. Myburgh JA, Smit JA, Browde S, Hill RRH: Transplantation tolerance in primates following total lymphoid irradiation and allogeneic bone marrow injection. I. Orthotopic liver allografts. *Transplantation* 29:401–404, 1980.
52. Smit JA, Hill RRH, Myburgh JA, Browde S: Transplantation tolerance in primates after total lymphoid irradiation and allogeneic bone marrow injection. III. Lymphocyte responsiveness and suppressor cell activity. *Transplantation* 30:107–110, 1980.
53. Myburgh JA, Smit JA, Browde S, Stark JH: Current status of total lymphoid irradiation. *Transpl Proc* 15 (1): 654–667, 1983.
54. Myburgh JA, Smit JA, Stark JH, Browde S: Total lymphoid irradiation on kidney and liver transplantation in the baboon: Prolonged graft survival and alterations in T cell subsets with low cumulative dose regimens. *J Immunol* 132:1019–1025, 1984.

55. Bentley FR, Sutherland DER, Najarian JS: Treatment of rat heart allograft recipients with postoperative total lymphoid irradiation (TLI). *J Surg Res* 32:360–363, 1982.
56. Bentley FR, Sutherland DER, Rynasiewicz JJ, Najarian JS: Synergistic effect of posttransplant total lymphoid irradiation and pharmacologic immunosuppression with low-dose anti-lymphocyte globulin or cyclosporine on prolongation of rat heart allograft survival. *Transpl Proc* 15:671, 1983.
57. Strober S, Hoppe RT, Levin B, Miller E, Girinsky T, Modry D, Sampson D: Immunological changes during the reduction and elimination of immunosuppressive drugs in human cadaver allograft recipients prepared with TLI. *Transpl Proc* 17, 1985, in press.
58. Sampson D, Levin BS, Hoppe RT, Bieber CP, Modry D, Girinski T, Kaplan HS, and Strober S: Total lymphoid irradiation abrogates cadaver graft rejection. Transpl Proc 17, 1985, in press.
59. Waer M, Vanrenterghem Y, Ang KK, Van Der Schueren E, Michielsen P, Vandeputte M: Comparison of the immunosuppressive effect of fractionated total lymphoid irradiation (TLI) vs. conventional immunosuppression (CI) in renal cadaveric allotransplantation. *J Immunol* 132:1041–1048, 1984.
60. Michielsen P, Vanrenterghem Y, Waer M, van der Schueren E, Gruwez J, Bouillon R, Vandeputte M: The use of pretransplant fractionated total lymphoid irradiation (TLI) in diabetic cadaveric kidney allograft recipients. *Transpl Proc* 17, 1985, in press.
61. Cortesini R, Renna Molajoni E, Monari C, Famulari A, Berloco P, Capua A, Marinucci G, Alfani D: Total lymphoid irradiation in clinical transplantation: Experience in 28 high risk patients. *Transpl Proc* 17, 1985, in press.
62. Bentley FR, Sutherland DER, Fryd DS, Kaufman D, Ascher NL, Simmons RL, Najarian JS: Renal allograft survival rates are similar for kidneys from sibling donors matched for zero versus one haplotype with the recipient. *Transplantation*, 1984, in press.
63. Gifford RM, Sutherland DER, Fryd DS, Simmons RL, Najarian JS: Duration of first renal allograft survival as indicator second allograft outcome. *Surgery* 88:611–618, 1980.
64. Hanto DW, Sakamoto K, Purtilo DT, Simmons RL, Najarian JS: The Epstein-Barr virus in the pathogenesis of posttransplant lymphoproliferative disorders: Clinical, pathologic and virologic correlation. *Surgery* 90:204–13, 1981.
65. Sutherland DER, Morrow CE, Fryd DS, Ferguson RM, Simmons RL, Najarian JS: Improved patient and primary renal allograft survival in uremic diabetic recipients. *Transplantation* 34:319–325, 1982.
66. Sutherland DER, Strand M, Fryd DS, Ferguson RM, Simmons RL, Ascher NL, Najarian JS: Comparison of Azathioprine–Antilymphocyte globulin versus cyclosporine in renal transplantation. *Am J Kidney Dis* 3:456–461, 1984.
67. Najarian JS, Fryd DS, Strand M, Canafax DM, Ascher NL, Payne WD, Simmons RL, Sutherland DER: A single institution randomized prospective trial of cyclosporine versus azathioprine–antilymphocyte globulin for immunosuppression in renal allograft recipients. *Ann Surg*, in press.
68. Strober S: Overview: Effect of total lymphoid irradiation of autoimmune disease and transplantation immunity. *J Immunol* 132:968–970, 1984.

50

Cyclosporin A as an Immunosuppressive Agent in Transplantation

R. Y. Calne

Cyclosporin A (CyA) is an immunosuppressive agent that has exciting major interest because of its potential. Borel discovered its *in vitro* and *in vivo* immunosuppressive properties in a screening program of fungal products. CyA is a cyclic peptide of 11 amino acids. CyA is highly soluble in alcohol and fat solvents but it is totally insoluble in aqueous solutions. Borel's[(1)] demonstration of prolongation of skin graft survival between mice differing for the H2 locus led David White, in my department, to suggest investigation of CyA in an organ allograft model. Our initial studies[(2)] showed that the agent prolongs survival of heterotopic hearts in rats across an AGB incompatability barrier.

The mechanism of action of CyA is not fully understood, but it appears to affect T cells at an early stage in their transformation. A subpopulation of T cells appears to be particularly susceptible to the drug.[(3)]CyA is relatively nontoxic to the bone marrow.

We also found that CyA prolongs survival of kidney grafts from unrelated donors in bilaterally nephrectomized mongrel dogs.(4) Rejection was effectively inhibited in animals. When 25 mg/kg per day are given, the median survival of 67 days was reached compared with 27 days for control animals treated with azathioprine, 5 mg/kg per day. Forty percent of the dogs developed jaundice and histologic changes consisting of focal necrosis and cholestasis of the liver; 35% became infected, the lungs being the usual site, and 25% died of rejection.

CyA has an even more powerful immunosuppressive effect in pigs receiving orthotopic heart grafts.[(5)] Donor and recipients were mismatched

R. Y. Calne • Department of Surgery, School of Medicine, Cambridge University, Cambridge CB2 2QQ, England.

for the MHC. Control animals received no immunosuppressive treatment and died of rejection with a median survival of 6 days. Although the animals treated with azathioprine and methylprednisone did not have improved survival rates, rejection was less prominent; infection was the usual cause of death.

Eight pigs were given 25 mg/kg per day of CyA, the dosage being reduced by approximately 50% every month. Three animals died of rejection on days 22, 43, and 72, respectively. In the remaining animals CyA was stopped between 125 and 197 days. The median survival of the eight pigs was in excess of 200 days. There were no obvious side effects and the animals appeared to thrive and grow rapidly. After CyA treatment was stopped, rejection occurred slowly in three pigs. Of the remaining two, one was killed 1 year later with no evidence of rejection in the heart graft. The other animal is still alive, more than a year after CyA treatment was stopped.

Green and Allison[6] investigated CyA in rabbits with kidney grafts and found that the drug produced long-term survivors after only 4 weeks of treatment. The CyA was dissolved in olive oil and given by mouth at a dose of 25 mg/kg per day. Green and Allison postulated that CyA might be causing a selective decloning of lymphocytes that had responded to the kidney grafts.

Similar profound prolongation was reported by Dunn *et al.*[7] using the same dose of CyA but administered by intramuscular injection in olive oil. The drug was stopped between 1 month and 55 days after grafting. In six rabbits the first kidney grafts were removed and second kidneys, from the same or third-party donors, were grafted. Untreated rabbits with grafted kidneys died from uremia with a median survival of 10.3 ± 1.4 days. Rabbits given CyA survived between 42 and 92 days. The rabbits that had their grafts removed between the thirty-ninth and sixty-fourth days when renal function was normal showed no rejection, and the second kidneys were not rejected. An unexpected finding was that the original donor and third-party kidneys did equally well. Biopsy of one of the third-party kidneys showed sustantial mononuclear cell infiltration after 1 week, but this had disappeared by the third week when another biopsy sample was taken. The kidney supported life for 70 days.

This nonspecific production of immunosuppression was difficult to explain. It is possible that the drug had remained as a depot in body fat, in cell membranes, or within cells. Alternatively, nonspecific T-cell impairment had resulted which permitted establishment of the new kidney.

In a small number of experiments in the Rhesus monkey, we found that CyA prolonged survival of kidney allografts (unpublished observations). Jamieson *et al.*[8] reported prolonged survival of heterotopic cardiac allografts in cynomolgus monkeys treated with CyA. We have also studied pancreatic allografts in the dog and have found that CyA prolonged survival nearly as well as kidney allografts in dogs.[9]

Thus, extensive animal studies performed in most of the common laboratory species with a variety of different organ grafts, all pointed to the powerful and relatively nontoxic immunosuppressive effects of CyA. We felt that these results were sufficiently encouraging to proceed to a pilot trial of the drug in clinical practice. Two reports have been published, the most recent data in November 1979.[10,11](Table 1).

Thirty-four patients received organs from cadaver donors, 32 were given kidneys, and two received orthotopic liver transplants. All these patients had previously received blood transfusions. Thirty-one of the renal allografts were first transplants; the remaining one was a second graft. A patient with diabetic nephropathy also received a pancreas allograft from the kidney donor. The body and tail of the pancreas was transplanted into the right iliac fossa using the technique of Dubernard *et al.*,[12]the duct having been injected with latex. One of the liver recipients also had juvenile-onset diabetes and received a heterotopic pancreas from the kidney donor. All recipients and donors were mismatched for HL-A A and B antigens. In most cases there were two or more mismatches. The DR matching of these cases is not yet available.

The dosage of CyA given varied from 25 mg/kg per day in seven patients to 10 mg/kg per day in six, but 21 patients received 17 mg/kg per day as a starting dose.[11] Twenty-six renal allografts are sustaining life, three now more than a year after grafting, and both pancreases and livers are also functioning. Twenty patients are off steroids, and of these 15 have never received additional immunosuppressive agents. There was only one acute rejection crisis evidenced by a swollen kidney, general malaise, and a high fever. Other rejection epsodes have presented as impairment of renal function. No kidney has been lost due to rejection.

1. *Nephrotoxicity*

An unexpected side effect of CyA encountered in clinical practice was nephrotoxicity, sometimes severe enough to produce complete anuria. The toxic effects were aggravated by poor initial function of the graft, although the brain death donors had intact circulations. Primary anuria had not been expected, yet there were six cases of primary nonfunction and nine of secondary anuria. There was insufficient histologic damage to explain the anuria in nine of the kidneys. Four patients had substantial rejection. Because the patients who had been deliberately hydrated and given mannitol all had good initial function, we decided to make this treatment part of our standard policy. Since then, 19 patients managed in this way have had primary diuresis. Three of them developed secondary anuria, with histologic evidence of severe rejection which responded to steroid treatment. The remaining 16 patients have functioning grafts with no need for additional steroids, and 11 have never received additional immunosuppressive agents.

2. *Infections and Malignancy*

In our original group of 16 patients who required only CyA there were two self-limiting viral infections, one by herpes simplex, and one by combined

Table 1. Details of Studies of Transplant Patients Treated with Cyclosporin A[a]

Case no.	Age, sex	Date of transplant, no. of HLA-B mismatches	Starting dose of CyA	Present dose of CyA	Other drugs	Outcome and present function
1	37 M	6/26/78 2	25	—	No	Transplant nephrectomy day 28, pyelonephritis in graft, on dialysis
2	30 F	7/1/78 3	25	12	No	Discharged day 22, 6/28/79, urea 8.9, creatinine 119
3	21 M	7/1/78 4	25	12.5	CM	Vascular rejection day 7, recovered function, discharged day 53, 9/6/79, urea 13.3, creatinine 287
4	27 M	7/14/78 3	25	—	CM Pred	CMV and varicella, died at 12/11 of sepsis, lymphoma found in jejunum
5	22 F	7/14/78 2	25	—	CM Pred	Marrow aplasia and septicemia, died after 139 days
6	46 M	8/4/78 2	25	—	CM Pred	Septicemia, died after 55 days
7	52 M	8/4/78 2	25	3	CM Pred	No initial function, 1 liter day 24, function improved with falling dose of CyA, CM stopped at 1 year, prednisolone now 5 mg, biopsy at 12/13: focal scarring and hypertensive changes, at 12/13, urea 21.8, creatinine 418
8	46 M	11/11/78 2	10	5	No	Good function, biopsy at 12/11: focal scarring and hypertensive changes, at 12/11, urea 18.7, creatinine 359
9	44 F	12/5/78 3	10	5	Pred	Oliguric day 0, diuresed day 9, 8/30/79, urea 29.9, creatinine 490, prednisolone now 15 mg
10	29 M	1/25/79 2	10	—	CM Pred	Diuresed day 1, oliguric day 4, good function till death at 12/8 from pneumocystis pneumonia
11	64 F	1/26/79 2	10	7	Pred	Diuresed day 1 then oliguria, good function, 8/30/79, urea 13.8, creatinine 135, prednisolone now 5 mg
12	54 M	2/28/79 2	17	—	Pred	Diuresed day 14, died at 12/4 septicemia and pneumonitis, lymphoma found in lungs

13	36 M	3/7/79 2	17	17	No	Diuresed day 1, good function, 9/13/79, urea 10.6, creatinine 256
14	57 F	3/19/79 1	17	—	CM Pred	Anuric, no function at any time, died day 75 septicemia and pulmonitis, candidiasis
15	59 M	4/23/79 2	17	12	Pred	Anuric, diuresed day 10, good function, 9/13/79, urea 10.9, creatinine 136
16	50 M	5/4/79 2	17	1.6	No	Diuresed day 16, good function, 9/19/79, lymphoma resected from 1st part of duodenum and lesser curve of stomach, urea 6.5, creatinine 141
17	31 M	5/4/79 1	17	12.5	Pred cover for asthma for 2/52	Diuresed day 1, good function, 9/6/79, urea 19.3, creatinine 255
18	39 F	5/19/79 1	17	15	No	Diuresed day 1, good function, 9/27/79, urea 6.9, creatinine 122
19	66 M	5/19/79 1	17	8.5	No	Diuresed day 1, good function, 9/13/79, urea 18.2, creatinine 163
20	12 F	5/30/79	17	10	No	Diuresed day 1, good function, 9/20/79, urea 6.8, creatinine 102
21	37 F	7/10/79 2	17	7	No	Diuresed day 1, good function, 9/13/79, urea 9.9, creatinine 181
22	52 M	7/10/79 2	17	6	SM 3 × 1 g	Diuresed day 1, good function, 9/21/79, urea 23.9, creatinine 280
23	59 F	8/2/79 2	17	5	SM 5 × 1 g	Diuresed day 1, biopsy day 42: moderate cellular rejection, 9/12/79, urea 14.7, creatinine 182, improving
24	50 M	8/2/79 2	17	5	Pred	Diuresed day 1, biopsy day 36: moderate cellular rejection, prednisolone now reduced to 25 mg, urea 19.5, creatinine 227, improving
25	17 F	8/5/79 2	17	14	Pred	Diuresed day 1, biopsy day 18: severe cellular rejection, prednisolone now reduced to 20 mg, urea 21, creatinine 329, improving
26	25 M	8/5/79 3	17	12.5	Pred	Diuresed day 1, biopsy day 21: severe cellular rejection, prednisolone now reduced to 15 mg, urea 10.4, creatinine 225

(Continued)

Table 1. *(Continued)*

Case no.	Age, sex	Date of transplant, no. of HLA-B mismatches	Starting dose of CyA	Present dose of CyA	Other drugs	Outcome and present function
27	55 F	8/18/79 + pancreas 4	17	13	No	Diuresed day 1, good function, urea 7.5, creatinine 97, glucose 5.4
28	29 M	9/4/79 2	17	15	SM 4 × 1 g	Diuresed day 1, biopsy day 13: moderate cellular rejection, function now: urea 54.4, creatinine 664, improving
29	50 F	9/10/79 (liver) Not done	10	8	No	Good function
30	68 M	9/17/79 2	17	17	No	Diuresed day 1, function now: urea 18.1, creatinine 287, improving
31	49 M	9/18/79	17	15	No	Diuresed day 1, function now: urea 26.8, creatinine 285, improving
32	25 M	10/3/79 (liver + pancreas) Not done	10	10	No	Good function
33	62 M	10/3/79 3	17	17	No	Diuresed day 1
34	44 F	10/3/79 3	17	17	No	Diuresed day 1

[a] CM, Cytimun; Pred, prednisolone; SM, Solu-medrone. (Reprinted from ref. 11, by kind permission of the editor of *Lancet*.)

herpes zoster and herpes simplex. CyA administration was stopped when another patient developed cytomegalovirus infection; steroids and Cytimun (a cyclophosphamide derivative) were used. One allograft developed a bacterial infection after biopsies and was removed. Another patient developed weight loss and anemia 4 months after grafting. A mucosal lymphoma in both the stomach and duodenum was found at endoscopy, and a partial gastrectomy was performed, with removal of the first part of the duodenum with the stomach. The lymph nodes were not involved in the growth, and the patient is back at work, and free from symptoms, on a greatly reduced dose of CyA (100 mg/day). Five of the six patients given steroids and Cytinum died of sepsis; a jejunal lymphoma was found in one of these patients. Of 11 patients given additional steroids, one died of sepsis and was found to have small lymphomatous deposits scattered throughout the lungs and liver.

Peroxidase staining of the three lymphomas suggested that they were all of B-cell origin, and the patient who had a gastroduodenal resection had developed a high titer of antibodies against the Epstein–Barr virus.

3. Other Side Effects

Most of the patients who received CyA developed liver function abnormalites, with raised blood level of bilirubin and alkaline phosphatase. About 50% had small rises in their serum transaminase levels. The two recipients of the liver grafts also had mild derangements of liver function, but in most patients function tended to return to normal as the dose of CyA was reduced. An increase in facial and arm hair occurred in most patients, and those with their own teeth developed temporary hypertrophy of the gums. Tremor, although usually mild and tending to resolve, was common in the early postoperative phase.

4. Renal Function

None of the 26 patients with life-supporting grafts has normal renal function. The lowest serum creatinine level is 97 mmoles/liter and urea 4.1 mmoles/liter. The patients who received additional steroids tend to have the least renal function, possibly because they have evidence of rejection. The highest serum creatinine is 470 mmoles/liter and urea 31 mmoles/liter. We have seen improved renal function following reduction of the CyA dosage. Most patients alive more than 6 months after transplantation are receiving between 10 and 12 mg/kg per day of CyA; one patient, who had the gastroduodenal resection, is being treated with 1.6 mg/kg per day.

Rejection occurred in two grafts when the dose of CyA was reduced.

5. Conclusions

Even after prolonged and careful assessment of a new drug in animals, its effectiveness in patients cannot be predicted, and there may be dangerous side effects. Our first clinical experience with CyA indicates these dangers. The most serious side effects were nephrotoxicity and lymphoma development. We know little of the pharmacodynamics of CyA, and the available radioimmunoassay is not reliable, so it has been impossible to correlate administered dose with serum levels. Because the agent is probably excreted to a large extent in the bile, changes in liver function could be critical in relation to blood levels attained of this fat-soluble compound. The optimum dose of CyA is not yet established, but it appears that 17 mg/kg per day is a compromise starting dose. The dosage is slowly reduced after the first 3 weeks, but whether it is necessary to continue the drug indefinitely is not yet known. In most animal species grafts were eventually rejected after cessation of CyA treatment, but as Green and Allison[(6)] showed in rabbits, the species differences are marked in this drug.

Powles *et al.*[(13)] have used CyA in the treatment of graft-versus-host disease in patients with bone marrow grafts. Initially they found rapid recurrence of cutaneous graft-versus-host disease after withdrawal of CyA treatment. If the treatment is continued for some months, the drug can, in most patients, be eventually stopped without recrudescence of the disease. The mechanism of action is not known, but CyA is a new type of agent which has a partially selective immunosuppressive action. The nephrotoxicity of CyA is unexplained. It appears to be rapidly reversible. In the acute stage it is not associated with morphologic changes in light or electron microscopy, and it appears that serious nephrotoxicity can be avoided if the patient is deliberately hydrated and given diuretics.

Our new policy is to withhold the first dose of CyA until it is clear at 6 hr after renal transplantation that the graft is functioning. Should the kidney not diurese, the patient is given conventional treatment with azathioprine and steroids. If secondary anuria occurs, we perform a renal biopsy, and if there is evidence of rejection, a course of steroids is given for a short period of time. If rejection continues, we will remove the graft or stop the CyA and change to azathioprine steroids. In six of our patients there was histologic evidence of deterioration of renal function, associated with rejection. These patients all responded well to additional steroid therapy. In three of the patients the steroids were stopped without recurrence of rejection.

Two patients received additional drugs to treat infections, but both died of sepsis, and lymphomas were found at postmortem. From this experience we feel that, if possible, CyA should be used alone, and the only additional drug that we are prepared to give is steroids. One other patient developed lymphoma but received no additional drugs. This patient is still alive. All three patients who developed lymphomas had impaired renal function in the early stages after transplantation. Malignant lymphoma is a well-known complication of conventional immunosuppressive regimens. In recipients of heart grafts for cardiomyopathy, the incidence is 18%. These patients were treated with high doses of azathioprine, steroids, and antithymocyte globulin.

CyA is an extremely powerful immunosuppressive drug and is the most effective agent yet used in patients receiving cadaveric renal allografts. It can be totally steroid sparing and therefore avoid both the cushingoid side effects, which can be distressing to patients, and the danger of joint destruction.

Consistently effective and safe immunosuppression is an elusive goal but so also have been attempts to produce donor-specific immunosuppression. It is probable that in the immediate future nonspecific pharmacologic agents that are highly selective against immune-reacting cells will still be required in clinical organ grafting. CyA is of interest because it is chemically different from any other previously described drug. Our clinical trial will continue with frequent review of patients so that side effects will be recognized as early as possible.

References

1. Borel JF: Comparative study of in vitro and in vivo drug effects on cell-mediated cytotoxicity. *Immunology* 31:631–641, 1976.
2. Kostakis AJ, White DJG, Calne RY: Prolongation of the rat heart allograft survival by cyclosporin A. *IRCS Med Sci* 5:280, 1977.
3. Gordon MY, Singer JW: Selective effects of cyclosporin A on colony-forming lymphoid and myeloid cells in man. *Nature* 279:433–434, 1979.
4. Calne RY, White DJG: Cyclosporin A—a powerful immunosuppressant in dogs with renal allografts. *IRCS Med Sci* 5:595, 1977.
5. Calne RY, White DJG, Rolles K, Smith DP, Herbertson BM: Prolonged survival of pig orthotopic heart grafts treated with cyclosporin A. *Lancet* 1:1183–1185, 1978.
6. Green CJ, Allison AC: Extensive prolongation of rabbit kidney allograft survival after short-term cyclosporin A treatment. *Lancet* 1:1182–1183, 1978.
7. Dunn DC, White DJG, Wade J: Survival of first and second kidney allografts after withdrawal of cyclosporin A therapy. *IRCS Med Sci* 6:464, 1978.
8. Jamieson SW, Burton NA, Bieber CP, Reitz BA, Oyer BE, Stinson EB, Shumway NE: Cardiac allograft survival in primates treated with cyclosporin A. *Lancet* 1:545, 1979.
9. McMaster P, Procyshyn A, Calne RY, Valdes R, Rolles K, Smith D: Prolongation of canine pancreas allografts with cyclosporin A (a preliminary report). *Transplant Proc* 12:275–277, 1980.
10. Calne RY, White DJG, Thiru S, Evans DB, McMaster P, Dunn DC, Craddock GN, Pentlow BD, Rolles K: Cyclosporin A in patients receiving renal allografts from cadaver donors. *Lancet* 2:1323–1327, 1978.
11. Calne RY, Rolles K, White DJG, *et al.*: Cyclosporin A initially as the only immunosuppressant in 34 recipients of cadaveric organs: 32 kidneys, 2 pancreases and 2 livers. *Lancet* 1:1033–1036, 1979.
12. Dubernard JM, Traeger J, Meyra P, Touraine HL, Tranchant D, Blanc-Brunat A: A new method of preparation of segmental pancreatic grafts for transplantation trials in dogs and in man. *Surgery* 84:633–639, 1978.
13. Powles RL, Barrett AJ, Clink H, Kay HEM, Sloan J, McElwain TJ: Cyclosporin A for the treatment of graft-versus-host disease in man. *Lancet* 2:1327–1331, 1978.

51

The Pretreatment Principle in Renal Transplantation as Illustrated by Thoracic Duct Drainage

Thomas E. Starzl, Richard Weil, III, and Lawrence J. Koep

In spite of all that has been achieved, renal transplantation still provides a flawed and unpredictable service. In the average American center in the decade of the seventies, less than half the recipients of first cadaver kidneys had graft function by the end of the first postoperative year. One reason may be neglect of what has been called the "forgotten pretreatment principle." It is that subject which is addressed here, with particular emphasis on thoracic duct drainage (TDD).

1. *Early Clues*

In 25 of our first kidney recipients, Wilson and Kirkpatrick[31] used preoperative skin testing and typhoid vaccination to assess cellular and humoral immune reactivity. Immunosuppressive therapy for those patients was with azathioprine to which prednisone was added only if rejection developed.[19,20] After transplantation, the patients previously classified as nonresponders had a mean rejection time of 14.8 days, compared to 4.3

Thomas E. Starzl • Department of Surgery, School of Medicine, University of Pittsburgh Health Sciences Center, Oakland Veterans Administration Medical Center, Pittsburgh, Pennsylvania 15213. ***Richard Weil, III*** • Department of Surgery, School of Medicine, University of Colorado, Denver, Colorado 80262. ***Lawrence J. Koep*** • Phoenix, Arizona 85006. This work was supported by research grants from the Veterans Administration, by Grants AM-17260 and AM-07772 from the National Institutes of Health, and by Grants RR-00051 and RR-00069 from the General Clinical Research Centers Program of the Division of Research Resources, National Institutes of Health.

days in the responders. These findings were not influenced by donor relationship. Wilson and Kirkpatrick concluded that

> These observations support the concept that impaired immunologic responsiveness in uremia is an important factor in successful human kidney transplantation. Furthermore, the difference in rejection times between the responsive and unresponsive groups suggests that the reactive group might benefit from additional immunosuppressive therapy prior to [transplantation]. . . .

Almost a decade later, the prognostic implication of the reactor-versus-nonreactor state of kidney recipients was reemphasized by the antibody studies of Opelz, Mickey, and Terasaki.[16] More recently, Jones *et al.*,[8] Thomas *et al.*,[27] and Opelz and Terasaki[15] came to the same conclusion from the results of *in vitro* phytohemagglutin, concanavalin A, and mixed-lymphocyte culture (MLC) tests all of which are expressions of T-lymphocyte reactivity. The MLC studies[15] were particularly illuminating. The MLC index using third-party lymphocytes was almost as predictive of the outcome after cadaveric kidney transplantation as when the stimulator cells were provided by the actual donor.

Although well known, the foregoing information has had surprisingly little influence on treatment practices. In the early days of our program almost all human kidney recipients were given azathioprine for 8–10 days before transplantation. The practice was based on analogous canine experiments in which average homograft survival was doubled thereby over that obtained when the drug was started on the day of operation.[19] Gradual abandonment of the policy of preoperative treatment of our patients with azathioprine, and often steroids may have been a systematic error inasmuch as other immunosuppressive adjuncts to condition the recipients were not being substituted. As cadaveric transplantation became more common, practical reasons made pretreatment difficult. The waiting period for a cadaver kidney was unpredictable, during which time extra infectious risks were introduced by giving azathioprine with or without prednisone. Furthermore, there were no accepted guidelines about the appropriate duration of such pretreatment. Worldwide, transplantation centers drifted into the practice of starting therapy on the day of grafting.

2. TDD and the Pretreatment Principle

The immunosuppressive procedure of TDD has provided an unusually analyzable example of the pretreatment principle and of the loss of much of the value of this procedure if its timing is wrong. TDD was given a trial in several centers 5–15 years ago[1–6,11–13,17,18,28,29] but was never accepted as a major therapeutic tool. This was because the scientific framework for its use in humans had not been worked out.

3. Contemporaneous TDD

Eighteen months ago we began a systematic trial with TDD in renal transplantation, starting the lymphoid depletion on the day of grafting along

Table 1. Rejection in First 2 Months of Cadaver Kidneys: Influence of TDD[a]

	Percent rejection		
	Contemporaneous TDD (17)[b]	3 Weeks pretreatment with TDD (13)	≥4 Weeks pretreatment with TDD (14)
Incidence rejection	41%	38%	7%
Irreversible rejection	24%	8%	0%
Deaths	0	1	2

[a] In 50 immediately precedent cadaveric recipients treated with azathioprine, prednisone, and sometimes ALG, the incidence of early rejection was 48%.[(22)]
[b] Data from ref. 22.

with azathioprine, prednisone, and sometimes antilymphocyte globulin (ALG).[(22,23)] The protocol was similar to that usually used by Franksson *et al.*[(5)] The results were somewhat better than in historical controls without TDD, but vigorous rejection was often encountered during the first month (Table 1). The most striking clinical observation was that if the TDD was continued, a second graft could often be performed after failure of the first.[(23)] It was obvious that TDD was being inappropriately used for the primary transplant. Data in these patients plus precise immunologic studies by Machleder and Paulus[(10)] in nontransplantation patients established that a pronounced immunodepressive influence of TDD was not established until about 3 weeks and that this effect deepened for another week or so. Kidneys in our early TDD series were being rejected during this uncovered 3 or 4 weeks and, in addition, "antibody storms" in the postoperative period were often seen[(23)] with a heavy representation of the so-called warm anti-T and anti-B cytotoxic antibodies of the IgG class.[(26)]

4. *Pretreatment with TDD*

To correct the flaw in therapeutic strategy,[(23)] a new series was begun using TDD in advance of cadaveric renal transplantation,[(24)] adding azathioprine and prednisone on the day of operation. This time, the presence of preexisting recipient antibodies was taken into consideration. These antibodies recently were characterized on the basis of their reactivity against homologous T and B lymphocytes at warm (IgG class) and cold (IgM) temperatures.[(26)] It has been accepted that warm anti-T antibodies cause hyperacute rejection,[(26)] but the significance of the other antibody varieties has remained controversial. Whatever their meaning, the cytotoxic antibodies could be construed as an index of the patients' immune reactivity, both by their presence before and by their development after transplantation. In the new treatment scheme, patients with no (or only cold) antibodies were scheduled for 3 weeks' preparation with TDD. Those possessing warm antibodies were scheduled for 35 days. If anti-T antibodies persisted and

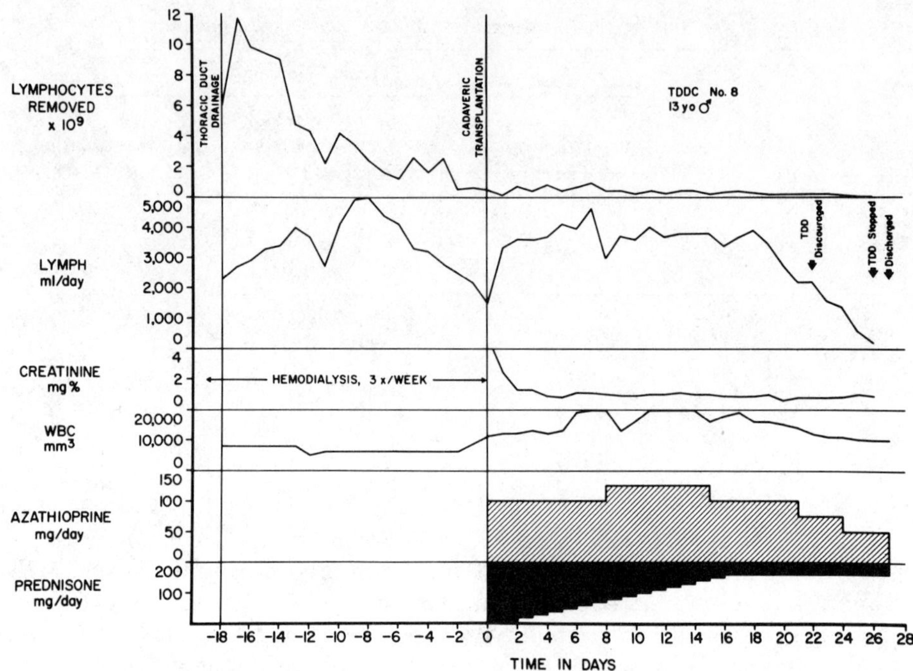

Figure 1. Example of short pretreatment with TDD. Although the patient had a perfect result, it is now known that the conditioning period was too brief. The drop in lymphocytes removed during the pretransplantation period was invariably observed. This finding was in contrast to our experience with TDD started on the day of transplantation in which the number of lymphocytes removed remained high. (The postoperative retention of TDD for about 3 weeks is still our policy.) The patient has had no evidence of late rejection.

reacted against the potential donors, it was shown earlier[(23)] that a low titer was necessary before proceeding in the face of a positive cross match. After 35 days, acceptance of cadaver donors whose positive cross matches were due to other kinds of antibodies was recommended.

The recipients in this new series represented a modern-day cross section of risk factors. Many of the patients were old with known coronary artery disease, three were diabetics, and three were undergoing retransplantation. Because the donor selection was random except for red-cell-group compatibility, the HLA and DR matches were all poor.[(24)] The results from the studies permitted precise conclusions about TDD pretreatment.

4.1. Pretreatment of 3 Weeks

Thirteen consecutive cadaver recipients of whom only one had preexisting warm anti-B antibodies had preoperative TDD for 17–28 days. The therapeutic approach is illustrated in Fig. 1. During the pretreatment period, the numbers of collected lymphocytes always fell markedly. After transplantation, the TDD was maintained for at least 3 more weeks.

Table 2. Broadly Reacting[a] Warm Anti-B Lymphocyte Antibodies 2 Weeks after Transplantation

TDD pretreatment for 3 weeks	7/13
TDD pretreatment ≥4 weeks	1/14

[a] Broadly reacting means reactivity against half or more of a 30-donor lymphocyte panel.

During follow-ups of 2–6 months, five of these patients (38%) had rejection, which in four instances was reversible (Table 1). The fifth patient was treated with prompt retransplantation. These patients retained a potent capacity for cytotoxic antibody production. Two weeks after transplantation 11 of the 13 had developed warm anti-B antibodies against a panel of 30 lymphocyte donors, and in seven cases the antibodies reacted against more than half the panel (Table 2). All five of the rejections were in these latter seven antibody-producing recipients. One patient died 1 month after transplantation from acute pancreatitis.

4.2. Pretreatment for 4 Weeks or Longer

Fourteen consecutive cadaveric recipients, of whom four had preexisting warm antibodies, had the longer pretreatment of 26–58 days. After 2–6 months only one (7%) patient had a rejection (Table 1) and that one was so minor as to be equivocal. At the same time, the capacity to generate all categories of cytotoxic antibodies was remarkably reduced. Even though 4 of the 14 recipients already had warm antibodies predating TDD, these tended to diminish during pretreatment, and only 1 of the 14 possessed broad reacting warm antibodies 2 weeks posttransplantation (Table 2).

Two patients died, one from a virus infection after 7 weeks, and the other at 2 months from a massive lidocaine overdosage given inadvertently by her family physician.

5. Long-Term Implications

In these patients, it remains to be seen if a delayed immunologic rebound will cause major kidney losses after discontinuance of TDD. However, Walker,[30] Johnson,[7] and Niblack[14] and their associates have not seen a catch-up deterioration of grafts in patients followed 2–5 years after preoperative and postoperative TDD. Late stability after earlier TDD was also reported recently by Kaplan.[9] It seems likely that the poorly understood change in host–graft relationship that has made clinical transplantation practical will be expedited rather than hindered by properly timed TDD. If so, improvements in early graft survival should be translated into better long-term results.

6. *Broader Implications*

If the pretreatment principle delineated by the foregoing experience is valid, it will influence other developments and practices in transplantation.

6.1. *Other Therapeutic Regimens*

It would be surprising if host conditioning, equivalent to that of chronic TDD, could not be achieved with other means over a period of several weeks. An obvious possibility is mechanical removal of lymphocytes from the peripheral blood (lymphapheresis), a procedure for which commercial instrumentation is already available. We have treated two liver recipients and one kidney recipient in this way. The procedures of total lymphoid irradiation[25] and thymectomy are variations on the same theme. So would be pretransplantation conditioning with powerful antilymphocyte sera and globulins, an approach that has been made impractical in patients by immune reactions to the heterologous protein.[21] It is clear that a sufficiently long conditioning period will be required.

Today, for the first time in years, there is the real prospect of better drugs for core immunosuppression, of which cyclosporin A is the most promising, as Calne has reported. (cf. Chapter 50, this volume). The potential value of pretreating with cyclosporin (or other drugs) or alternatively of combining drugs with preoperative lymphoid depletion is obvious. With any such conditioning effort, the use of the battery of *in vitro* immunologic tests now available should permit the curves of preoperative immunodepression to be quantitated for individual patients.

We have in fact treated four patients with cyclosporin for 24–42 days following TDD. The convalescence of these patients has been remarkably uncomplicated. Within 1 or 2 days after transplantation, maneuvers were begun to discontinue the TDD. No steroids or azathioprine were given. It will be interesting to see if cyclosporin itself can be substituted for TDD in the pretreatment period.

6.2. *Patient Selection and Histocompatibility*

In the past, renal recipients (particularly those needing cadaveric organs) always have been ruled by the donors, with the final decision about candidacy hinging mainly on the conventional negative cytotoxic cross match and, in most centers, to a lesser extent on HLA matching. With effective pretreatment by TDD, it has been possible to give weight to the recipient's wishes. Based on the antibody state, a rational decision has been possible about the duration of pretreatment and about the prospects for success without any consideration of tissue match. Once the TDD is instituted, the patient has been assured of transplantation and at a fairly predictable time. The ability to offer transplantation to cadaveric kidney recipients as an elective and planned undertaking has drastically changed our program. The numbers of consanguineous transplants have dwindled to less than 10% of the total as the prospective recipients have perceived the improved cadaveric situation. The number of cases that can be handled by our fixed-bed unit has substantially increased (60 in the last 7 months), in spite of the time investment for pretreatment which is more than canceled by the ability to discharge patients earlier after a homograft has been placed.

6.3. Other Organs

Improvements in immunosuppression should be applicable for other organs including the liver and heart. The direct application of these findings in liver recipients may pose special problems. Lymph drainage in patients with hepatic disease tends to be voluminous, particularly if ascites is present. Recently, we were forced to perform a liver transplant after only 18 days of TDD because the amount of lymph obtained per day had reached 25 liters, a volume so great that fluid management was becoming difficult. It may be that many of the liver recipients can have safer lymphoid depletion by lymphapheresis or by other kinds of preoperative conditioning discussed earlier. Certainly, pretreatment will be a major factor in patient care as our liver transplant program reopens.

7. Summary

Pretreatment with TDD markedly influences early graft survival and virtually eliminates early rejection, provided that the lymphoid depletion is for at least 4 weeks. Such preoperative recipient conditioning has improved the quality of patient service. It is probable that the pretreatment principle can be applied effectively while using other immunosuppressive measures including drugs.

References

1. Archimbaud, J. P., Banssillan, V. G., Berhardt, J. P., Revillard, J. P., Perrin, J., Traeger, J., Carraz, M., Fries, D., Saubier, E. C., Bonnet, P., Brochier, J., and Zech, P., 1960, Technique, surveillance et interet de drainage du canal theracique, effectue en vue d'une transplantation renale, *J. Chir.* **98:**211.
2. Fish, J. C., Sarles, H. E., Tyson, K. R. T., Remmers, A. R., and Ritzmann, S. E., 1969, The immunologic consequences of lymph lymphocyte depletion, *Surg. Forum* **20:**268.
3. Franksson, C., 1964, Survival of homografts of skin in rats depleted of lymphocytes by chronic drainage from the thoracic duct, *Lancet* **1:**1331 (letter to editor).
4. Franksson, C., and Blomstrand, R., 1967, Drainage of the thoracic lymph duct during homologous kidney transplantation in man, *Scand. J. Urol. Nephrol.* **1:**128.
5. Franksson, C., Lundgren, C., Magnusson, E., and Ringden, O., 1976, Drainage of thoracic duct lymph in renal transplant patients, *Transplantation* **21:**133.
6. Ianhez, L. E., Verginelli, G., Sabbaga, E., and Campos Frere, J. G., 1974, Thoracic duct drainage in human kidney allotransplantation, *Rev. Bras. de Pesquisas Med. Biol.* **7:**265.

7. Johnson, H. K., Niblack, G. D., Tallent, M. B., and Richie, R. E., 1977, Immunologic preparation for cadaver renal transplant by thoracic duct drainage, *Transpl. Proc.* **9:**1499.
8. Jones, A. R., Vaughan, R. W., Bewick, M., and Batchelor, J. R., 1976, Transformation of lymphocytes from patients awaiting cadaver renal transplants, *Lancet* **2:**529.
9. Kaplan, M. P., 1979, Thoracic duct drainage—an overview, *Dial. Transpl.* **8:**781.
10. Machleder, H. I., and Paulus, H., 1978, Clinical and immunological alterations observed in patients undergoing long-term thoracic duct drainage, *Surgery* **84:**157.
11. Martelli, A., and Ronomini, V., 1970, Thoracic duct fistula in human kidney transplantation, in: *Pharmacological Treatment in Organ and Tissue Transplantation* (A. Bertelli and A. P. Monaco, eds.), p. 140, Williams & Wilkins, Baltimore.
12. Murray, J. E., Wilson, R. E., Tilney, N. L., Merrill, J. P., Cooper, W. C., Birtch, A. G., Carpenter, C. B., Hager, E. B., Dammin, G. J., and Harrison, J. H., 1968, Five years' experience in renal transplantation with immunosuppressive drugs: Survival, function, complications, and the role of lymphocyte depletion by thoracic duct fistula, *Ann. Surg.* **168:**416.
13. Newton, W. T., 1955, The biologic basis of tissue transplantation, *Surg. Clin. North Am.* **45:**393.
14. Niblack, G. D., Johnson, H. K., Richie, R. E., Gonzalez, L., Locke, J., and Jackson, D., 1975, Preformed cytotoxic antibody in patients subjected to thoracic duct drainage, *Proc. Dial. Transpl. Forum* **5:**146.
15. Opelz, G., and Terasaki, P. I., 1977, Significance of mixed leukocyte culture testing in cadaver kidney transplantation, *Transplantation* **23:**375.
16. Opelz, G., Mickey, M. R., and Terasaki, P. I., 1972, Identification of unresponsive kidney-transplant recipients, *Lancet* **1:**868.
17. Sarles, H. E., Remmers, A. R., Jr., Fish, J. C., Canales, C. O., Thomas, F. D., Tyson, K. R. T., Beathard, G. A., and Ritzman, S. E., 1970, Depletion of lymphocytes for the protection of renal allografts, *Arch. Intern. Med.* **125:**443.
18. Sonoda, T., Takaha, M., and Kusunoki, T., 1966, Prolonged thoracic duct lymph drainage: Application for human homotransplantation, *Arch. Surg.* **93:**831.
19. Starzl, T. E., 1964, *Experience in Renal Transplantation*, pp. 131–138, Saunders, Philadelphia,
20. Starzl, T. E., Marchioro, T. L., and Waddell, W. R., 1963, The reversal of rejection in human renal homografts with subsequent development of homograft tolerance, *Surg. Gynecol. Obstet.* **117:**335.
21. Starzl, T. E., Porter, K. A., Iwasaki, Y., Marchioro, T. L., and Kashiwagi, N., 1967, The use of antilymphocyte globulin in human renal homotransplantation, in: *Antilymphocytic Serum* (G. E. W. Wolstenholme and M. O'Connor, eds.), pp. 4–34, Churchill, London.
22. Starzl, T. E., Koep, L. J., Weil, R., III, Halgrimson, C. G., and Franks, J. J., 1979a, Thoracic duct drainage in organ transplantation; will it permit better immunosuppression? *Transpl. Proc.* **11:**276.
23. Starzl, T. E., Weil, R., III, Koep, L. J. McCalmon, R. T., Jr., Terasaki, P. I., Iwaki, Y., Schroter, G. P. J., Franks, J. J., Subryan, V., and Halgrimson, C. G., 1979b, Thoracic duct fistula and renal transplantation, *Ann. Surg.* **190:**474.
24. Starzl, T. E., Weil, R., III, Koep, L. J., Iwaki, Y., Terasaki, P. I., and Schroter, G. P. J., 1979c, Thoracic duct drainage before and after cadaveric kidney transplantation, *Surg. Gynecol. Obstet.* **149:**815.
25. Strober, S., Slavin, S., Fuks, Z., Kaplan, H. S., Gottlieb, M., Bieber, C., Hoppe, R. T., and Grumet, F. C., 1979, Transplantation tolerance after total lymphoid irradiation, *Transpl. Proc.* **11:**1032.
26. Terasaki, P. I., Bernoco, D., Park, M. S., Ozturk, G., and Iwaki, Y., 1978, Microdroplet testing for HLA-A, -B, -C and -D antigens, *Am. J. Clin. Pathol.* **69:**108.
27. Thomas, F., Mendez–Picon, G., Thomas, J., and Lee, H. M., 1977, Quantitation of pretransplantation immune responsiveness by *in vitro* T-cell testing, *Transpl. Proc.* **9:**49.
28. Tilney, H. L., Atkinson, J. C., and Murray, J. E., 1970, The immunosuppressive effect of thoracic duct drainage in human kidney transplantation, *Ann. Intern. Med.* **72:**59.

29. Traeger, J., Touraine, J.–L., Archimbaud, J.–P., Malik, M.–C., and Dubernard, J.–M., 1978, Thoracic duct drainage and antilymphocyte globulin for renal transplantation in man, *Kidney Int.* **13**(suppl. 8):103.
30. Walker, W. E., Niblack, G. D., Richie, R. E., Johnson, H. K., and Tallent, M. B., 1977, Use of thoracic duct drainage in human renal transplantation, *Surg. Forum* **28:**316.
31. Wilson, W. E. C., and Kirkpatrick, C. H., 1964, Immunologic aspects of renal homotransplantation, in: *Experience in Renal Transplantation* (T. E. Starzl, ed.), pp. 239–245, Saunders, Philadelphia.

52

Thoracic Duct Drainage

Clinical Experience

Robert E. Richie, Gary Niblack, H. K. Johnson, and M. B. Tallent

Allograft rejection continues to be the major obstacle to obtaining a successful graft in spite of significant strides having been made in the areas of histocompatibility, organ preservation, and immunosuppression. At the Veterans Administration Medical Center and the Vanderbilt University Medical Center in Nashville, we have used thoracic duct drainage (TDD) as a means of immunologically preparing a select group of patients for transplantation. This report presents our clinical experience with this therapeutic modality during the past 10 years.

1. Historical Note

Gowans *et al.*[1] in 1962 showed that the primary immune response to sheep erythrocytes and tetanus toxoid in rats was impared by creating a thoracic duct fistula. Woodruff and Anderson[2] obtained prolongation of skin graft survival in rats with the use of antilymphocyte serum and TDD. In 1964, Franksson[3] reported the use of this modality in a renal transplant recipient.

Subsequently TDD was used in Boston[4] and Galveston,[5] and both transplantation groups concluded that there was definitely a benefit from its use, particularly when cadaver kidneys were used. Despite these favorable reports, there has not been widespread acceptance of this technique, possibly because of difficulty in establishing a fistula, lack of patient acceptance of long-term hospitalization, or difficulty in maintaining a fistula for a long period of time.

Robert E. Richie, Gary Niblack, H. K. Johnson, and M. B. Tallent • Transplantation Section, Surgery Service, Veterans Administration Hospital, and Department of Surgery, Vanderbilt University Medical Center, Nashville, Tennessee 37232.

Recently the group from Denver[6] has reported their experience with TDD in kidney recipients and concluded that it should be used as a pretreatment of all cases either with or without prior antibodies.

2. *Method and Materials*

Between August 1970 and December 1979, 81 patients at the Veterans Administration Medical Center and the Vanderbilt University Medical Center elected to receive TDD as immunologic preparation prior to receiving a renal transplant. This modality was offered to patients who were not doing well on dialysis, to patients who had previously rejected one or more cadaver grafts, and to patients who had been on dialysis for an extended period of time and had not received a transplant. Many of the patients selected were in the high-risk group, i.e., increased age, high percent reactive antibody to a defined lymphocyte panel (PRA), or known responders to histocompatibility antigens. The average length of time on dialysis was between 21 and 22 months. After admission to the hospital, all patients were started on a high-lipid diet. This consisted of 1 ounce of a mixture of one-half whipping cream and one-half water every 3 hr for the first 25 hr prior to operation. This was continued until 5 hr prior to the operation.

The cannulation of the thoracic duct was carried out under general anesthesia. A transverse superclavicular incision was made in the left side of the neck. Initially a rigid Teflon tip was inserted into the duct, and this was connected to a double-lumen silastic catheter which permitted infusion of heparin solution to prevent clotting of the lymph. More recently, the double-lumen Swan–Ganz catheter as advocated by the Denver group[7] has been used. The lymph was collected in sterile 600-ml blood transfer packs and stored in the refrigerator. The lymph was collected daily, centrifuged to remove the lymphocytes, cultured, frozen, and subsequently thawed and reinfused in order to maintain protein oncotic pressure and prevent protein depletion. The amount of lymph removed varied from 17 to 600 liters with an average of approximately 150 liters. As many as 100 billion lymphocytes may be removed. During the postdrainage period, immunologic activity was monitored by histoplasmin, *Candida*, and purified protein derivative (PPD) skin tests. Absolute lymphocyte counts were determined by the differential count, and T-lymphocyte levels were determined weekly by the number of cells forming spontaneous rosettes with sheep erythrocytes. In addition, serial cell-mediated lympholysis assays and serial mixed-lymphocyte cultures were done. When the patient was felt to be immunologically depressed, he received the first ABO compatible kidney with a negative cross match that became available, regardless of the HLA match. After the transplant, the drainage was continued for up to 2 weeks unless the duct clotted prior to that time. The period of drainage ranged from 2 weeks to a maximum of 6 months with the average being 6 weeks. After transplantation, the patients received the standard immunosuppression according to our routine protocol consisting of prednisone, 60 mg/day, and azathioprine, 100 mg/day. Rejection episodes were treated with infusions of 500 mg of Solu-medrol and graft irradiation. Only six patients have received antithymocyte serum.

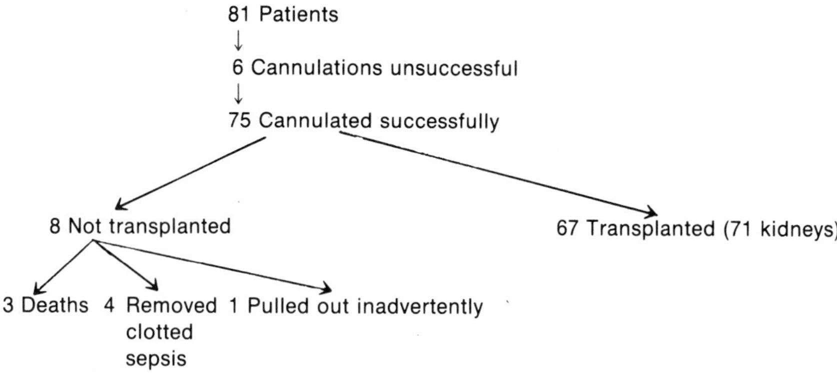

Figure 1. TDD patients, August 1970–December 1979.

3. Results

Eighty-one patients elected to undergo thoracic duct drainage (Fig. 1). In six instances the duct was not successfully cannulated. Seventy-five patients had successful cannulation of the thoracic duct. Eight patients were excluded from the study group: three died while undergoing drainage in preparation for a transplant, and their deaths were unrelated to the drainage procedure; in four patients, the drainage was terminated because of clotting or sepsis; and in another patient, the cannula was pulled out inadvertently during a dressing change and recannulation was not successful.

The remaining 67 patients received 71 transplants (Fig. 2). Only three received kidneys from living related donors. Forty-five were primary transplants and 22 were retransplants. There were eight deaths within 30 days of the transplant, with a resultant mortality rate of 12%. Twenty-one grafts were rejected during the 9-year period. Of this group, six patients received a second transplant and four are alive with a functioning graft. Fifteen patients were returned to dialysis, of whom ten are still alive. Ten patients

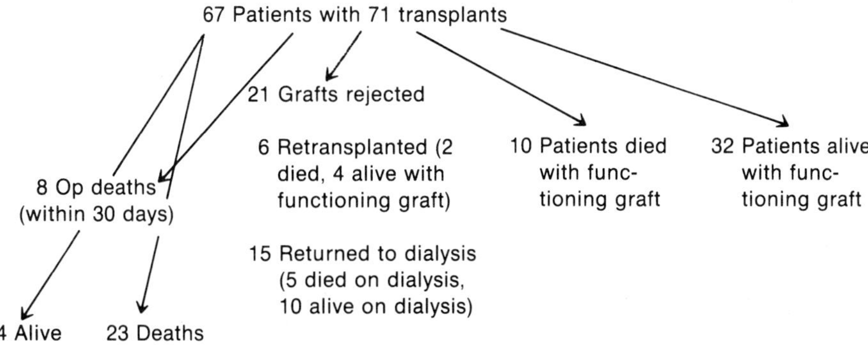

Figure 2. TDD in patients who received transplants, August 1970–December 1979.

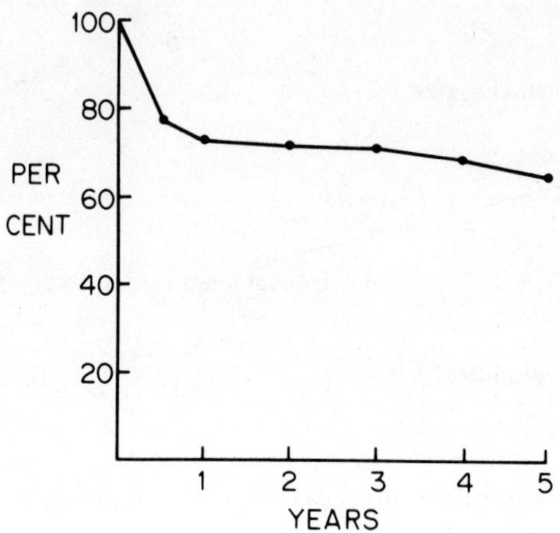

Figure 3. Actuarial graft survival of TDD patients who received renal allografts.

died with a functioning graft at intervals from 2 months to 7 years. Thirty-two patients are alive with a functioning graft at intervals of 2 months to 7 years.

Actuarial graft survival is 73% at 1 year and 71% at 3 years (Fig. 3 and 4). Patient survival is 79% at 1 year and 77% at 3 years. Of the patients included in these computations, all have been at risk for a least 1 year, and half for more than 3 years.

4. *Mortality*

During the 10-year period 23 of our 67 patients died. The eight deaths that occurred within 30 days of transplant were classified as operative deaths (Table 1). Four patients died of sepsis and one each of pancreatitis, cardiac

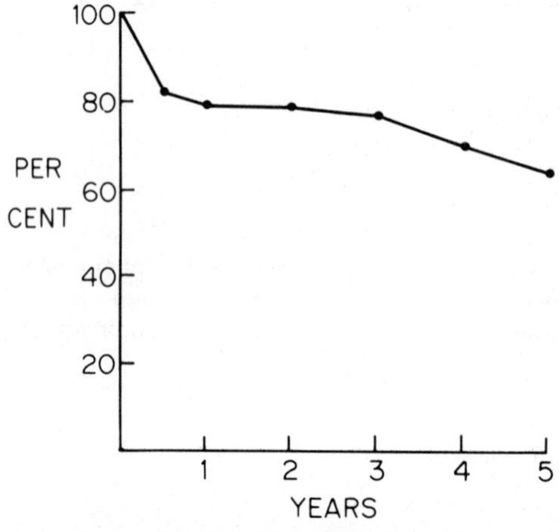

Figure 4. Actuarial patient survival of TDD patients who received renal allografts.

Table 1. TDD Patients Who Died in Postoperative Period after Transplant or after Return to Dialysis after Rejection of Transplant

Deaths in postoperative period	
Sepsis	4
Pancreatitis	1
Chronic active hepatitis with liver failure	1
Cardiac arrhythmia	1
Infarction of bowel	1
Total	8
Died on dialysis after rejection of kidney (2 months to 5 years)	5

arrhythmia, infarction of the bowel, and liver failure from chronic active hepatitis. Of those patients who rejected their kidney and had to be returned to dialysis, five died at intervals of 2 months to 5 years. Two of these deaths were felt to be related to the transplant and three were unrelated to the procedure.

Ten patients died with a functioning graft (Table 2). Myocardial infarction was the cause of death in two instances, at 7 years and 4 years post transplant, respectively. Complications of pancreatitis accounted for two deaths at 2 and 4 months, respectively. One patient succumbed to viral encephalitis at 3 years. Another patient refused to seek medical advice when he became ill and was admitted to his local hospital in a moribund condition. He subsequently died and an autopsy revealed crytococcal meningitis. One patient had an eye enucleation at 4 years after which he developed a *Pseudomonas* pneumonia which ultimately resulted in his death. Of two patients who died of sepsis at 6 months, one was a diabetic, and the other death occurred at 7 years of unknown causes.

5. Discussion

Our interest in this procedure initially stemmed from the clinical trials reported by the Boston and Galveston groups. It has been the philosophy

Table 2. TDD Patients Who Died with a Functioning Allograft

Died with functioning graft	
Myocardial infarction	2 (7 years and 4 years)
Pancreatitis	2 (2 months and 4 months)
Viral encephalitis	1 (3 years)
Cryptococcal meningitis	1 (4 years)
Complications of diabetes (pneumonia and sepsis)	1 (6 months)
Pneumonia, and *Pseudomonas*	1 (4 years)
Sepsis	1 (6 months)
Unknown	1 (7 years)
Total	10

of our program to try to utilize better HLA-matched kidneys; however, there is a group of patients in whom this is not possible. It is with this group of patients that we began to utilize TDD. Initially the logistical problem of handling the lymph was significant, as were establishing and maintaining the fistula for long periods of time. With experience and improvement in technique, however, these problems have been overcome.

With the use of immunologic parameters to monitor these patients, we have found that the drainage period may vary up to a month or 6 weeks, although lack of availability of kidneys has resulted in longer periods of drainage in some instances.

A major problem in transplantation is the highly sensitized patient. This may become more of a problem as increasing data show improved transplant results with preoperative blood transfusion. Nine of the patients who have received TDD in preparation for transplant received a kidney with a positive cross match. Seven of the nine had a successful transplant without a hyperacute rejection. Four of these seven have had long-term graft survival. Our understanding of the mechanisms involved is lacking, and we feel further investigation in this area is warranted.

TDD is an effective means of immunosuppression. Although the overall mortality may seem high, we believe that the operative mortality is acceptable in this group, many of whom are high-risk patients. We believe this procedure should continue to be offered to patients on a selected basis, and that further clinical trials are indicated.

References

1. Gowans JL, McGregor DD, Cowen DM: Initiation of immune responses by small lymphocytes. *Nature* 196:651, 1962.
2. Woodruff MFA, Anderson NA: Effect of lymphocyte depletion by thoracic duct fistula and administration of anti-lymphocytic serum on the survival of skin homografts in Rats. *Nature* 200:702, 1963.
3. Franksson C: Survival of homografts of skin in rats depleted of lymphocytes by chronic drainage from the thoracic duct. *Lancet* 1:1331, 1964.
4. Murray JE, Wilson RE, Tilney NL, Merrill JP, Cooper WC, Birth AG, Carpenter CB, Hager EB, Dammin GJ, Harrison JH: Five years' experience in renal transplantation with immunosuppressive drugs: Survival, function, complications, and the role of lymphocyte depletion by thoracic duct fistula. *Ann Surg* 168:416, 1968.
5. Fish JC, Sarles HE, Remmers AR, Tyson KRT, Canales CO, Beathard GA, Fukushima M, Ritzmann SE, Levin WC: Circulating lymphocyte depletion in preparation for renal allotransplantation. *Surg Gyn Obstet* 128:777, 1969.
6. Starzl TE, Weil R, Koep LJ, McCalmon RT, Terasaki PI, Iwaki Y, Schroter GPJ, Franks JJ, Subryan V, Halgrimson CG: Thoracic duct fistula and renal transplantation. *Ann Surg* 190:474, 1979.
7. Starzl TE, Koep LJ, Weil III, R, Halgrimson CG, Franks JJ: Thoracic duct drainage in organ transplantation: Will it permit better immunosuppression?, *Transplant Proc* 11:276, 1979.

53

Current Status of Induction of Specific Unresponsiveness to Organ Allografts

Anthony P. Monaco

Few, if any, purposeful attempts have been made to induce specific unresponsiveness to organ allografts in man. Nevertheless, there is an enormous experimental literature to show that attempts to induce unresponsiveness of some type in man are a reasonable undertaking. It is the purpose of this chapter to identify the principles and problems in the induction of unresponsiveness to allografts. No attempt will be made to review the enormous literature of this subject. Rather, experimental models developed and studied by our own group will be described to illustrate how clinical attempts for unresponsiveness induction could be undertaken.

In the early 1950s Medawar and colleagues[1] reported the induction of *actively acquired immunologic tolerance* to tissue allografts in mice. They showed that immunologically incompetent neonatal mice could be injected *in utero* or intravenously in the neonatal period with lymphoid cells from another inbred strain and that such mice, as adults, were specifically tolerant to skin grafts of the donor strain. Donor strain grafts survived indefinitely whereas third-party grafts were specifically rejected. Tolerant mice were lymphoid cell chimeras of both recipient and donor strains; second donor skin grafts were also tolerated indefinitely. Donor strain grafts could only be rejected when tolerant mice were "reequipped" with normal syngeneic lymphoid cells or syngeneic cells previously sensitized against the donor strain. F_1 hybrid cells were required to induce tolerance between strongly histocompatible recipient–donor strains to avoid graft-versus-host reactions.

A less profound type of unresponsiveness was produced by Kaliss[2] which he termed *immunologic enhancement*. He found that tumor grafts from one strain of mouse ordinarily rejected by another strain would grow

---

Anthony P. Monaco • Cancer Research Institute, New England Deaconness Hospital, Boston, Massachusetts 02115.

indefinitely if the recipient had previously been injected with a lyophilized preparation of the tumor (active enhancement) or had been injected with serum from a mouse that had previously rejected the tumor graft (passive enhancement). In contrast to actively acquired tolerance, in which there is absence of recipient antidonor immunologic reactivity, a definite host antidonor response is present in enhancement systems.

Numerous examples of actively acquired tolerance or enhancement models exist, many showing characteristics of these early prototypes. In general, it is appropriate to speak of models of specific unresponsiveness rather than tolerance or enhancement. Monaco *et al.*[3] were the first to show that a model of specific unresponsiveness very similar to that of Medawar's actively acquired immunologic tolerance to skin allografts could be induced in adult mice using antilymphocyte serum (ALS) and donor antigen. Highly immunosuppressed, ALS-treated, adult-thymectomized A/He mice were injected with large doses of (C3H/HexA/He)F_1 hybrid lymphoid cells and grafted with C3H/He skin. Such mice were shown to be specifically tolerant to C3H/He grafts, since they easily accepted second C3H/He grafts, but rejected third-party C57Bl/6 grafts. These mice were lymphoid cell donor–recipient chimeras and only rejected C3H/He grafts after being reequipped with normal syngeneic A/He lymphoid cells or syngeneic cells previously sensitized to C3H/He tissues. In short, such mice had all the characteristics of the actively acquired tolerance defined by Medawar. These mice did not show *in vitro* recipient antidonor cytotoxicity or serologic blocking factors as studied by the Hellstroms' technique.[4] Also, administration of Cytoxan to adult-thymectomized, ALS-treated mice prior to F_1 hybrid lymphoid cell injection did not prevent the induction of unresponsiveness.[5] Furthermore, all donor strain grafts were perfectly normal on histologic examination.[6] The induction of specific unresponsiveness in adult-thymectomized, ALS-treated mice with F_1 hybrid cells was defined as the *chimera model.* From the standpoint of clinical application, F_1 hybrid cells would never be available. When large doses of homozygous donor strain lymphoid cells were used for the induction of unresponsiveness, vigorous and fatal graft-versus-host reactions resulted. Use of nonreplicating cells (liver, epidermal, renal) failed to produce unresponsiveness.[7] Likewise, cell-free antigen[8] was only minimally effective.

However, when ALS-treated, adult-thymectomized mice were injected with normal, homozygous donor bone marrow cells, excellent unresponsiveness was induced. ALS-treated, adult-thymectomized A/He mice injected with 25 X 10^6 C3H/He bone marrow cells showed extraordinary unresponsiveness to C3H/He grafts. Such grafts survived for 150–250 days and second donor strain grafts also survived for very long periods, but not indefinitely.[9] Such mice were *not* chimeras. Furthermore, in spite of the fact that donor grafts were tolerated for almost the life of the animal, recipient antidonor cell-mediated immunity could be detected by the *in vitro* cytotoxicity method. Serological blocking factors capable of inhibiting cell-mediated immunity were found to be present during the time grafts were well tolerated. In spite of the presence of cell-mediated immunity and serologic blocking factors, administration of Cytoxan, an antibody suppressant, prior to bone marrow administration in this model did not abrogate the induction of unresponsiveness. Long-surviving skin allografts in this model were not normal on histologic examination. Although visually perfect, mild cell infiltration consistent with low-grade allograft rejection was present. It is clear that the techniques involved in this model, *the adult thymectomy, ALS, bone marrow model*—ALS treatment, adult thymectomy, donor bone marrow infusion—are all potentially clinically applicable.

The effect of varying the several parameters used in the second model were studied in a third model in which adult thymectomy was omitted.[10,11] Nonthymectomized, ALS-treated A/He mice received ALS on days −1 and +2 relative to C3H/He skin grafting on day 0 and were infused with low doses of homozygous lymphoid cells on day +8. At all doses tested, bone marrow cells were superior to splenocytes, lymph node cells, and thymocytes in specifically prolonging grafts in marrow-infused mice over that achieved in mice given ALS alone. At higher doses, up to 100 × 10^6 cells/per 30-g mouse, splenocytes were almost as effective as bone marrow cells. In the case of bone marrow, progressively increasing the dose did not increase the degree of unresponsiveness induced, so that a dose of 25–50 × 10^6 cells/30-g mouse was optimal. Higher doses decreased the amount of unresponsiveness produced. With lymph node lymphocytes, high doses of cell (>100 × 10^6 cells/30-g mouse) actually induced sensitization, i.e., shortened graft survival relative to that achieved with just immunosuppression (ALS) alone. The unresponsiveness induced with bone marrow and ALS alone was of shorter duration than that produced in ALS-treated, thymectomized mice, but was specific. The timing of bone marrow administration was critical; bone marrow had to be administered within a week after ALS treatment was terminated. Bone marrow given during ALS treatment sensitized patients, but bone marrow given later (2 or 3 weeks after ALS) failed to have any effect. The intravenous route was not obligatory for unresponsiveness induction. Direct intrasplenic injection of bone marrow to ALS-treated recipients was very effective. Splenectomy up to 2 hr after direct bone marrow injection abrogated unresponsiveness induction, suggesting that intrasplenic injection did not constitute merely an intravenous injection. Although grafts were well tolerated, recipients showed a high degree of antidonor cell-mediated immunity with corresponding serologic blocking factors present during the time of unresponsiveness. In contrast to the first two models, Cytoxan given before bone marrow abrogated induction of unresponsiveness, presumably by destroying cells that could produce serologic blocking factors necessary to achieve unresponsiveness. Cytoxan given after bone marrow augmented unresponsiveness, probably by an additive immunosuppressive effect. When examined histologically, grossly well-tolerated grafts on unresponsive ALS-treated, marrow-injected mice showed significant cellular infiltration with collagen destruction consistent with a progressive allograft rejection reaction. Recently, Gozzo *et al.*[12] showed that whole bone marrow was not necessary for induction of unresponsiveness. Fractions of whole bone marrow produced by bovine serum albumin gradients containing exclusively small lymphocytes were equally as effective as whole marrow in producing specific unresponsiveness. Obviously, ALS and donor-specific bone marrow can be applied clinically. ALS-treated dogs given donor-specific bone marrow showed marked prolongation of canine renal allograft survival over that achieved with ALS alone.[13]

These models of unresponsiveness illustrate the principles that may be used and problems that may be encountered in attempts to produce specific unresponsiveness in clinical organ transplantation. The techniques of the first model, using ALS, adult thymectomy, and F_1 hybrid lymphoid cells, are not practical because F_1 hybrid cells will never be available. On the other hand, the induction of chimerism is clearly *not* a requirement for induction of unresponsiveness, and the attainment of complete actively acquired tolerance with a chimeric state in humans is probably not a practical consideration. Complete and total specific unresponsiveness in the recipient to all antigens by which a donor-recipient pair differs is probably unnecessary for practical application of specific unresponsiveness induction. Ample experimental evidence exists to show that induction of unresponsiveness to many, but not all, the differing histoincompatible antigens results in prolonged graft survival which may be maintained by lower or minimal doses of nonspecific immunosuppression. In this context, adult thymectomy, ALS, and bone marrow, or just ALS and bone marrow, are practical techniques that could be applied for the clinical induction of specific unresponsiveness in clinical human allografting. Since both the second (thymectomized) and third (nonthymectomized) models were experimentally feasible, one might want to omit adult thymectomy in the human or, perhaps, attempt thymic ablation by pretransplant irradiation. In the case of living related transplants, antilymphocyte globulin could be administered prior to grafting. Donor marrow could be harvested at the time of donor nephrectomy and administered shortly after transplantation. If bone marrow infusion is to be delayed for a week or 2, it could be preserved by standard techniques or harvested at this later time from the living donor. In the case of cadaveric transplantation, organs and bone marrow will be harvested simultaneously. Bone marrow could be administered with the graft or preserved for later administration. The dose of bone marrow to be used could be extrapolated from previous canine experiments. Indeed, ALS treatment and bone marrow infusion has been used in one case of cadaveric renal transplantation by my colleagues and me.[14] Preserved donor-specific cadaver bone marrow was infused in an ALS-treated cadaveric renal allograft recipient. The patient, who was highly sensitized, survived with perfect renal function, rejection free for 8 months only to succumb to perforative sigmoid diverticulitis. This case demonstrated that specific donor marrow could be preserved and infused in cadaveric recipients without untoward effects.

The time is at hand in clinical renal transplantation for carefully controlled trails of induction of specific unresponsiveness in kidney transplant recipients. The goal of such studies should not be induction of complete recipient antidonor nonreactivity, although this would be a welcome result. Rather, attempts to induce specific unresponsiveness should be evaluated not only in increased patient and graft survival, but also in decreased levels of nonspecific immunosuppressive agents required to maintain graft survival or, better still, the elimination of certain drugs (i.e., steroids) which have profoundly morbid side effects. These attempts should involve the use of total lymphoid irradiation (TLI) and bone marrow[15] and ALG (with or without thymic ablation) and donor bone marrow.

References

1. Billingham RD, Brent L, Medawar PB: Actively acquired tolerance of foreign cells. *Nature* 172:603, 1953.
2. Kaliss N: Dynamics of immunologic enhancement. *Transpl Proc* 2:59, 1970.
3. Monaco AP, Wood ML, Russell PS: Studies on heterologous antilymphocyte serum in mice. III. Immunologic tolerance and chimerism produced across the H-2 locus with adult thymectomy and antilymphocyte serum. *Ann NY Acad Sci* 129:190, 1966.
4. Hellstrom I, Hellstrom KE: microcytotoxicity assays of cell-mediated tumor immunity and blocking serum factor, in: Bloom BR, Glade PR (eds): *In Vitro Methods in Cell-Mediated Immunity*. New York, Academic Press, 1976, pp 533–539.
5. Wood ML, Monaco AP: Differential effect of cyclophosphamide on states of specific allograft unresponsiveness in immunosuppressed mice. *Transplantation* 27:186, 1979.
6. Wood ML, Monaco AP: Models of specific unresponsiveness to tissue allografts in antilymphocyte serum (ALS) treated mice. *Transpl Proc* 10:379, 1978.
7. Monaco AP, Wood ML, Lytle B, Barrett I: Studies on heterologous antilymphocyte serum in mice. VI Further studies on tolerance. *Colloques Internationaux CNRS* 190:361, 1971.
8. Monaco AP: Immunological tolerance and enhancement in experimental and clinical renal transplantation, Mexico 1972. Basel Karger, 1974, *5th International Congress Nephrology*, in: *Proceedings* vol. 1, pp 99–109.
9. Wood ML, Heppner G., Gozzo JJ, Monaco AP: Mechanisms of augmented graft survival in mice after ALS and bone marrow infusion. *Transpl Proc* 5:691, 1973.
10. Monaco AP, Gozzo JJ, Wood ML, Liegeois A: Use of low doses of homozygous allogeneic bone marrow cells to induce tolerance with antilymphocyte serum (ALS): Tolerance by intraorgan injection. *Transpl Proc* 3:680, 1971.
11. Wood ML, Monaco AP, Gozzo JJ, Liegeois A: Use of homozygous allogeneic bone marrow for induction of tolerance with antilymphocyte serum: Dose and timing. *Transpl Proc* 3:676, 1971.
12. Gozzo JJ, Litvin DA, Monaco AP, Bhatnager YM: Fractionated bone marrow: Use of a lymphocyte containing fraction for skin allograft prolongation in ALS treated mice. *Transpl Proc* 13:592, 1981.
13. Caridis DT, Liegeois A, Barrett I, Monaco AP: Enhanced survival of canine renal allografts of ALS-treated dogs given bone marrow. *Transpl Proc* 5:671, 1973.
14. Monaco AP, Clark AW, Wood ML, Sahyoun AI, Codish SD, Brown RW: Possible active enhancement of a human cadaver renal allograft with antilymphocyte serum (ALS) and donor bone marrow: Case report of an initial attempt. *Ann Surg* 79:384, 1976.
15. Strober S, Slavin S, Fuks Z, Kaplan HS, Gottlieb M. Bieber C, Hoppe RT, Grumet FC: Transplantation tolerance after total lymphoid irradiation. *Proc* 11:1032, 1979.

54

Immunogenetics of HLA

Fritz H. Bach

The major approaches used for detection of major histocompatibility complex (MHC)-encoded antigens involve serologic methods; there are serologically detected determinants that are recognized on essentially all cells of the body and others that have an apparently more restricted tissue distribution.[1-3] In addition, there are cellular methods, studying activation of T lymphocytes in mixed leukocyte culture (MLC), that can be used to define MHC-encoded determinants. Here, also, determinants can be divided into two categories including those that activate much of the proliferative response in a primary mixed-leukocyte culture in which the donors of the responding and stimulating cells differ by an entire MHC, and those that are recognized by cytotoxic T lymphocytes.[4]

There is substantial evidence to suggest that determinants recognized serologically and those recognized by T lymphocytes are not identical. Conceptually, thus, we must deal with two methods of detection: serologic and cellular, with two different "types" of antigens recognized by each of the methods. In order to have a uniform nomenclature that allows us to refer to these various types of determinants in any species, specific designations must be used (Table 1). The designations differentiate between the serologically defined antigens found ubiquitously on essentially all cell surfaces, as the *S* determinant (SD) antigens, and the serologically detected antigens with a much more limited tissue distribution encoded by HLA-D related genes *D* related (DR). The antigens detected by T-lymphocyte reactivities are referred to as *L* determinants (LD) and *C* determinants (CD) as listed.

Fritz H. Bach • Immunobiology Research Center and Departments of Laboratory Medicine/Pathology and Surgery, University of Minnesota Hospitals, Minneapolis, Minnesota 55455.
This work was supported by NIH Grants AI 08439, CA 09106, CA 16836, and AI 15588. This chapter was an outgrowth of a paper presented in conjunction with those on immunosuppressive therapy of kidney transplants and was submitted after the 1980 conference. This is paper No. 224 from the Immunobiology Research Center, University of Minnesota, Minneapolis, Minnesota 55455.

Table 1. HLA—Detection of Antigens

	Region(s)	
Method	ABC	D
Serologic	SD	Dr (Ia-like)
Cellular	CD	LD

1. *HLA—The Major Histocompatibility Complex in Man*

A schematic representation of the HLA complex is shown in Fig. 1. In man, as in mouse, serologic and cellular methods have been used for the definition of the various antigens and molecules encoded by HLA genes. The HLA-A, -B, and -C loci code for antigens that are present on essentially all cells of the body and that show sequence homology with the H-2K/D antigens. The HLA-D locus was first defined using cellular techniques, i.e., proliferation in a primary MLC. Thus, the antigens associated with HLA-D that can be detected by serologic methods have been referred to as the DR antigens. The DR antigens are thought to be homologues of the Ia antigens in mouse.

Table 2 shows the presently recognized antigens of HLA, as detected both by serologic methods and by the primary mixed-leukocyte culture response to homozygous typing cells (HTCs).[3] The HLA-A and -B loci are markedly polymorphic with a continuing finer definition of determinants that can be recognized by different sera. The HLA-C locus does not appear to be as polymorphic as HLA-A and -B.

The HLA-D locus is formally defined by response in a primary mixed-leukocyte culture to HTCs. The HTC technique[5] involves the use of stimulating cells that are homozygous for HLA-D antigen(s). The rationale behind HTC testing is that if a given individual does not carry the antigen(s) present on the HTC, then there should be a strong response by the cells of that one individual to that particular HTC. If, on the other hand, a second individual does carry the antigen(s) present on that HTC, then there should be a relatively weak, or absent, response by the cells of that second individual to the same HTC.

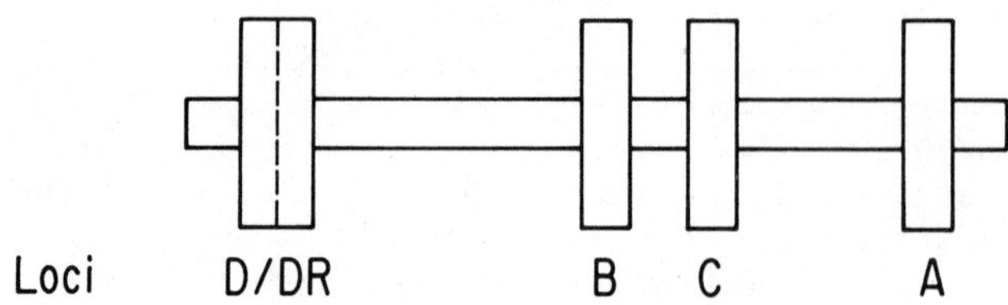

Figure 1. A schematic representation of the HLA complex.

Table 2. HLA-Encoded Antigens

W1	RW1	W4		W1	1	W19
W2	RW2	W6		W2	2	W23
W3	RW3			W3	3	W24
W4	RW4	5	W35	W4	9	W30
W5	RW5	7	W38	W5	10	W31
W6	RW6	8	W39	W6	11	W32
W7	RW7	12	W41		25	W33
W8		13	W42		26	W34
W9		14	W44		28	W36
W10		15	W45		29	W43
W11		17	W46			
		18	W47			
		27	W48			
		37	W49			
		40	W50			
		W16	W51			
		W21	W52			
		W22	W53			
			W54			

Although the results obtained with most HTCs, which are either genotypically or simply phenotypically homozygous for HLA-D, are not as "clean" as suggested by the prototype results given previously, it is possible to obtain useful information, and a number of different HLA-D antigens (or antigenic clusters) have been defined utilizing HTCs. These are listed as HLA-DW1 through DW11 in Table 2.

Seven different antigens that are associated with the HLA-D locus and have been recognized serologically are referred to as HLA-DRW1 through HLA-DRW7. A second series of HLA-DR antigens has been proposed that appears to be distinct from the series involving HLA-DRW1 through DRW7.

The relationship of the HLA-D to the HLA-DR antigens is not well elucidated. Whereas a given HLA-D antigen is most frequently found in a given population with a given HLA-DR antigen (for the sake of convenience, one refers, in most instances, to an individual having HLA-DW1 as also having HLA-DRW1), there is evidence to suggest that the determinants recognized by cellular response and serologically are different. This evidence is based both on a few putative recombinants within the HLA-D[3,6] region as well as the existence within Caucasians, and other populations, of associations between HLA-DR and HLA-D other than those most commonly found in the Caucasian population. Thus, for instance, in the Oriental population, the antigen HLA-DRW2 is frequently found with the D specificity referred to as DHO. Whereas this association is also found in the Caucasian population, the most common association in Caucasians with DRW2 is, again by convention, the DW2 specificity.

An additional method that has provided information about the HLA-D region has been primed LD typing (PLT).[7,8] This method uses "sensitization"

Table 3. PLT Response to HLA-D and -DR[a]

Sensitization MLC		Restimulation with:	
Responder	Stimulator	DRW2/DW2	DRW2/DHO
DRWX/DWX[b]	DRW2/DW2	++++	+++
DRWX/DWX	DRW2/DHO	+++	++++
DRW2/DHO	DRW2/DW2	+++	±
DRW2/DW2	DRW2/DHO	±	+++

[a] Adapted from ref. 9. Semiquantitative results obtained with PLT reagents sensitized either to both DRW2 and DW2 or DRW2 and DHO or presumably "only" to DW2 and DHO when the responding cell donor is DRW2 positive. The slightly greater restimulation response seen after sensitization to both DRW2 and either DW2 or DHO when the restimulating cell carries the sensitizing D antigen as well as DRW2 is difficult to establish with a high degree of confidence. However, the strong response to either DW2 or DHO when priming was done against the DW2 and DHO, respectively (when the responding cell donor was DRW2 positive), is clear.

[b] DRWX and DWX refer to any DR or D antigen other than DRW2 and DW2 or DHO.

of lymphocytes *in vitro* in a primary mixed-leukocyte culture in which donors of responding and stimulating cells differ by only a single HLA haplotype. The cells resulting 10 days following the initiation of the primary MLC are thought to represent "secondary-type" responding cells that will give a rapid proliferative response, measurable by 24 or 48 hr, to those antigens initially recognized by the responding cells on the stimulating cells during the sensitization phase. Although PLT reagents can respond to antigens other than those encoded by the HLA-D region, most of the responses are associated with HLA-D region encoded determinants.

PLT reagents can be prepared, each against a different HLA-D haplotype, and used to "define" primed LD (PL) antigens associated with HLA-D. A number of different PL antigens have been defined in this manner, most of which are highly associated with a given HLA-D antigenic cluster.

The PLT test can be used to detect both antigens associated with HLA-D and those associated with HLA-DR. This can be demonstrated by studying the situation in which DRW2 is associated with DHO in Orientals but primarily with DW2 in Caucasians. PLT reagents can be prepared against either the DRW2-DW2 or the DRW2-DHO complex and then tested for their responsiveness to each of these two types of stimulating cells. Under these conditions, there appears to be a clear response associated with DRW2. However the magnitude of the response is affected also by the presence of the priming D specificity on the restimulating cells. Further information regarding reactivity with D, or a factor associated with D, is obtained if priming is done against only DW2 or DHO, with respect to these determinants. Under these conditions the resulting PLT reagents react only with DW2 and not with DHO if primed to DW2 and vice versa.[9](Table 3).

A finer analysis of D-associated antigens is promised by the recent advent of cloning of PLT cells. Day 4 blasts are isolated from a regular MLC during the sensitization phase and then cloned in the presence of T-cell growth

Table 4. Proliferative Response of Noncloned PLT versus Limiting Dilution "Cloned" Alloactivated Cells

	Restimulating cells			
Responding cells	A_x	B_x	C_x	D_x
Original PLT	173	5,152	831	207
"Clones"[a]				
40-10E	543	6,000	536	375
40-7E	641	44,681	906	489
40-8E	576	3,842	2,313	710
40-4E	814	4,634	2,475	683
40-9D	881	999	993	742

[a] "Clones" were obtained from limiting dilution of day 4 MLC blast cells and were grown in Terasaki microtiter wells in the presence of feeder layers and TCGF. The cells were derived from wells that received on the average 40 cells/well at the time of dilution into Terasaki plates. 40-9D is an example of a clone giving no proliferative response.

factor (TCGF).[10] Under these conditions, presumed single precursor cells can be grown to large numbers. In many cases the resulting "monoclonal" PLT reagents give highly significant PLT-type responses providing a dissection of the D region hitherto unavailable with cellular reagents[11] (Table 4). The use of cloned PLT reagents must be considered at its inception, and thus much further analysis is needed to evaluate its practical usefulness.

2. *Cellular Response to MHC-Encoded Antigens*

Much of the interest relating to different "types" of antigens that are encoded by MHC genes is based on the differential response of helper T lymphocytes (T_h) and cytotoxic T lymphocytes (T_c) to antigens associated with different subregions of the MHC. The findings can be summarized[4] as follows: (1) HLA-D-region-encoded LD antigens are primarily responsible for activating the vast majority of the proliferating cells in a primary MLC where the donors of the responding and stimulating cells differ by the entire MHC. (2) The strongest cytotoxic responses are aimed at ABC-region-encoded CD antigens. (3) The combined presence of ABC region differences plus D-region-encoded difference on the stimulating cells results in the generation of a much stronger cytotoxic response than do ABC-region-encoded antigens alone. This phenomenon was referred to as LD–CD collaboration. The cellular counterpart to LD–CD collaboration is seen in the interaction of LD-responsive T_h and CD-responsive T_c. It is the combined response of T_h and T_c that leads to the strongest cytotoxic activity (Fig. 2). ABC region differences alone lead to cytotoxic responses in only some cases.[12]

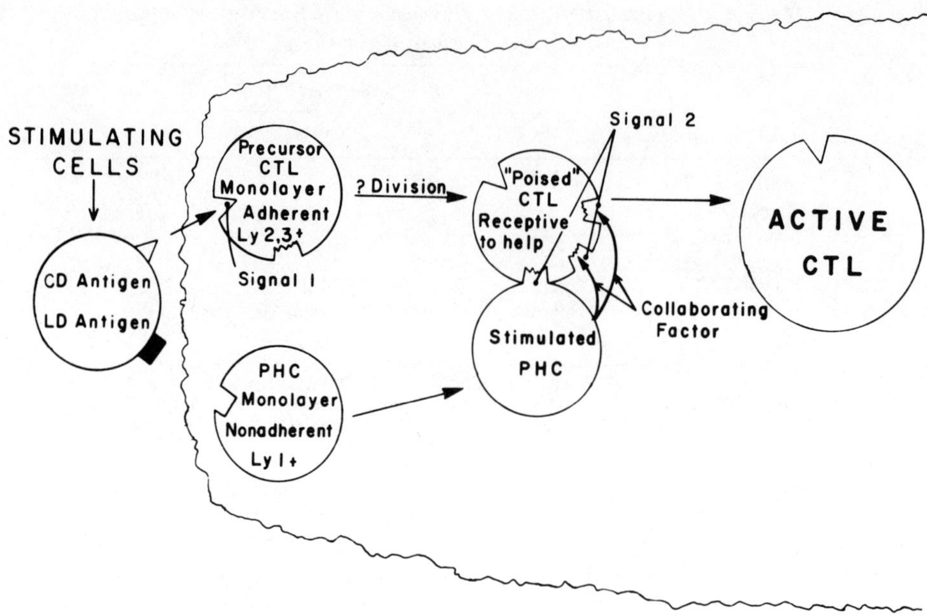

Figure 2. Cellular response to LD and CD antigens.[4]

3. *The Relevance of HLA Matching to Graft Survival*

A great number of studies have been performed attempting to relate degrees of matching for the HLA-A and -B antigens, as detected serologically, to the success of allograft survival. It would have to be concluded in the summary of all those studies that most centers, especially in the United States, fail to show a significant association between matching for the HLA-A and -B antigens although a few studies in the United States and several in Europe suggest such a correlation. In the United States, those centers that have found a correlation have recognized that the significance of that correlation is not very high.

During the last several years, attempts have been made to match for the HLA-D region to ask whether minimizing disparity for D-region-encoded antigens may correlate with graft survival. Two approaches have been taken: first, matching in primary MLC in living related donor–recipient combinations, and second, matching for the HLA-DR antigens for cadaver transplantation. Although these two types of approaches may not measure exactly the same determinants, certainly serologic typing for the HLA-DR antigens provides a convenient guide to other determinants usually found in association with the given DR antigen on the HLA-D haplotype. The results of both types of studies suggest that matching for the HLA-D region may have a highly significant effect on the outcome of graft survival.

It would be worthwhile to reserve final judgment until the results of a carefully planned, preferably prospective, trial are evaluated. This should certainly be performed with regard to kidney transplantation in the United States.

4. *Summary*

A variety of markers are associated with HLA genes that have allowed construction of the genetic map presented in Fig. 1. Primarily it has been the use of antisera that has allowed this dissection. In the process of performing such investigations, it has become apparent that there appear to be two types of antigens, differentiated initially on the basis of their tissue distribution. In addition, two "types" of antigens are differentially active in stimulating proliferating and cytotoxic cells.

References

1. Terasaki PI (ed): *Histocompatibility Testing 1970.* Copenhagen, Munksgaard, 1970.
2. Kissmeyer-Nielsen F (ed): *Histocompatibility Testing 1975.* Copenhagen, Munksgaard, 1975.
3. Bodmer WF, Batchelor Jr, Bodmer JG, Festenstein H, Morris PJ (eds): *Histocompatibility Testing 1977.* Copenhagen, Munksgaard, 1978.
4. Bach FH, Bach ML, Sondel PM: Differential function of major histocompatibility complex antigens in T-lymphocyte activation. *Nature* 259:273, 1976.
5. Mempel W, Grosse-Wilde H, Baumann P, Netzel B, Steinbauer–Rosenthal I: Population genetics of the MLC response: Typing for MLC determinants using homozygous and heterozygous reference cells. *Transpl Proc* 5:1529, 1973.
6. Reinsmoen N, Noreen H, Friend P, Giblett E, Greenberg L, Kersey J: Anomalous mixed lymphocyte culture reactivity between HLA-A, B, C, DR identical siblings. *Tissue Antigens* 13:19, 1979.
7. Sheehy, MH, Sondel PM, Bach ML, Wank R, Bach FH: LD (lymphocyte defined) typing: A rapid assay with primed lymphocytes. *Science* 188:1308, 1975.
8. Bach FH, Jarrett–Toth, EK, Benike CJ, Shih CY, Valentine EA: Primed LD typing: Reagent preparation and definition of the HLA-D region antigens. *Scand J Immunol* 6:469, 1977.
9. Reinsmoen NL, Noreen HJ, Sasazuki T, Segall M, Bach FH: Roles of HLA-DR and HLA-D antigens in haplotype-primed LD typing reagents, in Kaplan JG (ed): *The Molecular Basis of Immune Cell Function,* Proceedings of the 13th International Leucocyte Culture Conference. Amsterdam, Elsevier/North-Holland, 1979.
10. Morgan DA, Ruscetti FW, Gallo RC: Selective in vitro growth of T lymphocytes from normal human bone marrows. *Science* 193:1007, 1976.
11. Bach FH, Inouye H, Hank JA, Alter BJ: Human T lymphocyte clones reactive in primed lymphocytes typing and cytotoxicity. *Nature* 281:307, 1979.
12. Long MA, Handwerger BS, Amos DB, Yunis EJ: The genetics of cell mediated lympholysis. *J Immunol* 117:2092, 1976.

Nutritional Therapy in Chronic Renal Failure

55

Some Questions of a Clinical Nephrologist Concerning Nutritional Therapy and Patients with Chronic Renal Failure

William B. Blythe

This chapter poses some questions about nutritional therapy in patients with chronic renal failure.

The perspective is that of one who has taken care of pateints with chronic renal failure for a quarter of a century. Five major questions need to be answered: (1) How can renal disease that leads to chronic renal failure be prevented? (2) Once renal disease is established, how can the development of progressive renal failure be prevented or slowed? (3) Are there better alternatives to the treatment of end-stage chronic renal failure than dialysis and transplantation? (4) How can the effectiveness of dialysis and transplantation be improved? And last, (5) How can the cost of effective dialysis and transplantation be reduced?

These questions are arranged so that a clear answer to each question makes the questions that follow of little—or certainly lesser—importance.

Each of the questions is examined in the context of this group of chapters with the aim of attempting to determine whether there is a relationship between these questions and diet—or nutrition in the broadest sense—whether the relationship is thought to be trivial or faddish or real, or whether the relationship has reached the point that some answers to the broad questions might be found.

Regarding the first question, "How can renal disease that leads to chronic renal failure be prevented?" to my mind, there is a reasonable relationship

William B. Blythe • Division of Nephrology, Department of Medicine, University of North Carolina School of Medicine, Chapel Hill, North Carolina 27514.

between this question and nutrition in one area—salt intake and hypertension leading to chronic renal failure—and a nebulous relationship in two others—dietary factors involved in the development of nephrolithiasis and nephrocalcinosis which can cause chronic renal failure and dietary factors in the development of atherosclerosis which may lead to chronic renal failure in later life.

These last two relationships in the context of this chapter are to me, personally, intellectual quagmires which I, therefore, choose to avoid.

The first—that is, the possible relationship between salt intake and hypertension—I deem to be of more importance.

In my part of the world, the southeastern section of the United States, hypertension is the leading cause of chronic renal failure in patients undergoing chronic dialysis.

For the past 5 years, hypertension is judged to be the cause of chronic renal failure in 40–45% of the patients entering the chronic dialysis program at the North Carolina Memorial Hospital. These estimates agree closely with those of the other dialysis units in North Carolina and, I suspect, with all those in the Southeast. Thus, if hypertension could be eliminated as a cause of chronic renal failure, the dialysis population could be significantly reduced.

Now even though the evidence is far from conclusive regarding (1) the role of high salt intake in the development of hypertension and (2) the question whether control of blood pressure in hypertensive patients reduces the prevalence of chronic renal failure, I do believe that there is enough evidence from epidemiological studies to indicate that the incidence of hypertension is lower in populations that eat little salt, and this warrants a closer look.

As for immune diseases that cause chronic renal failure: to my knowledge, there have been no studies—or even speculations—that in any way implicate nutrition as an important element in the development of renal disease consequential to immune mechanisms.

Thus, it is not reasonable to believe—with our current understanding—that, with the possible exception of hypertension, studies involving nutrition are likely to afford an answer to the first question of how renal disease that leads to chronic renal failure might be prevented.

If this is the case, the second question, "How can the development of progressive renal failure be prevented or slowed down?" assumes paramount importance in a reasoned approach to the economic as well as therapeutic aspects of the management of patients with chronic renal failure.

In my judgment, the relationship between this question and nutritional therapy is most cogent, and I gather it is a major force in this subpart of the volume. I believe that it is in this area that some of the most exciting and promising investigation has been taking place in the recent past and will be occurring over the next decade. Two lines of investigation, in particular, are exciting to me, and I suppose the hope is that they may eventually reach some similar conclusions. The first is laboratory investigation which implicates nephron hyperfiltration (or some function thereof) in rats with reduced renal mass as being responsible for the progressive renal damage that occurs in this model, and the second is the finding that feeding low-protein diets may ameliorate or prevent the deterioration of renal function (Hostetter *et al.*, 1981). Whether the low-protein diet *per se*, or phosphate, or something else—or some combination of these factors—is responsible is as yet unclear, and I shall leave it to the experts to delineate the importance of these factors.

The second line of investigation includes those clinical studies in patients with chronic renal failure in which the effect on renal function of low-protein diets—or low-protein diets coupled with essential keto acids—or essential amino acids has been examined.

Protein restriction has been widely employed in the treatment of chronic renal failure, at least since the time of Richard Bright in the early nineteenth century. However, the accumulation of evidence that such dietary management might slow down the progression of renal failure, or have any beneficial affect at all on renal function, is, by and large, a recent phenomenon.

It might be of interest to examine why this might be the case. With the exception of studies by Addis and his colleagues (Addis, 1952), all the studies of Shannon *et al.*(1932), Van Slyke *et al.* (1935), and Pitts (1944) showed that feeding high-protein diets to animals increased glomerular filtration rate. All those studies were short term and, in the framework of our current understanding, might have been expected to turn out the way they did. The early studies of Kempner (1945), of Keutmann and McCann (1932), and of Bang (1949) in man with chronic renal disease, in which they found neither improvement nor deterioration in renal function as a consequence of low-protein diets, were flawed by the use of urea clearances as a measure of glomerular filtration rate. Early studies on the use of Giordano–Giovannetti type diets (Shaw *et al.*, 1965; Franklin *et al.*, 1967; Kopple *et al.*, 1968) in patients with chronic renal failure have shown that these diets do not result in improvement of renal function in patients with severe renal failure; however, none of these studies has actually confronted the question as to whether they slow the progression of chronic renal failure in patients with moderate reduction in glomerular filtration rate.

More recent clinical studies by several investigators, notably Walser, Mitch, and their colleagues (Walser *et al.*, 1979; Walser, 1980) and Bergstrom and his colleagues (Alvestrand *et al.*, 1980), have specifically examined the question of whether dietary modification might slow the progression of chronic renal failure.

I should, however, like to make two comments: first, from my vantage point as a clinical nephrologist concerned about the enormity of the problem of chronic renal failure with all its overtones, I believe that if nutritional therapy is to play a significant role in alleviating the problem it will be in the possible halting or slowing deterioration in renal function in patients with chronic renal failure; second, the sum of the evidence from all the animal studies coupled with the clinical studies does not allow me to make a judgment as to whether low protein *per se*, essential keto acids, essential amino acids, phosphate, the calcium–phosphate product, or something else might be the critical factors. If it is decided that a large clinical trial is to be undertaken, I hope that it is possible to design the study so that an answer might be forthcoming.

Regarding the third question, "Are there better alternatives to the treatment of end-stage chronic renal failure than dialysis or transplantation?" I do not know of any, and, I believe that even the most enthusiastic proponents of dietary therapy make no claims that nutritional therapy can substitute for dialysis therapy once renal function has deteriorated to a very low level. Thus, I think that it is not fruitful or realistic to expect an answer to this question from nutritional therapy.

Nutrition, I believe, is intrinsically involved in answers to the fourth question, "How can the effectiveness of dialysis and transplantation be improved?"

Several studies—by Kopple and colleagues and by others—indicate that malnutrition is common, in either subtle or overt forms, in patients undergoing chronic dialysis and that malnutrition is a major factor in morbidity in these patients.

It is less clear as to why there is such a high prevalence of malnutrition. Most investigators believe that it is the result of a combination of factors including anorexia secondary to uremia or to the disease causing the chronic renal failure. This is certainly an important area, and cognizance of it—and attention to it—certainly makes a difference. I do believe that one thing should be mentioned about it in this setting: to my knowledge, the proper use of low-protein diets *per se* cannot be thought of as a significant contributing factor. So I believe that the effectiveness of dialysis can be substantially increased by awareness and correction of malnutrition.

Regarding the last question, "How can the cost of effective dialysis and transplantation be reduced?" the major answer is to be found in the sociopolitical arena, but nutrition may play a role in that the number of hospitalizations for infections and related complications may be substantially reduced by elimination of malnutrition as a causative factor.

The use of amino acids or keto acids as supplements in patients undergoing chronic hemodialysis to reduce the number of dialyses that a given patient might require has been advocated by some authors. This, too, is an important area that might help to increase the effectiveness of dialysis as well as to reduce the cost. I doubt that it can be expected to play a major role.

In summary, then, I believe that the most exciting prospect for nutritional therapy in patients with chronic renal failure is the possibility that it may be used to slow the progression of chronic renal failure. This could be an important factor in the overall approach to therapy in these patients.

To prove that it works or that it can be done is a big issue with which I will not wrestle. In my judgment, it does warrant serious confrontation with pristine objectivity.

References

Addis, T., 1952, *Glomerular Nephritis*, Macmillan, New York.

Alvestrand, A., Ahlberg, M., Furst, P., and Bergstrom, J., 1980, Clinical experience with amino acid and keto acid diets, *Am. J. Clin. Nutr.* **33:**1654.

Bang, H. O., 1949, Influence of dietary protein on the function of diseased kidneys, *Acta Med. Scand.* (suppl. 234)**:**18.

Franklin, S. S., Gordon, A., Kleeman, C. R., and Maxwell, M. H., 1967, Use of a balanced low-protein diet in chronic renal failure, *J M A* **202:**477.

Hostetter, T. H., Olson, J. L., Rennke, H. G., Venkatachalam, M. A., and Brenner, B. M., 1981, Hyperfiltration in remnant nephrons: A potentially adverse response to renal ablation, *Am. J. Physiol.* **141:**E85.

Kempner, W., 1945, Compensation of renal metabolic dysfunction, *N. Carolina Med. J.* **6:**62.

Keutmann, E. H., and McCann, W. S., 1932, Dietary protein in hemorrhagic Bright's disease. I. Effects upon the course of the disease with special reference to hematuria and renal function, *J. Clin. Invest.* **11:**973.

Kopple, J. D., Sorensen, M. K., Coburn, J. W., Gordon, S., and Rubini, M. E., 1968, Controlled comparison of 20-g and 40-g protein diets in the treatment of chronic uremia, *Am. J. Clin. Nutr.* **21:**553.

Pitts, R. F., 1944, The effects of infusing glycine and of varying the dietary protein intake on renal hemodynamics in the dog, *Am. J. Physiol.* **142:**355.

Shannon, J. A., Jolliffe, N., and Smith, H. W., 1932, The excretion of urine in the dog. IV. The effect of maintenance diet, feeding, etc. upon the quantity of glomerular filtrate, *Am. J. Physiol.* **101:**625.

Shaw, A. B., Bazzard, F. J., Booth, E. M., Nilwarangkur, S., and Berlyne, G. M., 1965, The treatment of chronic renal failure by modified Giovannetti diet, *Q. J. Med.* **34:**237.

Van Slyke, D. D., Rhoads, C. P., Hiller, A., and Alving, A., 1935, The relationship of the urea clearance to the renal blood flow, *Am. J. Physiol.* **110:**387.

Walser, M., 1980, Does dietary therapy have a role in the predialysis patients? *Am. J. Clin. Nutr.* **33:**1629.

Walser, M., Mitch, W. E., and Collier, V. U., 1979, Essential amino acids and their nitrogen-free analogues in the treatment of chronic renal failure, in: *Controversies in Nephrology* (G. Schreiner, ed.), Georgetown University Press, Washington, D.C.

56

The Loss of Renal Enzymes

A Risk Factor for Nutritional and Metabolic Disorders

Hani B. Affarah, Rajender K. Chawla, Julie C. Bleier, Elbert P. Tuttle, and Daniel Rudman

1. Risk Factors for Nutritional Disorders in End-Stage Renal Disease

Malnutrition is a common problem in patients with end-stage renal disease (ESRD), regardless of the mode of therapy (Coles, 1972; Blumenkrantz *et al.*, 1976; Kopple, 1978; Bansal *et al.*, 1980). The risk factors for malnutrition may be divided into two categories: (1) extrinsic factors, such as restricted diets prescribed by the physician (Berlyne *et al.*, 1968; Sorenson and Kopple, 1968), catabolic illness (Nsouli *et al.*, 1979; Dobkin *et al.*, 1978), blood losses from the gastrointestinal tract (Linton *et al.*, 1977) and during hemodialysis (Longnecker *et al.*, 1974), and loss of protein (Blumenkrantz *et al.*, 1981) and amino acids (Kopple *et al.*, 1973) into the dialysate; and (2) intrinsic factors, such as hypophagia (Atkin-Thor *et al.*, 1978), malabsorption of nutrients (Merrill and Tasch, 1976), abnormal metabolism of nutrients (Spannuth *et al.*, 1977; Relman, 1972), and loss of renal enzymes which catalyze the utilization or degradation of nutrients including their conversion to physiologically essential compounds.

The extrinsic factors have been thoroughly described in the literature, but the intrinsic factors, with the exception of hypophagia, have not received enough emphasis. Loss of renal enzymes in ESRD, with resulting impairment

---

Hani B. Affarah, Rajender K. Chawla, Julie C. Bleier, and Elbert P. Tuttle • Clinical Research Facility and Division of Nephrology, Department of Medicine, Emory University School of Medicine, Atlanta, Georgia 30322. ***Daniel Rudman*** • Divison of Geriatric Medicine, Veterans Administration Medical Center, North Chicago, Illinois 60064. Supported by USPHS Grants RR39 and AM30589.

of renal synthetic and catabolic pathways, is an important risk factor for malnutrition and will be the focus of this chapter.

2. *Rationale for the Loss of Renal Enzymes as a Risk Factor for Malnutrition*

Most renal enzymes are well represented in other tissues of the body, mainly liver and skeletal muscle, and in ESRD the other tissues are often able to compensate for the loss of enzyme activity in the kidney. This compensation is not possible when the enzyme is present predominantly in the kidney and is inadequate when the reaction is dependent on the transport of the substrate to the renal enzyme. Thus, even though a particular renal enzyme may constitute only a minor portion of the body content of this enzyme, high renal blood flow and an efficient substrate-extracting process by tubular reabsorption and direct uptake from peritubular capillaries may enhance the functional significance of the enzyme in the kidneys compared to the same enzyme in other tissues. Therefore, the contribution of a particular renal enzyme to the whole-body rate of the corresponding reaction can be far greater than would be predicted from the amount of enzyme contained in kidney, liver, and muscle.

An example of the importance of the renal-extracting processes is the enzyme glutathione-insulin transhydrogenase, which inactivates insulin by cleaving its disulfide bonds (Varandani, 1973). The specific activity of this enzyme in the rat has been determined by Chandler and Varandani (1972); although the kidney has only 2% of the total transhydrogenase activity in the body, it is, nevertheless, a major site for degradation of insulin (Elgee *et al.*, 1954; Rubenstein and Spitz, 1968). In normal subjects, about 40% of the insulin secreted each day is believed to be degraded in the kidneys. The clinical significance of this process is further shown by the decline in the insulin requirements of diabetic patients who develop ESRD (Reaven *et al.*, 1974). The rate-limiting step in the degradation of insulin appears to be the delivery of the hormone to the renal insulin-degrading enzyme.

Despite the potential clinical importance of loss of renal enzymes, the literature supplies little quantitative information comparing specific enzyme activities between the kidney and other organs. Moreover, the few studies reported in this area were done mainly in animals and not in humans. A helpful type of circumstantial evidence concerning the quantitative contribution of renal enzymes to whole-body metabolism, however, comes from the patients with ESRD. Myoinositol metabolism illustrates this point. Blood levels of myoinositol are elevated in uremic patients. The rate-limiting enzyme in myoinositol degradation is myoinositol oxygenase, which is known to be present in the kidney. The clinical evidence concerning the accumulation of myoinositol in uremic plasma indicates that this renal enzyme is the main catalyst in the body for myoinositol oxidation.

Table 1. Enzymes That Are Localized Mainly in the Kidney[a]

1.	25-Hydroxycholecalciferol 1-monoxygenase (E.C. 1.14.13.13)
2.	Neutral peptidase
3.	Myoinositol oxygenase (E.C. 1.13.99.1)
4.	Renin (E.C. 3.4.99.19)
5.	Phosphoglycerate dehydrogenase, phosphoserine transaminase
6.	γ-Butyrobetaine hydroxylase (E.C. 1.14.11.1)
7.	Arginine:glycine amidinotransferase (E.C. 2.1.4.1)
8.	Urokinase
9.	Maleate hydralase (E.C. 4.2.1.31)
10.	5′-Acylphosphoadenosine hydrolase (E.C. 3.6.1.20)
11.	*N*-Acetyl-β-alanine deacetylase (E.C. 3.5.1.21)
12.	Aspartoacylase (E.C. 3.5.1.15)
13.	Postproline endopeptidase
14.	Peptidyl carboxyamidase (E.C. 3.14.15.2)
15.	Dipeptidase (E.C. 3.4.13.11)
16.	Aminoacyl-lysine dipeptidase (E.C. 3.4.13.3)
17.	L-3-Aminoisobutyrate aminotransferase (E.C. 2.6.1.22)
18.	Kynurenine aminotransferase (E.C. 2.6.1.7)
19.	γ-Glutamyltransferase (E.C. 2.3.2.2)
20.	Cysteamine dioxygenase (E.C. 1.13.11.19)
21.	*N*-Methylaminoacid oxidase (E.C. 1.5.3.2)
22.	Pyrroline-2-carboxylate reductase (E.C. 1.5.1.1)
23.	D-Aspartate oxidase (E.C. 1.4.3.1)
24.	16-α-Hydroxysteroid dehydrogenase (E.C. 1.1.1.147)
25.	D-2-Hydroxy fatty-acid dehydrogenase (E.C. 1.1.1.98)
26.	Lactaldehyde reductase (E.C. 1.1.1.55)
27.	L-Gulonate dehydrogenase (E.C. 1.1.1.45)

[a] From Dixon and Webb, 1979.

3. Scope of This Chapter

Although we realize that a renal enzyme with a low percentage of the total-body enzyme activity may play a significant physiologic role, for the purpose of this review we will focus only on those enzymes known to be highly concentrated in the kidney (Dixon and Webb, 1979). Table 1 lists 27 enzymes that have been found to be localized mainly in the kidney. For seven of these, available evidence indicates that the loss of the renal activity in patients with ESRD causes clinical repercussions; for these seven enzymes, we will discuss the biochemical properties, the reactions catalyzed, and the nutritional or metabolic consequences of their loss in ESRD.

4. Review of Seven Renal Enzymes the Loss of Which Causes Nutritional and Metabolic Disorders in ESRD

4.1. 25-Hydroxycholecalciferol 1-Monoxygenase

This enzyme mediates the conversion of the major circulating form of vitamin D, 25-hydroxycholecalciferol, to its metabolically active form, 1,25-

dihydrocholecalciferol. Both NADPH and molecular oxygen are required as cofactors for the enzymatic reaction (DeLuca, 1978). The activated form of this vitamin stimulates calcium transport in kidney, bone, and intestines (Walling, 1977; Raisz *et al.*, 1972; Levine *et al.*, 1978). Its precursor is predominantly synthesized in the liver from cholecalciferol, which in turn is either absorbed from the diet or is formed in the skin from photolysis of 7-dehydrocholesterol (Ponchon and DeLuca, 1969; Schacter *et al.*, 1965; Rauschkolb *et al.*, 1969).

In patients with ESRD, impairment of the key hydroxylation process prevents the synthesis of 1,25-dihydrocholecalciferol (Mawer *et al.*, 1973). This metabolic deficiency has been implicated in the pathogenesis of uremic osteodystrophy (Stanbury, 1977). The diets of such patients are now supplemented with the active form of vitamin D.

4.2. *Renal Neutral Peptidase*

This enzyme catalyzes the degradation of glucagon, the insulin B chain, and adrenocorticotropin (Varandani and Shroyer, 1977). The peptidase attacks peptide bonds which involve the amino terminus of hydrophobic amino acids, provided that the residue is not C terminal. It hydrolyzes tripeptides and polypeptides, but not dipeptides. In kidney, the enzyme is localized in the microsomal fraction of the brush border and is membrane bound.

Although several peptidases capable of degrading glucagon are present in most mammalian tissues, physiologic and clinical evidence indicates that the renal neutral peptidase is a major factor in glucagon clearance (Duckworth, 1976). This evidence is based on the following observations: In rats, the kidney normally extracts 40% of glucagon from the renal arterial blood, and the urinary excretion of glucagon accounts for less than 2% of the renal extraction (Bastl *et al.*, 1977). In addition, the plasma disappearance time of exogenous glucagon is slightly increased in patients with ESRD or after bilateral nephrectomy. These data suggest that glucagon is filtered through the glomerulus and then reabsorbed by the tubular epithelial cells, after which it undergoes catabolism through the neutral peptidase system (Lefebvre *et al.*, 1974).

Patients with ESRD have elevated levels of plasma glucagon (Bilbrey *et al.*, 1975) resulting from both a fall in the mass of renal tissue and a qualitative change in the renal handling of glucagon (Bastl *et al.*, 1977). This hyperglucagonemia contributes to malnutrition and azotemia because it promotes conversion of amino acids to glucose and urea in the liver (Salter *et al.*, 1960; Unger, 1971; Knochel *et al.*, 1975).

4.3. *Myoinositol Oxygenase*

This enzyme catalyzes the initial step in myoinositol degradation, which is the oxygenation of myoinositol to D-glucuronate (White *et al.*, 1973), half of which is further converted to D-glucose and D-glucuronolactone, and the remainder of which is completely oxidized to carbon dioxide and water (Clements and Diethelm, 1979). The enzyme is highly specific for myoinositol and is inactive toward L- or D-inositol (Charalampous, 1962).

Myoinositol is a water-soluble sugar alcohol that occurs in plants as phytic acid and in animal tissues as free myoinositol or as part of phospholipids (White *et al.*, 1973; Liveson *et al.*, 1977) and is well absorbed from the diet.

The kidney is the major regulator of fasting plasma myoinositol concentration and pool size in man via its role in myoinositol synthesis (Clements and Diethelm, 1979), glomerular filtration, nearly complete tubular reabsorption (Pitkanen, 1976; Hammerman *et al.*, 1980), and degradation. Evidence for the renal control of myoinositol catabolism is provided by bilaterally nephrectomized rats, who do not catabolize any 2-^{14}C-labeled myoinositol (Anderson and Coots, 1958; Lewin and Sulimovici, 1975). Uremic patients have a markedly elevated plasma myoinositol (mean ± S.D., 942 ± 180 μm) compared to normal subjects (63 ± 26 μm) (Pitkanen, 1972).

In the rat, high concentrations of myoinositol impair nerve conduction velocity (De Jesus *et al.*, 1974). Concentrations comparable to those found in uremic patients are toxic to dorsal root ganglia in tissue culture (Liveson *et al.*, 1977). Thus the loss of renal myoinositol oxygenase may be a factor in uremic neurotoxicity.

4.4. Renin

Renin is a glycoprotein protease that acts on an α_2-globulin substrate in plasma to release angiotensin I. The native intrarenal enzyme is synthesized and stored in membrane-bound cytoplasmic granules by cells at the vascular pole of the renal glomerulus. It is then converted by a sulfhydryl-containing enzyme to the circulating active form (Inagami *et al.*, 1977). Reninlike enzymes have been extracted from a variety of organs, including the adrenal glands (Ryan, 1967), brain (Ganten *et al.*, 1971), and uterus (Ferris *et al.*, 1967), but are inactive at physiologic pH and become active only after exposure to acid pH or to acid proteases (Reid *et al.*, 1978).

Through its production of angiotensin, renin influences blood volume, blood pressure, and sodium balance. In anephric patients, reninlike activity and angiotensin I are absent from the serum, and renin substrate concentration is elevated (Berman *et al.*, 1972). These observations confirm that the kidney is the major site of renin synthesis. When this system is lost or inhibited, the maintenance of blood pressure in response to acute hypovolemia or upright posture is impaired (Schambelan and Stockigt, 1979).

4.5. Enzymes of Serine Biosynthesis

These include phosphoglycerate dehydrogenase and phosphoserine transaminase. Serine is normally a nonessential amino acid which is synthe-

A. Enzymes of serine synthesis

1. Hydroxymethyltransferase
2. Phosphoglycerate dehydrogenase (PGDH)
3. Phosphoserine transaminase (PST)
4. Serine phosphatase (SP)

B. Pathways for serine synthesis

1. Glycine $\overset{(a)}{\rightleftharpoons}$ serine
2. 3-Phospho-D-glyceric acid $\xrightarrow{(b)}$ 3-Phosphohydroxypyruvic acid
   3-Phosphohydroxypyruvic acid $\xrightarrow{(c)}$ 3-Phosphoserine
   3-Phosphoserine $\xrightarrow{(d)}$ Serine

Figure 1. (A) Enzymes of serine synthesis. (B) Pathways for serine synthesis.

sized in the body by the two metabolic pathways shown in Fig. 1. One route utilizes hydroxymethyltransferase to catalyze the reversible addition of a hydroxymethyl group to glycine to form serine (Blakley, 1960; Coon *et al.*, 1974). Although approximately 90% of the specific activity for this enzyme is located in liver, only in the kidney does the equilibrium favor serine synthesis, and the renal production of serine using this pathway is responsible for less than 7% of the total body turnover of serine (Pitts and MacLeod, 1972). In the major pathway of serine biosynthesis (Fig. 1), the rate-limiting enzymes—viz., phosphoglycerate dehydrogenase and phosphoserine transaminase—are mostly localized in the kidney (Tanaka, 1965; Hayashi *et al.*, 1975).

Uremic patients on low-protein diets have a low dietary intake of serine; consequently, loss of the renal enzymes could predispose to a deficiency of the amino acid. Several workers have reported significantly low values of plasma serine in uremic patients as compared to normals. Alvestrand *et al.* (1978) reported plasma serine levels of 117 ± 15 μm in uremic patients on a protein-restricted diet and 199 ± 3 μm in normal subjects. In another study, the plasma serine levels in uremic patients on a diet consisting of essential amino acids as the only source of nitrogen were even lower (50 ± 6 μm) (Zimmerman *et al.*, 1979). These values indicate the reduced capacity of the body to synthesize optimal quantities of serine in uremia. Hyposerinemia in Zimmerman's uremic patients may also reflect inhibition of hepatic phosphoglycerate dehydrogenase by the high dietary intake of methionine, tryptophan, and threonine furnished by the essential-amino-acid diet (Mauron *et al.*, 1972). Thus, in some uremic patients, serine may become an essential amino acid that needs to be provided in the diet.

Besides being a component of most tissue proteins, serine is essential for the synthesis of phosphoglycerides (Bosch, 1974) and sphingolipids (Stoffel, 1971). Its carbon chain is utilized in the biosynthesis of cysteine, in hepatic gluconeogenesis (Lehninger, 1978), and in the biosynthesis of choline.

Whether the low plasma serine levels in ESRD affect any of these precursor functions of serine is presently unknown.

4.6. γ-Butyrobetaine Hydroxlyase

This enzyme catalyzes the last step in the biosynthesis of carnitine: the reaction of γ-butyrobetaine, α-ketoglutarate, and O_2 to yield L-carnitine, CO_2, and succinate. γ-Butyrobetaine hydroxylase is a soluble mitochondrial enzyme that binds several transition-metal ions, but only the ferrous ion is catalytically active (Lindstedt, 1967). The specific activity of the enzyme in human tissues has been found by Rebouche and Engel (1980) to be highest in the kidney, where activity is approximately 4 times higher than that in liver and brain. No activity is found in heart and muscle. The specific activities of the four enzymes of carnitine biosynthesis in humans are shown in Table 2.

Carnitine is essential for the transport of long-chain fatty acids into mitochondria where they are oxidized (Bremer, 1977). Four factors can contribute to carnitine depletion: substandard intake of dietary carnitine; substandard intake of lysine and methionine, the precursors for endogenous carnitine synthesis; loss of the capacity to synthesize carnitine because of liver and/or kidney failure; and loss of carnitine from the body during dialysis (Rudman *et al.*, 1977; Böhmer *et al.*, 1978).

Myopathy, fatty liver, and cerebral disorders are the consequences of a genetic carnitine deficiency (Vandyke *et al.*, 1975; Karpati *et al.*, 1975; Engel and Angelini, 1973). Decreased plasma and muscle contents of carnitine have been reported in hemodialysis patients (Böhmer *et al.*, 1978), and carnitine deficiency has also been related to the hypertriglyceridemia in patients on hemodialysis (Guarnieri *et al.*, 1980) and on chronic ambulatory peritoneal dialysis (Buoncristiani *et al.*, 1981). Thus carnitine deficiency may occur in uremic patients on dialysis, and correction by oral supplements of carnitine could be helpful (Guarnieri *et al.*, 1980).

4.7. Arginine: Glycine Amidinotransferase

This enzyme catalyzes the transfer of a guanidine group between arginine and glycine to yield ornithine and guanidinoacetic acid, which is the first and the rate-limiting step in the synthesis of creatine (Walker, 1979) (Fig. 2). In man, it occurs predominantly in the kidney and pancreas (Van Pilsum *et al.*, 1972). Creatine is formed in the next reaction by transfer of a methyl group from *S*-adenosylmethionine to guanidinoacetate; this irreversible step occurs primarily in the liver.

Synthesized creatine is released into the circulation and actively taken up against a concentration gradient by muscle and other tissues (Walker, 1979; Haughland and Chang, 1975). About 98% of the total-body creatine pool is within muscle (Hunter, 1928). This creatine pool is slowly saturable and has a relatively slow daily turnover rate of about 1.5–2% (Fitch *et al.*,

Table 2. Tissue Distribution of Carnitine Biosynthetic Enzymes

	γ-Butyrobetaine hydroxylase (pmoles/min per mg protein)	Distribution (percent of body content)	Aldehyde dehydrogenase (pmoles/min per mg protein)	Distribution (percent of body weight)	β-Hydroxy aldolase (pmoles/min per mg protein)	Distribution (percent of body content)	Me_3Lysine β_2 hydroxylase (pmoles/min per mg protein)	Distribution (percent of body content)
Kidney	1350	38	15,700	8	2.7	1	180	6.7
Liver	370	42	46,800	92	39	58	45	6.7
Brain	140	18	—	—	5	9	36	6.2
Muscle	—	—	—	—	1	32	25	80

1. Glycine + arginine $\xrightleftharpoons{\text{Glycine amidinotransferase}}$ Guanidinoacetate + ornithine
2. *S*-Adenosyl-methionine + guanidinoacetate $\xrightarrow{\text{Guanidinoacetate methyltransferase}}$ Creatine + *S*-adenosyl-homocysteine
3. Creatine + ATP $\xrightarrow{\text{Creatine phosphokinase}}$ Phosphocreatine + ADP

Figure 2. Pathway for creatine synthesis.

1968). Creatine is phosphorylated to yield phosphocreatine, which is a high-energy phosphate compound that serves as an intermediate in excitation–contraction coupling, modulates glycolysis, increases intracellular flux of potassium and phosphorus, and also acts as a cofactor in muscle growth (Walker, 1979).

Several studies undertaken by Goldman and Moss (1960) to determine whether uremia interferes with creatine synthesis demonstrated that chronic renal disease in rats reduced creatine synthesis both by loss of the renal enzymatic mechanisms and by interference with methylation in the liver. Extrarenal synthesis may increase to partially compensate for these inhibiting factors.

Muscle phosphocreatine levels in patients with ESRD have not been reported, although clinical symptoms experienced by uremic patients include fatigability (Cardenas and Kutner, 1982), muscle cramps (Merrill, 1965; Stewart *et al.*, 1972), and muscle wasting (Cohen *et al.*, 1980). Uremic myopathy is common, but its causes are uncertain (Cohen *et al.*, 1980). The usefulness of a creatine supplement in ameliorating this problem is unknown.

5. *Other Renal Enzymes*

The reactions catalyzed by the rest of the enzymes in Table 1 have been identified, but their physiologic significance is unclear, and therefore the consequences of losing the corresponding renal enzyme cannot presently be predicted.

6. *Implications for Treatment*

The intrinsic loss of renal enzymes in ESRD suggests a need to modify the exogenous intake of nutrients. Renal enzymes enable the kidneys to synthesize hormones, to process nutrients, and to convert certain substrates to a more readily utilizable or storable form. Loss of renal enzymes and the corresponding renal synthetic capacities in ESRD could lead to new nutrient requirements. 1,25-Dihydrocholecalciferol, carnitine, creatine, and serine are examples of nutrients that may need to be supplemented in the diet of some patients with ESRD.

Several renal enzymes participate in the degradation of nutrients and hormones. When these enzymes are lost in uremic patients, toxic accumulation of nutrients and hormones may ensue. The neurotoxicity of myoinositol, the hypercatabolic effect of glucagon, and the decrease in exogenous requirements of insulin are such consequences of the loss of renal enzymes.

References

1. Alvestrand, A., Bergström, J., Fürst, P. Germanis, G., and Widstam, U., 1978, Effect of essential amino acid supplementation on muscle and plasma free amino acids in chronic uremia, *Kidney Int.* **14:**323.
2. Anderson, L., and Coots, R. H., 1958, Metabolism of 2-^{14}C-myoinositol in the rat. *Biochim. Biophys. Acta* **28:**666.
3. Atkin-Thor, E., Goddard, B. W., O'nion, J., Stephen, R. L., and Kolff, W. J., 1978, Hypogeusia and zinc depletion in chronic dialysis patients. *Am. J. Clin. Nutr.* **31:**1948.
4. Bansal, V. K., Popli, S., Pickering, J., Ing, T. S., Vertuno, L. L., and Hano, J. E., 1980, Protein–calorie malnutrition and cutaneous anergy in hemodialysis maintained patients, *Am. J. Clin. Nutr.* **33:**1608.
5. Bastl, C., Finkelstein, F. O., Sherwin, R., Hendler, R., Felig, P., and Hayslett, J. P., 1977, Renal extraction of glucagon in rats with normal and reduced renal function, *Am. J. Physiol.* **2**(1)**:**F67.
6. Berlyne, G. M., Gaan, D., and Ginks, W. R., 1968, Dietary treatment of chronic renal failure, *Am. J. Clin. Nutr.* **21**(6)**:**547.
7. Berman, L. B., Vertes, V., Mitra, S., and Gould, A. B., 1972, Renin–angiotensin system in anephric patients, *N. Engl. J. Med.* **286**(2)**:**58.
8. Bilbrey, G. L., Faloona, G. R., White, M. G., Atkins, C., Hull, A. R., and Knochel, J. P., 1975, Hyperglucagonemia in uremia. Reversal by renal transplantation, *Ann. Intern. Med.* **82:**525.
9. Blakley, R. L., 1960, A spectrophotometric study of the reaction catalyzed by serine transhydroxymethylase, *Biochem. J.* **77:**459.
10. Blumenkrantz, M. J., Kopple, J. D., and VA cooperative Dialysis Study Participants, 1976, Incidence of nutritional abnormalities in uremic patients entering dialysis therapy, *Kidney Int.* **10:**514.
11. Blumenkrantz, M. J., Gahl, G. M., Kopple, J. D., Kamdar, A. V., Jones, M. K., Kessle, M., and Coburn, J. W., 1981, Protein losses during peritoneal dialysis, *Kidney Int.* **19:**593.
12. Böhmer, T., Bergrem, J., and Eiklid, K., 1978, Carnitine deficiency induced during intermittent hemodialysis for renal failure, *Lancet* **1:**126.
13. Bosch, H. V. D., 1974, Phosphoglyceride metabolism, *Ann. Rev. Biochem.* **43:**243.
14. Bremer, J., 1977, Carnitine and its role in fatty acid metabolism, *Trends Biochem. Sci.* **2:**207.
15. Buoncristiani, U., Di Paolo, N., Carobi, C., Cozzari, M., Quintaliani, G., and Bracaglia, R., 1981, Carnitine depletion with CAPD, in: *Advances in Peritoneal Dialysis*, pp. 441–445, Excepta Medica, Amsterdam.
16. Cardenas, D. D., and Kutner, N. C., 1982, The problem of fatigue in dialysis patients, *Nephron* **30**(4)**:**336.
17. Chandler, M. L., and Varandani, P. T., 1972, Insulin degradation II. The widespread distribution of glutathione–insulin transhydrogenase in the tissue of the rat, *Biochim. Biophys. Acta* **286:**136.
18. Charalampous, F. C., 1962, Inositol—cleaving enzyme from rat kidney, *Methods Enzymol.* **5:**329.
19. Clements, R. S., Jr., and Diethelm, A. G., 1979, The metabolism of myoinositol by the human kidney, *J. Lab. Clin. Med.* **93:**210.

20. Cohen, I. M., Griffiths, J., Stone, R. A., and Leech, T. 1980, The creatine kinase profile of a maintenance hemodialysis population: a possible marker of uremic myopathy, *Clin. Nephrol.* **13**(5)**:**235.
21. Coles, G. A., 1972, Body composition in chronic renal failure, *Q. J. Med.* **41**(161)**:**25.
22. Coon, C. N., Luther, L. W., and Couch, J. R., 1974, Effect of glycine and serine in synthetic amino acid diets upon glycine and serine metabolism in chicks, *J. Nutr.* **104:**1018.
23. De Jesus, P. V., Clements, R. S., and Winegard, A. I., 1974, Hypermyoinositolemic polyneuropathy in rats: A possible mechanism for uremic polyneuropathy, *J. Neurol. Sci.* **21:**237.
24. DeLuca, H. F., 1974, Vitamin D—1973, *Am. J. Med.* **57**(1)**:**1.
25. DeLuca, H. F., 1978, Vitamin D metabolism and function, *Arch. Intern. Med.* **138:**836.
26. Dixon, M., and Webb, E., 1979, *Enzymes*, 3rd ed., Academic Press, New York.
27. Dobkin, J. F., Miller, M. H., and Steigbigel, N. H., 1978, Septicemia in patients on chronic hemodialysis, *Ann. Intern. Med.* **88:**28.
28. Duckworth, W. C., 1976, Insulin and glucagon degradation by the kidney, II. Characterization of the mechanisms at neutral pH, *Biochim. Biophys. Acta* **437:**531.
29. Elgee, N. J., Williams, R. H., and Lee, N. D., 1954, Distribution and degradation studies with insulin-I^{131}, *J. Clin. Invest.* **33:**1252.
30. Engel, A. G., and Angelini, C., 1973, Carnitine deficiency of human skeletal muscle with associated lipid storage myopathy: A new syndrome. *Science* **179:**899.
31. Ferris, T. F., Gorden, P., and Murlow, P. J., 1967, Rabbit uterus as a source of renin, *Am. J. Physiol.* **212:**698.
32. Fitch, C. D., Lucy, D. D., Bornhofen, J. H., and Dalrymple, G. V., 1968, Creatine metabolism in skeletal muscle: creatine kinetics in man, *Neurology* **18:**32.
33. Ganten, D., Boucher, R., and Genest, J., 1971, Renin activity in brain tissue of puppies and adult dogs, *Brain Res.* **33:**557.
34. Goldman, R., and Moss, J. X., 1960, Creatine synthesis after creatinine loading and after nephrectomy, *Proc. Soc. Exp. Biol. Med.* **105:**450.
35. Guarnieri, G. F., Ranieri, F., Toigo, G., Vasile, A., Ciman, M., Rizzoli, V., Maracchiello, M., and Campanacci, L., 1980, Lipid-lowering effect of carnitine in chronically uremic patients treated with maintenance hemodialysis, *Am. J. Clin. Nutr.* **33:**1489.
36. Hammerman, M. R., Sacktor, B., and Daughaday, W. H., 1980, Myo-inositol transport in renal brush border vesicles and its inhibition by D-glucose, *Am. J. Physiol.* **239:**F113.
37. Haughland, R. B., and Chang, D. T., 1975, Insulin effect on creatine transport in skeletal muscle, *Proc. Soc. Exp. Biol. Med.* **148:**1.
38. Hayashi, S., Tanaka, T., Naito, J., and Suda, M., 1975, Dietary and hormonal regulation of serine synthesis in the rat, *J. Biochem.* **77:**207.
39. Hunter, A., 1928, *Creatine and Creatinine, Monographs on Biochemistry*, Longmans, Green, New York.
40. Inagami, T., Hirose, S., Murakami, K., and Matoba, F., 1977, Native form of renin in the kidneys, *J. Biol. Chem.* **252:**7733.
41. Karpati, G., Carpenter, S., Engel, A., Watters, G., Allen, J., Rothman, S., Klassen, G., and Mainer, O., 1975, The syndrome of systemic carnitine deficiency. Clinical morphologic, biochemical and pathophysiologic features, *Neurology* **25:**16.
42. Knochel, J. P., Blachley, J., and Carter, N. W., 1975, Hyperglucagonemia in experimental potassium adaptation, *Clin. Res.* **23:**432A.
43. Kopple, J. D., 1978, Abnormal amino acid and protein metabolism in uremia, *Kidney Int.* **14:**340.
44. Kopple, J. D., Swendseid, M. E., Shinaberger, J. H., and Umezawa, C. Y., 1973, The free and bound amino acids removed by hemodialysis, *Tr. Am. Soc. Artif. Intern. Organs* **19:**309.
45. Lefebvre, P. J., Luyckx, A. S., and Nizet, A. H., 1974, Renal handling of endogenous glucagon in the dog: Comparison with insulin, *Metabolism* **23**(8)**:**753.
46. Lehninger, A., 1978, *Biochemistry*, 2nd ed. New York, Worth.
47. Levine, B. S., Brautbar, N., and Coburn, J. W., 1978, Does vitamin D affect the renal handling of calcium and phosphorus? *Miner. Electrolyte Metab.* **1:**295.

48. Lewin, L. M., and Sulimovici, S., 1975, Distribution and metabolism of radioactive myoinositol in the male rat, *Isr. J. Med. Sci.* **11**(11):1178.
49. Lindstedt, G., 1967, Hydroxylation of γ-butyrobetaine to carnitine in rat liver, *Biochemistry* **6**(5):1271.
50. Linton, A. L., Clark, W. F., Dreidger, A. A., Werb, R. M., and Lindsay, R., 1977, Correctable factors contributing to the anemia of dialysis patients, *Nephron* **19**:95.
51. Liveson, J. A., Gardner, J., and Bornstein, M. B., 1977, Tissue culture studies of possible uremic neurotoxins: Myoinositol, *Kidney Int.* **12**:131.
52. Longnecker, R. E., Goffinet, J. A., and Hendler, E. D., 1974, Blood loss during maintenance hemodialysis. *Tr. Am. Soc. Artif. Intern. Organs* **20**:135.
53. Mauron, J., Mottu, F., and Spohr, G., 1972, Reciprocal induction and repression of serine dehydratase and phosphoglycerate dehydrogenase by proteins and dietary essential amino acids in rat liver, *Eur. J. Biochem.* **32**:331.
54. Mawer, E. B., Backhouse, J., and Taylor, C. M., 1973, Failure of formation of 1,25-dihydroxycholecalciferol in chronic renal insufficiency, *Lancet* **1**:626.
55. Merrill, J., 1965, *The Treatment of Renal Failure*, 2nd ed., Grune & Stratton, New York.
56. Merrill, R. H., and Tasch, R., 1976, Iron absorption in hemodialyzed patients, *Tr. Am. Soc. Artif. Intern. Organs* **22**:69.
57. Nsouli, K. A., Lazarus, M., Schoenbaum, S., Gottlieb, M. N., Lowrie, E. G., and Shocair, M., 1979, Bacteremic infection in hemodialysis, *Arch. Intern. Med.* **139**:1255.
58. Pitkanen, E., 1972, The serum polyol pattern and the urinary polyol excretion in diabetic and uremic patients, *Clin. Chim. Acta* **38**:221.
59. Pitkanen, E., 1976, Changes in serum and urinary myo-inositol levels in chronic glomerulonephritis, *Clin. Chim. Acta* **71**:461.
60. Pitts, R. F., and MacLeod, M. B., 1972, Synthesis of serine by the dog kidney *in vivo, Am. J. Physiol.* **222**(2):394.
61. Ponchon, G., and DeLuca, H. R., 1969, The role of the liver in the metabolism of vitamin D, *J. Clin. Invest.* **48**:1273.
62. Raisz, L. G., Trummel, C. L., Holick, M. F., and DeLuca, H. F., 1972, 1,25-dihydroxycholecalciferol: A potent stimulator of bone resorption in tissue culture, *Science* **175**:768.
63. Rauschkolb, E. W., Davis, H. W., Feinmore, D. C., Black, H. S., and Fabre, L. F., 1969, Identification of vitamin D_3 in human skin, *J. Invest. Dermatol.* **53**:289.
64. Reaven, G. M., Weisinger, J. R., and Swenson, R. S., 1974, Insulin and glucose metabolism in renal insufficiency, *Kidney Int.* **6**(suppl. I):S63.
65. Rebouche, C. J., and Engel, A. G., 1980, Tissue distribution of carnitine biosynthetic enzymes in man, *Biochim. Biophys. Acta* **630**:22.
66. Reid, I. A., Morris, B. J., and Ganong, W. F., 1978, The renin–angiotensin system, *Ann. Rev. Physiol.* **40**:337.
67. Relman, A. S., 1972, Metabolic consequences of acid–base disorders, *Kidney Int.* **1**:347.
68. Rubenstein, A. H., and Spitz, I., 1968, Role of the kidney in insulin metabolism and excretion, *Diabetes* **17**:(3):161.
69. Rudman, D., Sewell, C. W., and Ansley, J. D., 1977, Deficiency of carnitine in cachectic cirrhotic patients, *J. Clin. Invest.* **60**:716.
70. Ryan, J. W., 1967, Renin-like enzyme in the adrenal gland, *Science* **158**:1589.
71. Salter, J. M., Ezrin, C., Laidlow, J. C., and Gornall, A. G., 1960, Metabolic effects of glucagon in human subjects, *Metabolism* **9**:753.
72. Schacter, D., Finkelstein, J. D., and Kowarski, S., 1965, Metabolism of vitamin D. I. Preparation of radioactive vitamin D and its intestinal absorption in the rat, *J. Clin. Invest.* **43**:787.
73. Schambelan, M., and Stockigt, J. R., 1979, Pathophysiology of the renin–angiotensin system, *in: Hormonal Function and the Kidney* (D. Brenner and J. Stein, eds.), pp. 1–39. London, Churchill, Livingstone.
74. Sorenson, M. K., and Kopple, J. D., 1968, Assessment of adherence to protein-restricted diets during conservative management of uremia, *Am. J. Clin. Nutr.* **21**(6):631.

75. Spannuth, C. L., Jr., Warnock, L. G., Wagner, C., and Stone, W. J., 1977, Increased plasma clearance of pyridoxal 5′phosphate in vitamin B_6 deficient uremic man, *J. Lab. Clin. Med.* **90**(4):632.
76. Stanbury, S. W., 1977, The role of vitamin D in renal bone disease, *Clin. Endocrinol.* **7**:25S.
77. Stewart, W. K., Fleming, L. W., and Manuel, M. A., 1972, Muscle cramps during maintenance hemodialysis, *Lancet* **2**:1049.
78. Stoffel, W., 1971, Sphingolipids, *Ann. Rev. Biochem.* **40**:57.
79. Tanaka, T., 1965, Metabolic regulation of serine and gluconeogenesis in higher animals, *Tampakushitsu Kakusan Koso* **10**(7):668.
80. Unger, R. H., 1971, Glucagon physiology and pathophysiology, *N. Engl. J. Med.* **285**(8):443.
81. Vandyke, D. H., Griggs, R. C., Markesbery, W., and DiMauro, S., 1975, Hereditary carnitine deficiency of muscle, *Neurology* **25**:154.
82. Van Pilsum, J. F., Stephens, G. C., and Taylor, D., 1972, Distribution of creatine, guanidinoacetate and the enzymes for the biosynthesis in the animal kingdom, *Biochem. J.* **126**:325.
83. Varandani, P. T., 1973, Insulin degradation IV. Sequential degradation of insulin by rat kidney, heart and skeletal muscle homogenates, *Biochim. Biophys. Acta* **295**:630.
84. Varandani, P. T., and Shroyer, L. A., 1977, A rat kidney neutral peptidase that degrades B chain of insulin, glucagon, and ACTH: Purification by affinity chromatography and some properties, *Arch. Biochem. Biophys.* **181**:82.
85. Walker, J. B., 1979, Creatine: Biosynthesis, regulation and function, *Adv. Enzymol.* **50**:177.
86. Walling, M. S., 1977, Intestinal calcium and phosphate transport: Differential responses to vitamin D_3 metabolites, *Am. J. Physiol.* **233**:E448.
87. White, A., Handler, P., and Smith, E., 1973, *Principles of Biochemistry*, 5th ed. New York, McGraw–Hill.
88. Zimmerman, E. W., Meisinger, E., Weinel, B., and Strauch, M., 1979, Essential amino acid/Ketoanalogue supplementation: An alternative to unrestricted protein intake in uremia, *Clin. Nephrol.* **11**(2):71.

57

Can Low-Protein Diet Retard the Progression of Chronic Renal Failure?

Jonas Bergström, Marianne Ahlberg, and Anders Alvestrand

1. Introduction

Patients with advanced renal failure who exhibit symptoms of uremia may experience symptomatic relief concomitantly with a decrease in blood urea concentration when the dietary protein intake is reduced. Treatment with low-protein diet (LPD) in chronic uremia may significantly prolong life and postpone the mandatory time for start of chronic dialysis. Marked protein restriction (15–20 g protein per day) may be required to control uremia when glomerular filtration rate is reduced to 2–10% of normal. At such low protein intakes essential amino acids (EAA) or their N-free keto analogues (KAA) have to be furnished along with the diet to fulfill nutritional requirements and to prevent depletion of body protein (Bergström *et al.*, 1975; Walser, 1975).

It was suggested earlier that protein reduction not only affords symptomatic relief in patients with chronic renal failure but also may improve renal function (Levin and Cade, 1965) or may slow the rate of progression of renal failure (Kluthe *et al.*, 1971). Mitch *et al.* (1976) reported that, in most cases of chronic renal insufficiency, the reciprocal of serum creatinine declines linearly with time as renal failure progresses. This observation makes it possible to estimate the effect of therapy on progression. Using this method, Walser *et al.* (1979) showed that the progression of the renal insuffciency was halted or retarded in several patients when treatment with LPD supplemented with KAA was instituted. Similar results were reported by Barsotti *et al.* (1981), who measured creatinine clearance repeatedly in their patients.

Jonas Bergström, Marianne Ahlberg, and Anders Alvestrand • Department of Renal Medicine, Karolinska Institute, S-104 01 Stockholm, Sweden, and Huddinge University Hospital, S-141 86 Huddinge, Sweden.

Prompted by these observations we decided to make a retrospective analysis of our own patients with chronic renal failure who were treated with a protein-restricted diet (15–20 g/day) supplemented with EAA or KAA to find out whether the progression of renal failure had been influenced by this treatment.

2. *Material and Methods*

To evaluate progression of renal failure the inverse of serum creatinine was plotted against time. If the progression of renal disease is altered, the slope of the line (regression coefficient) will change. To include a patient in our study, the criteria were that the reciprocal of creatinine declined approximately linearly with time before the diet was changed and that there were at least eight creatinine determinations performed over a period of 200 days before as well as during LPD. Of all patients treated with LPD and EAA or KAA over the period 1975–1980, 17 fulfilled these requirements. The diagnoses were as follows: chronic glomerulonephritis in two patients, chronic pyelonephritis in three patients, analgesic nephropathy in two patients, congenital renal dysplasia in one patient, and polycystic kidney disease in nine patients.

Before the patients were switched to LPD they had either no protein restriction or were ordered a diet containing 60 or 40 g protein per day. The prescribed LPD diet contained 15–20 g protein per day (Noree and Bergström, 1975) and was supplemented orally in 14 cases with EAA (Aminess®, AB Vitrum, or a modified EAA preparation) (Alvestrand *et al.*, 1982), and in three cases with a KAA preparation containing the keto analogues of valine, isoleucine, leucine, and phenylalanine, the hydroxy analogue of methionine, and the amino acids threonine, lysine, histidine, and tryptophan (Ketoperlen®, Pfrimmer AG).

All patients received aluminum hydroxide gel or tablets before as well as during treatment with LPD, and the dose was adjusted to keep the plasma phosphate concentration within normal range (below 1.8 mmoles/liter). Oral calcium carbonate, 1–3 g/day, was given to most of the patients to prevent a negative calcium balance. Apart from a minor dose of vitamin D_3 (250 IU) included in a multivitamin preparation, no patients received vitamin D or its analogues.

The LPD which contained about 500 mg Na^+ per day was generally supplemented with NaCl powder, 2–4 g/day, to improve palatability. $NaHCO_3$ was given to prevent acidosis. We aimed at keeping the plasma bicarbonate concentration at or above 22 mmol/liter. Furosemide was given as required to prevent sodium overload and to control hypertension. Additional antihypertensive therapy was prescribed when indicated.

Each patient was checked at our outpatient clinic during the initial observation period as well as during treatment with LPD, usually by the

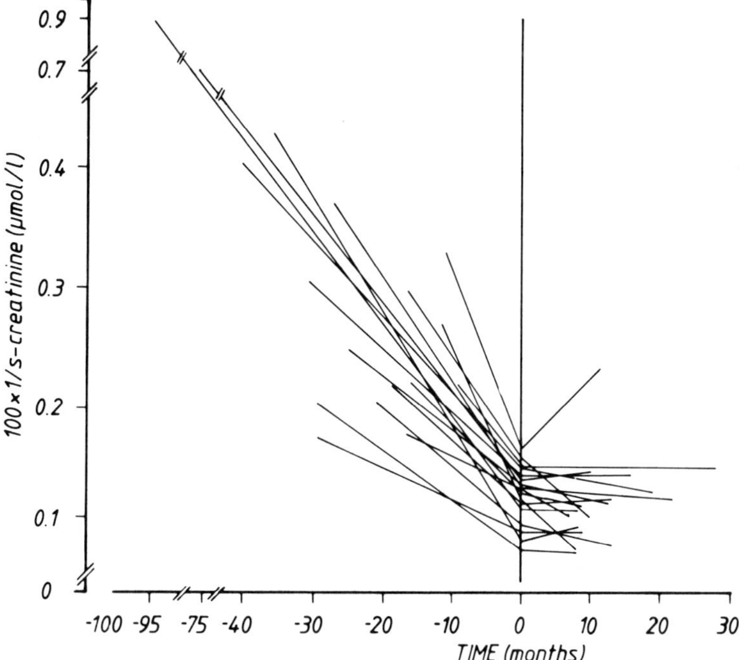

Figure 1. Regression lines of the reciprocal of the serum creatinine versus time in 17 patients before and during treatment with LPD supplemented with EAA or KAA. The patients were switched to LPD at time 0.

same physician. The principles for control of fluid and electrolyte balance and blood pressure were the same in both periods.

3. Results

Figure 1 shows the regression lines of the reciprocal of serum creatinine versus time in the 17 patients before and after introduction of the LPD. In most cases the slope of the regression line (regression coefficient) decreased markedly after switching to the LPD. The mean regression coefficient ±S.E.M. before LPD was -0.230 ± 0.026 and during LPD -0.022 ± 0.020 ($p < 0.001$). A typical curve in an individual case is seen in Fig. 2. In eight cases the improvement in renal function appeared to be associated with a decrease in serum phosphate, whereas in three cases progression of renal disease was retarded in spite of a significant increase in serum phosphate. In the whole group the plasma phosphate concentration was slightly lower during LPD (1.47 ± 0.29 mmoles/liter) than before (1.63 ± 0.24 mmoles/liter, $p < 0.052$). Plasma calcium was significantly higher during LPD (2.34 ± 0.11 mmoles/liter) than before (2.22 ± 0.15 mmoles/liter, $p < 0.001$), but the Ca X P product was not significantly different. Improved blood pressure control

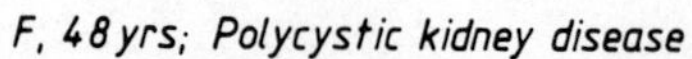

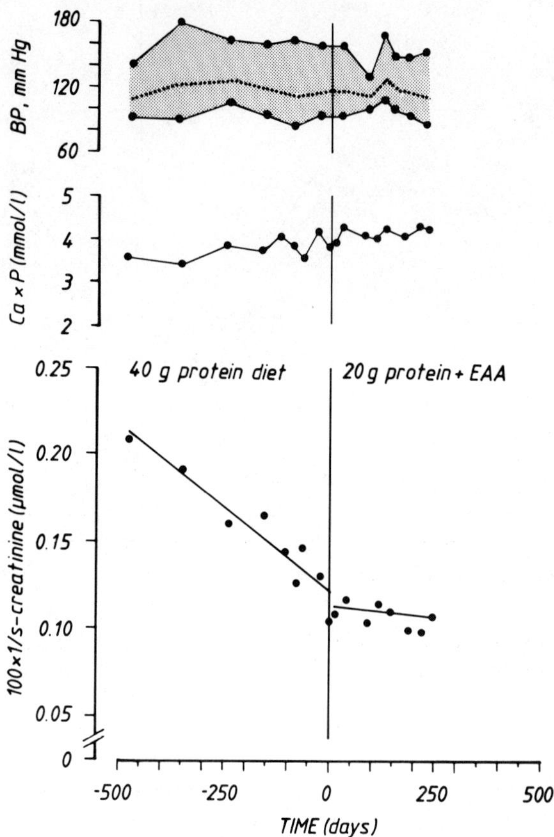

Figure 2. The reciprocal of the serum creatinine versus time in a patient treated with LPD and EAA. Blood pressure was not different and Ca × P product was higher during LPD than before.

may also influence the progression of renal disease. However, in these patients blood pressure control was not any better during than before LPD.

4. *Discussion*

The results of this study are in keeping with previous observations that LPD may slow the progression of chronic renal failure. However, our results must be evaluated with caution owing to the fact that the study was retrospective and thus was not conducted in a controlled manner. In most cases clinical and laboratory checkups were more frequent during treatment with LPD than before. There is, thus, a possibility that improved patient care during LPD with regard to control of hypertension, fluid and electrolyte

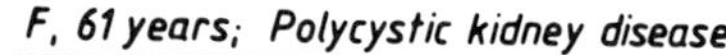

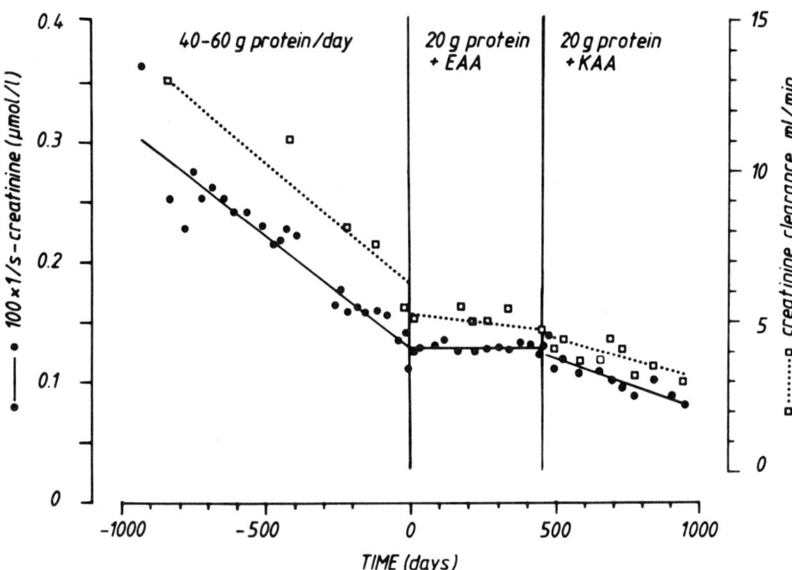

Figure 3. The reciprocal of the serum creatinine and creatinine clearance, respectively, versus time. In this patient progression of chronic renal failure was halted during LPD and EAA, but renal failure deteriorated further during a following period on LPD and KAA.

balance, infections, and other factors might have affected the results, although we found no evidence that this was the case. Furthermore, evaluation of renal function by following the reciprocal of serum creatinine is questionable since a decrease in muscle mass due to protein depletion and inactivity may reduce creatinine production, and extrarenal elimination of creatinine may be enhanced with the severity of renal failure (Mitch *et al.*, 1980). However, creatinine clearance data available in some of our patients (see Fig. 3) supported the validity of conclusions drawn from the curves of reciprocal of serum creatinine with time.

The mechanisms by which LPD may slow the progression of renal failure in man have not been elucidated. Since the phosphate content in LPD is generally low, it was suggested that improved control of serum phosphate might be involved (Walser *et al.*, 1979). In support of this explanation are reports in subtotally nephrectomized rats (Ibels *et al.*, 1978) and in rats with nephrotoxic serum nephritis (Karlinsky *et al.*, 1980) that a low-phosphate diet may prevent deterioration of renal function. However, Barrientos *et al.* (1982) did not find that improved control of serum phosphate by low-phosphate diet and 12 g aluminum hydroxide per day had any effect on progression of renal failure in patients with chronic renal disease. The protein content of their low-phosphate and control diets was not given. Our own data do not support the suggestion that improved control serum phosphate by LPD is the only mechanism by which LPD exerts its effect on progression of renal failure, since in some of our patients LPD had an effect in spite of enhanced phosphate retention.

Hostetter *et al.* (1982) have speculated that the final common outcome of chronic renal disease, i.e., predictable progression from mild renal insufficiency to end-stage renal failure independent of the etiology of the initial injury, depends on some critical loss of renal mass. Compensatory raised glomerular pressures and flows would underlie the ultimate sclerotic destruction of those nephrons which survive the initial renal insult. In partially nephrectomized rats severe restriction of dietary protein intake could partly prevent glomerular hyperfiltration and reduce the structural abnormalities in remnant glomeruli (Hostetter *et al.*, 1981). This effect was apparently not dependent on improved phosphate control since the phosphate contents of the LPD and control diet were comparable. These data suggest that protein restriction *per se* or some factor associated with protein restriction (except reduced phosphate intake) is operative. It should be pointed out that the effect of protein restriction on glomerular hyperfiltration in remnant nephrons was found in rats with experimental renal failure but that there is a lack of evidence that the same mechanism is operating in human renal disease. If this were the case, one might expect that switching to more marked protein restriction would result in an immediate decrease in glomerular filtration rate and, thus, an increase in serum creatinine, a phenomenon not observed by us or reported by others.

In conclusion, available clinical data from different groups, although anecdotal or not well controlled, strongly suggest that progression of end-stage renal failure in man may be retarded or halted by LPD supplemented with EAA or KAA. This may have important clinical implications in the future, especially if it can be shown that this principle of treatment is operative in early renal failure as well. Prospective, randomized studies are now required to confirm the present findings and to evaluate by which mechanisms protein restriction affects progression of renal failure.

References

Alvestrand, A., Fürst, P., and Bergström, J., 1982, Plasma and muscle free amino acids in uremia: Influence of nutrition with amino acids, *Clin. Nephrol.* **18:**297.

Barrientos, A., Arteaga, J., Rodicio, J. L., Alvarez Ude, F., Alcazar, J. M., and Ruilope, L. M., 1982, Role of control of phosphate in the progression of chronic renal failure, *Min. Elec. Metab* **7:**127.

Barsotti, G., Guiducci, A., Ciardella, F., and Giovannetti, S., 1981, Effects on renal function of a low-nitrogen diet supplemented with essential amino acids and ketoanalogues and of hemodialysis and free protein supply in patients with chronic renal failure, *Nephron* **27:**113.

Bergström, J., Fürst, P., and Noree, L. O., 1975, Treatment of chronic uremic patients with protein-poor diet and oral supply of essential amino acids, I. Nitrogen balance studies, *Clin. Nephrol.* **3:**187.

Hostetter, T. H., Olson, J. L., Rennke, H. G., Venkatachalam, M. A., and Brenner, B. M., 1981, Hyperfiltration in remnant nephrons: A potentially adverse response to renal ablation, *Am. J. Physiol.* **241:**F85.

Hostetter, T. H., Rennke, H. G., and Brenner, B. M., 1982, Compensatory renal hemodynamic injury: A final common pathway of residual nephron destruction, *Am. J. Kidney Dis.* **1**:310.

Ibels, L. S., Alfrey, A. C., Haut, L., and Huffer, W. E., 1978, Preservation of function in experimental renal disease by dietary restriction of phosphate, *N. Engl. J. Med.* **298**:122.

Karlinsky, M. L., Haut, L., Buddington, B., Schrier, N. A., and Altrey, A. C., 1980, Preservation of renal function in experimental glomerulonephritis, *Kidney Int.* **17**:293.

Kluthe, R., Oeschlen, D., Quirin, H., and Jedinsky, H. J., 1971, Six years experience with a special low-protein diet, in: *Uremia, International Conference on Pathogenesis, Diagnosis and Therapy* (R. Kluthe, G. Berlyne, and B. Burton, eds.), Georg Thieme, Stuttgart.

Levin, D. M., and Cade, R., 1965, Metabolic effects of dietary protein in chronic renal failure, *Ann. Intern. Med.* **4**:642.

Mitch, W. E., Walser, M., Buffington, G. A., and Lemann, J. Jr., 1976, A simple method of estimating progression of chronic renal failure, *Lancet* **2**:1326.

Mitch, W. E., Collier, V. U., and Walser, M., 1980, Creatinine metabolism in chronic renal failure, *Clin. Sci.* **58**:327.

Noree, L. O., and Bergström, J., 1975, Treatment of chronic uremic patients with protein-poor diet and oral supply of essential amino acids, II. Clinical results of long-term treatment, *Clin. Nephrol.* **3**:195.

Walser, M., 1975, Ketoacids in the treatment of uremia, *Clin. Nephrol.* **3**:180.

Walser, M., Mitch, W. E., and Collier, V. U., 1979, The effect of nutritional therapy on the course of chronic renal failure, *Clin. Nephrol.* **11**:66.

58

Evaluation of Amino Acid Requirements in Uremia by Determination of Intracellular Free-Amino-Acid Concentrations in Muscle

Jonas Bergström, Anders Alvestrand, and Peter Fürst

Many studies have documented abnormal plasma concentrations of amino acids in patient with chronic renal failure (Gulyassy *et al.*, 1968; Young and Parsons, 1969; Giordano *et al.*, 1970; Swendseid and Kopple, 1973). Typical findings are low concentrations of several essential amino acids and high concentrations of some nonessential amino acids. Certain abnormalities appear to be caused by renal failure whereas others, resembling those observed in subjects with low intake of protein and energy, may be related to malnutrition.

In uremia the distribution of some amino acids between the extra- and intracellular compartments is altered (Shear, 1969; Bergström *et al.*, 1978; Alvestrand *et al.*, 1978). Therefore, the plasma concentrations do not necessarily reflect the intracellular concentrations. Skeletal muscle contains the largest pool of free amino acids, and determination of the free-amino-acid concentration in muscle is therefore of particular interest in the study of amino acid metabolism in uremic patients. Bergström *et al.* (1978) reported low intracellular concentrations of threonine, valine, lysine, and tyrosine and increased concentrations of several nonessential amino acids in untreated uremic patients (Fig. 1). However, intracellular leucine and isoleucine concentrations were normal in the presence of reduced plasma concentrations of these amino acids.

The abnormalities among the branched-chain amino acids (BCAA) valine, isoleucine, and leucine persisted during long-term treatment with a

Jonas Bergström, Anders Alvestrand, and Peter Fürst • Department of Renal Medicine, Karolinska Institute, S-104 01 Stockholm, Sweden, and Huddinge University Hospital, S-141 86 Huddinge, Sweden.

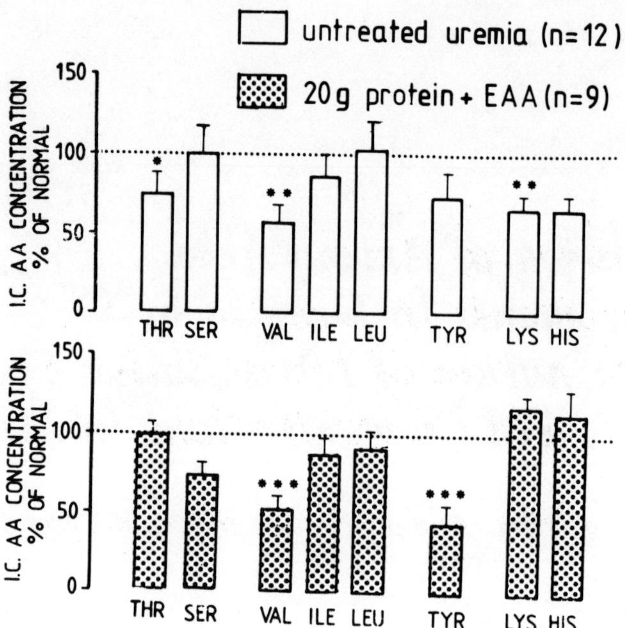

Figure 1. Selected muscle intracellular amino acids in patients with near end-stage renal failure, untreated, and long-term treated with 15–20 g protein per day, essential amino acids in Rose's proportion, histidine (EAA), mean ± S.E.

low-protein diet (16–20 g protein per day) (LPD) supplemented with an essential-amino-acid preparation providing 2–3 times the minimum requirements for normal man (Rose, 1949) and histidine (EAA) (Fig. 1).

Selective valine depletion in spite of a high intake of valine would require that this amino acid be preferentially catabolized. This might lead to a relative excess and an abnormal distribution of the other two BCAAs, a so-called amino acid antagonism (Fig. 2). It is of interest that the BCAA pattern in uremia partly resembles that of rats fed a low-protein diet containing an excess of leucine, in which case the antagonism results in impaired growth and reduced nitrogen utilization (Shinnic and Harper, 1977). Hence it is possible that uremic patients may require different proportions of the BCAA as compared to normals in order to optimize nitrogen utilization and to overcome the antagonism between the BCAA.

Low intracellular tyrosine concentrations also were observed after treatment with LPD plus EAA in Rose's proportions and histidine (Fig. 1). Reduced production of tyrosine from phenylalanine in uremia may underlie this abnormality (Young and Parsons, 1973; Tizianello *et al.*, 1980).

In an attempt to compensate for the depletion in muscle-free valine and tyrosine pools, a new amino acid formula (NAAF) was designed in which the relative proportion of valine was increased and tyrosine was added. The composition of Aminess® and the new formula is given in Fig. 3. The effects

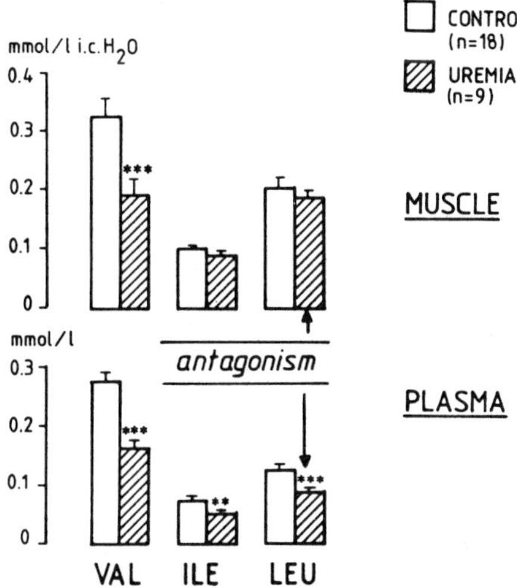

Figure 2. Branched-chain amino acid antagonism in uremic patients.

on muscle and plasma amino acid concentrations was studied in eight patients on long-term treatment (52–211 days) with LPD and NAAF (Fig. 4) (Alvestrand *et al.*, 1982).

With the new amino acid preparation intracellular valine and tyrosine concentrations were not significantly different from normal, although the intracellular tyrosine concentration was still to some extent reduced (Fig. 4).

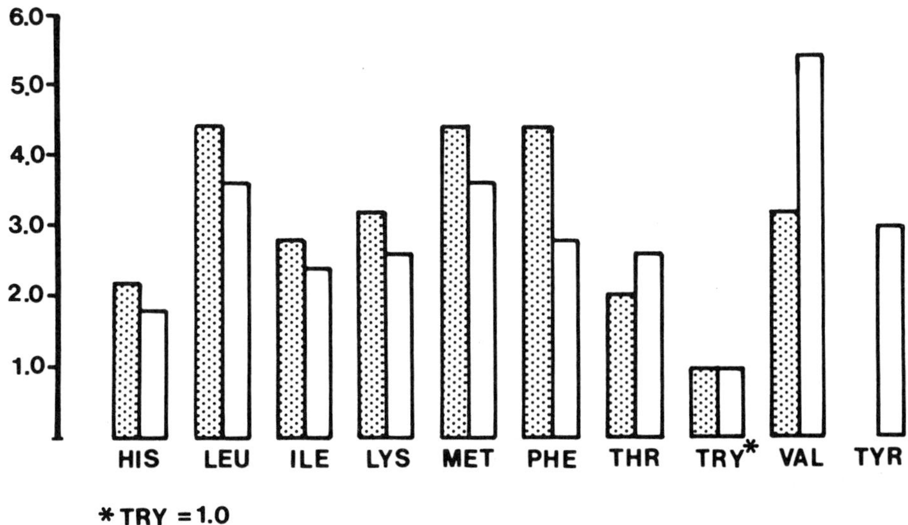

Figure 3. Comparison of the amino acid composition of Aminess® (stippled) and the new formula.

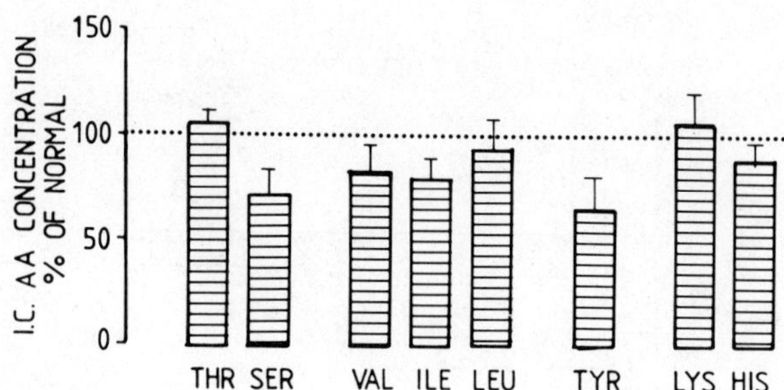

Figure 4. Muscle intracellular amino acids after long-term treatment with the modified amino acid preparation ($N = 8$).

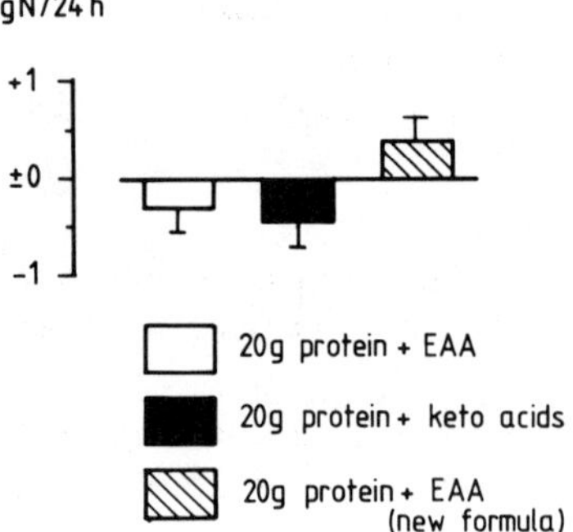

Figure 5. Nitrogen balance in patients treated with LPD supplemented with essential amino acids in Rose's proportions and histidine (EAA), with a preparation containing ketoanalogues and essential amino acids (Ketoperlen®, Pfrimmer AG), and with the modified amino acid preparation (EAA, new formula).

Our results suggest that the free-amino-acid inadequacy of uremia may be overcome with more adequate nutrition which takes the intracellular free-amino-acid abnormalities into consideration.

An obvious question is whether improvement of the intracellular amino acid profile in uremia is beneficial with regard to nitrogen utilization. We believe that this is the case since nitrogen balance in patients with chronic uremia on long-term treatment with LPD was better maintained by supplementation with NAAF than with EAA in Rose's proportions and histidine (Fig. 5) (Alvestrand *et al.*, 1983).

References

Alvestrand, A., Bergström, J., Fürst, P., Germanis, G., and Widstam, U., 1978, The effect of essential amino acid supplementation on muscle and plasma free amino acids in chronic uremia, *Kidney Int.* **14:**323.

Alvestrand, A., Fürst, P., and Bergström, J., 1982, Plasma and muscle free amino acids in uremia: Effect of nutrition with amino acids, *Clin. Nephrol.* **18:**297.

Alvestrand, A., Ahlberg, M., Fürst, P., and Bergström, J., 1983, Clinical results of long-term treatment with a low protein diet and a new amino acid preparation in patients with chronic uremia, *Clin. Nephrol.* **19:**67.

Bergström, J., Fürst, P., Noree, L. O., and Vinnars, E., 1978, Intracellular free amino acids in muscle tissue of patients with chronic uremia: effect of peritoneal dialysis and infusion of essential amino acids, *Clin. Sci. Mol. Med.* **54:**51.

Giordano, C., De Pascall, C., De Santo, N. G., Esposito, R., Cirilli, C., and Stangherlin, P., 1970, Disorder in the metabolism of some amino acids in uremia, in: *Proceedings of the 4th International Congress of Nephrology* (N. Alwall, F. Berglund, and B. Josephsson, eds.), p. 196, Karger, Basel.

Gulyassy, P. F., Peters, J. H., Lin, S. C., and Ryan, P. M., 1968, Hemodialysis and plasma amino acid composition in chronic renal failure, *Am. J. Clin. Nutr.* **21:**565.

Rose, E. C., 1949, Amino acid requirements of man, *Fed. Proc.* **8:**546.

Shear, L., 1969, Internal redistribution of tissue protein synthesis in uremia, *J. Clin. Invest.* **48:**1252.

Shinnic, F. L., and Harper, E. A., 1977, Effects of branched-chain amino acid antagonism in the rat on tissue amino acid and ketoacid concentration, *J. Nutr.* **107:**887.

Swendseid, M. E., and Kopple, J. D., 1973, Nitrogen balance, plasma amino acid level and amino acid requirements, *Tr. N.Y. Acad. Sci.* **35:**471.

Tizianello, A., DeFerrari, G., Baribotto, G., Gurreri, G., and Robando, C., 1980, Renal metabolism of amino acids and ammonia in subjects with normal renal function and in patients with chronic renal insufficiency, *J. Clin. Invest.* **65:**1162.

Young, G. A., and Parsons, F. M., 1969, The effect of peritoneal dialysis upon the amino acids and other nitrogenous compounds in the blood and dialysates from patients with renal failure, *Clin. Sci.* **37:**1.

Young, G. A., and Parsons, F. M., 1973, Impairment of phenylalanine hydroxylation in chronic renal insufficiency, *Clin. Sci. Mol. Med.* **45:**88.

59

Nutritional Management of Chronic Renal Failure for Two Purposes: Postponing Onset and Reducing Frequency of Dialysis

Ralph A. Nelson, C. F. Anderson, James C. Hunt, and Joyce Margie

1. Introduction

A program to offer nutritional support to patients with chronic renal failure (CRF) was developed in the early 1970s, representing a joint effort between disciplines of nutrition and nephrology for the purpose of postponing the need for dialysis or kidney transplantation.[1] Objectives of the program were

1. To retard or inhibit progression from chronic renal failure to end-stage renal disease (ESRD).
2. To keep patients working, out of the hospital, and living a useful life.
3. To postpone the psychosocial problems associated with entry into a dialysis or transplant program.
4. To save money.
5. To use available food or not to resort to highly purified mixtures of essential amino acids.

In the early 1960s, Giordano's work using essential amino acids opened a new era in nutritional support for chronic renal failure.[2] Later, Giovannetti

Ralph A. Nelson • Division of Research, Carle Foundation Hospital, and College of Medicine, University of Illinois, Urbana, Illinois 68101. ***C. F. Anderson*** • Department of Medicine, Mayo Medical School, Rochester, Minnesota 55905. ***James C. Hunt*** • University of Tennessee, Memphis, Tennessee 38163. ***Joyce Margie*** • Summit, New Jersey 07901.

and Maggiore developed a diet using foods deficient in protein for 5–10 days followed by supplementation with essential amino acids or egg albumin.[3] Diets developed in subsequent years by Shaw, Berlyne, and their associates were restricted to low-protein diets containing 18–21 g daily regardless of the body weight of the patient.[4,5]

The present program prescribed dietary protein at a level of 0.38 g/kg body weight. This figure was chosen because Scrimshaw and colleagues had shown that 0.38 g/kg of high-biologic-value protein would maintain nitrogen equilibrium in healthy young men if enough calories were consumed so that a small gain in body weight occurred daily.[6]

2. *Diet*

The diet program permitted individualization of meals and meal plans for patients with a variety of kidney disease. Recipes were developed that used available foods plus newly developed food products. Further, meal planning for the patients was integrated into meal planning for the family so that preparation of separate foods was kept to a minimum.[7,8]

The meal plan was divided into the following nine food groups:

1. Meat and meat substitutes
2. Milk and milk products
3. Bread and bread substitutes
4. Low-protein products
5. Fats
6. Vegetables
7. Fruits
8. Carbohydrate supplements
9. Beverages

2.1. *Calories*

The diet prescription and meal plans were developed for daily calorie levels between 2500 and 2600. For most patients, these calorie levels were sufficient to produce a daily gain in weight. When additional calories were required, nonprotein sources were added. When weight reduction was required (a rare occurrence), calorie-deficient diets were prescribed.

2.2. *Protein*

High-biologic-value protein was prescribed at 0.38 g/kg body weight. Eggs, meat, and milk products were considered as having the highest biologic value with bread, cereal, vegetables, and fruit having lower scores. However, it was also appreciated that a mixture of two sources of vegetable protein such as bread and peanut butter also gave a high-biologic-value protein source.

2.3. Fat

Fat content in the diet amounted to 30% of total calories. Foods low in cholesterol were chosen. Dietary cholesterol could easily be reduced to 300 mg/day or less for those patients with hypercholesterolemia. The polyunsaturated-to-saturated fatty acid ratio was 0.7. This permitted sufficient polyunsaturated fatty acids to be in the diet to meet essential-fatty-acid requirements while exerting a cholesterol-lowering effect.[9]

2.4. Carbohydrates

Carbohydrate content of the diet amounted to 65% of total calories. Complex carbohydrates were used as much as possible.

2.5. Minerals

Diets contained 20, 40, or 90 mEq sodium per day. Potassium content was 45 mEq/day for protein diets of 30 g or less. The diet was deficient in calcium and phosphorus.[10] However, low phosphorus content was considered advantageous in light of problems associated with phosphorus in this group of patients.

2.6. Vitamins

Diets were deficient in vitamin A, thiamine, niacin, riboflavin, and folic acid content.[8]

2.7. Trace Metals

Diets were deficient in iron (Fe), copper (Cu), magnesium (Mg), and zinc (Zn).[11]

2.8. Water

Fluid content of the diet was approximately 1500 ml total volume per day. Requirements of 1 ml water per kilocalorie were easily met. Patients who could form urine easily were instructed to drink enough water to make 2 liters of urine per day.

2.9. Supplements

1. *Nonprotein sources of calories.* A carbohydrate supplement was used to increase daily calories without changing total protein content. In those patients with elevated serum triglycerides, a fat supplement was substituted.[8]
2. *Calcium supplement* was ordered in relation to serum and dietary calcium.[7]

3. *Vitamin and trace metals.* A prenatal vitamin preparation was prescribed which contained daily recommended or suggested allowances of vitamins and trace elements.

Thus, an 80-kg man would be prescribed the following daily diet:

Calories:	2600 plus carbohydrate supplement to bring total level to 3000
Protein:	30 g
Fat:	85 g, P/S ratio 0.7, cholesterol less than 300 mg/day
Carbohydrate:	410 g plus carbohydrate supplement of 400 calories/day
Sodium:	90 mEq
Potassium:	45 mEq
Calcium:	400 mg
Phosphorus:	575 mg
Vitamins:	Deficient in water and fat-soluble vitamins
Trace minerals:	Deficient in Mg, Fe, Cu, Zn

Calcium, vitamin, and trace mineral supplements were added.

3. Patients

Fifteen patients who desired the nutrition support program were entered regardless of their associated diseases or complications due to chronic renal failure (Table 1). The patients were treated for hypertension with salt-controlled diets (90, 45, and 27 mEq/day) and drugs if necessary. When indicated, calcium supplements, phosphate binders, and uric-acid-lowering agents were administered.

The rationale for the diet prescription was discussed with each patient by a physician and by a nutritionist. Adherence to the diet was assessed by 7-day food diaries and a 24-hr urine collection for total nitrogen and sodium on the seventh day of the diet diary.

An indirect, but objective, method for determining compliance to the dietary prescription was utilized by comparing nitrogen excretion in urine with calculated nitrogen intake from the 7-day food diary. In our experience, a diary is considered accurate if nitrogen calculated from dietary records is ± 2 g of the nitrogen excreted in the urine.[12]

4. Evaluation of Nutrition Support Program

4.1. Longevity on the Diet

The length of time patients remained on the program varied between 12 and 78 months. None of the patients died. The decision about entry into transplant and/or dialysis programs was reached by discussions between

Table 1. Patients with Chronic Renal Failure

Diagnosis of primary renal disease	Sex	Number	Age
Chronic glomerulonephritis with hypertension	F	2	Range: 30–53 years
Congenital polycystic kidney disease with hypertension	F	2	Average: 41
Fibromuscular dysplasia of renal arteries and hypertension	F	1	
Chronic pyelonephritis, renal papillary necrosis, and kidney atrophy	F	1	
Chronic glomerulonephritis with renal hypertension	M	3	Range: 22–59 years
Congenital polycystic kidney disease (one of whom had renal hypertension)	M	2	Average: 46
Renal hypertension and renal atrophy	M	1	
Progressive glomerulonephritis with renal hypertension	M	1	
Chronic pyelonephritis and renal hypertension	M	1	
Primary hypertension and hypertensive renal disease	M	1	

patients and their attending physician. There were no emergency transfers from the nutrition program to the transplant or dialysis program.

After 1 year, 14 of the 15 patients remained in the nutrition support program. After 24 months, 12 patients continued in the program. After 36 months, six patients remained in the program, and after that, three people continued up to 54 months with one individual remaining on the program for 6½ years.

4.2. Adherence to the Diet

Results of the interviews between the patient, physician, and nutritionist indicated that patients were adhering well to the diet. Food diaries revealed daily calorie intakes between 1800 and 3600, an average protein intake of 0.44 g/kg body weight (range between 0.35 and 0.55), and a sodium intake averaging 51 mEq/day.

Diet diaries were judged to be reliable since nitrogen intake calculated from them was within ± 2 g of 24-hr total nitrogen excretion in urine.[12] In fact, there was no statistical difference between calculated nitrogen and sodium intake from diet records and daily nitrogen and sodium in urine.

4.3. Clinical Response

Patients noted an improved sense of well-being. Body weight increased in ten, remained constant in one, and decreased slightly in four patients. Of

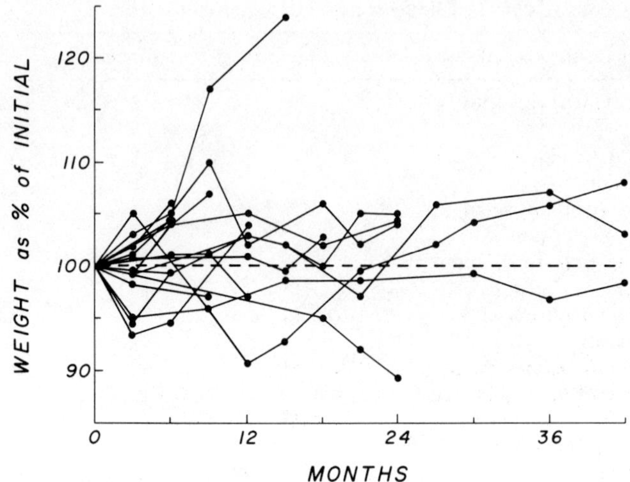

Figure 1. Change in body weight while on diet therapy.

the three patients who remained in the program the longest, two had increased their body weight and one demonstrated a slight reduction of approximately 2% from starting level (Fig. 1).

At the start of the study, excretion of creatinine in urine was 1068 ± 151 mg/24 hr. While patients were on the diet, creatinine excretion averaged 951 ± 125 mg/day. This difference was not statistically significant.

Body composition using dilution of the isotope D_2O in total body water[13] was performed in five patients before and while they were on the diet. Data indicated no significant differences in lean body mass or in body fat measurements. For instance, lean body mass was 51.8 kg at the start and 50.6 kg after 10 months on the diet. Body fat was 14.9 ± 3.2 kg at the start and 16.3 ± 3.5 kg 10 months later.

Blood values (in means) of patients entering the program revealed anemia (hematocrit 32%, hemoglobin 11 g/dl), normal serum proteins but depressed serum albumin (2.91 g/dl), elevated creatinine and urea (7.7 and 135 mg/dl, respectively), and normal calcium, sodium, and potassium. Serum phosphorus was slightly elevated (5.5 mg/dl). Creatinine clearance determined in nine patients at the start of the study averaged 10 ml/min per 1.73 m^2.

While on the diet, blood urea varied between 100 and 188 mg/dl for more than 24 months (Fig. 2). After 1 year, creatinine was 8.3 mg/dl and after 2 years, 11 mg/dl (Fig. 3). Essentially no change in serum creatinine was noted in the three patients who remained with the program 42–78 months (Fig. 3). The urea-to-creatinine ratio decreased from 17 to 12 and remained at 12 or more than 2 years (Fig. 4). At the time of dialysis, serum creatinine was 16.3 (range 8–24) and serum urea was 188 (range 125–260) mg/dl.

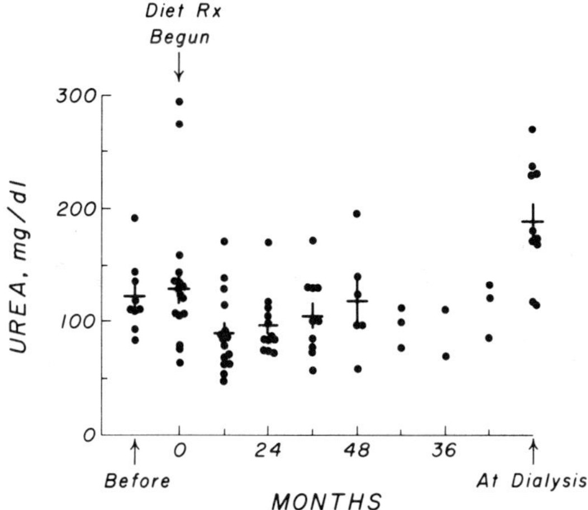

Figure 2. Blood urea (mean ± S.E.) and diet therapy.

While on the program, hematocrit remained fairly constant (varying from 31.5% to 34.3%) although at the time of dialysis it was 24%. Similarly, for hemoglobin, values ranged between 10.4 and 11.8 whereas at the time of dialysis it was 7.2 g/dl. Total proteins varied between 6.92 and 7.21, and at dialysis, they were 6.8 g/dl. Albumin increased, ranging between 3.32 and 3.82, and at the time of dialysis, it was 3.5 g/dl. Phosphorus varied between 4.0 and 5.7 and was 5.9 mg/dl at dialysis. Calcium varied between 9.2 and 9.3 and was 9.4 mg/dl at dialysis.

Serum sodium was 136 meq/dl and potassium 4.9 mEq/dl at the time of dialysis. Both remained within normal limits during the dietary program.

Metabolism, as judged by the basal metabolic rate, remained within normal limits (Table 2). Although no changes occurred in the metabolic rate

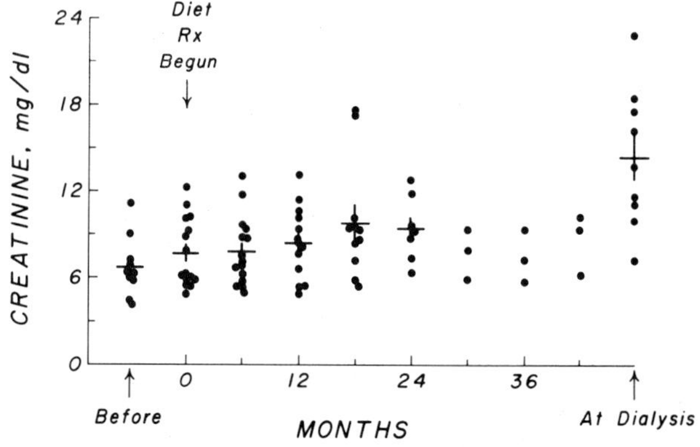

Figure 3. Serum creatinine (mean ± S.E.) and diet therapy.

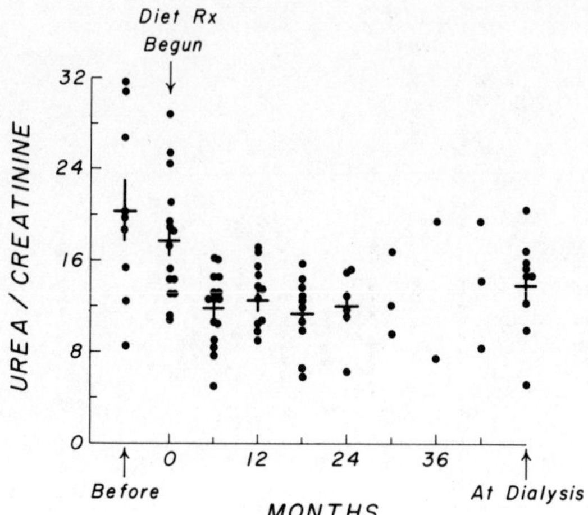

Figure 4. Urea/creatinine ratios (mean ± S.E.) and diet therapy.

or total calories expended per hour, there was a significant decrease in the amount of protein used in basal metabolism. It decreased from 15% to 10% of total calories. Carbohydrate and fat increased slightly representing the dietary substitution of carbohydrates and fat for protein.

5. Discussion

It is difficult to compare clinical results of this diet with results of other diets which have used essential amino acids and/or alpha-keto-acid substitutions. However, it was clear that this nutritional support program accomplished most of its goals for the patients who chose to follow it. While in the program, hospitalization was not required and patients remained working and saved money. All but one patient received at least 12 months of benefits while 12 of 15 patients remained in the program at least 2 years.

Three patients showed no change in their serum creatinine for 42–78 months. This finding supported experience of others (reviewed by Walser) in that nutritional intervention, along with appropriate drug therapy, can

Table 2. Metabolic Data before and during Diet (10 Patients)[a]

	Rate	Total calorie	Percent of calories from		
			CHO	Fat	Protein
Before diet	−7	63	27	58	15
During diet	−9	63	29	61	10[b]

[a] Mean values.
[b] Significant when $p < 0.01$.

retard or even arrest progression of chronic renal disease.[14] Johnson and associates followed 27 patients with early chronic renal failure.[15] They showed in patients who were treated with protein-restricted diets, phosphate binders, and calcium supplements, for hypertension and hyperuricacidemia, that renal osteodystrophy was prevented and serum creatinine remained nearly constant. These patients had several forms of renal disease including diabetic nephropathy.[15] In contrast, Ahlmen showed that 70% of similar patients with serum creatinine of 5 mg/dl and who were given no specific therapy had died or had started dialysis after 12 months.[16]

Most patients in this study improved nutritionally and gained weight while demonstrating an increase in serum albumin.

Dietary compliance appeared related to motivational factors such as being able to remain at work to save money, and to stay away from complicated procedures that appeared life threatening to them and their families. There were other factors as well. For instance, patients experienced an almost immediate sense of well-being once they became adjusted to the diet. Since most patients were encouraged to eat at least 2600 kcal/day, the diet was much easier to follow than a weight-reduction diet, for instance.

The ratio of blood urea to creatinine declined during diet therapy. Without restriction of protein, urea and creatinine ratios tend to remain constant or increase. Our studies of hibernating bears have shown that for bears to hibernate successfully, urea-to-creatinine ratio must decrease from between 30 to 40 to less than 10.[17] In this study, the urea-to-creatinine ratio in many of the patients decreased below 10. We presumed this to be beneficial, signifying that more successful handling of nitrogenous end products was operative.

Patients were removed from the study pending decision between the patient and his attending physician. None of the patients were removed from the study for emergency purposes. Some patients eventually found the program tiresome, others became candidates for transplantation, and others felt, along with the attending physician's advice, that perhaps it would be better to go onto dialysis. The worsening in laboratory values prior to dialysis reflected these factors along with probable progression of renal failure.

On the other hand, some patients preferred to stay on the diet as long as possible. In one patient, creatinine clearance became less than 3 ml/min. However, he continued to work as a steelworker and had taken a trip to Australia prior to entering a transplant program. It was necessary to convince this patient to enter the transplant program.

Feeding dietary protein at levels of 0.38 g/kg body weight per day along with a balanced 2600-calorie diet postponed the need for dialysis or transplantation in 15 patients for periods of time up to 78 months. The diet proved safe if its low protein content was coupled with adequate calorie intake which induced a slight daily incremental increase in body weight. Compliance was excellent. No patients died. All eventually entered transplantation and dialysis programs as an elective choice.

Table 3. Examples of a Diet Prescription[a]

Insensible water loss	672 g/day
Metabolic water	192 g/day
Water in food	460 g/day
Energy	1900 kcal/day
Protein	20 g/day
Fat	88 g/day
Carbohydrate	249 g/day
Sodium	46 mEq/day
Potassium	18 mg/day
Phosphorus	351 mg/day
Calcium	180 mg/day
Vitamins	Deficient in vitamin A, thiamine, riboflavin, niacin, and vitamin C
Trace minerals	Deficient in Mg, Cu, Fe, Zn

[a] Average values.[19] Calcium supplement and vitamin and trace metal supplement added to supply daily recommended or suggested allowances.

6. *Nutritional Management to Reduce Frequency of Dialysis*

Diets were further refined for people already on dialysis for the purpose of reducing the number of dialyses required each week[18,19](Table 3). In one sense, this program gave the worst of two possible worlds to the patient: a highly restricted diet and dialysis. Nevertheless, the program appealed to patients both on a short-term (anephric patients awaiting kidney transplantation) and on a long-term basis (patients on home dialysis programs).

Development of the diet prescription was based on two objectives: maintenance of body hydration so that hemodialysis was not required for fluid overload and reduction of formation of catabolic products of protein metabolism to a minimum so that dialysis could be postponed safely. These two objectives were felt to be of prime importance because of previous experience working with hibernating bears. Bears hibernate for 3 months at a normal body temperature and burn 4000 kcal/day. They neither eat, drink, urinate, nor defecate during this time. Body hydration remains within normal limits, and total body urea gradually decreases. Dehydration and uremia do not occur unless the bear cannot hibernate. Giving urea to bears who are successfully hibernating causes urine formation and dehydration.[17] It was decided, therefore, to prescribe as much as possible a diet program that would maintain hydration and slow urea formation.[18]

6.1. *Water*

Body hydration was maintained within normal limits in anephric patients by equating daily production of metabolic water plus water consumed in food with daily insensible water loss (Fig. 5). To do so, insensible water loss

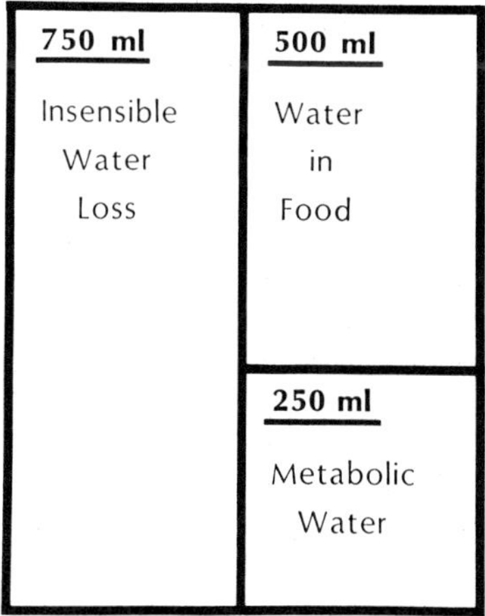

Figure 5. Water balance on restricted diet.

was measured while patients reclined in a fasting state on a Brookline metabolic bed scale. This bed measures, in grams per minute, weight loss which is mostly due to insensible water loss. Metabolic water production was calculated using indirect calorimetry. Water allowed in food was determined by the difference in insensible and metabolic water. For instance, in an individual who lost approximately 750 ml of water per day through insensible pathways and manufactured 250 ml of metabolic water, a diet containing 500 ml of water was prescribed. This usually left no free water except sips for medication. Fecal water loss (approximately 100 mg/day) was ignored although it tended to balance out water taken for medications. Exercise had no appreciable effect on water balance since the increase in insensible water loss was balanced by a corresponding increase in metabolic water production.

Formulas were developed to calculate insensible water loss and metabolic water production without the need to resort to complicated measurements.[18]

6.2. *Protein*

Although it was calculated that essential-amino-acid requirements could be met in patients losing no nitrogen via their urine with as low as 1–1½ eggs per day,[20] all patients were given the equivalent of two eggs a day. With the addition of other foods, protein intake amounted to 18–22 g/day and met daily essential-amino-acid requirements.

6.3. *Safety*

Initially, the diet was give for only 3–6 weeks in anephric patients awaiting kidney transplation.[18] In these patients, dialysis was safely postponed for periods of between 7 and 10 days. Body weight remained almost unchanged between dialyses, and patients appeared to be in a good clinical state. They were ambulatory and remained out of the hospital. Blood values before each dialysis averaged creatinine 24 mg/dl, urea 142 mg/dl, potassium 5.4 mEq/liter, and pH 7.33. Sodium concentration remained within normal limits. The amount of water in red blood cells was normal although plasma water was slightly increased from 92 to 95 ml water per milliliter plasma. Patients were satisfied with the program. The program was successful in allowing patients to save money while they awaited their kidney transplants.

Diet safety was then assessed in five patients on home dialysis.[19] To judge safety, the effect of protein and water restriction and infrequent dialysis on peripheral nerve function was assessed.

Five patients were studied in a crossover design so that each patient received 6 months on the conventional diet program and 6 months on the restricted-diet-and-dialysis program. The control diet consisted of 50 g of protein for females and 70 g of protein for males per day along with 60–100 mEq/day of potassium and 90 mEq/day of sodium. The experimental diet was described for anephric patients.[18]

There was no demonstration of any worsening of peripheral nerve function when the frequency of hemodialysis was markedly curtailed and diet severely restricted. Hemodialysis was reduced from 25.9 to 9.6 m^2-hr/wk (number of hours of dialysis per week times surface area of dialyzer). Despite this marked reduction in dialysis, orthodromic nerve action potentials were unchanged. Although a slight but significant reduction in muscle action potential was noted in the diet–dialysis restriction period, there was an equally slight but significant increase in conduction velocity of motor nerves in this group. Considering net effects, it was concluded that no clinical change in peripheral nerve function occurred.[19]

Body weight of patients on the restricted diet was not significantly different from body weight when they were dialyzed routinely.

Serum creatinine was elevated significantly in patients on the restricted program and averaged 15.8 versus 11.0 mg/dl on the control diet. Sodium, potassium, and calcium were within normal limits, and serum phosphorus was slightly, but not significantly, higher (5.2 mg/dl) on the restricted diet.

Serum cholesterol was 183 and triglyerides 139 mg/dl while on the restricted diet as compared to 208 and 170 mg/dl, respectively, on the control diet.

Patients on the restricted diet complained that they disliked both the excessive use of eggs and the diet. They felt thirsty and tired. However, when the study was finished and the patients returned to their home dialysis program, all chose to return to the restricted diet and infrequent dialysis program.

7. Summary

Complex medical facilities are not required to instruct patients properly in a restricted-diet–dialysis program. The program has proved safe for use for at least 6 months.

References

1. Nelson RA, Anderson CF, Hunt JC, Margie JD: Use of minimal levels of protein and maximum levels of calories as a diet prescription for chronic renal failure; clinical response and nutrient utilization in metabolism. Unpublished poster seminar. First International Congress on Nutrition in Renal Disease. Wurzburg, Germany, May 1977.
2. Giordano C: Use of exogenous and endogenous urea for protein synthesis in normal and uremic subjects. *J Lab Clin Med* 62:231–246, 1963.
3. Giovannetti S, Maggiore Q: A low-nitrogen diet with proteins of high biological value for severe chronic uremia. *Lancet* 1:1000–1003, 1964.
4. Shaw AB, Bazzard FJ, Booth EM: The treatment of chronic renal failure by a modified Giovannetti diet. *Q J Med* 34:237–253, 1965.
5. Berlyne GM, Shaw AB, Nilwarangkur S: Dietary treatment of chronic renal failure: Experiences with a modified Giovannetti Diet. *Nephron* 2:129–147, 1965.
6. Scrimshaw NS, Young VR, Huang, PC, Thanangkal O, Cholakos BV: Partial dietary replacement of milk protein by nonspecific nitrogen in young men. *J Nutr* 98:9–17, 1969.
7. Anderson CF, Nelson RA, Margie JD, Johnson WJ, Hunt JS: Nutritional therapy for adults with renal disease. *JAMA* 223:68–72, 1973.
8. Margie JD, Nelson RA, Anderson CF, Hunt JD: *The Mayo Clinic Renal Diet Cookbook.* New York, Western, 1974, p 307.
9. Briones ER, Palumbo PJ, Kottke BA, Ellefson RD, Nelson RA: Nutrition, metabolism and blood lipids in humans with type II-A hyperlipoproteinemia. *Am J Clin Nutr* 26:259–263, 1973.
10. Committee on Dietetics, Mayo Clinic: *Mayo Clinic Diet Manual.* Philadelphia, Saunders, 4th ed. 1971, pp 77–86.
11. Pennington JA: *Dietary Nutrient Guide.* Westport, Connecticut, 1976, pp 228–269.
12. Huse DM, Nelson RA, Briones ER, Hodgeson PA: Urinary nitrogen excretion as objective measure of dietary intake. *Am J Clin Nutr* 27:771–773, 1974 (Letter to the editor).
13. Nelson RA, Hayles AB, Wahner HW: Exercise and urinary nitrogen excretion in two chronically malnourished subjects. *Mayo Clin Proc* 48:459–555, 1973.
14. Walser M: Nutritional therapy of renal failure: current status future directions. *Postgrad Med* 71:9–14, 1982.
15. Johnson WJ, Goldsmith RS, Jowsey J, Frohnert PP, Arnaud CD: The influence of maintaining normal serum phosphate and calcium on renal osteodystrophy, in Norman AW, Schaefer K, Grigoleit HG, von Herrath D, Ritz E (eds): *Vitamin D and Problems Related to Uremic Bone Disease.* New York, Walter de Gruyter, 1975, p 513.
16. Ahlmen J: Incidence of chronic renal sufficiency. A study of the incidence and pattern of renal insufficiency in adults during 1966–71 in Gothenberg. *Acta Med Scand* (suppl 582): 1, 1975.
17. Nelson RA: Protein and fat metabolism in hibernating bears. *Fed Proc* 39:2955–2958, 1980.
18. Nelson RA, Anderson CF, Donadio JV Jr, Frohnert PP, Johnson WJ: Water balance and the frequency of hemodialysis in anephric patients. *Tr Am Soc Artif Intern Organs* 18:91–97, 1972.
19. Dyck PJ, Johnson WJ, Nelson RA, Lambert EH, O'Brien PC: Uremic neuropathy, III, Controlled study of restricted protein and fluid diet and infrequent hemodialysis versus conventional hemodialysis treatment. *Mayo Clin Proc* 50:641–649, 1975.
20. Hegsted DM: Normal protein requirements in man, in Berlyne GM (ed): *Nutrition in Renal Disease.* Edinburgh, E & S Livingston, 1968, pp 1–16.

60

A Progressive Encephalopathy in Children with Renal Failure in Infancy

Thomas E. Nevins, Alberto Rotundo, Lawrence A. Lockman, S. Michael Mauer, and Alfred F. Michael

1. Introduction

Most of the chapters in this volume relate to the nutritional state of adult patients with end-stage renal disease. Dr. Holliday has addressed the contribution of undernutrition to poor statural growth in children with developing uremia. This chapter expands upon his and outlines the devastating effects of chronic renal insufficiency (CRI) on the developing central nervous system (CNS) of infants.

More than 30 years ago Roosen-Runge (1949) recognized an association between abnormal cerebral and renal cortices. Clinically we have recognized profound CNS dysfunction in children with uremia but did not appreciate its frequency. In 1972 Alfrey *et al.* first described a progressive, usually fatal syndrome including disturbed speech, dementia, myoclonus, asterixis, and convulsions occurring in adult patients on chronic hemodialysis. More recently Baluarte and co-workers (1977) reported a similar encephalopathy in five uremic children who were not receiving dialysis. During 1980, an additional six children with a similar clinical picture were documented in the literature (Bale *et al*, 1980; Nathan and Pedersen, 1980; Geary *et al.*, 1980). As we have seen more infants in chronic renal failure, the magnitude and frequency of CNS dysfunction was striking.

Thomas E. Nevins, Alberto Rotundo, Lawrence A. Lockman, and Alfred F. Michael • Department of Pediatrics, University of Minnesota Health Sciences Center, Minneapolis, Minnesota 55455. ***S. Michael Mauer*** • Department of Pediatric Nephrology, University of Minnesota Health Sciences Center, Minneapolis, Minnesota 55455.

Table 1. Frequency of the Five Major Findings in the 20 Patients with CNS Abnormalities

Developmental delay[a]	19/20	(95%)[b]
Microcephaly	15/20	(75%)
Hypotonia	13/20	(65%)
Seizures	13/20	(65%)
Dyskinesia	11/20	(55%)

[a] Delay was assessed by Denver Developmental Screen and either Bayley Scales of Infant Development or the Stanford–Binet Intelligence Scale.
[b] Number in parentheses is the appropriate percentage.

2. Patients

Retrospectively, we studied 23 patients with CRI appearing in the first year of life (Rotundo *et al.*, 1982). All these infants had a persistent elevation of serum creatinine in the range of 1.1–7.6 mg/dl. Patients were identified by reviewing hospital records at the University of Minnesota Hospitals between 1968 and 1980. In addition, records were reviewed from the Divisions of Pediatric Nephrology, Urology, and Transplant Surgery. Twenty-three children with CRI were identified. Nineteen of the patients were boys and four were girls, probably reflecting the frequency with which obstructive uropathy leads to CRI. None of our patients had severe birth asphyxia, prematurity, head trauma, or other nonrenal syndromes as possible etiologies for CNS dysfunction.

3. Results

Remarkably, 20 of the 23 children, or 85% had significant CNS dysfunction. Their syndrome was composed of five major findings: developmental delay, microcephaly, hypotonia, seizures, and dyskinesia (Table 1). Of our 20 patients, 18 had at least three of these major findings. In all patients the CNS problem was noted after their presentation with renal disease but before dialysis or renal transplantation was required. The typical sequence of events recorded in the medical record was first CRI, then decreased velocity of head growth, followed by seizures, dyskinesia, and still later hypotonia and developmental delay. The microcephaly appears to be an acquired problem. All six children with head circumferences measured in the first 2 months of life were normal. By 6 months of age six of nine patients had head circumferences below 2 standard deviations from the mean for age, and eventually 15 of 20 patients had abnormal head circumferences. This observation seems particularly ominous. Dyskinesia was evidenced by one or more of these signs: chorea, ataxia, myoclonus, or tremor.

Finally, these patients have a poor prognosis. In our series 11 of the 20 have died. Four deaths occurred following transplant; two patients rejected their grafts, another patient developed varicella, and one died with normal renal function. Three additional patients were transplanted, and they appear to have stable neurologic status.

These observations raise questions about the etiology of this syndrome that cannot be answered by our retrospective study. Some of our patients had normal levels of parathyroid hormone. None of our patients had begun dialysis when their CNS symptoms appeared. Finally, although aluminum has been implicated in dialysis dementia (Alfrey, 1972), 4 of our 20 patients had not received any aluminum salts before CNS dysfunction was noted. No factors clearly predicted which children would develop neurologic signs.

4. *Therapy*

In general, our patients received standard conservative therapy. Parents were advised to give a diet of adequate calories and high-biologic-value protein, but no routine assessment was made of either overall nutrition or the adequacy of the actual diets. In addition, vitamin D, diuretics, iron, folate, multiple vitamins, and aluminum hydroxide were prescribed as required. In spite of our recommendations, these patients, by any of the parameters discussed in this volume, had some degree of nutritional deprivation. Many of them were ill, often hospitalized for long periods, and most had one or more operative procedures.

As noted earlier, seven of these patients eventually received renal transplants. In all, three patients have had too brief a follow-up period, two patients showed no improvement in CNS function, and two patients are clinically much better. Presently, we are systematically evaluating the intelligence and performance of all children before and after transplantation.

In summary, our present therapy for CRI in young children is unsatisfactory in view of the remarkable CNS morbidity in this group. We hope that earlier diagnosis and intervention will improve their poor prognosis.

5. *Future Studies—Ethics*

Since children are minors and unable to choose for themselves, any studies with children will inevitably raise questions of propriety. However, as indicated earlier, our current therapy is flawed both by a high mortality [an experience shared by others (T. M. Barratt *et al.*, Chapter 36, this volume)] and by severe CNS morbidity. In this light, we believe ethical concerns require us to offer children and their parents any additional therapy or new therapeutic combinations that may be expected to have a reasonable risk–benefit ratio.

6. *Study Design*

Although we do not believe children should be excluded from studies for ethical reasons, we do recognize that children are different. Since children possess dynamic, growing systems, they may offer unique opportunities to study the benefits of any intervention over a relatively short time frame. Because there are only a few diseases leading to CRI in children, a fairly homogeneous study group with a defined natural history is available.

But certainly none of us would be satisfied with a therapy that restored or preserved renal function at the expense of CNS function. Along this tack, the work of Teschan *et al.* (1979) is tantalizing. As discussed, he has applied noninvasive computerized electroencephalographic (EEG) techniques which promise a quantitative measure of CNS integrity. These electroneurologic techniques coupled with careful nutritional measurements, age-appropriate psychometric examinations, and anthropomorphic and growth velocity measurements offer quantitative tools to measure the results of any clinical trial in uremic children.

7. *Conclusion*

In conclusion, renal transplantation (S. Michael Mauer *et al.*, Chapter 33, this volume), pediatric dialysis (Michel Broyer *et al.*, Chapter 35, this volume), and nutritional interventions are available to virtually all children independent of age or size. It is now our responsibility to define the roles of these modalities and refine our overall therapeutic strategy so that future children will have an opportunity to live happy and productive lives.

References

Alfrey, A. C., Mishell, J. M., Burks, J., Contiguglia, S. R., Rudolph, H., Lewin, E., and Holmes, J. H., 1972, Syndrome of dyspraxia and multifocal seizures associated with chronic hemodialysis, *Tr. Am. Soc. Artif. Organs* **18:**257.

Bale, J. F., Jr., Siegler, R. L., and Bray, P. F., 1980, Encephalopathy in young children with moderate chronic renal failure, *Am. J. Dis. Child.* **134:**581.

Baluarte, H. R., Gruskin, A. B., Hiner, L. B., Foley, C. M., and Grover, W. D., 1977, Encephalopathy in children with chronic renal failure, *Proc. Clin. Dial. Transpl. Forum* **7:**95.

Geary, D. F., Fennell, R. S., Andriola, M., Gudat, J., Rodgers, B. M., and Richard, G. A., 1980, Encephalopathy in children with chronic renal failure, *J. Pediatr.* **96:**41.

Nathan, E., and Pedersen, S. E., 1980, Dialysis encephalopathy in a nondialyzed uraemic boy treated with aluminum hydroxide orally, *Acta Paediatr. Scand.* **69:**793.

Roosen-Runge, E. C., 1949, Retardation of postnatal development of kidney in persons with early cerebral lesions, *Am. J. Dis. Child.* **77:**185.

Rotundo, A., Nevins, T. E., Lipton, M., Lockman, L. A., Mauer, S. M., and Michael, A. F., 1982, Progressive encephalopathy in children with chronic renal insufficiency in infancy, *Kidney Int.* **21:**486.

Teschan, P. E., Ginn, H. E., Bourne, J. R., Ward, J. W., Hamel, B., Nunnally, J. C., Musso, M., and Vaughn, W. K., 1979, Quantitative indices of clinical uremia, *Kidney Int.* **15:**676.

Contributors

Nancy D. Adams, Division of Nephrology, University of Connecticut School of Medicine, Farmington, Connecticut 06032

Hani B. Affarah, Clinical Research Facility and Division of Nephrology, Department of Medicine, Emory University School of Medicine, Atlanta, Georgia 30322

Marianne Ahlberg, Department of Renal Medicine, Karolinska Institute, S-104 01 Stockholm, Sweden, and Huddinge University Hospital, S-141 86 Huddinge, Sweden

Anders Alvestrand, Department of Renal Medicine, Karolinska Institute, S-104 01 Stockholm, Sweden, and Huddinge University Hospital, S-141 86 Huddinge, Sweden

C. F. Anderson, Department of Medicine, Mayo Medical School, Rochester, Minnesota 55905

Allen I. Arieff, Nephrology Service, Department of Medicine, Veterans Administration Medical Center, and University of California School of Medicine, San Francisco, California 94121

Fritz H. Bach, Immunobiology Research Center and Departments of Laboratory Medicine/Pathology and Surgery, University of Minnesota Hospitals, Minneapolis, Minnesota 55455

T. M. Barratt, Department of Nephrology, Institute of Child Health, London WC1N 1EH, England

William M. Bennett, Division of Nephrology, Department of Medicine, Oregon Health Sciences University, Portland, Oregon 97201

Jonas Bergström, Department of Renal Medicine, Karolinska Institute, S-104 01 Stockholm, Sweden, and Huddinge University Hospital, S-141 86 Huddinge, Sweden

Jay Bernstein, Department of Anatomic Pathology, William Beaumont Hospital, Royal Oak, Michigan 48072

C. P. Bieber, Los Altos Hills, California 94022

Julie C. Bleier, Clinical Research Facility and Division of Nephrology, Department of Medicine, Emory University School of Medicine, Atlanta, Georgia 30322

William B. Blythe, Division of Nephrology, Department of Medicine, University of North Carolina School of Medicine, Chapel Hill, North Carolina 27514

Jeffrey E. Bonadio, Department of Pathology, University of Washington, Seattle, Washington 98195

Michel Broyer, Hôpital des Enfants Malades, 75730 Paris 15, France

Felix Brunner, Registry Committee of the EDTA, St. Thomas Hospital, London SE1 7EH, England

Hans Brynger, Registry Committee of the EDTA, St. Thomas Hospital, London SE1 7EH, England

R. Y. Calne, Department of Surgery, School of Medicine, Cambridge University, Cambridge CB2 2QQ, England

Rajender K. Chawla, Clinical Research Facility and Division of Nephrology, Department of Medicine, Emory University School of Medicine, Atlanta, Georgia 30322

Russell W. Chesney, Department of Pediatrics, University of Wisconsin Center for the Health Sciences, Madison, Wisconsin 53792

Allen W. Cowley, Jr., Department of Physiology and Biophysics, University of Mississippi Medical Center, Jackson, Mississippi 39216

Robert E. Cronin, Veterans Administration Medical Center, University of Texas Southwestern Medical School, Dallas, Texas 75216

Raymond Donckervolke, Registry Committee of the EDTA, St. Thomas Hospital, London SE1 7EH, England

Andrew P. Evan, Department of Anatomy, Indiana University School of Medicine, Indianapolis, Indiana 46223

Federico M. Farin, Department of Pathology, University of Washington, Seattle, Washington 98195

J. Fay, Department of Nephrology, Institute of Child Health, London WC1N 1EH, England

Ronald M. Ferguson, Departments of Surgery and Therapeutic Radiology, University of Minnesota, Minneapolis, Minnesota 55455

Richard N. Fine, Division of Pediatric Nephrology, UCLA Center for Health Sciences, Los Angeles, California 90024

David S. Fryd, Department of Surgery, University of Minnesota Health Sciences Center, Minneapolis, Minnesota 55455

Peter Fürst, Department of Renal Medicine, Karolinska Institute, S-104 01 Stockholm, Sweden, and Huddinge University Hospital, S-141 86 Huddinge, Sweden

Patricia Gabow, Department of Medicine, Denver General Hospital, Denver, Colorado 80204

Mark H. Gardenswartz, Department of Medicine, University of Colorado Health Sciences Center, Denver, Colorado 80262

Kenneth D. Gardner, Jr., Department of Medicine, University of New Mexico School of Medicine, Albuquerque, New Mexico 87131

F. John Gennari, Department of Medicine, University of Vermont College of Medicine, Burlington, Vermont 05405

Thomas P. Gibson, Section of Nephrology/Hypertension and Department of Medicine, Northwestern University Medical School, Northwestern Memorial Hospital, and Veterans Administration Lakeside Medical Center, Chicago, Illinois 60611

Richard J. Glassock, Department of Medicine, UCLA School of Medicine, and Department of Medicine, Harbor-UCLA Medical Center, Torrance, California 90509

Jan P. Goldberg, Department of Medicine, University of Colorado Health Sciences Center, Denver, Colorado 80262

Thomas A. Golper, University of Oregon Health Sciences Center, Portland, Oregon 97201

Frank A. Gotch, Franklin Hospital Hemodialysis Center, San Francisco, California 94114

M. S. Gottlieb, Division of Clinical Immunology (CIA), Department of Medicine, UCLA Center for the Health Sciences, Los Angeles, California 90024

Jared Grantham, Department of Medicine, University of Kansas School of Medicine, Kansas City, Kansas 66103

Richard W. Gray, Departments of Medicine and Biochemistry and the Clinical Research Center, Medical College of Wisconsin and Milwaukee County Medical Complex, Milwaukee, Wisconsin 53226

Warren E. Grupe, Division of Nephrology, The Children's Hospital, Boston, Massachusetts 02115

William E. Harmon, Division of Nephrology, The Children's Hospital, Boston, Massachusetts 02115

Malcolm A. Holliday, Department of Pediatrics, School of Medicine, University of California, San Francisco 94110

Joseph H. Holmes, Department of Medicine, University of Colorado School of Medicine, Denver, Colorado 80204

R. T. Hoppe, Department of Radiology, Stanford University Medical Center, Stanford, California 94305

Keith Hruska, Renal Division, Jewish Hospital of St. Louis, St. Louis, Missouri 63110

James C. Hunt, University of Tennessee, Memphis, Tennessee 38163

Claude Jacobs, Registry Committee of the EDTA, St. Thomas Hospital, London SE1 7EH, England

H. K. Johnson, Transplantation Section, Surgery Service, Veterans Administration Hospital, and Department of Surgery, Vanderbilt University Medical Center, Nashville, Tennessee 37232

H. S. Kaplan (deceased)**,** Department of Radiology, Stanford University Medical Center, Stanford, California 94305

D. N. S. Kerr, Royal Postgraduate Medical School, Hammersmith Hospital, London W12 OHS, England

Paul D. Killen, Department of Pathology, University of Washington, Seattle, Washington 98195

Tae H. Kim, Departments of Surgery and Therapeutic Radiology, University of Minnesota, Minneapolis, Minnesota 55455

C. M. Kjellstrand, Division of Nephrology, Department of Medicine, Hennepin County Medical Center, Minneapolis, Minnesota 55415

Saulo Klahr, Renal Division, Department of Medicine, Washington University School of Medicine, St. Louis, Missouri 63110

Lawrence J. Koep, Phoenix, Arizona 85006

S. H. Koretz, Institute of Clinical Medicine, Syntex Research, Palo Alto, California 94304

B. L. Kotzin, Division of Rheumatology, Department of Internal Medicine, Medical Center, Denver, Colorado 80220

Peter Kramer, Registry Committee of the EDTA, St. Thomas Hospital, London SE1 7EH, England

Stephen M. Krane, Department of Medicine, Harvard Medical School, and Medical Services (Arthritis Unit), Massachusetts General Hospital, Boston, Massachusetts 02114

Jacob Lemann, Jr., Departments of Medicine and Biochemistry and the Clinical Research Center, Medical College of Wisconsin and Milwaukee County Medical Complex, Milwaukee, Wisconsin 53226

Lawrence A. Lockman, Department of Pediatrics, University of Minnesota Health Sciences Center, Minneapolis, Minnesota 55455

Edmund G. Lowrie, National Medical Care, Waltham, Massachusetts 02154

Friedrich C. Luft, Renal Section, Department of Medicine, Indiana University School of Medicine, Indianapolis, Indiana 46223

Mart Mannik, Division of Rheumatology, Department of Medicine, University of Washington, Seattle, Washington 98195

Joyce Margie, Summit, New Jersey 07901

Kevin Martin, Renal Division, Department of Medicine, Washington University School of Medicine, St. Louis, Missouri 63110

S. Michael Mauer, Department of Pediatric Nephrology, University of Minnesota Health Sciences Center, Minneapolis, Minnesota 55455

Alfred F. Michael, Department of Pediatrics, University of Minnesota Health Sciences Center, Minneapolis, Minnesota 55455

Anthony P. Monaco, Cancer Research Institute, New England Deaconness Hospital, Boston, Massachusetts 02115

Richard S. Muther, Division of Nephrology, Department of Medicine, Oregon Health Sciences University, Portland, Oregon 97201

John S. Najarian, Departments of Surgery and Therapeutic Radiology, University of Minnesota, Minneapolis, Minnesota 55455

Ralph A. Nelson, Division of Research, Carle Foundation Hospital, and College of Medicine, University of Illinois, Urbana, Illinois 68101

Thomas E. Nevins, Department of Pediatrics, University of Minnesota Health Sciences Center, Minneapolis, Minnesota 55455

Gary Niblack, Transplantation Section, Surgery Service, Veterans Administration Hospital, and Department of Surgery, Vanderbilt University Medical Center, Nashville, Tennessee 37232

Viggo Kamp Nielsen, Neuromuscular Laboratory, Department of Neurology, University of Pittsburgh, School of Medicine, Pittsburgh, Pennsylvania 15261

I. S. Parkinson, Department of Clinical Biochemistry, Royal Victoria Infirmary, Newcastle upon Tyne NE1 4LP, England

D. P. (King) Paulnock, Department of Medical Microbiology, University of Wisconsin Medical School, Madison, Wisconsin 53706

George A. Porter, Department of Medicine, University of Oregon Health Sciences Center, Portland, Oregon 97201

Gerald M. Reaven, Department of Medicine, Stanford University School of Medicine, and Geriatric Research, Education and Clinical Center, Veterans Administration Medical Center, Palo Alto, California 94304

B. A. Reitz, Department of Surgery, Johns Hopkins Medical School, Baltimore, Maryland 21218

Robert E. Richie, Transplantation Section, Surgery Service, Veterans Administration Hospital, and Department of Surgery, Vanderbilt University Medical Center, Nashville, Tennessee 37232

S. P. A. Rigden, Department of Paediatrics, Guy's Hospital, London SE1 9RT, England

Alberto Rotundo, Department of Pediatrics, University of Minnesota Health Sciences Center, Minneapolis, Minnesota 55455

Daniel Rudman, Division of Geriatric Medicine, Veterans Administration Medical Center, North Chicago, Illinois 60064

Jon I. Scheinman, Department of Pediatric Nephrology, Duke University Medical Center, Durham, North Carolina 27710

Robert W. Schrier, Department of Medicine, University of Colorado Health Sciences Center, Denver, Colorado 80262

Neville Selwood, Registry Committee of the EDTA, St. Thomas Hospital, London SE1 7EH, England

Stanley Shaldon, Department of Nephrology, University Hospital, Nîmes-Montpellier, France

Donald J. Sherrard, Dialysis Unit, Veterans Administration Medical Center, Seattle, Washington 98108

Richard L. Simmons, Departments of Surgery and Therapeutic Radiology, University of Minnesota, Minneapolis, Minnesota 55455

Eduardo Slatopolsky, Renal Division, Department of Medicine, Washington University School of Medicine, St. Louis, Missouri 63110

Shimon Slavin, Departments of Surgery and Therapeutic Radiology, University of Minnesota, Minneapolis, Minnesota 55455

Nancy S. Spinozzi, Division of Nephrology, The Children's Hospital, Boston, Massachusetts 02115

Thomas E. Starzl, Department of Surgery, School of Medicine, University of Pittsburgh Health Sciences Center, Oakland Veterans Administration Medical Center, Pittsburgh, Pennsylvania 15213

Gary E. Striker, Department of Pathology, University of Washington, Seattle, Washington 98195

S. Strober, Division of Immunology, Department of Medicine, Stanford University Medical Center, Stanford, California 94305

David E. R. Sutherland, Departments of Surgery and Therapeutic Radiology, University of Minnesota, Minneapolis, Minnesota 55455

M. B. Tallent, Transplantation Section, Surgery Service, Veterans Administration Hospital, and Department of Surgery, Vanderbilt University Medical Center, Nashville, Tennessee 37232

Steven L. Teitelbaum, Division of Bone and Mineral Metabolism, and Department of Pathology and Laboratory Medicine, The Jewish Hospital of St. Louis, Washington University School of Medicine, St. Louis, Missouri 63110

F. Gary Toback, Department of Medicine, University of Chicago Pritzker School of Medicine, Chicago, Illinois 60637

Elbert P. Tuttle, Clinical Research Facility and Division of Nephrology, Department of Medicine, Emory University School of Medicine, Atlanta, Georgia 30322

Robert L. Vernier, Department of Pediatrics, University of Minnesota Health Sciences Center, Minneapolis, Minnesota 55455

M. K. Ward, Department of Medicine, Royal Victoria Infirmary, Newcastle upon Tyne NE1 4LP, England

Richard Weil, III, Department of Surgery, School of Medicine, University of Colorado, Denver, Colorado 80262

Dan J. Welling, Departments of Pathology and Physiology, University of Kansas Medical Center, Kansas City, Kansas 66103

Larry W. Welling, Veterans Administration Medical Center, Kansas City, Missouri 64128

Curtis G. Wickre, Division of Nephrology, Department of Medicine, Oregon Health Sciences University, Portland, Oregon 97201

Curtis B. Wilson, Department of Immunopathology, Research Institute of Scripps Clinic, La Jolla, California 92037

Jan Winberg, Department of Pediatrics, Karolinska Hospital, S-104 01 Stockholm, Sweden

Antony Wing, Registry Committee of the EDTA, St. Thomas Hospital, London SE1 7EH, England

Index